THE ROUTLEDGE COMPANION TO HEALTH HUMANITIES

The health humanities is a rapidly rising field, advancing an inclusive, democratizing, activist, applied, critical, and culturally diverse approach to delivering health and well-being through the arts and humanities. It has generated new kinds of interdisciplinary research, knowledge, and communities of practice globally. It has also acted to bring greater coherence and political force to contributions across a range of related disciplines and traditions.

In this volume, a formidable set of authors explore the history, current state, and future of the health humanities, in particular how its vision of the arts and humanities:

- Promotes creative public health.
- Opens new routes to health and well-being.
- Informs and drives better health care.
- Interrogates relationships between ill health and social equality.
- Develops humanist theory in relation to health and social care practice.
- Foregrounds cultural difference as a resource for positive change in society.
- Tests the humanity of an increasingly globalized health-care system.
- Looks to overcome structural and process obstacles to cross-disciplinary ventures.
- Champions co-construction, co-design, and mutuality in solving health and well-being challenges.
- Showcases less familiar, prominent, or celebrated creative practices.
- Includes multiple perspectives on the value and health benefits of the arts and humanities not limited to or dominated by medicine.

Divided into two main sections, the *Companion* looks at "Reflections and Critical Perspectives," offering current thinking and definitions within health humanities, and "Applications," comprising a wide selection of applied arts and humanities practices from comedy, writing, and dancing to yoga, cooking, and horticultural display.

Paul Crawford is Professor of Health Humanities in the Faculty of Medicine and Health Sciences at the University of Nottingham, UK.

Brian Brown is Professor of Health Communication at De Montfort University, UK.

Andrea Charise is an Assistant Professor in the departments of English and Interdisciplinary Centre for Health and Society at the University of Toronto Scarborough, Canada.

ROUTLEDGE COMPANIONS TO LITERATURE SERIES

For more information on this series, please visit: www.routledge.com/literature/series/RC4444

THE ROUTLEDGE COMPANION TO HEALTH HUMANITIES

*Edited by Paul Crawford, Brian Brown and
Andrea Charise*

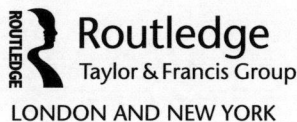

LONDON AND NEW YORK

First published 2020
by Routledge
4 Park Square, Milton Park, Abingdon, Oxon OX14 4RN
605 Third Avenue, New York, NY 10017

First issued in paperback 2023

Routledge is an imprint of the Taylor & Francis Group, an informa business

British Library Cataloguing-in-Publication Data
A catalogue record for this book is available from the British Library

Library of Congress Cataloging-in-Publication Data
A catalog record has been requested for this book

ISBN: 978-1-03-257034-1 (pbk)
ISBN: 978-1-138-57990-3 (hbk)
ISBN: 978-0-429-46906-0 (ebk)

DOI: 10.4324/9780429469060

Typeset in Bembo
by Swales & Willis, Exeter, Devon, UK

Publisher's Note
The publisher has gone to great lengths to ensure the quality of this reprint but points out that some imperfections in the original copies may be apparent.

In Memoriam

Professor Ronald Carter (1947–2018)

CONTENTS

Contents

Contents

Contents

Contents

BOXES, FIGURES, AND TABLE

Boxes

Figures

Table

ACKNOWLEDGEMENTS

We are grateful for permission from individual contributors to this volume for the use of their own tables, figures, and images in Chapters 3, 12, 15, 24, 28, 40, 56, and 59. For the image used in Chapter 19, the contributing author claims fair use as applied with trans- formative purpose that differs from the original, and amounts to a fraction of a full-length video advertisement. We would wish to thank Aimee O'Neill for permission for the two images of the bathroom murals (before and after) in Chapter 22. We are also grateful to Jamie O. Crawford for his editorial advice in collating this volume.

Professor Crawford wishes to send his heartfelt thanks to the Arts and Humanities Research Council, UK for their stalwart support in developing the field of health humanities.

CONTRIBUTORS

Brian Abrams is an Analytical Music Therapist and Fellow of the Association for Music and Imagery, and serves as Associate Professor of Music and Coordinator of Music Therapy at Montclair State University in the United States. He has been a music therapist since 1995, with experience across a wide range of clinical contexts.

Jon Allard is a Researcher and Academic Lead for Cornwall Partnership NHS Foundation Trust, United Kingdom. He also has an Honorary Fellow position with Plymouth University. He has published a number of health-care research papers and is particularly interested in qualitative research, NHS teamworking, and mental health care.

Gail Allsopp MBChB MRCS FRCGP is a Professional Actor, General Practitioner, and Associate Professor of primary care at the University of Nottingham, United Kingdom. She uses creativity within her medical and academic career, drawing on a wealth of experience. Formally trained at the Bristol Old Vic Theatre School, she has worked in theater, TV, radio, and film across the United Kingdom and Europe.

Elaine Argyle is a Senior Researcher at the University of Nottingham, United Kingdom, and a dually registered health and social care professional. She has worked on many projects relating to the arts and health. These have focused on the mediums of theater, music, museum resources, painting, drawing, and ceramics.

Cariad Astles is a Puppetry Trainer, Researcher and Performer. She is Course Leader for the BA Puppetry at the Royal Central School of Speech and Drama and Lecturer in Drama at the University of Exeter, United Kingdom, and also President of the UNIMA Research Commission. She specializes in training, puppets, and objects in health care, and in directing puppetry.

Jacqueline M. Atkinson is Emeritus Professor of Mental Health Policy and Honorary Senior Research Fellow University of Glasgow, Institute of Health and Wellbeing, United Kingdom. She is a Chartered Psychologist, Fellow of the British Psychological Society, and lifelong quilter.

Olivia Banner is Assistant Professor of Critical Media Studies at the University of Texas at Dallas, United States. Her book, *Communicative Biocapitalism: The Voice of the Patient in Digital Health and the Health Humanities*, was published in 2017.

Charley Baker is an Associate Professor in Mental Health in the School of Health Sciences at the University of Nottingham, United Kingdom. She has written and spoken internationally on the portrayal of mental health in literature and self-harm. Charley has research interests that span the health humanities.

Raymond Barfield is a Pediatric Oncologist at Duke University, United States, interested in the role of the humanities and the arts in the formation of physicians. He has published several books of fiction, poetry, and philosophy. Forthcoming books include *Dante's New Moon* (poetry) and *The Practice of Medicine as Being in Time* (philosophy).

Phillip Barrish is the Tony Hilfer Professor of American and British Literature at the University of Texas at Austin and Associate Director for Health and Humanities at the University of Texas Humanities Institute, United States. The author of three scholarly books, his current work focuses on literary engagements with health care as a system.

Heike Bartel is Associate Professor in German at the University of Nottingham, United Kingdom, and Fellow of Nottingham's Institute of Mental Health. She has led the AHRC-funded interdisciplinary research network "Hungry for Words" about male eating disorders. She has published widely on contemporary, modern, and eighteenth-century poetry, prose, and women's writing.

Josie Billington is Professor in English Literature and Deputy Director of the Centre for Research into Reading, Literature and Society, University of Liverpool, United Kingdom. She has published extensively on the power of literary reading to influence health, including *Is Literature Healthy?* (2016) and *Reading and Mental Health* (2019).

Alex Bishop is an Educationalist with over ten years' experience in learning and organizational development in corporate settings. A keen music fan and avid concertgoer with eclectic tastes, Alex has been published online and in print for rock music magazine *Get Your Rock Out*.

Alan Bleakley is Emeritus Professor of medical education and medical humanities at Plymouth University Medical School, United Kingdom. He is an internationally recognized academic and author in the fields of medical education and medical humanities and a widely published poet.

Lisa Boivin, PhD Candidate at the University of Toronto, Canada, is a member of the Deninu Kue First Nation in Northwest Territories. The image *Sharing Bioethics* (discussed in the chapter "Indigenous Health Humanities") is her original artwork; it has been previously published in the Canadian Medical Association Journal (2018).

Lydia Bracken, BCL, LLM, Barrister-at-Law, PhD, is a Lecturer in the School of Law, University of Limerick, Ireland. Lydia's research interests are in the areas of children's rights and family law, with a particular focus on "non-traditional" and "new" family forms.

Frances Cadd is a Doctoral Researcher at the University of Nottingham, United Kingdom, specializing in Modern British History. Her PhD research examines the work of British nurse and campaigner Avis Hutt (1917–2010), investigating the connections between nursing, the peace movement, and the political Left in the twentieth century.

Brian Callender is a Practicing Clinician at the University of Chicago, United States, with an academic focus on the health humanities, particularly the clinical applications of graphic medicine. He has taught the courses "The Body in Medicine and Performing Arts" and "Graphic Medicine: Concepts and Practice" (with MK Czerwiec).

Havi Carel is Professor of Philosophy at the University of Bristol, United Kingdom. She is the author of *Illness* (3rd edition 2018), *Phenomenology of Illness* (2016), and *Life and Death in Freud and Heidegger* (2006), as well as numerous papers. She co-leads the Life of Breath project, funded by Wellcome.

Gretchen Case is an Associate Professor and Chief of the Medical Ethics and Humanities Program at the University of Utah School of Medicine, United States, where she teaches arts and humanities. Her research addresses the many intersections of performance and health care, with particular emphasis on medical education.

Sydney Cheek-O'Donnell is an Associate Professor in the Department of Theatre and the Associate Dean for Research in the College of Fine Arts at the University of Utah, United States. Her current research focuses on the use of theater techniques and story to improve communication and well-being.

Stephen Clift is Director, Sidney De Haan Research Centre for Arts and Health Canterbury Christ Church University, United Kingdom. He has worked in the field of arts, well-being, and health since the late 1990s and has led a program of research on the value of creative arts participation for well-being and health since 2005.

Jonathan Coope is Research Fellow on a mental health and theater project he co-devised, based in a *basti* in Pune, India, funded by the Global Challenges Research Fund (GCRF), Arts and Humanities Research Council (AHRC), and Medical Research Council (MRC). At De Montfort University, United Kingdom, Jonathan teaches postgraduate courses on "Leading Change for Sustainability," "Medical Leadership, Education and Research," and "Acting Skills for New Lecturers."

Betsan Corkhill is a Lifestyle Health Coach who specializes in working with people living with long-term health problems, particularly pain. She is a passionate advocate for a whole-person approach to health and is an expert on the use of therapeutic knitting for improving health, wellness, and managing illness.

Allison Crawford, MD, PhD, is a psychiatrist and Associate Professor in the Departments of Psychiatry, Dalla Lana School of Public Health, and English at the University of Toronto. Her PhD dissertation, *Where Sickness Comes From: Reading and Unsettling Medicine in the Canadian Arctic*, was completed at the University of Toronto (2017). She works in circumpolar communities in Canada and internationally, and uses arts-based methods in community engagement, research, and teaching.

MK Czerwiec, RN, MA, also known as the Comic Nurse, MK Czerwiec, RN, MA, is the creator of *Taking Turns: Stories from HIV/AIDS Care Unit 371* (2017), co-author of the *Graphic Medicine Manifesto* (2015), and editor of *Menopause: A Comic Treatment* (forthcoming). With Ian Williams, Matthew Noe, and Alice Jaggers, she manages Graphic Medicine, a website that explores the interaction between the medium of comics and the discourse of health care.

Sayantani DasGupta originally trained in pediatrics and public health, and teaches in the Graduate Program in Narrative Medicine, the Institute for Comparative Literature and

Society, and the Center for the Study of Ethnicity and Race, all at Columbia University, New York, United States. She is also a writer of children's fiction.

Philip Davis is Professor of English Literature, University of Liverpool and Director of The Centre for Research into Reading Literature and Society, United Kingdom. He is author of *Reading and the Reader* (2013) and has published on literature and brain imaging. He is launching a series with on Bibliotherapy and Wellbeing.

Tomi D. Dreibelbis is Instructor in Public Health Sciences and Senior Director, Educational Affairs at Penn State College of Medicine, Hershey, Pennsylvania, United States.

Nehal El-Hadi is a Visiting Scholar at the City Institute at York University, and Sessional Faculty at the University of Toronto Scarborough, Canada. Her research explores the relationships between body, place, and technology, and she advocates for the responsible, accountable, and ethical treatment of user-generated content in journalism, planning, and health care.

Daisy Fancourt is a Senior Research Fellow in at University College London, United Kingdom. She specializes in psychoneuroimmunology and epidemiology, focusing on the effects of social and community participation, with a particular interest in the effects of arts and culture on health. She is also a BBC New Generation Thinker and World Economic Forum Global Shaper.

Rebecka Fleetwood-Smith has a background in fashion and textile design. Her concern with the psychological aspects of clothing ownership led her to complete an MA in Psychology for Fashion Professionals at London College of Fashion, United Kingdom. She is currently a PhD student exploring the significance of clothing and textiles to people with dementia.

Claire Garabedian is a professional cellist specializing in historical performance, a Certified Music Practitioner (MHTP), and an experienced researcher focusing on how the arts benefit people with dementia and in palliative care. She has presented her work throughout the United Kingdom, Europe, and the United States, including at the Hay Festival and on BBC Radio 4.

Danny George is an Associate Professor in the Department of Humanities, Penn State Hershey College of Medicine, United States.

Anna Greenwood is an Associate Professor in Medical History at the University of Nottingham, United Kingdom. She has published widely on the operation of Western medicine in colonial contexts and the utility of history in what are traditionally non-historic disciplines. She is co-director, with Paul Crawford, of the Health Humanities Research Priority Area in Nottingham and a member of the International Health Humanities Network.

Brenda Hall has more than 35 years of health-care leadership experience, completing her doctoral degree in medical humanities from Drew University. Dr. Hall is a National Malcolm Baldrige Award Board Examiner and serves as Vice Chair of the Mid-Atlantic Alliance for Performance Excellence for Hospitals in Pennsylvania, Delaware, and New Jersey, United States.

Emily Haslam-Jones is a yoga teacher based in Nottingham, United Kingdom, who is interested in the embodiment of emotions and the use of yoga as a tool for resilience and for processing traumatic and adverse experience.

Susan Hogan is Professor of Arts and Health at the University of Derby, and a Professorial Fellow at the Institute of Mental Health, University of Nottingham, United Kingdom. Her latest books are *Art Therapy Theories* (2016), *Gender Issues in International Arts Therapies Research* (2019), *Gender and Difference in the Arts Therapies: Inscribed on the Body* (2019), and *The Maternal Tug: Ambivalence, Identity and Agency* (forthcoming).

Kate Holland is a Senior Research Fellow in the Faculty of Arts and Design at the University of Canberra, Australia. Her research focuses on different contexts and dimensions of health communication, including media representations, journalistic practices, and the communication practices of health organizations, academics, activists, and people with lived experience.

Sara Houston is Principal Lecturer in Dance Studies at University of Roehampton, United Kingdom. Her research focuses on community dance, in particular with marginalized populations. Houston's work on dancing with Parkinson's won her the BUPA Foundation Prize, 2011 and she was finalist for the National Public Engagement Awards in 2014.

Jeffrey Huffman is Assistant Professor of English in the Graduate School of Nursing Science, St. Luke's International University, Tokyo, Japan. He is a doctoral candidate in education (applied linguistics) at Temple University, United States. His research interests are second-language reading, language testing, Nursing English, study abroad, and the health humanities.

Rick Iedema is Professor and Director of the Centre for Team-based Practice and Learning in Health Care at King's College London, United Kingdom. Recent publications include *Visualising Health Care Improvement* (2013), *Communicating Quality and Safety in Health Care* (2015), and *Video Reflexive Ethnography in Health Research and Healthcare Improvement* (2019).

Ikem Ifeobu is a Mathematics Teacher turned Educationalist. His main research interests are centered around various aspects of educational sociology and psychology, with particular focus on innovation in educational and social policy and practice.

Mami Inoue is Professor of English in the Graduate School of Nursing Science and Director of the Center for Academic Resources, St. Luke's International University, Japan. She has co-authored textbooks on Nursing English. She is a member of the Kanto Branch editorial board of the English Literary Society of Japan.

J. Lauren Johnson is a Registered Psychologist and is the founder of the Therapeutic Film-making Institute in Edmonton, Canada. Although she is currently working in private practice, she previously held positions at a world-class cancer hospital and in various First Nations health centers in northern Alberta.

Melanie Jordan is an Assistant Professor in the School of Sociology and Social Policy at the University of Nottingham, United Kingdom, undertaking research in prison health care, prison architecture, criminal justice system mental health, sex offenders, sexual abuse survivors, police, and modern slavery offenders.

Emma Joyes completed her doctorate at the School of Health Sciences, University of Nottingham, United Kingdom, in 2019. Her doctoral research explored recovery and creative practice within forensic mental health. Emma has worked on various national and international research and evaluation projects across the fields of health care, mental health, and criminal justice.

Paul Kadetz is Deputy Director of the Center for Global Health, Zhejiang University, China, and an Associate of the China Centre for Health and Humanity, University College London, United Kingdom. He has published the co-edited volume *Handbook of Welfare in*

China (2017) and co-authored the volume *Creating Katrina, Rebuilding Resilience: Lessons from New Orleans on Vulnerability and Resiliency* (2017).

Travis Chi Wing Lau received his PhD in English at the University of Pennsylvania and is a Postdoctoral Teaching Fellow at the University of Texas at Austin, United States. He specializes in eighteenth- and nineteenth-century British literature, the history of medicine, medical humanities, and disability studies.

Christina Lee is an Associate Professor in the School of English, University of Nottingham, United Kingdom. Her research interests include definitions of illness, health, and impairment in Early Medieval England and the cultural implications of illness and the experiences of the affected. She has published on leprosy, trauma, and disability, as well as medical textiles. As part of a group of arts/science researchers (the "AncientBiotics") she examines the efficacy of medieval remedies.

Susan Levy is Senior Lecturer in Social Work in the School of Education and Social Work, University of Dundee, United Kingdom. Her research focuses on disability, difference, and citizenship, with a particular interest in the use and impact of the arts in social work and the intersections with health care.

Bradley Lewis is an Associate Professor at New York University's Gallatin School of Individualized Study, United States. He is affiliated with NYU's Disability Studies minor, Department of Social and Cultural Analysis, and Department of Psychiatry. His books include *Narrative Psychiatry: How Stories Shape Clinical Practice* (2011) and *Depression: Integrating Science, Culture, and Humanities* (2012).

Lydia Lewis is based at the Institute of Education, University of Wolverhampton, United Kingdom. Her work focuses on theoretically informed, applied sociological research and knowledge exchange with third-sector organizations. She has developed a program of research on education and mental health, with a particular focus on adult community learning.

Lan A. Li is a Filmmaker and Historian of the body focusing on global East Asia. Her written work includes a long visual history of mapping meridians and a transnational history of numbness. She is currently Assistant Professor in the Department of History and Medical Humanities Program at Rice University, United States.

Alastair Macdonald is Senior Researcher in the School of Design at Glasgow School of Art, United Kingdom. With a product design background, he is a full-time researcher with expertise in the interdisciplinary and participatory co-development of health and care interventions, using evidence-based, mixed method, and design-led iterative prototyping approaches.

Drew Luan Matott received his MFA in Book and Paper Arts from Columbia College-Chicago (2008) and his BFA in Printmaking from Buffalo State College (2001), United States. The Founder and Director of the Peace Paper Project, Drew is a Master Papermaker with an expertise using traditional papermaking as a form of social engagement and community activism. Since 2009, he has taught and exhibited internationally and completed numerous artist residencies.

Colin Macduff is Senior Research Fellow in the School of Design at Glasgow School of Art and Visiting Reader in the School of Nursing and Midwifery at Robert Gordon

University, Aberdeen, United Kingdom. Colin has extensive experience in nursing and in the development of arts and humanities approaches within health care.

Peter Meineck is Professor of Classics in the Modern World at New York University, Affiliated Professor at the Tisch School of the Arts at NYU, the founder of Aquila Theatre and Assistant Chief of the Bedford Fire Department in New York, United States. Recent publications include: *Theatrocracy: Greek Drama, Cognition and the Imperative for Theatre* (2018) and *Classics and Cognitive Theory* (2019).

Gretchen Miller is a Registered Board Certified Art Therapist and Advanced Certified Trauma Practitioner. She has developed Peace Paper Project coursework and workshops, and provides consultation to art therapists and students seeking to learn about the therapeutic qualities of papermaking as a form of trauma intervention, personal transformation, social action, and recovery.

Hilary Moss is Senior Lecturer in Music Therapy at the Irish World Academy of Music and Dance, University of Limerick, and formerly the Director of the National Centre for Arts and Health, Dublin, Ireland. She works at the interface of arts and health-care services, bringing together clinicians, arts practitioners, and service users to improve health and well-being.

Shane Neilson is a Poet, Physician, and Critic who completed his PhD in English and Cultural Studies at McMaster University, Canada, in 2018. Shane's latest book, *New Brunswick*, was published in the spring of 2019. He is currently completing a postdoctoral position at McMaster University as part of the $50,000 Talent grant awarded by SSHRC in 2018.

Rosie Perkins is a Reader in Performance Science at the Royal College of Music (RCM) and an honorary Research Fellow at Imperial College London, United Kingdom. Rosie's research focuses on arts-in-health and performers' career development, and she is program director for the RCM's ground-breaking MSc in Performance Science.

Elvira Perez Vallejos is an Associate Professor of Mental Health and Digital Tech at the National Institute for Health Research (NIHR) Nottingham Biomedical Research Centre, United Kingdom. She is interested in the ethical challenges embedded in digital solutions for mental health and the development of new mental health interventions that incorporate creative practices.

Aimie Purser is Lecturer in Sociology at the University of Nottingham, United Kingdom. Her research explores the ways in which dance and other somatic practices can both ameliorate and illuminate the human condition.

Santiago Quesada-García is an Associate Professor in the Department of Architectural Design, University of Seville, Spain; member of the PhD Faculty Board of the doctoral program in Biomedicine, Translational Research and New Technologies in Health in the Faculty of Medicine of Malaga, Spain; and main Researcher of the Healthy Architecture and City Research Group. His main lines of research are architecture and Alzheimer's, Ambient Assisted Living (AAL), and Ambient Intelligence (AmI) in architecture.

Carla Rice is a Canada Research Chair in Care, Gender, and Relationships and a Full Professor at the University of Guelph, Canada. Dr. Rice is the Founder/Director of the Re•Vision Centre for Art and Social Justice and seeks to explore how communities can use arts-informed research to advance social inclusion and justice by challenging stereotypes.

Lisa Richardson (Anishnaabe/Scottish) is a clinician-educator in the Division of General Internal Medicine and practices at the University Health Network in Toronto, Ontario. She is an Associate Professor in the Department of Medicine. Her scholarly interest lies in the integration of critical and Indigenous perspectives into medical education and she is a Centre Researcher at the Wilson Centre. She is the Strategic Lead in Indigenous Health for the Faculty of Medicine at the University of Toronto and she co-chairs the Indigenous Health Committee for the Royal College of Physicians and Surgeons of Canada.

Javier Saavedra is at the Department of Experimental Psychology of the University of Seville, Spain. He is also Research Fellow in the Andalusian Foundation for the Social Integration of People with Mental Illness, studying the recovery of people with schizophrenia. He is a member of the International Health Humanities Network and the Madness and Literature Network. He is also the founder of the "Art and Psychology Seminar" at the University of Seville.

Steven Schlozman is Assistant Professor of Psychiatry, Harvard Medical School, a psychiatrist at Massachusetts General Hospital, and Co-Director, the Clay Center for Young Healthy Minds, United States. He directs the psychiatry curriculum for the Health Science and Technology Program at Harvard Medical School and MIT. He also teaches film at Harvard.

Lorenzo Servitje is Assistant Professor of Literature and Medicine at Lehigh University, United States. His current book project, *Medicine Is War*, traces the metaphorical militarization of medicine in the nineteenth century. His articles have appeared in *Literature and Medicine* among other journals.

Curie Scott is a Senior Lecturer at Bournemouth University, United Kingdom. She facilitates creative workshops and is a coach, painter, and origami artist. After qualifying as a medical doctor with a pharmacology degree, she moved into Health Education. Her PhD investigated what happens when adults draw to think about their future ageing.

Susan Merrill Squier is Brill Professor Emerita, Penn State University, United States, and Visiting Fellow at Freie Universität, Berlin, Germany. Her books include *Epigenetic Landscapes* (2017), *Poultry Science, Chicken Culture* (2010), *Liminal Lives* (2003), *Babies in Bottles* (1994), and (with MK Czerwiec et al.), *Graphic Medicine Manifesto* (2015). She co-edits the Graphic Medicine book series at Penn State Press. Susan Squier is Founding President of the Graphic Medicine International Collective, incorporated as a nonprofit 501c3 organization with the mission "To guide and support the uses of comics in health."

Jenny Tillotson is a Sensory Designer and founder of eScent (Sensory Design & Technology Ltd). She is a Churchill Fellow, a member of Cambridge Neuroscience, United Kingdom, a Royal Society of the Arts Fellow, and an Associate of the British Society of Perfumers. Jenny holds a degree from Central Saint Martins and a PhD from the Royal College of Art, and has won AHRC and ERDF awards in the field of well-being, design, and entrepreneurship.

Victoria Tischler is a Chartered Psychologist whose research interests focus on creativity and mental health and multisensory approaches to dementia care. She is co-executive editor of the journal *Arts and Health*. She serves on the scientific advisory board for Boots UK archive and is a trustee for the charity Paintings in Hospitals, United Kingdom.

Marina Tsaplina is a performing artist, patient activist, and Kienle Scholar in health humanities. Her research is in object ontology, puppetry animation, and indigenous/traditional ways of knowing. Her pedagogy *Embodiment and Puppetry* focuses on cultivating embodiment and training the imagination in illness, care and healing. Her work serves clinicians, medical students, and disability communities.

Pablo Valero-Flores is an Architect and expert in the rehabilitation of buildings. He also has expertise in town and country planning. Since 2015, he has worked as a researcher on the Designing for the Absence of Memory project as part of the Healthy Architecture and City Research Group affiliated with the PhD medicine program at the University of Malaga, Spain.

Olaf Werder holds a Senior Lectureship and Directorship in Health Communication at the University of Sydney, Australia, where he also leads a research node in health humanities. His work focuses on understanding how people communicate and understand health to identify community-collaborative pathways for system changes and improved health outcomes.

Aaron Williamon is Professor of Performance Science at the Royal College of Music, Untied Kingdom, where he directs the Centre for Performance Science. His research focuses on skilled performance and applied scientific initiatives that inform music learning and teaching, as well as the impact of music and the arts on society.

Mike Wilson is Professor of Drama at Loughborough University, United Kingdom, where he leads a research team in Applied Storytelling to bring new knowledge and voices into the fields of health, education, environmental policy, and social justice. He is currently working on UKRI-funded projects in India, Colombia and Kenya, as well as Europe. He has published widely on storytelling in its many forms.

Edward J. Wright is Lecturer in Sociology and Criminology at Nottingham Trent University, United Kingdom. He has diverse interests as a criminologist and sociologist, such as time, embodiment, identity, knowledge acquisition and production, consumer capitalism and consumption, and inequality. These interests reflect and inform the research projects in which Edward has been involved, respectively concerning white-collar boxing, imprisonment, "modern slavery", and capoeira.

INTRODUCTION

Global health humanities and the rise of creative public health

Paul Crawford

Introduction

Health humanities is a fast-growing field of research, education, and practice that has generated a more inclusive, democratizing, and applied approach to arts and humanities in health care, health, and well-being. Its rise over the past 13 years represents an interdisciplinary departure from the longer-established tradition of medical humanities. However, it seeks to enjoin the medical humanities as well as fields such as arts and health, expressive therapies, community arts, and social prescribing to work more collaboratively to advance creative public health.

To date, multiple networks, research units, projects, and taught courses in health human-ities have emerged worldwide. Importantly, this "burgeoning" (Purser, 2017) field has brought diverse academics, creative practitioners, and health, social care, and education professionals to work more closely with the public to find new applications and social innovations through the arts and humanities in an interdisciplinary and non-hierarchical way. As such, the field has shifted beyond medical conceptions of health and well-being, rejecting a pecking order for who controls or mandates the application of the arts and humanities to improve the human condition.

As Crawford and Brown (2020: 41) write, the health humanities offer a "superordinate evolution" that advances innovation, mutuality, and dialogue between congruent traditions. In this way, it seeks to inspire, not to control or govern innovation. Klugman (2017: 419) goes so far as to suggest that health humanities may even "stave off the decline of the broader humanities" in higher education where STEM subjects (typically defined as science, technology, engineering and mathematics/medicine) are deemed to more clearly tie in with employment opportunities. Skylar (2017) reports how health humanities is informing medical training in new and compelling ways: providing a focus on the use of arts and humanities to foreground the perspectives of patients, their families, and social conditions or environments.

Here, I present a brief overview of health humanities as an increasingly global field, outlining its origins, definitions, critical reception, praxis and creative public health. I also provide a summary of the very many excellent contributions to this important volume from new and leading voices in the field.

1

Origins

In 2006, I consulted with the Arts and Humanities Research Council UK (AHRC) on developing a much broader application of the arts and humanities to health care, health, and well-being than that currently available in fields such as medical humanities. The earliest field description and definition for the health humanities, a term previously only loosely applied, followed in a paper presented at the Economic and Social Research Council Business Seminar held at BioCity Nottingham, United Kingdom in 2007 (Crawford, 2007) and in the first peer-reveiewed field description (Crawford et al., 2010). The latter coincided with the launch of the International Health Humanities Conference at Nottingham University, UK (August 6–8). By 2011, the International Health Humanities Network, funded by the AHRC, spearheaded multiple symposia and workshops worldwide. In 2015, the Health Humanities Consortium in the United States launched and agreed to co-produce the International Health Humanities Conference series, held every two years up to this point. The fourth International Health Humanities Conference was hosted that same year at the University of Colorado, and subsequent events have been hosted annually.

Since these early days, health humanities research units have emerged across the United Kingdom, Europe, United States, Canada, Australia, Africa, India, China, Japan, and other territories. These developments have led to a rapid growth in undergraduate and postgraduate programs in the field. Berry et al. (2016) identified 57 baccalaureate Health Humanities programs instituted in the United States alone. In 2014, the first undergraduate Health Humanities curriculum was launched in Canada at the University of Toronto Scarborough (Charise, 2017), with a Canadian Association for Health Humanities appearing in 2018. In the United Kingdom—where the focus of health humanities has been on applied, inclusive research, health and well-being innovation innovation, and activism—dedicated educational initiatives have only recently started to emerge, with a Masters in Health Humanities at University College London and the University of Edinburgh, and others in the pipeline.

Alongside the early work in field description, networking, and the formation of research units and university courses, a first manifesto for the field (Crawford et al., 2015) and a first reader (Jones et al., 2014) have been published. In addition, a wide range of articles and commentary papers have been written, debating the nature and work of the field, including approaches to or evaluations of teaching programs (e.g., Charise, 2017; Jones, 2014; Klugman, 2017; Peterkin and Skorzewska, 2018; Rubens, 2017; Skylar, 2017; Tsevat et al., 2015). In 2020, there will be a major new health humanities-led series called "Arts for Health" with Emerald and a much-anticipated *Encyclopedia of Health Humanities* (Crawford and Kadetz, forthcoming). Such field-defining publications mark a consolidation of relevant scholarly discussion alongside this current volume.

Field consolidation of the health humanities has also benefited from increased levels of funding from grant-awarding bodies and the support and sponsorship of multiple and high-profile institutions. In the United States, the field has found favor with OppNet and National Institutes of Health, while in the United Kingdom, health humanities has attracted the support of UK Research and Innovation and several of its Research Councils, major charities, and prominent organizations such as the British Library, the Science Museum, and the Royal Society for Public Health to name but a few. In the United Kingdom, health humanities research has featured in important government reports and been celebrated in the launch in 2020 of new national awards for both the medical humanities and health humanities, supported by the Arts and Humanities Research Council and Wellcome Trust. These more substantially funded awards replaced the earlier Health Humanities Medal which ran in 2018 (AHRC/UKRI, 2020).

For many, the shift to health humanities has been a radical and welcome move. Despite the clear collaborative approach of the field (Crawford, 2015), the development has presented a challenge to some established or more specialist movements anxious to maintain their prominence, status, or funding. For some, health humanities has provoked a kind of replacement anxiety. Yet the magic of health humanities has been its openness to all movements valuing the contribution of the arts and humanities to advancing health care, health, and well-being. In this sense, health humanities has proven to be a valuable integument for diverse individuals, groups, and organizations to make a difference in this work. As we witness above in the way that health humanities has gathered global momentum as a field, it is so much more than a switch in nomenclature. With a more public-savvy mission, the field has spurred a broadening in the scope, inclusion, or application of previously established and more narrowly configured disciplines. As Jones et al. (2017: 932) argue, the move to health humanities is not simply a matter of semantics and "splitting hairs." Given the range of subjects, health professions, stakeholders, and practice environments it involves, health humanities is a "more encompassing, contemporary, and accurate label" (Jones et al. 2014: 6).

Since 2006, health humanities has gained traction both in re-describing, expanding, and generating a much more encompassing vision for applied arts and humanities for health and well-being. It has proposed and foregrounded the recognition of the arts and humanities as a major force for public health—as such, we might call this creative public health. In short, the field has welcomed and promoted inclusion in its work from all sectors and communities. It has challenged the privileging of professional expertise over lived experience and lay perspectives, and widened the pedagogic bandwidth for how the arts and humanities can inform multi-professional training and service development related to health and well-being. It has demonstrated how practices in the arts and humanities can act as a shadow health and social care service to any nation, albeit not necessarily led by medicine. It has pursued the development of a stronger evidence base for the application of both the arts and humanities to improve health and well-being. Finally, and importantly, it has inspired new, active communities worldwide, broadening out from Western perspectives, increasing in cross-cultural sensitivity and dynamism. It is particularly welcome to note how various scholars have begun to interrogate and deepen this move (Gutierrez and DasGupta, 2015), including (in this volume) DasGupta, El-Hadi, Crawford (A.), Boivin, and Richardson. Indeed, the salience of health humanities for diverse international health challenges has been noted by Stewart and Swain (2016: 2587) in referring to "global health humanities," and the recent emergence of research and education networks across the African continent.

Definitions

The health humanities adopt an interdisciplinary, inclusive, applied, democratizing, and activist approach to the arts and humanities in informing and transforming health care, health, and well-being. It is a field "engaging with the contributions of those marginalized from the medical humanities" (Crawford et al., 2010: 4). As such, health humanities has moved beyond a predominating concern with training health professionals through the arts and humanities, and a privileging of a medical, biomedical, or scientific frame or lens above that of the expertise of the public, non-medical, or non-science contributions, and challenges mechanistic or reductive routes to "injecting" the arts and humanities as a kind of treatment. Importantly, it has fractured the expert to non-expert dynamic, revealing faultlines in the project of professional "injectables," treatments, or interventions over grassroots self- and community help and more open access to the benefits of social and cultural assets, that is, creative public health. As such, health humanities strives to bring the public to thera-peutic uses of the arts and humanities. It champions creative, non-professional, or non-expert solutions to health and well-being challenges among service users, informal carers, and self-caring individuals or groups. It values co-design, co-creativity, and co-learning over privileged direction and control in maintaining or recovering the best possible lives while living with, or having experienced, poor health. It also seeks to advance compassionate environments for health care, health, and well-being, not least for practitioners who face continual exposure to trauma (Crawford et al., 2015, 2010). As Purser (2017: 2) notes, such early definitions point to a field that "calls for a reimaging of the boundaries of health and healing, so that our intellectual and therapeutic focus might escape the physical and, perhaps more importantly, the epistemological constraints of the clinical."

In terms of its application in education, Charise (2017: 433) confirms: "One of the innov-ations of Health Humanities is its radically interdisciplinary approach, which differs from con-ventional health education by foregrounding subjects that generally value aesthetics, social experiences, and interpretive methods over quantitative and/or biomedical modes of investi-gation." She identifies health humanities as an open and diverse "undergraduate, pre- or non-health-professional field of study," and more broadly, a "vibrant site of public learning and activism" (Charise 2017: 444). As the field develops, it is the latter—activism—which could prove the field's greatest aspect; that is, activism for public health through the arts and human-ities. The rise of creative public health seems ever more relevant as nations realize that clinical or clincally sanctioned assets are not the only route to enhancing the health of populations. In this way, health humanities loosens itself from educational and training contexts to drive note-worthy research underpinning social change. In a very compelling and powerful way, health humanities is a "free-form and viral movement" that can inform and transform ways of seeing or conceiving health care, health, and well-being (Crawford et al. 2015: 19).

Critical reception

The health humanities feature in critical discussions in the literature, for example, Jones (2014) and Jones et al. (2014). Atkinson et al. (2015) consider it a "post-disciplinary" field of study, while various commentaries have pointed to it, essentially, as the "new kid on the block" or as a competing terminology for particular kinds of research and teaching. Of course, its recep-tion and utilization continues to evolve across different territories with diverse infrastructure and cultures for how the arts and humanities can conceive, drive, and transform health and well-being. For example, Charise (2017) notes that the health humanities may require or create different resources and approaches in unique cultures and contexts: for instance, in research funding. She flags the conventionally narrow-track, discipline-segregated research activities in the United States and Canada, where it can be challenging for any interdisciplinary field to secure funding geared to particular academic silos and rigid concepts. As a result, health humanities will always have to adapt and respond to the different cultural emphases that apply. To date, across North America the educational or pedagogic aspect remains dominant, as with medical humanities and bioethics, yet enriched by new and more open dimensions as to how education in this field is not solely focused on medical trainings and how the social aspects of the arts and humanities inform and shape new visions for health care, health, and well-being. In the United Kingdom and elsewhere in Europe, China, India and Australia, however, applied research or praxis for human benefit and democratizing and activist approaches are to the fore, with educational initiatives running alongside.

Praxis

Research in the health humanities has led to a variety of practical applications in terms of the health and well-being of the public, health care innovation, pedagogic developments, and policy influence. It is beyond the scope of this short chapter to review this work in full, but a couple of examples from recently funded programs should suffice in alerting the reader to its potential for social impact and change. In a recently completed AHRC-funded study, "Creative Practice as Mutual Recovery," 14 separate projects examined how a selection of different creative practices in the arts and humanities can help with promoting good mental health and well-being. It explored how this is possible within and between groups of health service users, family carers, arts practitioners and health, social care and education professionals, in a shared experience termed "mutual recovery."

One of the projects at the Royal College of Music, for example, found that a ten-week program of group drumming reduced depression by as much as 38% and anxiety by 20%, while improving social resilience by 23% and mental well-being by 16% (Fancourt et al., 2016). This is creative public health in action, adding to a raft of evidence for how the arts and humanities can promote mutual recovery without the need for a prescription as such. Importantly, mental health service users co-designed the program from start to finish. In a separate investigation of how medieval medical remedies can tackle antibiotic resistance, AncientBiotics forges new possibilities for application of historical texts to contemporary public health such as dealing with infections (Harrison et al., 2015). In the pages below, there are many other wonderful offerings of applied research and practical work to advance public health by creative means.

This volume highlights the very rich and diverse possibilities with health humanities. It comprises two parts—reflections and applications—to capture a sample of the critical thinking about health humanities and examples of how knowledge and practices in the arts and humanities can apply themselves to multiple contexts of health care, health, and well-being. It is important to acknowledge that the 65 individual chapters represent only a small part of the rich body of theory and practice in the field of health humanities worldwide. We have avoided trying to totalize in any sense this flow of activity, but hope that the current volume illuminates and points to debate, innovation, and new, exciting trends.

In Part I, "Reflections and critical perspectives," we find several threads of the latest thinking about health humanities. Some of these chapters may reprise familiar ground, but many provoke with less familiar and by no means unitary approaches to the topic. This section features reflections on cross-cultural and indigenous perspectives (A. Crawford, Boivin, Richardson, Das-Gupta, El-Hadi); the genealogy of recovery (Brown); challenges and constraints in relation to austerity (Charise); health-care systems (Barrish); clinical settings (Joyes and Baker); and visualizing health care (Macduff); digital contexts (Banner); post-conflict resolution (Meineck); medicine within health humanities (Allsopp); graphic medicine (Squier); the sublime (B. Lewis); the role of creatives (Tischler); co-design (Macdonald); advocacy (Levy); the role of imagination (Tsaplina and Barfield); historicizing anti-vaccination (Lau); the semiotics of drug advertising (Servitje); neoliberalization and biomedicine (Neilson); sensation and culinary texts (Li); creative adult education (Lewis); zombie health care (Schlozman); and the objectified patient (Hall and Kadetz). In addition, there are critical perspectives on the potential for health humanities beyond the United States, Canada, the United Kingdom, and Europe, in terms of Japan (Huffman and Inoue), Australia (Werder and Holland), and Africa (Ifeobu).

In Part II "Applications," this volume offers a firework display of multiple, contemporary, and surprising routes for the application of the arts and humanities to health care, health, and well-being. The tone here is a long way from "injectables," yet it combines notice of both quantitative and qualitative evidence alongside illustrative cases. This section presents lively and inspiring accounts of how the arts or humanities contribute to health care, health, and well-being through the following: theater (Iedema, Case, Cheek O'Donnell, Tsaplina, Astles, Meineck); gallery and museum visiting (Saavedra); literature and reading (Bartel, Baker, Davis, Billington, Meineck); storytelling (Rice, Bleakley, Wilson, Allard); visual arts (Hogan, Scott, Argyle, Tischler, Johnson, Czerwiec, Callender); fashion and textiles (Fleetwood-Smith, Cork-hill, Atkinson, Tillotson); music (Perkins, Fancourt, Williamon, Garabedian, Baker, Bishop, Abrams); singing (Clift, Abrams); dancing or movement (Houston, Jordan, Wright, Purser, Perez-Vallejos, Haslam-Jones); architecture (Quesada-García, Valero-Flores, Moss); horticultural arts (Coope); cooking (George, Dreibelbis); paper making (Matott and Miller); history (Greenwood); biography (Cadd); ancient texts (Lee); philosophy (Carel); and law (Bracken).

In all, we have tried to live up to the inclusiveness at the heart of health humanities by inviting a selection of new writers with unique and developing voices among more established and leading practitioners, academics, and commentators committed to the application of the arts and humanities to health care, health, and well-being.

We have aimed to encourage different kinds of reflections, critical perspectives, and accounts of application without insisting upon a standard presentation of these. Such offerings are by no means exhaustive, but they do indicate the rich and diverse ways that health humanities is emerging worldwide, and how our conceptions of what we hold as belonging to the arts and humanities must remain open—not least in relation to the less privileged or obvious areas of practice such as cooking, horticulture, knitting, quilting, and so forth.

Furthermore, this volume seeks to give emphasis to another core feature of the health humanities, that is, "appliedness." This volume offers an entry point for many different and versatile ways that the arts and humanities can be relevant to a wide range of physical and mental health challenges.

It is particularly pleasing to see a variety of contributions that come to us, "low carbon," from all around the globe. We welcome the focus on different social and cultural contexts for health humanities and fresh insights into how to develop new opportunities for innovation.

To sum up, we are beginning to see the maturation of health humanities as an energetic, robust, applied, and inclusive field: one that signals a more co-created and co-operative vision for how the arts and humanities can stand as an interdisciplinary, and not solely medicalized, shadow health care service to any nation. Working beyond the control of traditional hierarchies of professional knowledge and practice, health humanities is an evolving, game-changing field that attracts different arts and humanities traditions to work more closely with the public to advance health care, health, and well-being. Whether we are considering education, research, or practice, this field is opening medical and non-medical visions of how to improve human health through innovative cultural care. It continues to open up new possibilities for creative public health.

References

AHRC/UKRI (2020). Medical humanities awards 2020. 11/01/2020. https://ahrc.ukri.org/docu ments/calls/medical-humanities-awards-application-guidance/

Atkinson, S., Evans, B., Woods, A. and Kearns, R. (2015). 'The Medical' and 'Health' in a Critical Medical Humanities. *Journal of Medical Humanities*, 36: 71–81.

Berry, S.L., Lamb, E.G. and Jones, J. (2016). Health Humanities Baccalaureate Programs in the United States. Center for Literature and Medicine, Hiram College. www.hiram.edu/images/pdfs/center-litmed/HHBP_8_11_16.pdf. 14/12/2019.

Charise, A. (2017). Site, Sector, Scope: Mapping the Epistemological Landscape of Health Humanities. *Journal of Medical Humanities*, 38: 431–444.

Crawford, P. (2007). Health Humanities Innovation. *Knowledge Transfer from Medical Professionals to Industry: An ESRC Business Seminar*. Biocity, Nottingham. 28 November.

Crawford, P. (2015). Health Humanities: We're Here to Collaborate, Not to Compete. *The Guardian Higher Education*. www.theguardian.com/higher-education-network/2015/mar/30/health-humanities-here-to-collaborate-not-compete

Crawford, P. and Brown, B. (2020). Health Humanities: Democratising the arts and humanities applied to healthcare, health and wellbeing. In A. Bleakley, ed., *Handbook of Medical Humanities*, Routledge, 401–409.

Crawford, P., Brown, B., Baker, C., Tischler, V. and Abrams, B. (2015). *Health Humanities*. Palgrave: London.

Crawford, P., Brown, B., Tischler, V. and Baker, C. (2010). Health Humanities: The Future of Medical Humanities? *Mental Health Review Journal*, 15(3): 4–10.

Crawford, P. and Kadetz, P. eds. (Forthcoming). *Encyclopedia of Health Humanities*. Springer Nature: New York.

Fancourt D., Perkins, R., Ascenso, S., Carvalho, O.A., Steptoe, A. and Williamson, A. (2016). Effects of Group Drumming Interventions on Anxiety, Depression, Social Resilience and Inflammatory Immune Response among Mental Health Service Users. *Plos One*, org/10.1371/journal.pone.0151136

Gutierrez, K. A. and DasGupta, S. (2015). The Space that Difference Makes: On Marginality, Social Justice and the Future of the Health Humanities. *Journal of Medical Humanities*, 37(4): 435–448.

Harrison, F., Roberts, A.E.L., Gabrilska, R., Rumbaugh, K.P., Lee, C. and Diggle, S.P. (2015). A 1000 Year Old Antimicrobial Remedy with Anti-Staphylococcal Activity. *mBio*, 6: 3. 10.1128/mBio.01129-15

Jones, T. (2014). "Oh, the Humanit(ies)!" Dissent, Democracy, and Danger. In V. Bates, A. Bleakley and S. Goodman, eds., *Medicine, Health and the Arts: Approaches to the medical humanities*, Routledge: London. 27–38.

Jones, T., Blackie, M., Garden, R. and Wear, D. (2017). The Almost Right Word: The Move from *Medical* to *Health* Humanities. *Academic Medicine*, 92(7): 932–935.

Jones, T., Wear, D. and Friedman, L.D. (2014). *Health Humanities Reader*. Rutgers University Press: New Brunswick, N.J.

Klugman, C.M. (2017). How Health Humanities Will Save the Life of the Humanities. *Journal of Medical Humanities*, 38: 419–430.

Peterkin, A.D. and Skorzewska, A. (2018). *Health Humanities in Post-Graduate Medical Education*. Oxford University Press: Oxford.

Purser, A. (2017). Dancing Intercorporeality: A Health Humanities Perspective on Dance as a Healing Art. *Journal of Medical Humanities. Open Access*, https://doi.org/10.1007/s10912-017-9502-0

Rubens, A. (2017). Uniting the Pre-Health Humanities with the Introductory Composition Course. *Journal of Medical Humanities*, 38: 361–371.

Skylar, D. (2017). Health Humanities and Medical Education: Joined by a Common Purpose. *Academic Medicine*, 92: 1647–1649.

Stewart, K.A. and Swain, K. (2016). The Art of Medicine: Global Health Humanities: Defining an Emerging Field. *Lancet*, 388(10060): 2586–2587.

Tsevat, R.K., Sinha, A.A., Gutierrez, K.A. and DasGupta, S. (2015). Bringing Home the Health Humanities: Narrative Humility, Structural Competency, and Engaged Pedagogy. *Academic Medicine*, 90(11): 1462–1465.

PART 1

Reflections and critical perspectives

1

THE HEALTH HUMANITIES, GENEALOGIES OF HEALTH CARE, AND THE CONSOLATION OF UNDERSTANDING

Towards a critique of "recovery" in mental health

Brian Brown

Introduction

Understanding ideas, practices, and sensibilities that shape the present is greatly aided by recognizing where they came from. What may look commonplace or taken for granted nowadays may not have always looked this way. Having a grasp of the stories behind our present-day ideas may help us to critically evaluate them and decide whether, and to what extent, we wish to allow them purchase on our everyday lives. Understanding that things have not always been this way will help us become discerning, self-aware, critical consumers of currently fashionable nostrums and practices. Indeed, as Michel Foucault (1926–1984) argued, phenomena become "things" by virtue of being embedded in a grid of language. One of the capabilities of health humanities is to take forward the critical interrogation of concepts and commonplaces in health care. This can be seen in work that attempts to rethink health care from perspectives in anthropology, sociology, or philosophy, which reposes how we visualize the human condition, and explores how evidence may derive from creative practice (Crawford et al., 2014). This kind of awareness demands more than just the traditional history of ideas, but rather a genealogy of ideas.

"Genealogy" in this sense comes from German philosopher and cultural critic Friedrich Nietzsche's (1844–1900) use of the term, and his implementation of the idea, most famously in *Genealogy of Morals* (first published in 1887). Here he sought to untangle the origin of notions of morality. At that point, many intellectuals, inspired by Darwin's then fashionable evolutionary theory, had tried to explain actions that were moral or altruistic in terms of how they benefitted others, or contributed to the well-being of the group. As Paul Ree's

On The Origin of the Moral Sensations (1877) described, an action that contributes to the group's survival, in this view, comes to be seen as moral, altruistic, or desirable. Nietzsche disagreed with this position. Through his detailed knowledge of classical languages, he argued that what came to be seen as morality was in fact closely aligned with the interest of powerful people and elite groups. For example, in ancient Greek the term for "bad" also meant "worthless" or "ill-born"; even in present day language we might describe a desirable course of action as "noble." Powerless people, by contrast, were apt to adopt a "slave morality," in which they believed that they would get their rewards in the hereafter. Thus, morality could be argued to derive from particular political, social, and linguistic arrangements. Hence, when a particular course of conduct is recommended as a good way to behave, Nietzsche invites us to consider whose interests this is likely to serve, and who is likely to benefit.

In the twentieth century, this approach was taken up with some enthusiasm by Michel Foucault, who developed genealogy as a historical perspective and investigative method. In this view, genealogy offers an intrinsic critique of the present by enabling the development of critical skills for exploring and analysing the links between knowledge, power, and human subjectivity in contemporary society. Allied to this, a genealogical approach invites us to consider how our existence has been shaped by historical forces. In this respect we might be interested in how patterns of power predispose us to see crime as a result of some sort of deficiency on the part of the criminal, or in why poverty is often seen as the fault of the poor for not making themselves sufficiently attractive to employers. A genealogical approach can help us understand how the limits of what people think is possible have come into existence, such as why psychiatry became a part of medicine, why sexuality became subject to medical expertise, or why punishment became concerned with the reform of the wrongdoer. Once the limits of those worldviews have been exposed, it is also possible to reveal the spaces of freedom people can yet experience and the changes that can still be made (Foucault, 1970).

Foucault's relevance to the genealogical approach in the health humanities is well known in light of his expositions of madness, sexuality, and selfhood. For example, how did madness come to be a medical matter? In *Madness and Civilisation* (1965) Foucault argues that the category of "madness" arose as a result of a process of confinement of deviants that began at the start of the Age of Reason: vagrants, the immoral, the blasphemous, and, of course, those deemed mad. As a consequence, doctors gained a key role in the process and in the development of asylums, which provided the opportunity to classify, compare, and attempt to cure those who appeared to lack reason. Moreover, confinement ensured that doctors were in a privileged position to dispense wisdom about the issue, and ensure that their voices were the dominant ones wherever the management of the boundary between normality and abnormality was at stake. This view supervened over former approaches to the issue, where deviance was assumed to be freely chosen, or the result of supernatural or spiritual forces, or where confinement was concerned with protecting society. Now, confinement of the mad involved study, classification, and attempts at cure.

There have of course been many critiques of Foucault's work, especially where his historical examples are concerned. Was the ship of fools to which he alludes ever a real ship or was it an imaginary notion? Foucault has also been criticized for his "tunnel vision" focus on the West and his failure to acknowledge empire and colonialism (Stoler, 1995). Similarly, there have been many critiques and revisions of Foucauldian thinking from a feminist perspective—if women are turned into "docile bodies," how are we to understand or facilitate resistance (Fraser, 1989)? If subjectivity itself is merely an effect of power, how are we to make sense of the experiences and stories of people in oppressed groups who are increasingly demanding to be heard (Hartsock, 1990)? Nevertheless, the overall argument concerning the way intellectual life in the human sciences is conditioned by sociohistorical forces and interests has gained traction in many quarters, not least in medicine itself.

It is often difficult to distinguish genealogical approaches from the intersecting, but often distinct, practice of history itself. The exact practice of a genealogical method is hard to pin down. Foucault himself has this to say:

> Genealogy is grey, meticulous, and patiently documentary. It operates on a field of entangled and confused parchments, on documents that have been scratched over and recopied many times ... Genealogy ... requires patience and a knowledge of details and it depends on a vast accumulation of source material. Its "cyclopean monuments" are constructed from "discreet and apparently insignificant truths and according to a rigorous method"; they cannot be the product of "large and well-meaning errors." In short, genealogy demands relentless erudition. Genealogy does not oppose itself to history as the lofty and profound gaze of the philosopher might compare to the molelike perspective of the scholar; on the contrary, it rejects the metahistorical deployment of ideal significations and indefinite teleologies. It opposes itself to the search for "origins."
>
> *(Foucault, 1980: 139–140)*

The history of systems of thought proposed by Foucault is concerned not so much with determining whether the knowledge systems of the human sciences were true, but rather with contextualizing and historicizing notions of truth, knowledge, and rationality. He examined their conditions of emergence, how and why a society in a given era considers some things knowledge, how and why some procedures are judged to be rational and others not. A genealogy of ideas would also attempt to trace the paths of idea dissemination. Ideas diffuse over both time and space in a way that leaves a trace along the path those ideas have taken. Over time, ideas undergo modification in the process of descent, and in space ideas go through adaptive radiation. These processes are not separate from each other, but instead occur simultaneously.

A genealogy of recovery

To illustrate the value of genealogy, let us consider a project I was recently involved in. The United Kingdom's Arts and Humanities Research Council supported a project entitled "Creative Practice as Mutual Recovery" (2013–2018), which was concerned with a variety of creative activities and their impact on recovery in mental health. A part of this project was a study of the genealogy of the notion of recovery itself. In contemporary mental health practice, the usual starting point is a definition of recovery provided by Anthony (1993: 15):

> [A] deeply personal, unique process of changing one's attitudes, values, feelings, goals, skills, and/or roles. It is a way of living a satisfying, hopeful, and contributing life even within the limitations caused by illness. Recovery involves the development of new meaning and purpose in one's life as one grows beyond the catastrophic effects of mental illness.

Yet what is less frequently explored is the intellectual and practical history of the *idea* of recovery. The idea can be traced to the "training of the will" advocated by Abraham

Low (1950) and the quasi-religious approach to alcohol problems promoted by "Dr Bob" and "Bill W" in founding Alcoholics Anonymous (AA). Interestingly, both of these antecedents took a "medical model" approach to the problems they were addressing. Here I use the term "medical model" to denote a view that human troubles can be defined as illnesses and disorders that are susceptible to diagnosis and treatment and have a basis in underlying physical factors. The idea of alcoholism as an "illness," and even a disease, has been pervasive in AA, and while Low was keen to promote self-help and non-hospital alternatives for his patients, he remained firmly in charge and the distinction between being well and alcoholism's various forms of "illness" remained unchallenged.

From a genealogical point of view, I am not saying that the promoters of contemporary recovery policy and practice have deliberately created the movement from the insights of Low, or Bill and Bob. What I would suggest instead is that the process reflects what Nikolas Rose, and before him Foucault, would see as the "capillary" nature of power and influence. Power, they would suggest, has a capillary quality because of its ability to take different forms—from physical violence, to persuasion and expertise, to ideas that are simply ready-to-hand—at different points in its circulation through the social fabric. The practices of recovery are locally implemented and are true in a much more particular sense than if they had resulted from the imposition of some wide-ranging ulterior instruction. They are made up and realized in practice without any explicit history—which is perhaps why the quote from Anthony (1993) is so widely used. This focus on the interior quality of recovery, as critics (e.g. Harper and Speed, 2012) have asserted, can itself be a source of friction between clients and health professionals. As one of our participants remarked:

> Pete: I wasn't getting on well with it and I kept saying to my key worker I'm not getting on well with it, and she said to me, you know what she said to me, was that 'you're not psychologically minded'.
>
> *(Brown and Baker, 2018: 9)*

In a sense, the practice of recovery-oriented work in mental health involves the curation of a particular kind of mindset, further elaborated by Irene:

> Irene: I got the sense that they were teaching me how to recover. And most of it was useful. But the thing was it was all on their terms, you know. Living with your illness and all that. So all their ideas didn't change, it was us that had to change.
>
> *(Brown and Baker, 2018: 9)*

This represents what Peter Miller describes as the "calculating self," the continual process of reorganizing and reconfiguring consciousness and the self. This might include activities such as personal growth, well-being and therapy, investing in training and education so as to make oneself attractive to employers, or even changes in how we dress, speak or appear. In our case it is possible to see the origins of this process in early twentieth-century self-help such as AA or Recovery Inc. This, says Miller, is peculiar to the modern age and is part of this task of shaping subjectivity and forms of personhood (Miller and Rose, 2008). While this offers new possibilities for acting on oneself and on the actions of others, it does not always work seamlessly. The "technologies," as Foucault calls them, with which personhood can be shaped are never fully effective, perhaps through the cultivation of counter-discourses that were evident in our study activity. Some participants had experience of compulsory hospitalization, but even in these cases some of them formulated narratives of resistance:

> James: I've been reading about hospitals, I've been scouring the internet and some of the stuff you find is pretty horrendous. There was that mid Staffordshire case and that other place in Wales recently and that care home that was on the telly, and it is all pretty awful, so it makes you wonder whether putting people in hospital does them any good at all after all.
>
> *(Brown and Baker, 2018: 10)*

For James, who had described his experience of compulsory hospitalization earlier in the interview, it is as if understanding problems in the health-care system itself provides an intelligible way of framing the difficulties that he personally had experienced. Identifying the problems as systematic and frequent meant that obstacles to recovery could be understood less as the participant's fault and more as being a societal problem.

Consequently, understanding the emergence of a discourse of recovery, and illuminating its more coercive histories, makes these kinds of experience on the part of participants more intelligible. Rather than glitches in the operation of the therapeutic process, apprehending the discursive genealogy of recovery exposes and reprises enduring tensions in the way care practices have been organized, and its conceptual structures formulated. Indeed, without being formally steeped in this way of thinking about things, it was as if some participants were working towards this kind of analysis themselves. Perhaps through a growing incredulity at the terms used by staff to describe them and their difficulties—"you've got to walk before you can run," "you'll make yourself ill again," or the "not psychologically minded" comment above—they were placing their unease in a wider sociohistorical context. This was underscored by those who were familiar with conflict and service delivery problems elsewhere in the health-care system. These activities of critique, analysis, and deconstruction in themselves appeared to help participants in this study make sense of what was happening to them—perhaps by indicating points of release from the enmiring language and practice of conventional, hospital-based mental health care.

More broadly, a genealogical approach can help us understand how approaches like "recovery" in mental health have been brought to visibility as a result of social, intellectual, and rehabilitative practice; and, furthermore, what the conceptual antecedents of recovery are, and how this understanding might help us define its form and function in the present. For example, recovery approaches often advocate acceptance of the limits imposed by an underlying "illness" whose ontology often goes unchallenged. That is, in practice recovery often involves accepting the notion of mental disorder rather than deconstructing or challenging it. In addition, recovery approaches often focus on interior psychological life and encourage clients to think of a division between the illness, which remains in medical hands, and the psychosocial recovery, which is in the hands of the client. These aspects have not come about by accident but rather have been systematically built into these approaches for the best part of a century.

The friction participants experienced between the health-care system and the poverty of therapeutic ambition resonates with a variety of Foucault-inspired scholarship on mental health issues. As Parker et al. (1995) describe them, the human service professions are concerned with ascribing pathological identities to vulnerable people. This is associated with the persistence of a deficit model of the client, which has been particularly robust across time and in differing health-care contexts. In other words, depression is often seen as a failure of

15

attitudes, cognition, or neurotransmitters; autism as a failure to develop a theory of others' minds; or an episode of schizophrenia an example of the client's failure to adequately monitor their relapse profile. At the same time, where people consider social context, nowadays it is not likely to be in terms of radical collective action and politics, but instead with a focus on interpersonal processes such as support and education (which are often closely aligned with overtly medicalized concepts of distress and illness). The notion that one can culture and cultivate the self through therapy, healing, and self-help today seems to travel effortlessly across a vast range of territories and care contexts (Illouz, 2008). Other approaches, for example, thinking about human misery through the lens of structural inequalities, seem rather more difficult to get to grips with. This may reflect the fact that such thinking would be more troubling to elite groups and powerful interests as it might point to their role in sustaining human misery. The genealogical approach can help us to reflect on how some ways of thinking are somehow easier to do and fall more readily to hand than others.

Genealogies of ideas and the consolation of understanding

In summary, a genealogical approach to understanding health can help to show us how present-day ideas and practices have come about. They are often not self-evident, but have emerged through struggles, debates, and conflict where some interests have prevailed. Through the example of "recovery" approaches in mental health described above, I have attempted to show how thinking about the practice and ideology of health care in this way can open up the possibility of alternatives and help to grasp and place in context resistance, failure, and context in the present day. The latter are not just the result of people not getting the message or having poor "health literacy," or of failures of compliance. Rather, they may represent the beginnings of a more informed scepticism towards present-day practice. A genealogical approach can also enable us to trace how health-care practice is as much about gaining purchase on the management of identities as it is about the nature and structure of services. The genealogical approach then allows us to examine the degree of consilience between the variety of practices that seek to manage health, formulate health risks, operationalize and shape desirable conduct, and specify a desired mindset on the part of citizens and health practitioners, because, as Rose puts it, these practices "spread out over a variety of surfaces." We can examine the nature and limits of new healthy identities that are encouraged and promoted through publicity, educational materials, therapeutic interventions, and the wider culture.

A genealogical approach of this kind implies that current notions in and around health and illness are but a small set of a much larger variety of options, and that alternatives may be present around the corner. Understanding the origins and family trees of what is happening to us in health care can offer the consolation of understanding, even when health care itself seems crass or ineffective. Awareness of the genealogical histories of these tendencies in the health and social care disciplines will make it easier for those in distress, their careers, and health-care providers to decide whether a course of action is genuinely helpful to them and which aspects, if any, they wish to retain.

References

Anthony, W.A. (1993). Recovery from Mental Illness: The Guiding Vision of the Mental Health Service System in the 1990s, *Psychosocial Rehabilitation Journal*, 16(4): 11–23.
Brown, B. and Baker, S. (2018). The Social Capitals of Recovery in Mental Health, *Health*, DOI: 10.1177/1363459318800160.

Crawford, P. Brown, B., Baker, C., Tischler, V. and Abrams, B. (2014). *Health Humanities*. London: Palgrave.

Foucault M. (1965). *Madness and Civilization: A History of Insanity in the Age of Reason*. Howard R, trans. New York: Vintage.

Foucault, M. (1970). *The Order of Things*. London: Tavistock Publications.

Foucault, M. (1980). Nietzsche, Genealogy, History. In D.F. Bouchard, ed, *Language, Counter-Memory, Practice: Selected essays and Interviews by Michel Foucault*. Ithaca, NY: Cornell University Press: 139–164.

Fraser, N. (1989). *Unruly Practices: Power, Discourse and Gender in Contemporary Social Theory*. Cambridge: Polity Press.

Harper, D., and Speed, E. (2012). Uncovering Recovery: The Resistible Rise of Recovery and Resilience, *Studies in Social Justice*, 6(1): 9–25.

Hartsock, N. (1990). Foucault on Power: A Theory for Women? In: L.J. Nicholson, ed, *Feminism/Postmodernism*. London and NY: Routledge: 157–175.

Illouz, E. (2008). *Saving the Modern Soul: Therapy, Emotions and the Culture of Self-Help*. Berkeley, CA: University of California Press.

Low, A. A. (1950). *Mental health Through Will Training*. West Hanover, MA: Christopher Publishing House.

Miller, P., and Rose, N. (2008). *Governing the Present: Administering Economic Social and Personal Life*. Cambridge: Polity Press.

Parker, I., Georgaca, E., Harper, D., McLaughlin, T. and Stowell-Smith, M. (1995). *Deconstructing Psychopathology*. London: Sage.

Stoler, A.L. (1995). *Race and the Education of Desire: Foucault's History of Sexuality and the Colonial Order of Things*. Durham, NC: Duke University Press.

2

ON APPLYING THE ARTS AND HUMANITIES IN AUSTERE TIMES

Andrea Charise

Introduction

For almost two centuries, arguments regarding the *value* of the arts and humanities have opposed the rallying rhetoric of "utility" with its supposed antithesis, the preservation of "arts for art's sake." Sore spots persist: resistance to the arts' "instrumentalization" (Belling, 2010) is often soaked through with economic and social privilege (Small, 2013). At the same time, recent decades have also witnessed disciplines traditionally considered as detached from the arts and humanities—including computing, technology, and, of course, medicine —rebranding their work as compatible with, even indebted to, the knowledge, skills, and aptitudes conventionally associated with aesthetic traditions (e.g., close reading, narrative, storytelling, and creativity, to name just a few).

In the context of health and medicine, anxieties regarding the *application* of the arts and humanities are usually evident in references to their status as a "handmaiden" to clinical education, training, and practice (Bleakley, 2015: 50): a strikingly gendered metaphor that asserts the apparently unidirectional flow of such interdisciplinary business. In fact, the proliferation of labels for this field and its cognate practices—including medical humanities, health humanities, arts and/in/for health, and art therapy—imply ongoing tensions concerning the applied versus critical (or theoretical) shading of the creative arts and humanities within health and health-adjacent settings. The stakes are high: if health humanities' applied value is, as some critics have asserted, an "inoculation" against both the "decline of the broader humanities" and medicine's own "hidden curriculum" (Klugman, 2017), then it presents a key opportunity to counteract diminishing funding and social support for arts and humanities programs in academic and community spheres alike. Alongside other interdisciplinary arts and humanities fields such as digital humanities, applied theater, creative writing, and critical pedagogy, the twenty-first-century ascendance of health humanities suggests its tenuously fortunate situation within a Western cultural context increasingly sceptical of non-STEM research fields and education pathways.

In 1959, C.P. Snow published *The Two Cultures and the Scientific Revolution*: a canonical, if controversial, statement on the divergent "cultures" of arts and science (Snow, 1959). Sixty years later, it seems important to recall that Snow's lecture was less concerned with *disciplinary* knowledges than with the competing epistemologies of practice, work, and labour engendered by *theoretical* versus *applied* science (the latter was "the real stuff," to cite Snow's own fighting words). More recently, from the emergence of arts-based "social pre-scription" in the United Kingdom and Canada (Bickerdike et al., 2017), to the growth of health humanities baccalaureate programs across North America (Berry et al., 2017), there exist pressing new reasons to consider the matter of application within this field.

Current debates regarding health humanities as an "applied" practice may therefore be said to reflect a longstanding concern in the arts and humanities more generally: as Michael Bérubé (2003: 23) observes, artists and humanists are "generally ambivalent about the idea of defending their enterprises in terms of social utility." Furthermore, the rhetorical conver-gence of interdisciplinarity with vacuous allusions to "innovation," "relevance," and indeed "application" (Callard and Fitzgerald, 2015; Campion, 2018) makes health humanities a rea-sonable target for critical misgivings. Layered onto this, however, is the newly fraught matter of doing health humanities within the neoliberal climate of austerity in the second decade of the twenty-first century. Those notoriously slippery terms require some rough-and-ready definition: I use "neoliberalism" to describe an economic system in which a market paradigm is radically extended throughout personal and public life, including the pri-vatization or international decentralization of traditionally public or social services (educa-tion, health, transportation, and so on). Austerity frequently aids in neoliberalism's expansion by converting aspects of the social economy into marketable commodities premised on the claim that, in doing so, such practices will control costs and reduce public debt (Monbiot, 2016; Verhaeghe, 2014).

This chapter reflects on my own experience as a health humanities researcher in the midst of such times, with a particular focus on "empathy training" as an application of arts and humanities in the health context. From these experiences I share my thoughts on revisiting the commitments of our field, its emphases, and future directions—for applying our work, ourselves, and our critical solidarities.

Applying empathy

Although enhancing empathy—defined in the *Oxford English Dictionary* as "the ability to understand and appreciate another person's feelings, experience, etc.," or by the well-known phrasing "the capacity to place oneself in another's shoes" (Bellet and Maloney, 1991)—is a decent, if moralized, ideal, there exist important critiques of empathy training as a motivat-ing concern for health humanities. On one hand, research shows that empathy decline in health professionals (and related issues like ethical or moral "erosion") is associated with clin-ical training (Batt-Rawden et al., 2013). Contributing factors include work-related and vic-arious trauma, long hours, and sleep deprivation (Chen et al., 2007). In response to calls for improving "compassionate" and "humanized" health care, since the mid-1990s, arts- and especially narrative-based training to enhance empathy has been integrated in a range of clinical education and practice environments (Charon, 2006; Charon et al., 2016).

At the pre-professional level, "empathy training" describes one of the three main approaches to teaching and learning health humanities (Jones et al., 2014). But, in so far as empathy training constitutes a *raison d'être* of health humanities, a cautious approach seems wise "for a field that claims to offer access to the perspectives of those marginalized in med-ical practice and education, as well as an effective means of inculcating empathy" (Garden, 2015: 79). Alan Bleakley calls it a "weasel word," one that "carr[ies] authority, but this is false or hollow. It creates an impression of certainty but actually carries a good deal of ambiguity" (2015: 85). In a similar vein, Rebecca Garden (2015: 79) echoes feminist science studies scholar Donna Haraway when she warns that an uncritical focus on empathy presents a "serious danger of romanticizing and/or appropriating the vision of the less powerful while claiming to see from their positions." To this critique of empathy training as an application of the arts, I would add the potential alignment of arts- and humanities-based interventions with neoliberal ideology (which typically involves the marketization of public goods like health). As a partial case study of these issues, I turn now to a recent project where I was involved as both a researcher and facilitator.

"H is for hospital": narrative training for nursing empathy

Following the usual institutional research ethics process, our goal was to assess the perceived impact of an arts-based narrative training intervention (namely, reflective writing and comics drawing) involving nurses at a major urban Canadian pediatric rehabilitation hospital. At first we intended to deploy a small-scale "narrative medicine"-style initiative (Charon, 2006) simply for the purpose of introducing an arts-based activity into the nursing workplace. However, meaningful institutional support—not to mention funding that enabled the hiring of a research assistant—was forthcoming only when we explicitly reoriented the intervention's purpose as a means of promoting nursing empathy. While it was not our plan to so overtly instrumentalize the project, these pragmatic concerns helped us direct our applied initiative. The study began.

I will not repeat the results here (see Adamson et al., 2018) except to say that we were permitted to recruit eight pediatric rehabilitation nurses for a once-weekly, 90-minute narrative training session over six weeks. (Our decision to use the language of narrative *training* rather than narrative *medicine* to describe this application of close reading, attentive listening, and reflective writing is in keeping with research encouraging such inclusiveness [Crawford et al., 2010]). In addition to the facilitated sessions, participants completed a pre- and post-intervention interview to assess their sense of the intervention's impact. Our discovery of narrative training's "triple benefit"—meaning the enrichment of nurses' empathy for patients and families, for their peers, and for themselves—meaningfully extended the existing research with a significantly under-researched group of nursing professionals.

Following the conclusion of the study, some personal reflections emerged for me that were not, for various reasons, reflected in the article. For one, I noted how several participants voiced how institutionally driven empathy directives seemed to confuse the boundaries of compassionate care with abusive behavior in the workplace. As one nurse remarked:

> You want to be able to stand up for yourself, but I find that it's hard to figure out that line with [patient- and] family-centered care. Professionally, too, right? You want to be able to assert yourself, to stand up for yourself, but just finding the line to keep it professional, to keep it therapeutic, that's hard. I haven't quite figured that one out yet. So that's why I try everything to avoid that situation ... I think it damages a little piece of you.
>
> *(Participant interview transcript, unpublished)*

Here, institutional commitment to "patient-and family-centered care"—whose principles include Respect and Dignity, Information Sharing, Partnership, and Collaboration (IPFCC, 2019)—is squarely at odds with the extension of those very principles to health-care providers, in this case nurses. Another participant voiced a similar assessment of the dilemma presented by codifying empathy in the health-care setting: "We [nurses] are here to heal, but at what cost?" Written and visual narratives generated during the intervention included being compared to "waitresses" and housekeepers ("a daily change of the parents' [bed] sheets? Please. Do you do that at your house?"), and a confusion of nurses' institutional/residential and professional/domestic roles—as reflected in the often-repeated phrase, "H is for hospital, not hotel."

With an awareness and appreciation for the extreme emotional demands placed on parents in the pediatric rehabilitation setting, nurses also articulated a critical impasse between the marginalized status of patients and families on one hand, and the poor treatment of nurses caring for those people on the other. As one observed:

> Nursing always was, when I first—[I'm] not that saying we didn't have families that yelled at you, or swore at you, or whatever, but it was not as bad. But in the last four or five years, I've really noticed a kind of a change and it's not been a really—we still have amazing parents that are really very, very thoughtful, very sweet ... but you've got their expectations, and then when you hear from the hospital about, you know, the "client" business. What happened to the "patient"? Why can't it be a "patient"? ... "Client" is what you refer to anybody outside [the hospital].
>
> *(Participant interview transcript, unpublished)*

While debate concerning health-related labeling has existed since the mid-1970s (Scheff, 1974; Sjöström, 2017), nurses voiced renewed concern about "user"-focused language: "Hospital language of 'clients' and 'service' has changed the respect for nurses. That's the part that's really bothered me in the last ten years." That the idiom of "patient" has been usurped by the consumerist rhetoric of "clients"—effectively uniting sick people under "the community of all customers," to use Theodor Adorno's phrasing—is indicative of a fractured workplace where latent solidarities between health-care "users" and "providers" are effectively neutralized (Adorno, 1978).

This transformation of language could very well track alongside the uptake of empathy training within the neoliberalized health care setting. How to conduct and report this kind of research while remaining alert to the ideological realities of compulsory empathy? This prospect was bolstered by another study finding, namely a subtheme that emerged exclusively post-intervention. The subtheme "Renewal of professional purpose" was used to describe how the narrative training intervention prompted participants' own recognition of the significance of their role as nurses, by counteracting the grinding diminishments of interprofessional discord, workloads, and the challenges of providing complex care ("the once-a-week [narrative training intervention] really brings you back to the purpose of my role, or one of the most important aspects of my role"). Of course, "renewal of professional purpose" was a remarkable and undeniably uplifting finding (Hawthorne and participant reactivity effects notwithstanding), given the dire portrait of nursing work conveyed in pre-intervention interviews and early sessions (e.g., "Instead of my job being a good thing it's just about working your butt off").

To be clear: this project was one of the most satisfying moments of my own career as a researcher. I was moved to learn that the pleasurable sessions spent reading, writing, and making art with these nurses had the further result of improving our participants' relationship to work to some extent. Yet here was a moment where theory and application crashed together for me as a researcher and arts facilitator. Despite the earnest and, I think, meaningful impact of this work (as revealed by member-checking eight months after the study's conclusion), I suspect there is a risk of such initiatives being appropriated to cushion the effects of funding cuts to public health and the social institution of health care. Is it unreasonable, or simply realistic, to anticipate that a low-risk, low-cost intervention like narrative training may be implemented as a form of institutional window-dressing: as a means to innovate new ways for employees to work more and more contentedly alongside compassion fatigue, moral erosion, empathy decline, and burnout? To be blunt: narrative training, or any kind of arts- and humanities-inspired application, is not the solution to the effects of funding cuts, overwork, and dysfunctional healthcare working environments. The remedy, by contrast, is simple and devastatingly uncreative: fundamental system change that works to guarantee, promote, and protect the well-being of a hospital community.

"We heard health care": health humanities' austere activism

Critical discussions of empathy have yet to grapple with the difficult intersectional realities of systemically disenfranchised health workers (nurses, for one, but probably also a vast range of allied health providers and care staff), and other power-compromised roles within the health-care environment (patients most obviously). In the study just described, nurses' untheorized reflections were enabled by a highly applied activity; yet their words powerfully outline the conceptual infrastructure of health care at the present time, as well as the function of arts and humanities within this setting. Moreover, it is through the materials of the arts and humanities that we might investigate different perspectives on the underlying causes of similar trends: in this case, why the "demanding" patient (or their families) may be a consequence of an increasingly austere, precarious, and inaccessible health-care system—a system whose signs include the normalization of oppositional day-to-day patient–care provider interactions.

As a literary scholar, I hold on to my inclination to locate texts that engage and represent these phenomena—not simply for the purposes of performing endless feats of academic productivity (journal articles, book chapters, etc.) but by making use of their logics in the public and private ways available to me as a citizen. At the risk of collapsing important differences that exist between geographically specific health systems (see Phillip Barrish's work on this topic in this volume and elsewhere, 2016), I want to share some provocative examples that exemplify the inventive bridging of theory and application around matters of health in the twenty-first-century context of neoliberalism and the austerity climate it has engendered.

American works include Ann Cvetkovich's extraordinary memoir and critical essay *Depression: A Public Feeling* (2012), Chang-Rae Lee's dystopian novel *On Such a Full Sea* (2014), and Lionel Shriver's *So Much for That: A Novel* (2010)—an especially clear-eyed vision of the human and economic costs of illness, health, and treatment within the United States' private health insurance model. The frantic, diminishing hopes of the Obama-era undertaking of a government-run health insurance option is captured in award-winning poet, essayist, and playwright Claudia Rankine's "The Health of Us" (2016; an earlier audio version was published as "We Heard Healthcare" in 2011). Its opening lines read:

> We heard health care and we thought public option
> we thought reaching across the street across the lines
> across the aisle was the manifestation of not a red state
> not a blue state but these united states
>
> *(Rankine, 2016, ll. 1–4)*

In the United Kingdom, Harry Leslie Smith's memoirs—*Harry's Last Stand* (2014) and *Don't Let My Past Be Your Future: A Call to Arms* (2017)—illuminate his early life of poverty prior to the implementation of the National Health Service (NHS) in 1948. (With the exception of some services, the NHS provides free—that is, tax-funded—health care at the point of use for all United Kingdom residents.) Yet Smith's final years (he died in November 2018 at the age of 95) were spent sounding the alarm concerning what he saw as the return of the squalid miseries of pre-1948 British society: poverty, poor housing, the rise of fascism, and inaccessible health care.

Illuminating precisely the abysmal conditions Smith identifies, Ken Loach's recent Palme d'Or-winning film *I, Daniel Blake* (2016) stars Daniel John as a 59-year-old widowed carpenter who is denied welfare support following a heart attack. A contemporary update of the mid-nineteenth-century genre known as the "condition of England" or "protest" novel, such works engage directly with the social unrest provoked by growing class antagonism and economic precarity. Although a physician's diagnosis is that Daniel is unfit to return to work, he is apparently well enough to pass the government's "work capability assessment." The economically depressed location of Newcastle upon Tyne becomes the site of this conflict (the film includes documentary-like scenes of long food-bank queues and derelict government housing).

I, Daniel Blake's relentless examination of Daniel's Kafkaesque entrapment between the states of health and illness offers some unyielding lessons for health humanities at the present time. The film opens with approximately three minutes of black screen; as the credits run, the viewer can only listen to the spoken exchange between Daniel and "Amanda," an early- to mid-twenties-sounding (white) female (voice) tasked with establishing his eligibility for Employment Support Allowance. During a tediously long list of standardized questions ("Can we just talk about me heart?"), Daniel loses patience:

[Daniel Blake]: Can I ask you a question? Are you medically qualified?
[Amanda]: I'm a health care professional appointed by the Department of Work and Pensions to carry out assessments for Employment and Support Allowance.
[DB]: But there was a bloke out in the, er, in the waiting room, he says that you work for an American company.
[A]: Our company's been appointed by the Government.
[DB]: Are you a nurse? Are you a doctor?
[A]: I'm a health care professional.

This exchange establishes the film's indictment of social services radically abstracted from local, community-based kinship and "care webs" (Piepzna-Samarasinha, 2018). An American subcontractor becomes the synecdoche for the insinuation of private interests into the British welfare state, and Amanda's coolly vague qualifications as "health care professional" further signal how insecure the denotative and connotative meanings of "health" have become in the newly globalized twenty-first-century context. As with the nurses' objection to the collapsing of "hospital" and "hotel" in the study described earlier, *I, Daniel Blake* asks viewers to be awake to how an increasingly austere health-care environment thrives on the deliberate linguistic confusion of categories, roles, and responsibilities that once described the care of a community of sick people.

As the film progresses, Daniel becomes increasingly trapped between the theory and practice of "application": a word that is both a trigger and a motif for *I, Daniel Blake*'s portrait of the incessant evaluation, assessment, and escalating bureaucracy of the contemporary welfare state and, by extension, neoliberalized health care. Neither sick nor well enough to receive state benefits, Daniel's waking hours are fully occupied applying for jobs that he is unable to take until his appeal is decided. The insistently bleak, grey color-grading of Daniel's life is broken up only by the sporadic respite of his recreational wood-carving and listening to classical music; but even these brief moments of aesthetic relief are subject to monetizing forces. His beloved late wife's record collection is juxtaposed with the tinny, ear-splitting substitute that accompanies hours of waiting for call-center representatives; when Daniel's modest apartment and belongings are finally repossessed, the agent encourages him to name his price for his last, beautifully carved wooden fish mobile (Daniel refuses).

The film's evacuation of the aesthetic by exasperating consumerist proxies (music/muzak, mobiles/mobile phones, assistance/application) mirrors Daniel's own inexorable dehumanization. He dies in the bathroom of a government office minutes before he is able to appeal his case, and the film concludes with Daniel's own manifesto being read aloud at a pauper's funeral by his younger friend Katie (herself an impoverished, starving single mother):

> I am not a client, a customer, nor a service user … I am not a national insurance number, nor a blip on the screen … My name is Daniel Blake. I am a man, not a dog. As such, I demand my rights. I demand you treat me with respect. I, Daniel Blake, am a citizen, nothing more and nothing less. Thank you.

I, Daniel Blake's condemnation of the abstraction of application is at the heart of its scathing indictment of neoliberalism and the enabling conditions of austerity. Neither the theory nor application (literally and figuratively understood) of a chronically marketized society are capable of ensuring its constituents' most basic claims to a healthy, dignified life.

Conclusion

Clearly, the stale terms of a theory–application divide are not a productive driver for health humanities, nor does it make much sense to maintain such partition when mapping the future directions of the field. The forceful disjointing of theory and application—redolent as it is with class stigma and economic barriers to access—is perhaps inevitable in an interdisciplinary field that constructs its conceptual horizon from two deeply hierarchal professions; yet the persistence of such a fissure in health humanities seems especially rotten at a time when private and public health-care systems throughout the developed world appear to be in a state of acute system distress. The relatively apolitical work of medical/health humanities thus far has effectively ignored or, at the very least, left itself unprepared to defy its own entanglement in hierarchal intellectual inheritances and practice environments: the hospital and university perhaps most of all.

This reality exerts real pressure on the familiar, congratulatory claim of art's "humanizing" effect on health-care delivery. Is enhancing empathy the way that narrative training—or similar arts- and humanities-based applications—actually works? While some creative labors and outcomes may indeed be intended to enhance or provoke empathy (as remains the impetus for protest art such as *I, Daniel Blake*), the fact remains that the arts are rarely intended for the didactic purposes of moral reflection. It feels like an old joke now: if exposure to the arts really did have a humanizing effect, then English literature departments would be the most humane places on the planet. In the health context, perhaps arts and humanities interventions only appear to work because they extract, and temporarily shield, health-care workers from a toxic, even wounding, workplace environment. (And if this should prove to be the case, would that actually diminish the value of such applications of the arts and humanities in the health-care setting? I am less and less inclined to think so myself.)

As I have argued elsewhere (Charise, 2017), health humanities will only realize its promise by recognizing, and being legible to, the multiplicity of sites and communities where such work is needed, shaped, and experienced. In 2020, one ambient condition is neoliberalism and the lived effects of austerity. As the examples in this chapter show, the most pressing realities facing health care today—the issues that unite its workers, patients, and formal and informal care providers—actually require deeply untheoretical solutions: living wages, reliable housing, employment, respite from work, nutritious food, clean water, dignity. The neoliberal conditions of austerity reveal the structural limits of mere theorization. The purposive "application" of arts and humanities is, in turn, not the accumulation of uni-dimensional exemplars. Rather, such applications should be understood as unearthings of possibility that make health humanities a viable, because essentially dignifying, endeavor.

In keeping with a broader turn toward the "post-critical" (Felski, 2015), the arts and humanities in austere times must be infused with advocacy and alive to activism. What our work demands is a sustained, cross-sector alertness to the intrinsic entanglement of theory and practice. Only then can we actively create the conditions for the real stakes of our efforts: the realization of meaningfully improved states of physical, emotional, occupational, and social wellness, and the elevation of dignity for all. To the extent that humility is an emergent "god term" in this field (alongside empathy, compassion, reflection, and others), health humanities practitioners must decenter the longstanding elevation of theory in university-driven academic arts and humanities work. If there is an upside to late capitalism and the neoliberal policies it has so thoroughly engendered, it is its provision of a vital arena to prove health humanities' validity, substance, collective mandate, and ethics. For our field to realize its transformative potential we must face, and respond directly to, the difficult truths that underlie the arts and humanities' appeal within the health setting.

References

Adamson, K., Sengsavang, S., Charise, A., Wall, S., Kinross, L. and Balkaran, M. (2018). Narrative Training as a Method to Promote Nursing Empathy Within a Pediatric Rehabilitation Setting. *Journal of Pediatric Nursing: Nursing Care of Children and Families*, 42: e2–e9.

Adorno, T. (1978). *Minima Moralia*. (E.F.N. Jephcott, trans.ed.). London: Verso.

Barrish, P. (2016). Health Policy in Dystopia. *Literature and Medicine*, 34(1): 106–131.

Batt-Rawden, S.A., Chisolm, M.S., Anton, B. and Flickinger, T.E. (2013). Teaching Empathy to Medical Students: An Updated, Systematic Review. *Academic Medicine*, 88(8): 1171–1177.

Bellet, P.S. and Maloney, M.J. (1991). The Importance of Empathy as an Interviewing Skill in Medicine. *JAMA*, 266(13): 1831–1832.

Belling, C. (2010). Commentary: Sharper Instruments: On Defending the Humanities in Undergraduate Medical Education. *Academic Medicine*, 85(6): 938–940.

Berry, S., Jones, T. and Lamb, E. (2017). Health Humanities: The Future of Pre-Health Education is Here. *Journal of Medical Humanities*, 38(4): 353–360.

Bérubé , M. (2003). The Utility of the Arts and Humanities. *Arts and Humanities in Higher Education*, 2(1): 23–40.

Bickerdike, L., Booth, A., Wilson, P.M., Farley, K. and Wright, K. (2017). Social Prescribing: Less Rhetoric and More Reality. A Systematic Review of the Evidence. *BMJ Open*, 7: e013384.

Bleakley, A. (2015). *Medical Humanities and Medical Education: How the Medical Humanities Can Shape Better Doctors*. London: Routledge.

Callard, F. and Fitzgerald, D. (2015). *Rethinking Interdisciplinarity across the Social Sciences and Neurosciences*. London: Palgrave.

Campion, C. (2018). Whither the Humanities? Reinterpreting the Relevance of an Essential and Embattled Field. *Arts and Humanities in Higher Education*, 17(4): 433–448.

Charise, A. (2017). Site, Sector, Scope: Mapping the Epistemological Landscape of Health Humanities. *Journal of Medical Humanities*, 38(4): 431–444.

Charon, R. (2006). *Narrative Medicine: Honoring the Stories of Illness*. New York, NY, US: Oxford University Press.

Charon, R., Dasgupta, S., Hermann, N., Marcus, E.R., Colon, E.R., Spencer, D. and Spiegel, M. (2016). *The Principles and Practice of Narrative Medicine*. Oxford University Press.

Chen, D., Lew, R., Hershman, W. and Orlander, J. (2007). A Cross-Sectional Measurement of Medical Student Empathy. *Journal of General Internal Medicine*, 22(10): 1434–1438.

Crawford, P., Brown, B., Tischler, V. and Baker, C. (2010). Health Humanities: The Future of Medical Humanities? *Mental Health Review Journal*, 15(3): 4–10.

Cvetkovich, A. (2012). *Depression: A Public Feeling*. Durham, NC: Duke University Press.

Felski, R. (2015). *The Limits of Critique*. Chicago: University of Chicago Press.

Garden, R. (2015). Who Speaks for Whom? Health Humanities and the Ethics of Representation. *Medical Humanities*, 41: 77–80.

Institute for Patient- and Family-Centered Care (IPFCC) (2019). www.ipfcc.org. Accessed March 1, 2019.

Jones, T., Wear, D. and Friedman, L.D. eds. (2014). *Health Humanities Reader*. New Brunswick, N.J: Rutgers University Press.

Klugman, C.M. (2017). How Health Humanities Will Save the Life of the Humanities. *Journal of Medical Humanities*, 38(4): 419–430.

Loach, K. (2016). *I, Daniel Blake*. Film.

Lee, C.-R. (2014). *On Such a Full Sea*. New York: Penguin.

Monbiot, G. (2016). *How Did We Get into This Mess? Politics, Equality, Nature*. London: Verso.

Piepzna-Samarasinha, L.L. (2018). *Care Work: Dreaming Disability Justice*. Vancouver: Arsenal Pulp Press.

Rankine, C. (2016). The health of us. *Literary Hub*, November 16. Accessed March 1, 2019. https://lithub.com/the-health-of-us/.

Scheff, T. (1974). The Labelling Theory of Mental Illness. *American Sociological Review*, 39(3): 444–452.

Shriver, L. (2011). *So Much for That*. London: Fourth Estate.

Sjöström, S. (2017). Labelling Theory. In: *Routledge International Handbook of Critical Mental Health* ed. Bruce M. Z. Cohen (Abingdon: Routledge, 28 Sep 2017), Routledge Handbooks Online (Accessed 23/11/2019).

Small, H. (2013). *The Value of the Humanities*. Oxford: Oxford University Press.

Snow, C.P. (1993). *The Two Cultures*. Cambridge: Cambridge University Press.

Smith, H.L. (2014). *Harry's Last Stand: How the World my Generation built is falling down, and What We Can Do to Save it*. London: Icon Books.

Smith, H.L. (2017). *Don't Let my Past Be Your Future: A Call to Arms*. London: Constable.

Verhaeghe, P. (2014). *What About Me? The Struggle for Identity in a Market-Based Society*. Trans. Jane Hedley-Prole. Melbourne, London: Scribe.

3

CREATIVE PRACTICES IN CHALLENGING PLACES

Emma Joyes and Charley Baker

Introduction

This chapter provides a critical perspective on the application of the promotion of creative practice within forensic mental health (FMH) and mental health services, with its promise of improvements in recovery for patients. Recent research findings are introduced that illustrate the challenges faced with the introduction of creative practice and its potential for supporting recovery within challenging places, such as in high-secure or forensic mental health settings. The chapter has two sections, in the first an introduction to FMH is provided, followed by a brief history of creative practice and mental health. The challenges of implementing creative practices within the secure mental health environment is considered. The second section introduces an example of current practice provided by the first author that illuminates these challenges.

Forensic mental health in the United Kingdom

FMH is a specialism which involves the assessment and treatment of individuals with mental illness who engage in or are at risk of offending-related behavior (Mullen, 2000). The containment of the individual serves to protect the public (Sugarman and Dickens, 2015) while also providing care to the patient. Often the person within FMH is detained under the Mental Health Act (1983/2007), providing the legal basis and limitations for containment within various levels of secure settings, and limits to treatment approaches that can be applied without a person's consent. An overly custodial approach to care has been argued to underpin repeated, and much publicized, scandals of both abuse of patients and public safety concerns (Sugarman and Dickens, 2015). Furthermore, professional boundary violations, such as personal self-disclosure, are common within FMH care. Such violations become complicated in the landscape of inequalities of power between staff and patients, which are further complicated by attachment issues, and can lead to more severe violations, such as personal relationships (Adshead, 2012).

Individuals in contact with such services are referred to as offenders, patients, service users, mentally disordered offenders, and sometimes "deviants" (Prins, 2005), demonstrating the potential challenge society at large might have with equating offending behavior with a need for compassionate care and treatment rather than incarceration and punishment (Seymour, 2010). A multitude of professions now work within the field of FMH (Soothill et al., 2008); therefore these terms are used interchangeably within and across FMH services and the criminal justice system. In this chapter, the term "patient" will be adopted, although the authors recognize that "person" may be a preferred nominal within creative approaches.

Before the closure of the large asylums in 1960s, mental health services tended to offer little stimulation to patients. This lack of stimulation was argued to lead to institutional neurosis, a disease consisting of symptoms such as "apathy, loss of interest, lack of initiative, and sometimes a characteristic posture and gait result[ing] from institutional life" (Barton, 1966: 5). The advancement of psychiatric drugs and social and political campaigns contributed to the closure of the asylums (Killaspy, 2006), and FMH became influenced by the recovery movement motivated by the fundamental rights of people with mental illness. This also followed developments in sociological thought around the negative implications of labeling (Thornicroft, 2006). The aim of the recovery movement was "to afford people with serious mental illnesses the rights, opportunities and resources needed to lead meaningful and productive lives" (Davidson et al., 2010: 3). The recovery movement challenged notions of clinical recovery: the focus moved from recovery equating "cure" or symptomatic remission towards a more *personally defined* recovery journey, one that considers well-being from the perspective of the individual rather than the clinician (Slade, 2010).

The clinical recovery approach has some roots in the oft-noted, problematic, and sometimes disturbing history of psychiatry (Porter, 2002; Shorter, 1997). By the beginning of the nineteenth century, William Tuke implemented a new philosophy for institutional life for the mental health patient in England and pioneered the moral treatment movement (Duncan, 2006). As a result, modern life within institutions for the mental health patient often includes a range of activities (Borthwick et al., 2001). While some of these activities focus on activities of daily living (e.g., shopping, cooking, and budgeting), others will focus on leisure activities (such as sport), and some activities involve creative practices (e.g., cultural visits and art practices). There may be a crossover with art therapy practices, which may include creative art making, drama, dance or music, and what we might usefully see as creative activity whose therapeutic value lies in the space and time employed in enjoyable activities without a necessarily directly applied therapeutic aim. The premise of engaging in such activities is argued to promote well-being *and* hold therapeutic value (Holder, 2001). Engagement in creative activities and their contribution to health and well-being is well documented (Crawford et al., 2013); however, their effectiveness is suggested to be underevidenced (Daykin et al., 2013). This has been suggested to be due to ineffective and inappropriate measures, lack of scientific rigour, and potentially biased accounts or accounts with a vested interest in demonstrating value (Meekums and Daniel, 2011). The authors of this chapter acknowledge both our own backgrounds and our preferences towards both compassionate care and the use of creative approaches to enhance well-being and recovery. While it is argued that there is a lack of scientific evidence assessing the value of creative practices, there is a vast amount of literature that explores the positive value of engaging in the arts (Stickley, 2012). Additionally, engagement in creative practices *without* a specific psychotherapeutic aim has the potential for enjoyment-focused engagement without progress needing to be measured in terms of *clinical* recovery.

Research has found that engaging in creative practices can build communities and contribute to well-being through what has been referred to as "mutual recovery" (Crawford et al., 2015). As such, literature supports the notion that engaging in creative practices, such as capoeira (Jordan et al., 2018), art workshops (Hogan, 2015; Lewis et al., 2016), group drumming (Fancourt et al., 2016; Perkins et al., 2016), clay workshops (Argyle and Winship, 2015), comedy workshops (Barker and Winship, 2016), creative art gallery workshops (Saavedra et al., 2017a, 2017b), musical jamming (Callahan et al., 2017), storytelling (Wilson, 2018), Kundalini yoga workshops

(Pérez et al., 2016), story and music sharing (Wang et al., 2017) can lead to mutual recovery among participants. Such literature claims that engaging in creative practices can promote social connectedness, one of the key proponents of personal recovery, as suggested by the CHIME framework (Leamy et al., 2011). Occupational therapy utilizes activities to mediate interaction and communication to promote socialization (Hagedorn, 1995). The aims, then, are aligned here with a range of diverse approaches.

There are, though, significant challenges with regards the implementation of creative and health humanities–informed practices within forensic and secure settings. The Department of Health (1999) promotes the use of least restrictive possible practices, and creative approaches are certainly possible and practiced within FMH settings, for example, art therapy (Banks, 2012), literature groups (Cocking and Astill, 2004), and dance movement psychotherapy (Batcup, 2013); however implementation has not been clearly defined or measured. Applying recovery principles to the secure setting is highly challenging due to the conflicting nature of a restricted and locked environment versus the promotion of independent decision making, for example the emphasis on empowerment and choice (Drennan and Alred, 2012). Anthony (1993: 1) suggests that recovery means "taking charge of one's life even if one cannot take complete charge of one's symptoms." In fact, the forensic setting has been suggested to be *the* most challenging institution to apply recovery principles (Drennan and Wooldridge, 2014). The challenges are multilayered. The security of the environment, which is governed by perceptions of potential risk that underpin mental health and crime policy in England and Wales, is challenged in the face of recovery principles. Additionally, the restrictions of institutional life can impede upon notions of agency for the patient. The culture of risk management that necessarily underpins daily life within secure mental health services can restrict access to creative activity materials, such as musical instruments and drawing or painting materials. While the secure features of mental health environments have been suggested to facilitate psychological security (Adshead, 2002), such features have also been argued to conflict recovery principles (Drennan and Wooldridge, 2014; Mann et al., 2014).

Creative practice in challenging places: an applied example

The first author conducted an ethnographic research project within one FMH hospital in the United Kingdom, exploring creative practice. The study was conducted over a nine-month period with a total of 28 participants (14 staff, 14 patients) successfully recruited to the study. This resulted in over 150 hours of observations and 11 interviews (three staff, eight patients). The research program, entitled "Creative Practice as Mutual Recovery" (CPMR), was driven by a core, central belief: that creative practices could foster and connect communities in a way that enhances mental health and well-being. The CPMR program has found that engaging in creative practices facilitates social connectedness and mutuality among participants within a voluntary context (Argyle and Winship, 2015; Barker and Winship, 2016; Callahan et al., 2017; Fancourt et al., 2016; Hogan, 2015; Jordan et al., 2018; Lewis et al., 2016; Perkins et al., 2016; Saavedra et al., 2017a, 2017b; Wang et al., 2017; Wilson, 2018). However, barriers to engagement occurred when levels of agency were challenged (Pérez et al., 2016). Notions of agency within the FMH environment are also complex. It is, therefore, argued that the FMH environment can present challenges to notions of mutuality through a culture of risk-focused core policies, necessary to maintain safety for all but presenting challenges in terms of both the trust necessary for people to undertake arts-based activities and the risk assessments needed for their involvement to be practically and emotionally safe.

The Art in forensic mental health vignette (Box 3.1) highlights the complexities of creative practice within the secure environment.

Box 3.1 **Arts in forensic mental health vignette**

I met Dave, a patient at Westmarch Hospital, during one of the art sessions; we sat in the ward dining area, the table and chairs were bolted to the floor. We colored in an image provided by Siobhan (the occupational therapist) and introduced ourselves. Another patient came over to the table and asked Siobhan if this was art. She explained it was. He sat and began coloring in one of the images and asked Siobhan if she could make sure that his attendance was noted as his partici-pation had been raised as an issue during his ward round session. She reassured him that this would be noted on his file. The session was interrupted by an impromptu community meeting, which involved all patients on the ward. The smoking ban had recently been implemented on the NHS site and it had become known to the staff that there was a lighter on the ward. Another amnesty opportunity had arisen, but when no one came forward, the staff informed the patients that if the lighter was not found then, there would need to be room searches, including their bedrooms. This sparked great tension among those who were attending the art session, who felt that this was unfair; this was marked by verbal swearing—the coloring quickly subsided.

The art sessions were run on the ward; the location of the art sessions meant that patients could join in at any time, but this also meant that there could be distractions on the ward, as identified in the above vignette. The *relational security* (Department of Health, 2010) that the art session had the potential to offer was viewed as secondary to the risk of the lighter on the ward, indicating that *procedural security* (Department of Health, 2010) was viewed as most (or more) important within this context.

The research process so far in this project reveals key aspects of institutional life that influ-ence participation within creative practice. The risk-averse culture was found to restrict par-ticipation at the hospital—the art session described in the Art in forensic mental health vignette was interrupted by security procedures implemented by staff, informed by wider institutional and organizational policy. That is, the interruption was necessary in terms of policy, but gives one example of a challenge to full engagement with arts-based activities, meaning that the consistency of participation necessary for building secure and therapeutic relationships risks becoming a truncated process. In addition, the client group dynamic posed interpersonal challenges for patients—at times racism experienced by patients led to the avoid-ance of community engagements. Other patient interpersonal conflicts led to the avoidance of particular individuals through non-participation in the occupational therapy timetable.

Conclusion

While the aforementioned project explores arts-based experiences in FMH, there is scope for a wider consideration of practices that might be affirming and enjoyable, creating space for staff and people in the FMH units to mutually benefit. One such example might be shared reading aloud in groups (Davis, 2009; Davis et al., 2016)—this particular approach could theoretically both enhance perspectives of risk and also enhance empathy through discussion around individ-ual characters' situations. In female prison settings, this approach has been found to potentially augment approaches that enhance well-being (Billington et al., 2016).

There are further gaps in research around staff participation in creative practices—whether, for example, nursing staff who are the named professional for an individual could participate in specific activities as a way of building a therapeutic relationship. Such work is likely already taking place across different environments, although capturing the value of this work remains a priority in health humanities-informed research and practices in challenging settings.

References

Adshead, G. (2002). Three Degrees of Security: Attachment and Forensic Institutions. *Criminal Behaviour and Mental Health*, 12(2): 31–45.

Adshead, G. (2012). What the Eye Doesn't See: Relationships, Boundaries and Forensic Mental Health. In A. Aiyegbusi and G. Kelly, eds, *Professional and Therapeutic Boundaries in Forensic Mental Health Practice*. London: Jessica Kingsley Publishers: 13–35.

Anthony, W.A. (1993). Recovery From Mental Illness: The Guiding Vision of the Mental Health System in the 1990s. *Psychosocial Rehabilitation Journal*, 16(4): 11–23.

Argyle, E. and Winship, G. (2015). Creative Practice in a Group Setting. *Mental Health and Social Inclusion*, 19(3): 141–147.

Banks, L. (2012). Free to Talk About Violence: A Description of Art Therapy with a Male Service User in a Low Secure Unit. *International Journal of Art Therapy*, 17(1): 13–24.

Barker, A.B. and Winship, G. (2016). Recovery is No Laughing Matter—or Is It? *Mental Health and Social Inclusion*, 20: 167–173.

Barton, R. (1966). *Institutional Neurosis*. Bristol: John Wright & Sons.

Batcup, D.C. (2013). A Discussion of the Dance Movement Psychotherapy Literature Relative to Prisons and Medium Secure Units: Body, Movement and Dance in Psychotherapy. *International Journal for Theory, Research and Practice*, 8(1): 5–16.

Billington, J., Longden, E. and Robinson, J. (2016). A Literature-Based Intervention for Women Prisoners: Preliminary Findings. *International Journal of Prisoner Health*, 12(4): 230–243.

Borthwick, A., Holman, C., Kennard, D., Mcfetridge, M., Messruther, K. and Wilkes, J. (2001). The Relevance of Moral Treatment to Contemporary Mental Health Care. *Journal of Mental Health*, 10(4): 427–439.

Callahan, K., Schlozman, S., Beresin, E. and Crawford, P. (2017). The Use of Music in Mutual Recovery: A Qualitative Pilot Study. *Journal of Applied Arts and Health*, 8: 103–114.

Cocking, A. and Astill, J. (2004). Using Literature as a Therapeutic Tool with People with Moderate and Borderline Learning Disabilities in a Forensic Setting. *British Journal of Learning Disabilities*, 32: 16–23.

Crawford, P., Lewis, L., Brown, B. and Manning, N. (2013). Creative Practice as Mutual Recovery in Mental Health. *Mental Health Review Journal*, 18: 55–64.

Crawford, P., Brown, B., Baker, C., Tischler, V. and Abrams, B. (2015). *Health Humanities*. London: Palgrave Macmillan UK.

Davidson, L., Rakfeldt, J. and Strauss, J. (2010). *The Roots of The Recovery Movement in Psychiatry: Lessons Learned*. Chichester: John Wiley & Sons.

Davis, J. (2009). Enjoying and Enduring: Groups Reading Aloud for Wellbeing. *Lancet*, 373(9665): 714–715.

Davis, P., Magee, F., Koleva, K., Tangeras, T., Hill, E., Baker, H. and Crane, L. (2016). *What Literature Can Do*. Liverpool: University of Liverpool. Online: www.liverpool.ac.uk/media/livacuk/instituteofp sychology/researchgroups/crilswhatliteraturecando.pdf (Accessed 10/9/2018).

Daykin, N., De Viggiani, N., Pilkington, P. and Moriarty, Y. (2013). Music Making for Health, Well-being and Behaviour Change in Youth Justice Settings: A Systematic Review. *Health Promotion International*, 28: 197–210.

Department of Health. (1999). *A National Service Framework for Mental Health*. London: Department of Health.

Department of Health. (2010). *See, Think, Act: Your Guide to Relational Security*. London: Department of Health.

Drennan, G. and Alred, D. (2012). *Secure Recovery: Approaches to Recovery In Forensic Mental Health Settings*. London: Routledge.

Drennan, G. and Wooldridge, J. (2014). *Making Recovery a Reality in Forensic Settings: Implementing Recovery through Organisational Change Briefing*. Paper 10. www.imroc.org/wpcontent/uploads/2016/09/10imroc-briefing-10-making-recovery-a-reality-in-forensic-settings-final-for-web.pdf (Accessed 7/9/2018).

Duncan, E.A.S. ed., (2006). *Foundations for Practice in Occupational Therapy*. 4th edn. Edinburgh: Elsevier Churchill Livingstone.

Fancourt, D., Perkins, R., Ascenso, S., Carvalho, L.A., Steptoe, A. and Williamon, A. (2016). Effects of Group Drumming Interventions on Anxiety, Depression, Social Resilience and Inflammatory Immune Response Among Mental Health Service Users. *Plos ONE*, 11(3): 1–16.

Hagedorn, R. (1995). *Occupational Therapy: Perspectives and Processes*. New York: Churchill Livingstone.

Hogan, S. (2015). Mothers Make Art: Using Participatory Art to Explore the Transition to Motherhood. *Journal of Applied Arts and Health*, 6(1): 23–32.

Holder, V. (2001). The Use of Creative Activities Within Occupational Therapy. *British Journal of Occupational Therapy*, 64: 103–105.

Jordan, M., Wright, E.J., Purser, A., Grundy, A., Joyes, E., Wright, N., Crawford, P. and Manning, N. (2018). Capoeira for Beginners: Self-Benefit For, and Community Action by, New Capoeiristas. *Sport, Education and Society*, 1–14.

Killaspy, H. (2006). From the Asylum to Community Care: Learning from Experience. *British Medical Bulletin*, 79–80(1): 245–258.

Leamy, M., Bird, V., Le Boutillier, C., Williams, J. and Slade, M. (2011). Conceptual Framework for Personal Recovery in Mental Health: Systematic Review and Narrative synthesis. *British Journal of Psychiatry*, 199(6): 445–452.

Lewis, L., Ecclestone, K., Spandler, H. and Tew, J. (2016). *Mutuality, Wellbeing and Mental Health Recovery: Exploring The Roles of Creative Arts Adult Community Learning and Participatory Arts Initiatives: Research Briefing (Short Version)*. University of Wolverhampton. Available: www.wlv.ac.uk/connected communities (Accessed 17/9/2018).

Mann, B., Matias, E. and Allen, J. (2014). Recovery in Forensic Services: Facing the Challenge. *Advances in Psychiatric Treatment*, 20: 125–131.

Meekums, B. and Daniel, J. (2011). Arts with Offenders: A Literature Synthesis. *Arts in Psychotherapy*, 38: 229–238.

Mullen, P.E. (2000). Forensic Mental Health. *British Journal of Psychiatry*, 174: 307–311.

Pérez, E., Ball, M., Brown, P., Crepaz-Keay, D., Haslam-Jones, E. and Crawford, P. (2016). Kundalini Yoga as Mutual Recovery: A Feasibility Study Including Children in Care and Their Carers. *Journal of Children's Services*, 11(4): 1–22.

Perkins, R., Ascenso, S., Atkins, L., Fancourt, D. and Williamon, A. (2016). Making Music for Mental Health: How Group Drumming Mediates Recovery. *Psychology of Well-Being*, 6(11): 1–17.

Porter, R. (2002). *Madness: A Brief History*. Oxford: Oxford University Press.

Prins, H. (2005). *Offenders, Deviants or Patients?* London: Routledge.

Saavedra, J., Arias, S., Crawford, P. and Pérez, E. (2017a). Impact of Creative Workshops for People with Severe Mental Illness: Art as a Means of Recovery. *Arts and Health*, 10(3): 241–256.

Saavedra, J., Pérez, E., Crawford, P. and Arias, S. (2017b). Recovery and Creative Practices in People with Severe Mental Illness: Evaluating Well-Being and Social Inclusion. *Disability and Rehabilitation*, 40(8): 1–10.

Seymour, L. (2010). *Public Health and Criminal Justice: Promoting and Protecting Offenders' Mental Health Public Health and Wellbeing*. London: Centre for Mental Health. www.centreformentalhealth.org.uk/ public-health-and-criminal-justice (Accessed 17 September 2018).

Shorter, E. (1997). *A History of Psychiatry*. New York: John Wiley and Sons.

Slade, M. (2010). Mental Illness and Well-Being: The Central Importance of Positive Psychology and Recovery Approaches. *BMC Health Services Research*, 10(26): 1–14. 10.1186/1472-6963-10-26

Soothill, K., Rogers, P. and Dolan, M. eds, (2008). *Handbook of Forensic Mental Health*. London: Willan.

Stickley, T. ed., (2012). *Qualitative Research in Arts and Mental Health: Context, Meanings, and Evidence*. Ross-on-Wye: PCCS Books.

Sugarman, P. and Dickens, G.L. (2015). The Evolution of Secure and Forensic Mental Healthcare. In G.L. Dickens, P.A. Sugarman and M.M. Picchioni, eds, *Handbook of Secure Care*. London: Royal College of Psychiatrists Publications: 1–14.

Thornicroft, G. (2006). *Actions Speak Louder: Tackling Discrimination Against People with Mental Health Problems*. London: Mental Health Foundation.

Wang, C., Hua, Y., Fu, H., Cheng, L., Qian, W., Liu, J., Crawford, P. and Dai, J. (2017). Effects of a Mutual Recovery Intervention on Mental Health in Depressed Elderly Community-Dwelling Adults: A Pilot Study. *BMC Public Health*, 17(4): 1–10.

Wilson, M. (2018). Some Thoughts on Storytelling, Science and Dealing with a Post-Truth World. *Storytelling, Self and Society*, 13(1): 120.

4

VISIONARY MEDICINE

Race, health, power, and speculation

Sayantani DasGupta

Introduction

A young African American woman named Nish enters a roadside museum of medical horrors in the middle of the American Southwest. In this so-called "Black Museum," Rolo Haynes, a former biotechnological snakeoil salesman, curates "authentic criminologic artifacts." The ethically dubious medical trials Haynes once recruited for include a neurological transmission device that allows one person to feel another's pain, as well as a device that transfers the consciousness of one human being into another. But the museum's pièce de résistance is the exhibit behind the final curtain: the zombie/ghost-like consciousness of an African American man named Clayton Leigh, who was wrongly convicted of murder and executed. In order to provide for his wife and daughter, Leigh sold Haynes his consciousness in the moment of his death. Now, Leigh is perpetually trapped in a limbo-like existence where museum-goers get to execute him again and again, and voyeuristically take pleasure from the spectacle of Black pain. The tagline that the biotechnology charlatan Haynes uses is that Leigh is "always on, always suffering" (Brooker, 2017).

Interestingly, "Black Museum," the last episode of the fourth season of the television program *Black Mirror*, aired in 2017, the same year that Jordan Peele's horror blockbuster *Get Out* was released. *Get Out*'s protagonist Chris is almost trapped into a similar zombie-like existence by the machinations of his white girlfriend's upper crust Connecticut family—including her psychotherapist mother and neurosurgeon father. Chris's potential fate is not a disembodied consciousness like Leigh, who has his spirit imprisoned and controlled by outsiders, but a hyperembodiment where Chris' body is sold at auction to the highest (white) bidder and taken over from the inside out, such that his consciousness would be mostly removed, and he would be a mere spectator in his own body and life (Peele, 2017).

It is significant that in both narratives, the representatives of white supremacy wield medicine and biotechnology as their tools of subjugation. Yes, both "Black Museum" and *Get Out* see medical racism thwarted (spoiler alert!). Chris narrowly escapes after killing his would-be torturers, and Nish, who turns out to be Leigh's daughter, enacts revenge by poisoning Haynes, executing his trapped consciousness, and finally burning down the entire museum. Yet the power of these stories for students of the health humanities is as lenses through which to examine medicine's historic and present-day complicity in the dehumanization, subjugation, and torture of bodies of color. It is in this context that I teach both

"Black Museum" and *Get Out* in a senior undergraduate seminar called "Visionary Medicine: Racial Justice, Health and Speculative Fiction."

Medicine's role in constructing "race"

Medicine cannot imagine more racially just futures until it grapples honestly with its racially unjust past and present: its complicity in, dependence on, and enacting of racial violence. Institutional medicine has historically built its practices upon bodies of color, and has in fact been integral to creating notions of biologically different races. Consider the pseudosciences of biological anthropology. The fact that biological "scientists" once determined the different and inferior head size of people of different "races," comparing people of color to animals, reads like science fiction now. Yet it was medical science like this that that led to the justification of slavery as an institution, and the development of medical diagnoses such as drapetomania, a mental illness that caused slaves to run away, introduced in 1851 by Samuel A. Cartwright and based on entirely manufactured racial differences in temperament and biology (Roberts, 2015). It is this history that underlies the very title of Peele's *Get Out*, a film in which already zombified Black elders desperately warn the character Chris to run away, to get out from the modern-day plantation and its human auction.

The fallacy of race as a meaningful, biologically, or genetically based category has been established by many scholars, including Dorothy Roberts who has argued:

> The way doctors practice medicine continues to promote a false and toxic view of humanity. There's a failure of imagination when it comes to race. What would happen if doctors stopped treating patients by race? Suppose they rejected an 18th century classification system, and incorporated instead the most advanced knowledge of human genetic diversity and unity: that human beings cannot be categorized into biological races? What if instead of using race as a crude proxy for ... some more important factor, doctors investigated that more important factor? What if doctors joined the forefront of a movement to end the structural inequities caused by racism, not by genetic difference?
>
> *(Roberts, 2015)*

Rejecting race as a meaningful category does not, of course, imply rejecting racism as a real lived experience that deeply impacts health. By urging her listeners to challenge the boundaries of race as a genetic category, Roberts is calling for a focus not on some imagined biological differences between people of different skin tones and hair textures, but on structural inequities and their impact on lived experience.

In her essay, "Race and/as Technology; or, How to do Things to Race," techno-Orientalist scholar Wendy Chun asks, "To what extent can race be considered a technology and mode of medicalization?" (Chun, 2012: 39). Rather than a portrayal of some sort of knowledge or truth that makes visible exterior traits somehow innate, she notes that "race has historically been a tool of subjugation ... a mapping tool, a means by which origins and boundaries are simultaneously traced and constructed, and through which the visible traces of the body are tied to allegedly innate invisible characteristics" (Chun, 2012: 40). Race, she argues, is not just used as a technology of medicalized domination: it is a technology of medicalized domination.

From medical experimentation to medical imperialism

Texts like "Black Museum" and *Get Out* clearly evoke recollections of medical experimentation upon marginalized bodies. From J. Marion Sims, often considered the "father of modern gynecology," who developed the first pelvic speculum through acts of brutal unanesthetized surgery upon enslaved African American women (Lerner, 2003), to the bioethical travesties of the Tuskegee syphilis experiments and the Johns Hopkins/Kennedy Krieger Institute's lead paint experiments (Markowitz and Rosner, 2013, Reverby, 2000), to imagined "racial differences" in pain thresholds, racial violence is undoubtedly embedded into the very foundations of medical research itself. Teaching about this history alongside science and speculative fiction texts helps to contextualize both in the health humanities classroom.

Other sorts of texts, including outer space exploration stories, help students understand medicine's investment in colonialism, war, and empire building. Indeed, I start the semester in my "Visionary Medicine" class by playing Captain Kirk's *Star Trek* exhortation to "seek out new worlds and new civilizations ... to boldly go where no man has gone before" (Roddenberry, 1966). It is critical in such a classroom to examine white supremacy in its multiple facets—while anti-Black racism has justified enslavement and driven capitalism, settler colonialism has justified the genocide of Native people and takeover of land, while Orientalism has justified war against perceived foreign "aliens" and histories of imperialism and colonialism (Smith, 2006).

Consider how imperialists of the nineteenth and twentieth centuries conflated and justified "the power to govern" with "the power to heal." Throughout the European empires of the eighteenth and nineteenth centuries, there was a reliance on the idea of "imperial cleanliness," which is "development by sanitation ... colonising [sic] by means of the known laws of cleanliness rather than by military force" (Bashford, 2003). In the words of Dominique Laporte:

> If the history of modernity can ... be written as a triumph of cleanliness over bodily refuse, then so too could the European colonization of Africa and India. The sanitary crusade of the nineteenth century is central to the violent project of empire. Western medicine, with its emphasis on personal hygiene, functioned (and in some arenas still functions) as colonialism's benevolent cover.
>
> *(Laporte, 2000: 37)*

Who gets to imagine themselves into the future?

Not only does traditional medicine's past and present reveal its racial value systems, but so too do its speculations about the future. Who is allowed to imagine themselves into the future? Indeed, the US and European eugenics movements of the twentieth century can be understood as acts of racial speculation—imagining a certain kind of futurity based on the celebration of white, able-bodied reproduction in things like "fitter families contests," alongside the sterilization or killing of racialized or disabled "undesirables" (Olusoga, 2007). And even if "undesireables" were not actively killed, their deaths from man-made things such as the 1943 Bengal Famine were considered just as well. Remember that it was Winston Churchill who blamed the famine that killed upward of 2 million Indians on the fact that "beastly" Indians "bred like rabbits" (Tharoor, 2016). And one need not go back so far in history. It was only recently that the southern US state of North Carolina began the process

35

of reparations for the thousands of predominantly young, African American, and poor women forcibly sterilized by order of the state's Eugenics Board as recently as the late 1970s. These coercive state actions were envisioned as scientifically sound ways to "protect" the future and reduce the burdens upon the welfare state, by literally preventing future children of color from being born (Sharpiro, 2016). Similar coerced sterilizations occurred in Los Angeles County Hospital through the 1970s among predominantly Latinx immigrant populations (Tajima-Peña, 2015), and we can even think about certain modern-day anti-teenage pregnancy campaigns targeting women of color as descendants of that tradition.

Visionary medicine

In the context of medicine's racially violent past, present, and future speculations, how can the health humanities imagine a more racially just future: a future invested in the health and well-being of all people? I coin the term "Visionary Medicine" with a nod to what Walidah Imarisha, co-editor of *Octavia's Brood: Science Fiction Stories from Social Justice Movements*, calls "visionary fiction," a practice "defined by its insistence on imagining freer and more liberated worlds or critiquing injustice, rather than uncritically recreating the power structures of the world as we know it in fantastical garb" (Imarisha, 2015: 4) Imarisha adds, "Whenever we try and envision a world without war, without violence, without prisons, without capitalism, we are engaging in speculative fiction. All organizing is science fiction" (3). Although the class I teach draws initially from mainstream science fiction texts (see Pasco et al., 2016), the bulk of our syllabus includes films, stories, and theory by Indigenous creators and creators of color grappling with issues of health and futurity.

In this way, the "Visionary Medicine" seminar is inspired by Afrofuturism, which sociologist Alondra Nelson defines as not only a way to understand "diasporic Black artistic production but also as an epistemology, a way of thinking about the subject position of Black people … that is both alienating and about alienation … The alien comes to figure quite centrally … the outsider figure. It's about aspirations for modernity and having a place in modernity. It's about speculation … It's about imagining the impossible, a better place, a different world" (Nelson, 2010).

By drawing from not only Afrofuturist, but also Native, Asian American, and Latinx futurist texts, this class seeks to imagine more racially just medical futures. For health humanities students and teachers, this requires exercising and teaching for radical imagination by delving into such non-traditional texts, teaching "high" theory alongside popular culture, and creating a pedagogy of discomfort in our classrooms (Boler, 2004). In other words, recognizing that for racial injustice and white supremacy to be challenged and dismantled is undoubtedly an uncomfortable, complex, and long-term process, one that requires us to challenge ourselves and each other along the way, searching for innovative new ways of thinking and teaching that reject traditional teacher–student power dynamics, canonical ideas, and easy answers.

Importantly, when I talk about future speculation, radical imagination, and visionary medicine, I am not necessarily talking about utopianism or certainly any kind of imagined and artificial "post-racialism." Rather, I turn to a perspective of transgressive or critical dystopianism. I draw here from Jessica Langer who has suggested that utopianism is akin to colonialism, it cannot abide or include difference, and that actually beneath the "violence and cacophony" of dystopian narratives is a "positive hybridity" and "potential for subversion" of oppressive norms (Langer, 2011). Similarly, Thomas Moylan suggests that critical dystopias "take on the present system and offer not only astute critiques of the order of things, but also explorations of the oppositional spaces and possibilities from which the next round of political activism can derive imaginative sustenance and inspiration" (Moylan, 2000: xv). Thus, the Black vengeance fantasy of "Black Mirror" imagines Nish acting not alone, but with the consciousness of her deceased mother implanted in her brain: an image that literalizes the notion of modern-day revolution being guided by our ancestors. This is similar to Chris being urged to "get out" by the elders who have suffered before him, and this intergenerational connection and community is a theme that resonates again and again in the stories of multicultural futurists.

Ultimately, "Black Museum" and *Get Out* can be read as indictments of not only bio-technological medicine, but the health humanities as well, a field in which we often seek to empathetically "take the perspective of others." Yet there is no neurotechnological or narrative "in" into another's consciousness, embodiment, or experience. For the health humanities field to expect such empathetic access is a kind of voyeurism, just as demanding revealing first-person narratives from an ill person is to demand the performance of pain. If anti-racist work is to be a part of the health humanities, our task is not to "listen for the voices of the voiceless," an orientation which ignores medicine's own investment in racist violence and white supremacy. Rather, our task is to examine our own personal and institutional complicity in the silencing and marginalization of certain lived experiences in favor of others, and to listen harder, listen differently, listen better. Like Nish and Chris, we must make room to hear the voices of African American, Native, Asian American, and Latinx elders and contemporaries, getting out of our pedagogical and practical comfort zones, and burning our comfortably held assumptions to the ground.

References

Bashford, A. (2003). *Imperial Hygiene: A Critical History of Colonialism, Nationalism and Public Health.* Houndsmills: Palgrave Macmillan.

Boler, M. (2004). Teaching for Hope: The Ethics of Shattering World Views. In: D. Liston and J. Garrison, eds, *Teaching, Learning and Loving: Reclaiming Passion in Educational Practice.* New York: Routledge: 117–131.

Brooker, C. (2017) Black Museum. *Black Mirror.* Episode 6, Season 4. Channel 4, Netflix.

Chun, W.H.K. (2012). Race and/as Technology or How to Do Things to Race. In: L. Nakamura and P.A. Chow-White, eds, *Race After the Internet.* New York: Routledge: 38–60.

Imarisha, W. and Brown, A.M. (2015). *Octavia's Brood: Science Fiction Stories from Social Justice Movements.* Chico, CA: AK Press.

Langer, J. (2011). *Race, Culture, Identity and Alien/Nation: Postcolonialism and Science Fiction.* New York: Palgrave Macmillan.

Laporte, D. (2000). *History of Shit.* Cambridge, MA: MIT Press.

Lerner, B.H. (2003) Scholars Argue Over Legacy of Surgeon Who Was Lionized, Then Vilified. *The New York Times.* Oct 28. [cited 2017 Sept 17] www.nytimes.com/2003/10/28/health/scholars-argue-over-legacy-of-surgeon-who-was-lionized-then-vilified.html (accessed 18/2/2019).

Markowitz, G. and Rosner, D. (2013). *Lead Wars: The Politics of Science and the Fate of America's Children.* Oakland, CA: University of California Press.

Moylan, T. (2000). *Scraps of the Untainted Sky: Science Fiction, Utopia, Dystopia.* New York: Routledge.

Olusoga, D. producer, director (2007). *Scientific Racism: The Eugenics of Social Darwinism.* London: BBC.

Nelson, A. (2010). What is Afrofuturism? [cited Mar 2015] Available from: www.youtube.com/watch?v=IFhEjaal5js

Pasco, J.C., Anderson, C. and DasGupta, S. (2016). Visionary Medicine: Speculative Fiction, Racial Justice and Octavia Butler's "Bloodchild." *Medical Humanities,* 44 246–251.

Peele, J. (2017). *Get Out.* Universal City, CA: Universal Pictures.

Reverby, S. (2000). *Tuskegee's Truths: Rethinking the Tuskegee Syphilis Study.* The University of Chapel Hill, NC: North Carolina Press.

Roberts, D. (2015). The Problem with Race-Based Medicine. TEDMED. Nov 2015 [cited 2016 Mar 14]. Available from: www.ted.com/talks/dorothy_roberts_the_problem_with_race_based_medicine? language=en

Roddenberry, G. (1966). *Star Trek*, the original series. Los Angeles, CA: Desilu Productions.

Sharpiro, D.S. (2016). *The State of Eugenics*. USA: Brown Doggy Pictures.

Smith, A. (2006). Heteropatriarchy and the Three Pillars of White Supremacy. https://loveharder.files. wordpress.com/2009/08/andrea-smith.pdf (accessed 18/2/2019).

Tajima-Peña, R. (2015). *No Mas Bebés*. Los Angeles, CA: Renee Tajima-Peña and Virginia Espino d/b/a Moon Canyon Films.

Tharoor, S. (2016). *An Era of Darkness: The British Empire in India*. New Delhi: Aleph.

5

DIGITAL LIFE AND HEALTH HUMANITIES

Olivia Banner

Introduction

Health humanities is only just starting to address the infiltration of digital media into the management, care, and practices of health. It is of paramount importance that health humanities does so now: the health-care industries will be, and are being, overtaken by emerging technologies, with for-profit corporations embedding their products into health care, as IBM's Watson, Apple's HealthKit, and Verily's Study Watch make apparent. The ethical stakes are high: for example, Britain's National Health Service allowed Google access to millions of patient records for the stated aim of medical discovery, a use of data that abrogated principles of informed consent and patient privacy (Hodson, 2016). The political stakes are high too: technology enthusiasts envision a day when AI-enhanced robots will substitute for human physicians (e.g., Jaiprakash et al., 2016), perhaps leading to a "doctorless hospital." Yet thus far, we have multiple examples of bias in artificial intelligence (AI), from AI bots (e.g., Microsoft's Tay) that, shortly after being released into the human datasphere, spew out the racist and misogynist vitriol they "learn" from humans, to AI meant to improve efficiency in hiring, policing, and sentencing that simply replicates the racist biases present in the datasets from which they "learn" (e.g., Angwin et al., 2016; Buolamwini and Gebru, 2018). Will AI "doctors" that learn from medically racist datasets repeat that racism? What should be the orientation of the health humanities in this emerging landscape? Will focusing on developing skills of empathy and listening suffice?

Of course, digital interventions into health are not solely happening through corporations "from above"; digital networks have profoundly affected how health happens "from below." Grassroots efforts to organize outside of established health-care infrastructures for education, knowledge-building, and activism have happened for decades through the digital public-building the Internet enables. It is not a historical accident that during the period of the Internet's birth and growth, medicine moved toward "patient-centered care": digital networks were helping patients organize and pressure medicine to center the patient (for example, by forming individual disease forums in the 1990s, and post-2000, through the e-Patient movement [e.g., Miah and Rich, 2008]). While in the 1990s patients used networks to share information and build knowledge outside of medicine, the technology industries were developing methods to monetize that sharing, methods that were fully realized by 2004, when the Internet was restructured as Web 2.0 (Banner, 2017). In our post-Web 2.0

era, online patient communications are bought and sold via data brokers. Patient voices, in other words, have become economically valuable.

To think about the patient voice today, then, requires more than simply learning how to "listen" to it. Today, it requires comprehending the digital media matrix in which it is often embedded, a media matrix spun out of informatic capitalism, the technology industries, and what sociologists have labeled "biomedicalization" (Clarke et al., 2003), a paradigm in which research is joined to clinical practice via the technologies integrated into the health-care experience. In other words, methods from other humanities fields with rich histories of analyzing technology and media are urgently needed to grasp the technological transformation of medicine occurring today. If medical humanities arose in the 1970s in part to address the technologization of medicine occurring then, the digitalization of medicine—and of patient life—happening now requires a different kind of health humanities, one attuned to technology and media not only as tools (how health-care professionals typically view technology) or as methods of representation (how media are typically viewed), but rather as technoculture. "Technoculture," a concept familiar to science and technology studies and critical media studies, describes how technology and media emerge out of a cultural context that shapes them. For these fields of study, technology is never neutral, is never free of ideology: it cannot arise independent of the perspectives and worldviews of those who develop it.

Once we understand them as co-produced by cultural forces, we can approach medical technologies and health media using analytical tools similar to those the humanities brings to bear on art and literature. For example, we might analyze the technocultural production of health on the world's seventh-most visited website, Wikipedia, a site heavily consulted by physicians and patients alike. As technoculture, Wikipedia can—indeed must—be analyzed for how it structures knowledge according to the perspective of those who develop it. In a sense, Wikipedia invites us to do so, for it includes entries that explain its own problem with systemic bias (Wikipedia, 2018d). The entries note that it is mostly white men located in Europe and the United States who edit Wikipedia, and because of this, Wikipedia's entries reflect their interests and perspectives. But one might ask additional questions about Wikipedia, such as how the "five pillars" that undergird knowledge construction on the site themselves reflect those people's perspectives: what feminist philosophers of science such as Donna Haraway (1988) and Sandra Harding (1991) have long articulated as "situated knowledge" that nevertheless proclaims itself objective, the god's eye view from nowhere. One of these pillars is "neutrality," which Wikipedia explains the site accomplishes by including "multiple points of view" on a topic, forbidding editors' opinions, interpretations, or personal experiences, and requiring that editors draw on and cite reliable, authoritative sources (Wikipedia, 2018c). In its guidelines about entries on medicine and health, Wikipedia requires that those authoritative sources be from peer-reviewed academic science and medicine journals. Yet what happens with a page about a topic in which patient-generated knowledge contradicts that of established medicine? Or an entry about a topic that directly *challenges* medicine's models?

I refer here to "disability." In February of 2016, students in my "Disability and Media" class analyzed Wikipedia's disability entry (Wikipedia, 2018a). At that time, the entry began with a list of "disabilities" that used medical terminology for diagnosing human differences. Students determined that it therefore used what disability studies scholars call the "medical model of disability" (Shakespeare, 2006), a model in which physical/mental differences designated abnormal are viewed as requiring repair or cure. While the entry included sections that touched on how living with disabilities impacted a person's social mobility and wealth,

40

these were placed toward the bottom of the page, and so the medical framework for disability was given prime importance. For disability studies scholars, the arrangement of information to privilege medicine's conceptualization of disabled lives is not surprising: it simply reflects that the medical model for disability is culturally hegemonic. In the culturally subordinated understandings of disability drawn from disability studies and activism, disability is created by a *disabling society*: one that is not designed for people with bodies and minds designated abnormal. Since the 1960s and 1970s, a rich vein of disability activism has reshaped how the West addresses disability, not only by advancing such key pieces of law as the Americans with Disabilities Act, but also by intervening in cultural discourses of pity, charity, dependence, and other tropes that reiterate a general medicalized attitude that, unless "healthy" and "able," a life is not worth living. Knowing this, my students and I worked to edit Wikipedia's "Disability" entry to reflect this culturally subordinate, patient-generated kind of knowledge—a way of defining "disability" that diverges from the medical model. We had a vast store of disability studies scholarship to draw on, and so when our edits were contested by other Wikipedia editors, we were able to defend our changes using appropriate citational practices. This is not true for other kinds of knowledge; for example, at the time of this writing, the Wikipedia entry on Chinese medicine is categorized within a subheading of "fringe medicine and conspiracy theories" (Wikipedia, 2018b). The fact that, thus far, no collective voice of editors has emerged to contest how Chinese medicine is categorized attests to the way in which Internet access affects how knowledge is represented on the site; if China's Internet were not restricted by its government censors, perhaps these pages would be quite different.

Wikipedia is a not-for-profit, open-source platform for knowledge that assigns copyleft copyrights: in other words, it encourages its users to share and reuse its content. We might contrast this to for-profit, proprietary platforms for knowledge production about health: patient networking sites where any knowledge generated from participation with the site ultimately is meant to circulate within the constrained channels of market capitalism. These sites serve a vital function for patients adrift in a broken health-care system. They allow patients to communicate among each other, share information about treatments and symptoms, tell each other their patient stories, and lend each other support—in this, they allow patients to circulate patient-generated knowledge about their conditions. But as a technocultural formation, such sites can be analyzed in relation to broader cultures of health, including the economics of a health-care system that leads patients to such sites. Health care in the United States (and indeed elsewhere in the Western world) is a neoliberal system of austerity, which requires that patients assume "responsibility" for their health, for navigating the arcane maze of the system itself, for fighting with an insurance system designed to deny them benefits, and in which doctors too are overwhelmed. Coupled with a paternalistic, racist system where many patients, especially women and people of color, are not recognized or validated by medical authorities (e.g., Dusenbery, 2018; Ray, 2019), and where allopathic treatment is simply out of financial reach, the "voice" patients record on patient networking websites should be understood as growing out of larger austerity logics endemic to health care in the West. Of course frustrated people turn to networks that allow them to communicate with other people experiencing similar frustrations.

In other words, patient networking platforms, as technoculture, are produced by a for-profit culture of health that makes their use an inevitability. But even more so, the largest patient networking site, PatientsLikeMe, is produced by a for-profit health-care system in which every part of research, treatment, and care is monetized and that is greedily forming new markets from the recent turn to "big data" as an economic paradigm. PatientsLikeMe partners with pharmaceutical companies, pharmacy chains, and health insurance companies to sell them the data it gathers from patients using its platform for vital communications, an economic logic I have elsewhere termed "communicative biocapitalism" (Banner, 2017). Biocapitalism—where value is located in new markets in organs, tissues, and DNA—now pounces on "the patient voice" as a market.

Understanding how the patient voice circulates within the digital sphere can only help the health humanities to critically approach emerging patient technologies. These examples help illuminate that the patient voice is now a technocultural formation: a dominant cultural trope around which technologies are developed, those technologies themselves shaped by cultural forces such as inequities in participation in STEM cultures, economic paradigms, and gendered dynamics. As health humanities continues to expose future carers to humanistic perspectives, educating them in paying attention to the nuances of technology as culture can help them better prepare for their own digital futures, whether as professionals or when they are, if not now, then eventually, patients.

References

Angwin, J., Larson, J., Mattu, S. and Kirchner, L. (2016). Machine Bias. *ProPublica*, May 23. Available online at www.propublica.org/article/machine-bias-risk-assessments-in-criminal-sentencing (Accessed 18/2/2019).

Banner, O. (2017). *Communicative Biocapitalism: The Voice of the Patient in Digital Health and the Health Humanities*. Ann Arbor: University of Michigan Press.

Buolamwini, J. and Gebru, T. (2018). Gender Shades: Intersectional Accuracy Disparities in Commercial Gender Classification. *Proceedings of Machine Learning Research*, 81: 1–15. Available online at http://proceedings.mlr.press/v81/buolamwini18a/buolamwini18a.pdf. (Accessed 19/2/2018).

Clarke, A.E., Shim, J.K., Mamo, L., Foskett, J.R. and Fishman, J.R. (2003). Biomedicalization: Technoscientific Transformations of Health, Illness, and US Biomedicine. *American Sociological Review*, 6(2): 161–194.

Dusenbery, M. (2018). *Doing Harm: The Truth about How Bad Medicine and Lazy Science Leave Women Dismissed, Misdiagnosed, and Sick*. New York: HarperCollins.

Haraway, D. (1988). Situated Knowledges: The Science Question in Feminism and the Privilege of Partial Perspective. *Feminist Studies*, 14(3): 575–599.

Harding, S. (1991). *Whose Science? Whose Knowledge? Thinking from Women's Lives*. Chapel Hill, NC: Cornell University Press.

Hodson, H. (2016). Revealed: Google AI Has Access to Huge Haul of NHS Patient Data. *New Scientist*, April 29. Available online at www.newscientist.com/article/2086454-revealed-google-ai-has-access-to-huge-haul-of-nhs-patient-data/ (Accessed 18/2/2019).

Jaiprakash, A., Roberts, J. and Crawford, R. (2016). Robots in Healthcare Could Lead to a Doctorless Hospital. *The Conversation*, February 8. Available online at https://theconversation.com/robots-in-health-care-could-lead-to-a-doctorless-hospital-54316 (Accessed 18/2/2019).

Miah, A. and Rich, E. (2008). *The Medicalization of Cyberspace*. London: Routledge.

Ray, K. (2019) Giving Students a Contemporary Example of Medical Racism Using Black Patients' Testimonials. In O. Banner, N. Carlin and T.R. Cole, eds, *Teaching Health Humanities*, New York: Oxford University Press: 129–141.

Shakespeare, T. (2006) The Social Model of Disability. In L. Davis, ed, *The Disability Studies Reader*, 2nd ed. New York: Routledge: 197–204.

Wikipedia. (2018a). *Disability*. https://en.wikipedia.org/wiki/Disability. Last edited October 2, 2018. (Accessed 16/10/2018).

Wikipedia. (2018b). *Traditional Chinese Medicine*. https://en.wikipedia.org/wiki/Traditional_Chinese_medicine. Last edited October 13, 2018. (Accessed 16/10/2018).

Wikipedia. (2018c). *Wikipedia: Five Pillars*. https://en.wikipedia.org/wiki/Wikipedia:Five_pillars. Last edited September 15, 2018. (accessed 16/ 10/2018).

Wikipedia. (2018d). *Wikipedia: Systemic Bias*. https://en.wikipedia.org/wiki/Wikipedia:Systemic_bias, last edited October 13, 2018, (Accessed 16/10/2018).

6

THE PALIMPSEST

Black and ethnic minority perspectives in health humanities

Nehal El-Hadi

Introduction

In this chapter, I make the case for a social justice-oriented approach to health humanities that implicates this field in narratives of fairness and justice through informing the (attempted) provision of equitable health care. The radical interdisciplinarity of the field of health humanities means that its scholars, researchers, academics, and practitioners can choose to be unfettered by the historical complicity of the academic disciplines that inform it (the humanities writ large, anthropology, medicine, and so on). In recognition of the distinctions other scholars have made between medical and health humanities (Atkinson et al., 2015), here I use the term "health humanities" to also include the medical humanities, as the claims I make are germane to both. Like a palimpsest, theoretical and methodological approaches can retain the contributions of the academic disciplines that contribute to health humanities, but the field can address and extract approaches that problematize marginalized populations.

Health humanities can do this in the following three ways: (1) by acknowledging and confronting the violently racist histories of medical and scientific knowledge; (2) by intentionally, deliberately, and carefully including works produced by racialized, marginalized, and oft-excluded individuals that explore narratives of the experiences of illness, disease, and the health-care encounter; and (3) by imagining possibilities for equitable health-care research, practices, and delivery. My own work in this field explores the second of these—what I have termed *the production of presence*, which is the creation, management, and distribution of content and stories that center the marginalized individual and reflect the being-in-the-world of marginalized groups. In deliberately authentic and representative ways, these produced narratives then counter dominant hegemonic discourses of everyday life by providing alternate retellings and imaginings of everyday lived experiences.

In the introduction for her autopathographical book, Audre Lorde writes in *The Cancer Journals* that when a woman is diagnosed with breast cancer, "the weave of her every day existence is the training ground for how she handles crisis" (Lorde, 1980: 3). What Lorde refers to as the weave of existence is threaded by the subjecthood of the patient, a subjectivity produced by ethnicity, race, class, culture, language, faith, age, and so on. For Black women, how they handle the "crisis" and its diagnosis is complicated by their subjectivity in

43

the health care encounter. Using Black women's experiences and narratives of the medical/health-care encounter, I suggest that health humanities has an obligation to include and respectfully consider depictions of the lived experiences of *all* individuals, and a responsibility to address social inequality in medical and health care practice.

The acknowledgement of pasts

The relationships between medicine and health-care research and provision and racialized and marginalized communities have run the gamut—from problematic (and often violent and fatal) racism to life-changing and life-saving. For example, experiments on African American women held in slavery inform contemporary gynecology (Kapsalis, 1997). This section is not intended to be a catalog of examples; rather, here I highlight two well-known cases in the humanities of the depiction and portrayal of different historical examples.

Sarah (Saartjie) Baartman was a South African Khoikhoi woman who, in the early 1800s, was exhibited in Europe, paraded as the "Hottentot Venus," the attraction being her supposedly exaggerated bottom. Baartman died young of disease, and her remains—including her dissected pelvis—were displayed at the *Jardin des plantes de Paris* until 2002 when they were returned to South Africa (Crais and Scully, 2010). In death, Baartman's story provoked many retellings, such as the 2010 French-language film *Black Venus* by Tunisian-French filmmaker Abdellatif Kechiche (who also wrote and directed *Blue is the Warmest Colour*, 2013). Baartman has also been referenced in several poems and plays, as well as both William Makepeace Thackeray's *Vanity Fair* (1847) and James Joyce's *A Portrait of the Artist as a Young Man* (1916). From the perspective of health humanities, Baartman's history reflects racist scientific attitudes of the time, including direct linkages between her exploitation and medical racism as indicated by an entry in the *Dictionnaire des science médicale* (1819), written by the French physician Nicolas Philibert Adelon. In it, Adelon referred to Black women having larger genitalia as a reflection of their primitivity (Bickford, 2016: 120). Considering Baartman's legacy, Katherine McKittrick describes her as "the analytical template through which racist pornography, the grotesque, and the lewd seduction of black female popular-culture figures can be understood in relation to a history of racial imprisonment, bodily dismemberment, sexism, and white supremacy" (2010: 118).

A more recent case was popularized by the 2017 HBO film *The Immortal Life of Henrietta Lacks*, based on the 2010 book of the same name by Rebecca Skloot. Henrietta Lacks was an African American woman living in Baltimore who died of cancer in 1951; cells from her cancer were removed and grown and sold by laboratories for medical research purposes, without permission from or compensation to the surviving members of her family. In addition to the book, its dramatization, and an earlier BBC documentary, the story has been referenced in television shows and has provided the material for countless debates about the ethics of biological material and, more recently, genetic material; in 2013, scientists decoded and published the entire sequence (Landry et al., 2013). The sequence was removed from the public sphere at the request of the family, but, as Skloot wrote in an article for the *New York Times*, "[t]he Lackses' experiences over the last 60 years foretold nearly every major ethical issue raised by research on human tissues and genetic material." Hip-hop poet Saul Williams' poem *The Mother of Resurrection* was written about Henrietta Lacks and her cells, which are still used in research.

The effects of medical racism for Black women in western countries are well documented, anecdotally and scientifically (Prather et al., 2018). These historical examples, and others, contain lessons for the health humanities—accessing these narratives and using the lessons in them can help teach compassion and awareness. Acknowledging the racist history of medicine is a crucial part of addressing current health inequities.

The production of presence

Tennis champion Serena Williams had a near-death experience after giving birth to her daughter. "I almost died after giving birth to my daughter, Olympia," she wrote for CNN. com in February 2018, "[a]ccording to the Centers for Disease Control and Prevention, black women in the United States are over three times more likely to die from pregnancy or childbirth-related causes" (Williams, 2018). Less than a year later, Tressie-McMillam Cottom published a heartbreaking narrative about her miscarriage, her experience under-scoring the (deadly) challenges experienced by Black women when seeking treatment: "When the medical profession systematically denies the existence of black women's pain, underdiagnoses our pain, refuses to alleviate or treat our pain, health care marks us as incompetent bureaucratic subjects. Then it serves us accordingly" (2019).

These experiences are not uncommon, especially in the United States; study after study after study documents the medical racism experienced by Black and racialized women. For example, a recent review of maternal morbidity indicated that "[t]he findings of this study also support the need for enhanced screening and timely treatment for racial and ethnic minority women with chronic physical health conditions and particularly for women with multiple chronic conditions" (Admon et al., 2018: 1165). What McMillan-Cottom and Wil-liams' narratives do, however, is provide personalized narratives that are useful resources to include in health humanities curricula. In their investigation into the historical causes of health inequities for African American women in the United States, Prather et al. write that "[a]ddressing sexual and reproductive health through a historical lens and ensuring the implementation of culturally appropriate programs, research, and treatment efforts will likely move public health toward achieving health equity, which will benefit the health of African American women" (Prather et al., 2018: 256–257).

In an article by Hoffman et al. examining racial bias in pain assessment and treatment, the researchers found that "many white medical students and residents hold beliefs about biological differences between blacks and whites, many of which are false and fantastical in nature, and that these false beliefs are related to racial bias in pain perception" (2016: 4299). In my own research into online narratives, I found that social media networks, forums, per-sonal websites, and blogs were rich sites of narratives for all kinds of human experiences. Specifically, these online platforms provided the sites for the production of presence, while user-generated content—albeit anecdotal in quality—was able to provide "local instantiation and specific detail" (Frank, 2009: 107) for the research. Focusing on the experiences of Black women when seeking emergency treatment for chronic pain conditions, I found countless examples of narratives I had not come across elsewhere. While disparities in the experience of disease and provision of health care have been well documented at the inter-sections of race and gender, what I found to be disheartening were the personalized retell-ings of traumatic racist experiences in seeking care.

Elsewhere, I have collected autopathographies of Black women diagnosed with breast cancer to illustrate how these first-person narratives are able to inform a more compassionate and inclu-sive approach to disease management and treatment (El-Hadi, 2018), because "[h]ealth care practitioners and researchers can no longer afford to overlook the relationship between Black women's physical health and their psychosocial experiences" (Lawson, Rodgers-Rose and Rajaram, 1999: 288), especially when those experiences turn out to be deadly.

The imagining of futures

The increasing popularity of the genre of Afrofuturism imagines and presents Black futures in response to current social, political, technological, and environmental disparities. The genre of Afrofuturism began with African American expression, but "[a]lthough contemporary Black speculative thought has roots at the nexus of nineteenth century scientific racism, technology, and the struggle for African self-determination and creative expression, it has now matured into an emerging global phenomenon" (Anderson, 2016: 228). The voices of Black women in this genre are particularly strong, with authors such as Octavia Butler, Nalo Hopkinson, Nnedi Okorafor, and N.K. Jemisin, musical artists like Erykah Badu and Janelle Monae, and filmmakers like Frances Bodomo, Wanuri Kahiu, and Ava DuVernay to name a few. In the tradition of speculative fiction and science fiction, Afrofuturism works not only deal with Black protagonist in near and distant future settings, but also present fictionalized possibilities for Black people in the future.

In her introduction to *Medicine and Ethics in Black Women's Speculative Fiction*, Esther Jones writes that:

> Black women writers have long been aware of the complex nexus of personal health, larger societal problems and the challenge of locating the kind of medical care that attends to their needs as whole persons, as articulated in the lack of respect for a worldview centered on spiritual and religious factors that inform issues of wellness and illness … Speculative fiction is one place where black women can be portrayed as self-actualized and strategies for survival are expressed. It is where radical forms of medical and social justice are imagined. Black women speculative writers theorize difference, then, through their literature, challenging skewed notions and dominant misperceptions of blackness and womanhood, disease and pathology, social illness and personal health, while writing new prescriptions for how to relate humanely and ethically across differences.
>
> *(Jones, 2016: 4–6)*

These "new prescriptions," deliberately radical in their intent, and as an example of what cultural products by Black women can contribute, imagine new possibilities. Afrofuturist texts addressing current health inequities provide fertile ground for health humanities. An example of this can be found in a reading of Octavia Butler's vampire novel *Fledgling* that interprets it as a "novel about HIV/AIDS [that] transforms our understandings not only of the pandemic but of the practice of narrating illness" (Fink, 2010: 416). Another example lies in Kenyan artist Wangechi Mutu's 2005 collage series titled "Histology of the Different Classes of Uterine Tumour," where Mutu uses nineteenth-century medical illustrations as the background.

In these renderings of Black futures that comment on and are informed by history lie possibilities to engage with the health humanities that acknowledge that the current health disparities experienced by Black women are the culminating result of centuries of various oppressions. Including Afrofuturist texts contributes to the health humanities "as a vibrant site of public learning and activism" (Charise, 2017: 440). What Afrofuturist texts can provide is the possibility of hope: that existing health inequities *can* be addressed, and future health crises *might* be averted.

Scriptio superior

As health humanities becomes more integrated with medical education, there is an opportunity for responsible inclusivity and practices that respect the contributions of racialized and marginalized people to scientific knowledge—as both researchers and research subjects. There is a growing body of resources to help educators "teach [students] through art and literature" (Mohanna, 2006: 249), as a way to produce compassion and empathy. Metzl and Roberts write that many health-related factors previously attributed to culture or ethnicity also represent the downstream consequences of decisions about larger structural contexts, including health-care and food delivery systems, zoning laws, local politics, urban and rural infrastructures, structural racisms, or even the very definitions of illness and health (2014).

This complexity can be understood and communicated through the health humanities; studying the narratives of Black women can provide evidence and examples. The radical interdisciplinarity of health humanities means that useful tools of analysis can be employed from academic disciplines such as critical race studies, Black geographies, cultural studies, film studies, and women's and gender studies.

Discriminatory treatment of patients due to race, gender, and sexuality has been well documented. Examining the documentary and fictional representations of these experiences can serve to inform medical and health-care practice and delivery. An understanding of the health disparities faced by Black women would help to address some of these inequities for other groups as well within the context of health-care provision.

So what can a health humanities approach offer to these narratives? First of all, scholarship that engages with the narratives of (actual and imagined) Black women can help with the documentation and archiving of historical experiences with medicine and health care. Second, including contemporary narratives of Black women's experiences can, in effect, teach empathy and compassion in health care by personalizing data. And finally, in attempting to address current health disparities that are shaped by complex historical factors, a health humanities approach to futures-oriented texts can inform the imagination and generation of solutions to existing health-care disparities. In acknowledging historical trauma while conscious of the discriminatory practices of the past, and in careful and deliberate inclusive practices in curriculum development and delivery, health humanities has the opportunity to affect future health-care practice for the better.

References

Admon, L.K., Winkelman, T.N., Zivin, K., Terplan, M., Mhyre, J.M. and Dalton, V. K. (2018). Racial and Ethnic Disparities in the Incidence of Severe Maternal Morbidity in the United States, 2012–2015. *Obstetrics and Gynecology*, 132(5): 1158–1166.

Anderson, R. (2016). Afrofuturism 2.0 and The Black Speculative Arts Movement: Notes on a Manifesto. *Obsidian*, 42(1/2): 228.

Atkinson, S., Evans, B., Woods, A. and Kearns, R. (2015). The 'Medical' and 'Health' in a Critical Medical Humanities. *Journal of Medical Humanities*, 36(1): 71–81.

Bickford, A.L. (2016). *Southern Mercy: Empire and American Civilization in Juvenile Reform, 1890–1944*. Toronto: University of Toronto Press.

Charise, A. (2017). Site, Sector, Scope: Mapping the Epistemological Landscape of Health Humanities. *Journal of Medical Humanities*, 38(4): 431–444.

Crais, C. and Scully, P. (2010). *Sara Baartman and the Hottentot Venus: A Ghost Story and a Biography*. Princeton, NJ: Princeton University Press.

El-Hadi, N. (2018). The Production of Presence: The Internet and First-Person Illness Narratives. *Geo-Humanities: Space, Place, and the Humanities*, 4(2): 315–321.

Fink, M. (2010). AIDS Vampires: Reimagining Illness in Octavia Butler's "Fledgling.". *Science Fiction Studies*, 37(3): 416–432.

Frank, A.W. (2009). Why I wrote … The Wounded Storyteller: A Recollection of Life and Ethics. *Clinical Ethics*, 4(2): 106–108.

Hoffman, K.M., Trawalter, S., Axt, J.R. and Oliver, M.N. (2016). Racial Bias in Pain Assessment and Treatment Recommendations, and False Beliefs about Biological Differences between Blacks and Whites. *Proceedings of the National Academy of Sciences*, 113(16): 4296–4301.

Jones, E.L. (2016). *Medicine and Ethics in Black Women's Speculative Fiction*. New York: Springer.

Kapsalis, T. (1997) Mastering the Female Pelvis: Race and the Tools of Reproduction. In T. Kapsalis, ed, *Public Privates: Performing Gynecology From Both Ends of the Speculum*, Durham, NC: Duke University Press: 31–60.

Landry, J.J., Pyl, P.T., Rausch, T., Zichner, T., Tekkedil, M.M., Stütz, A.M., Jauch, A., Aiyar, R.S., Pau, G., Delhomme, N., Gagneur, J., Korbel, J.O., Huber, W. and Steinmetz, L.M. (2013). The Genomic and Transcriptomic Landscape of a HeLa Cell Line. *G3: Genes, Genomes, Genetics*, 3(8): 1213–1224.

Lawson, E.J., Rodgers-Rose, L. and Rajaram, S. (1999). The Psychosocial Context of Black Women's Health. *Healthcare for Women International*, 20(3): 279–289.

Lorde, A. (1980). *The Cancer Journals*. San Francisco: Aunt Lute Books.

McKittrick, K. (2010). Science Quarrels Sculpture: The Politics of Reading Sarah Baartman. *Mosaic: A Journal for the Interdisciplinary Study of Literature*, 43(2): 113–130.

McMillan Cottom, T. (January 8, 2019). I Was Pregnant and in Crisis. All the Doctors and Nurses Saw Was an Incompetent Black Woman. *TIME Magazine*. Retrieved from http://time.com/5494404/tressie-mcmillan-cottom-thick-pregnancy-competent/(Accessed 18/2/2019).

Metzl, J.M. and Roberts, D.E. (2014). Structural Competency Meets Structural Racism: Race, Politics, and the Structure of Medical Knowledge. *Virtual Mentor*, 16(9): 674–690.

Mohanna, K. (2006). Education for Life: Teaching Medicine Using Art and Humanities. *British Medical Journal*, 332(7556): s249–s250.

Prather, C., Fuller, T.R., Jeffries IV, W.L., Marshall, K.J., Howell, A.V., Belyue-Umole, A. and King, W. (2018). Racism, African American Women, and Their Sexual and Reproductive Health: A Review of Historical and Contemporary Evidence and Implications for Health Equity. *Health Equity*, 2(1): 249–259.

Williams, S. (February 20. 2018). Serena Williams: What My Life-threatening Experience Taught Me About Giving Birth. *CNN*. Retrieved from www.cnn.com/2018/02/20/opinions/protect-mother-pregnancy-williams-opinion/index.html (Accessed 18/2/2019).

7

REPRESENTATIONS OF MEDICAL AND HEALTH DELIVERY PARADIGMS

Phillip Barrish

Introduction

I begin with what may seem a provocative statement. As a field, the health humanities pays too much attention to individual experiences of illness and healing. Put less provocatively, the health humanities—including my own subfield, which I would describe as literature, health, and medicine—should pay more attention to health care as a system, which would include, among other elements, delivery and funding paradigms, governmental and institutional policies and practices, and personnel whose roles range well beyond patient and provider. Most existing work in literature, health, and medicine draws on literature and other expressive culture as a resource for understanding the illness experience or analyzes literary representations of medical practitioners or, less frequently, uses literary-critical methods to unpack biomedical discourse and its cultural effects. Narrative medicine, too, is a project primarily aimed at the interface between patient and provider. This is all immensely valuable and important work, and there are excellent historical, ethical, and pragmatic reasons for the field to have placed those who are ill and those who care for them front and central.

Over the past several decades, scholarly agendas in the medical and health humanities have tended to be more directly motivated by the exigencies of teaching, as well as practicing, the health professions than is typical in other humanities fields. The modern incarnation of the medical humanities took off from within medical schools and is still predominantly centered there, at least institutionally. In this context, the humanities tend to be valued for the lessons they can teach, and the skills and sensibilities they can help develop, regarding one-to-one human relationships, and above all the relationship between patient and health-care provider. Put spatially, the learning and insights produced in the health humanities classroom are designed to anticipate what students will encounter in clinical spaces, whether that be a consulting room or a hospital bedside. Yet I am convinced that literature and related forms of expressive culture also have much to teach us about what we might think of as the less visible spaces, the beams, hallways, thresholds, and wire conduits, so to speak, that help determine what occurs (or does not occur) in clinical spaces.

My interest in thinking about representations of health care as a system goes back to about 2011 and a confluence of things then happening more or less simultaneously in three different areas of my life: intellectual, civic, and familial. As will be clear, the latter two were specific to my location in the United States, with its notoriously convoluted, inefficient, and inequitable system for funding and distributing health care, but I would be surprised if many living in other countries have not had related experiences. Intellectually, I discovered the field of medical or health humanities, in part spurred by the planned opening of a new medical school at my university. I found the field revelatory and inspiring in many ways. But I also sensed there were some important dimensions of health and health care that the field was underemphasizing. This feeling was no doubt connected to events then transpiring in the public sphere and in my personal life. Publicly, major provisions of the Patient Protection and Affordable Care Act (ACA), also known as Obamacare, were moving closer to national implementation, having been passed by Congress and signed into law by President Obama in 2010. I had followed the political battles swirling around the ACA since before the law had been formally proposed, fascinated and often enraged by the sheer difficulty involved in trying to extend what I saw as a basic human right to more Americans. The 2012 presidential election, as well as upcoming congressional elections in 2014, only heightened the vitriolic and often misleading public debate surrounding the ACA. Although I myself have pretty good health insurance through my employer, my father's situation at the time helped bring home to me the stakes of what was being fought over.

Some years prior to my father Norman Barrish's death in 2014, I took over the management of his finances, which he was no longer capable of handling. He was already residing in a senior living facility in New York City, where I grew up, although I have lived in Texas for the past 20 years. It soon became clear that my father's pension and social security income could not possibly cover the increasing amount of in-home care he required. I learned that Medicare, the US government's health insurance plan for people over 65, includes quite limited home-care benefits. The only way to pay for the long-term home care my father needed was to get him accepted into Medicaid, a hybrid state and federal program that is supposed to provide health coverage for the indigent. But it turned out that, as is still the case for millions of people all over America, the income that was *in*sufficient to meet my father's health needs was high enough to disqualify him for Medicaid. That is to say, he wasn't indigent enough. After a convoluted year-long process that at the time I compared to applying simultaneously for a home mortgage and for tenure at a research university, a way was found to preserve enough of my father's income to pay his non-health expenses (through something called a "community trust") while also enrolling him in Medicaid. This solution was entirely legal, but I was still left with the uncomfortable feeling of having helped my father game the system in a way that would not have been possible for someone with fewer resources to put into navigating the multiple bureaucracies involved. Regardless, his successful enrollment in Medicaid made a meaningful difference to the quality of my father's last 18 months of life. Importantly, this difference was not directly tied either to the specific nature of his interactions with health providers or, as far as I could tell, to how he understood his illness—that is, to the usual foci of the health humanities. But it was nonetheless qualitative, relational (most literally, it allowed him to form a relationship with an empathic home-care provider whose wages Medicaid paid; the sad meagerness of those wages, which we did our best to supplement, is a crucial aspect of my larger point here), and deeply human. The qualitative, the relational, the human—the experience helped bring home to me how inseparable the ins and outs of health policy and funding are to what health humanists, and humanists in general, care most about.

The fact that he was in New York and I lived and worked in Texas meant that I was not able to be present as often as I wished I could be at my father's doctor appointments or, even worse, at his increasingly frequent trips to the emergency room, which often resulted in his spending a few days or more in the hospital. I spent a lot of time traveling back and forth and at least as much time feeling guilty when I could not travel. I was also very lucky that he had a life partner, Barbara, who despite health problems of her own did her best to be with him on those occasions. Nonetheless, I started to believe, or maybe I needed to believe, that the endless paperwork I was dealing with, and the back-and-forth communications not so much with doctors as with other people working in their offices or in hospital administrative departments, as well as ongoing communication with a paralegal whose expertise I relied on, with my father's accountant, and with some New York state and city government offices—I started to believe that all of this infrastructure, as frustrating and tedious as it sometimes was, was a crucial part of the care my father received and/or did not receive.

I began looking for works of literature that would speak to these dimensions of health care in what I hoped were interesting or fruitful ways. The first literary text I zeroed in on was a novel from 1900 called *The Web of Life*, by a once well-known American writer named Robert Herrick (Herrick, 1900). I loved how the title of Herrick's book takes a phrase often used as a metaphor for *natural* ecologies—the web of life—to instead portray medicine as an evolving *social* network of interests, institutions, funding models, and professional cultures. Here are some examples of the interrelated developments on which *The Web of Life* offers a critical perspective: one, the increasing pervasiveness of a strictly monetary fee-for-service model that incentivized doctors to provide more, and more expensive, forms of treatment; two, the multiplication of medical specialties, which, in dividing the human body into what Herrick (1911: 404) elsewhere called "numerous small principalities" ("the eye and the ear, the nose and the throat, the feet, the head, the heart, the skin, the lungs, the intestines"), each with its own "special priest," pushed medical costs further upward; three, the advent of newly bureaucratized medical offices filled with both sophisticated technology and clerks, which some people, including doctors, worried would undermine the personal dimension of medical care; and four, the use of poor people's bodies, alive and dead, for medical training and medical research, with the research leading to journal articles that helped doctors gain prestigious consulting positions at hospitals. The web of life indeed.

To put it mildly, I was astonished to find all of these facets of modern medicine not only depicted, but also *wrestled* with, in a novel first published in 1900. It was a time in the United States when so-called "orthodox" or establishment medicine, generally allopathic in approach, found itself beset financially and culturally by a broad range of alternative practices, ranging from homeopathy to hydrotherapy to Christian Science. Many Americans found these alternative approaches to be at least as effective as, and often more pleasant than, what the medical establishment offered them. Arguably, the most significant reasons for orthodox medicine's achievement by the 1920s of a hegemonic position in American health care—and the orthodox profession's attendant rise in status, authority, and profitability—were scientific and technical. By that I mean that orthodox medicine finally developed more effective tools for treating illness and injury than other approaches had at their disposal. But in addition to scientific advances there were also meaningful cultural, institutional, and affective dimensions of orthodox medicine's rise to what sociologist Paul Starr has called professional sovereignty. *Those* dimensions are what Robert Herrick's novel seeks to explore using the tools of fiction. The fictional prism also allows Herrick to probe both benefits and costs of the US medical sector's transformation from a chaotic but relatively egalitarian, relatively democratic space, energized from the bottom up, to a twentieth-century American health-care system that was, and is, notably more centralized, rationalized, and hierarchical. Herrick's novel begins by critiquing the features of modern medical professionalism that I listed above (fee for service, etc.), but gradually finds itself acknowledging if not the desirability, then the practical necessity, of the orthodox profession's dominance (Barrish, 2014).

In addition to realist novels such as Herrick's (and, for a more recent example, Lionel Shriver's 2010 *So Much for That*), I have found that dystopian speculative fiction also offers rich grounds—aesthetic, affective, and analytic—for probing not only the workings, but also the *feel* of what I have come to think of as health care's political economy. Speculative fiction is replete with representations of future societies that have been deformed by the use—or misuse—of advanced biomedical technologies including, for example, genetic engineering, cloning, organ transplantation, and increasingly sophisticated machine–human interfaces. But I have been more interested (Barrish, 2016, 2018) in works whose future dystopias are shaped just as much by issues of health-care access, distribution, and funding, in literary works such as Korean American novelist Chang-Rae Lee's recent *On Such a Full Sea* (2014) and films such as South African director Neill Blomkamp's *Elysium* (2013). Speculative fiction has been useful to my interests because of how it encourages readers, first, to develop an analytic understanding of the social structures of a given fictive world, and second, to view those social structures as contingent. As critic Tom Moylan (2000: 5–6) has noted, what appears in realist fiction—and, I would add, in personal narratives—

> to be the taken-for-granted background (the setting) is actually in [science fiction]
> the foreground (or driving force behind the total creation); for before a story can
> be followed or a character understood, the fictive world must itself be indulged in,
> grasped.

Speculative science fiction forces us to begin by attending to the systems—not merely scientific or technological, but also social, economic, and political—by which the portrayed society is organized, at least initially even over individual characters or plot. In foregrounding fictional modes of social organization that in crucial ways differ from our own, the genre further encourages us to recognize the material and ideological systems that subtend society as produced, rather than fixed or natural.

It is not the role of imaginative narrative, or of art as such, to provide explicit directions for how to solve a problem, or for that matter how to cure an illness or injury. Even in clinical settings, where narrative medical practices focus on personal non-fictional stories, the healing effects of such practices can be indirect or appear in unanticipated ways. One common benefit is that, "through the act of telling their stories, patients are able to distance themselves from their illness and provide space to reflect on what is happening to them and how their life stories are changing" (Engel et al., 2008: 222). Any analogy between fiction and the effects that narrating their own experience can generate for an individual patient will be loose at best. Still, fictional health policy narratives may also provide a "space to reflect" as we wrestle with how to create a more just and equitable system for funding and distributing the best health care of which we are collectively capable, whether within a given nation state or globally.

References

Barrish, P. (2014). The Sticky Web of Medical Professionalism: Robert Herrick's *The Web of Life* and the Political Economy of Healthcare at the Turn of the Century. *American Literature*, 86(3): 583–610.

Barrish, P. (2016). Health Policy in Dystopia. *Literature and Medicine*, 34(1): 106–131.

Barrish, P. (2018). Environmental Illness and the Future of Healthcare: Chang-Rae Lee's *On Such a Full Sea*. *Journal of the Medical Humanities*. 40(3): 297–313. (Online First).

Engel, J.D., Zarconi, J., Pethtel, L.L. and Missimi, S.A. (2008). *Narrative in Healthcare: Healing Patients, Practitioners, Profession, and Community*. Boca Raton, FL: Radcliffe Publishing (CRC Press).

Herrick, R. (1900). *The Web of Life*. New York: Macmillan.

Herrick, R. (1911). *The Healer*. New York: Macmillan.

Moylan, T. (2000). *Scraps of the Untainted Sky: Science Fiction, Utopia, Dystopia*. Boulder, Colo: Westview Press.

8

POST-CONFLICT RESOLUTION AND THE HEALTH HUMANITIES

The Warrior Chorus program

Peter Meineck

Introduction

"Warrior Chorus" is a military veteran–civilian public engagement, dialogue, and perform-ance program established in New York in 2012 by Aquila Theatre and New York Univer-sity. Since 2010, the Warrior Chorus program has used ancient Greek literature and drama to facilitate community, discussion, and presentations on the experience of veterans in America. Funded primarily by the National Endowment for the Humanities, this program grew directly from an earlier national public program called "Ancient Greeks/Modern Lives," which toured to one hundred underserved communities in the United States with a performance and discussion program based around Homer's *Iliad*. As the program developed, it became clear that members of the veteran community gravitated towards this material as a means to start to discuss their experiences of combat, post-conflict issues, and the relation-ship between American democracy, the military, and war.

Background

The close connections between ancient Greek texts and the experience of war and homecom-ing have been apparent since antiquity, including the works of Homer, Thucydides, and Xenophon. These intersecting themes became particularly resonant in the twentieth century as a greater number of Americans were exposed to ancient Greek material through more widely available publications, translations, and theatrical productions. In the mid-1990s, United States Veteran's Administration psychiatrist Jonathan Shay published *Achilles in Vietnam* (1995), which used Homer's *Iliad* as a means to approach certain clinical aspects he was observing in the veterans under his care. These included the so-called "berserker state" (explosive rage), post-deployment social isolation, and the subcategory of post-traumatic stress disorder (PTSD) known as combat trauma (PTSD had itself only been admitted into the Diag-nostic and Statistical Manual of Mental Disorders in 1980).

Shay's influential work was followed by his *Odysseus in Vietnam* in 2003, which focused on the issues of veteran homecoming and post-war reconciliation as reflected in Homer's *Odyssey* (Shay, 2003). These works led in turn to a number of scholars seeking to identify whether the signs and symptoms of combat trauma and PTSD could be discerned in ancient literature, such as Larry Tritle's *From Melos to Mai Lai* (2000), Tritle himself is a Vietnam combat veteran, and the collected volume *Combat Trauma and the Ancient Greeks* (Meineck and Konstan, 2014). In a similar vein, Nancy Sherman's *Afterwar* (Sherman, 2015) used Sophocles' tragedy *Philoctetes* as an example of the effects of *moral injury*, a condition defined by the National Center for PTSD as "a construct that describes extreme and unprecedented life experience including the harmful aftermath to such events" (Maguen and Litz, 2019). These events are interpreted as injurious if they "transgress deeply held moral beliefs and expectations" (Litz et al., 2009: 696).

Warrior Chorus puts this research into practice, applying Shay's insight that Greek drama was in its time created by combat veterans, performed by combat veterans, for an audience of combat veterans. This is an applied humanities-based public program that uses Greek texts as the basis for the exploration of themes such as ethics at war, women and war, the return of the warrior, and the meaning of democracy. The program has three centers—New York, Los Angeles, and Texas—where between 12 and 48 veterans at each location are paid to join a weekly program consisting of a discussion and reading group led by a veteran and a scholar, an artistic exploration and creation phase, and a final public presentation phase. The objective of the program is to train veterans to lead their own public programming in order that their voices be heard directly by the American public to try to make Americans more literate about the human costs of war. Although Warrior Chorus is not intended as a therapy-based program, the community of veterans it creates and the value it places in their opinions of classical material has been often reported as providing important mental health benefits to the participants involved (Zusi, 2016).

The capstone of the program is a series of performances. These take several forms and are curated based on the interests and skill sets of the veteran participants. For example, members of the 2015–2016 Los Angeles group expressed a desire to use film in their public programming, which ultimately took place in five sites in the LA area, including museums and public libraries. The veterans developed several themes based on a number of Greek plays that dealt with issues central to their experiences, such as Sophocles' *Ajax* (veteran suicide), *Philoctetes* (injury and social isolation), and Aeschylus' *Agamemnon* (the ethics of military leadership). The veteran members then created several short films that engaged these themes, and were then able to offer public screenings followed by audience discussion.

In 2016–2017, the New York group based their final presentations around staged readings of both ancient works and new pieces they had written inspired by them, based on their own experiences. These public, semi-staged readings were professionally directed and a scholar was part of the discussion group. They were performed to large audiences at venues including the Metropolitan Museum of Art, Federal Hall, and John Jay Homestead. As the program progressed, chorus members became more proficient at performance skills and presentation, and subsequently presented a full-length dramatized version of this work, entitled *Our Trojan War*, at the Brooklyn Academy of Music in April 2017.

New directions

Many participants in the Warrior Chorus program have gone on to pursue careers in the arts and humanities, including working as playwrights, actors, poets, and producers, with several going back into education to study advanced degree programs. The program itself has also developed through responding to the needs of the community it serves, placing veterans in leadership positions with creative control of the work produced. This was exemplified in the 2018 New York program, where veterans used their own dramatic writings and presented them to audiences alongside performances of scenes from ancient works. Additionally, at a time of increasing and troubling polarization in American political and ethical life, Warrior Chorus groups have become more interested in using the program to advance questions of democracy, service, and leadership. One motivator for this expanded scope of practice may be the reality that, in the United States, the American veteran is perhaps one of the very few people in the cultural landscape that may be able to induce dialogue from people of both sides of the current polarized political culture. For example, Warrior Chorus has been placed into service for humanities advocacy, including several trips to Washington, DC, to present work to members of both congressional houses and, in 2014, a presentation at the Obama White House. In this way, the veteran members are redeployed as warriors for the humanities, using the ancient material and reflections on their own experiences to help bring people together in civil discourse.

The initial aim of the Warrior Chorus was to be a humanities program that helped Americans better understand veterans through ancient texts and was never envisioned as a therapy-based or mental health program. However, it has provided both a therapeutic environment for its participants (as reported by them; see Boston, 2019; National Public Radio, 2014) and also been deployed in health environments, such as presentations at US Department of Veterans Affairs (VA) hospitals and for their staff, in medical schools, and in workshops with professional care staff who work in the field. In July 2015 the program also traveled to Greece, where its members worked alongside refugees in Athens, staging non-verbal workshops based on ancient drama. Several members of this refugee group came from Afghanistan, Iraq, and Syria and had only ever encountered American service personnel in military or administrative roles. Likewise, the veterans had not had the opportunity work on arts and humanities with people from the countries in which they served. The whole experience was a deeply moving one for all, and led to the program expanding its definition of "veteran" to include all those affected by war: soldiers, civilians, and people of all ages and every background.

Aquila Theatre's Warrior Chorus is not the only program that uses Greek literature with veterans, although it is the first on a national scale. There have been several programs inspired by Aquila's public programs and Shay's work more generally. Among the most well-known is Theater of War, a for-profit venture run by the enterprising Brian Doerries who has documented his work in a book of the same name. Doerries's program employs celebrity actors in readings of Greek plays, followed by a panel discussion and moderated town hall-style audience response session. Some criticisms of this approach has been the lack of veteran input in conceiving and managing the project, the for-profit business structure, the tightly controlled narrative of the moderator, and the focus only on PTSD of veterans. While PTSD is a real issue amongst many veterans it is a complex one: it is not restricted to veterans, and not all veterans suffer from it.

Opportunities and challenges

Although it is compelling to suggest that experiencing Greek drama can provide a form of cathartic healing, the realities are, of course, far more complicated. The risk is that in order to generate much needed publicity for these kinds of programs, veterans can be marginalized and their multifaceted experiences, backgrounds, and health issues oversimplified and perhaps even objectified. This kind of oversimplification of program messaging is not really the fault of programs such as Theatre of War, whose work has exposed many people to both ancient drama and the issue of veteran post-traumatic stress. Rather, it is that the funding structures currently available for health humanities-oriented public programs in the United States seem to demand this type of one-dimensional approach; to use a corporate term derived from the worlds in which most of the foundations and individual donors inhabit, programs like these are rewarded for being "on-message."

Part of the problem here may be the legal structure of the non-profit, individual donor and foundation world in the United States, where tax breaks are offered in return for charitable donations or costs can be written off as marketing expenses for a particular initiative. Although government funding for the arts and the humanities is very low in the United States, and not without its own problems, it is at least a source of money somewhat divorced from the needs of corporations or private donors. Moreover, national funding opportunities can effectively support a program that promotes more intensive veteran involvement and that uses the humanities to explore issues that are, by their very nature, complex, difficult, and resistant to nuanced public dialogue.

From the inception of the Warrior Chorus program it was a primary intention to foster active dialogue between members of the veteran community and the general public. Although the United States is a major military power, less than 1% of its population is serving at any one time, even though as of 2016, according to the VA there are more than 20.4 million veterans in America, representing less than 7% of the total population. This means that most Americans have never served in the military and have no first-hand knowledge of war and homecoming; yet, in a democracy, this same population is responsible for voting for the leaders who may take the country to war. The need for such a program therefore remains urgent.

Recruitment

In the Warrior Chorus's case, two different audiences need to be recruited for such work to succeed: veterans and the general public. Initially, large veterans groups were approached, such as the American Legion and the Veterans of the Iraq and Afghanistan Wars, but due to their size these organizations were not particularly responsive (although some were supportive) to a grassroots humanities program. Direct veteran recruitment was initially difficult, but was developed from the ground up by first reaching out to smaller, local existing groups such as NYU's informal Warrior Writers programs and to professors who knew of particular GI Bill students (veterans who have earned college tuition because of their military service) who might be interested in or would benefit from such a program. Starting small and scaling up was the key; evidently, veterans were attracted to the program mainly by word of mouth from other veterans or by attending the initial public programming. Partnerships with local veteran groups were also invaluable, and as the program grew to a national scale it was found that these same grassroots techniques could be applied locally. Another key to recruitment was placing veterans at the heart of the program right from the start: as consultants, program coordinators, and then partnering them with a local scholar. Scholars also needed to be trained to work with veterans, and attended several sessions to learn about the veteran community and the program themes as they related to their own areas of expertise.

The second component of success was the recruitment of the public's support for the Warrior Chorus. The program partnered with cultural institutions such as museums, theaters, and public libraries that already had a good record of audience outreach and could place those resources into service drumming up audiences for the program events. Social media was also employed, both through normal modes of amplification such as Facebook announcements, Twitter and Instagram feeds, and blog posts, but also by piggy-backing on existing veteran networks. Aquila Theatre also developed a web-based app called YouStories where veterans could engage with the program material, and then upload their own video responses that were collected by the Veterans section of the American Folklife Center at the Library of Congress.

Finally, the humanities content itself, in the form of texts by ancient Greek authors such as Homer, Sappho, Aeschylus, Sophocles, Euripides, and Aristophanes, proved to be an essential resource in the success of the program. Most audience members probably had only a small amount of knowledge about these works and many may have not known them at all, but Warrior Chorus exploited their reputation as "classics" to focalize the program's themes. Although the cultural products of ancient Greece and Rome have been historically favored—often at the expense of the works of other cultures, and variously used to justify colonialism, slavery, elitism, and patriarchy—it is this very use (and sometimes abuse) of classical material that has made them influential. Salvatore Settis describes the classics as a mirror we hold up to our natures, advancing that every era has invented a different idea of the 'classical' to create its own identity (Settis and Cameron, 2006), a way in which we seek to know more about ourselves by reflecting on another culture from a different time. Therefore, the kind of authority some sections of American culture places in classical work can be exploited to act as a sounding board for the issues that face the veteran community and, by extension, America today. In addition, audiences hearing these works for the first time often report being shocked at their subversiveness and emotional power, and the ways in which they can seem to give voice to marginalized groups, including prisoners, slaves, refugees, and elderly individuals (Seigel, 2015; Sherman, 2017). This is consistent with Shay's portrayal of the role of ancient Greek drama, which appears to have offered a kind of cultural therapy to its fifth-century Athenian audience—all men, all citizens, all with experience serving in the Athenian military, which was actively at war.

For much of the fifth century, Athens was under a state of siege from the Persians or the Spartans and, as a result, suffered a terrible mass-casualty plague, a series of debilitating military disasters, and bouts of political anarchy. One theory of the purpose of ancient drama is that the catharsis it offered was an affective and psychological one, providing a place where the Athenian voting public could empathize with others, reflect on alternate perspectives, and feel deeply and jointly as a community traumatized by almost constant war (Shay, 1995). As a result, Greek dramatic literature tackles very difficult themes by placing the experiences of the warrior, homecoming, and issues of hospitality to strangers front and center. As the success of the Warrior Chorus program continues to demonstrate, such an uncompromising art form can be highly effective in health humanities programs aimed at members of the veteran community.

References

Boston, M. (2019). Veteran Takes the Stage as a Great Trojan of the Past. *USC News*, October 26. https://news.usc.edu/109811/veteran-takes-the-stage-as-a-great-trojan-of-the-past/ (Accessed 17/1/2019).

Litz, B.T., Stein, N., Delaney, E., Lebowitz, L., Nash, W.P., Silva, C. and Maguen, S. (2009). Moral Injury and Moral Repair in War Veterans: A Preliminary Model and Intervention Strategy. *Clinical Psychology Review, 29*: 695–706.

Maguen, S and Litz B. (2019). *Moral Injury in the Context of War*. Washington, DC: Veterans Administration Healthcare: National Center for PTSD. www.ptsd.va.gov/professional/treat/cooccurring/moral_injury.asp (Accessed 18/1/2019).

Meineck, P. and Konstan, D., eds, (2014). *Combat Trauma and the Ancient Greeks*. New York: Springer.

National Public Radio. (2014). Veterans' 'Philoctetes' Puts Modern Spin on Ancient Greek Play. May 29, 2014. www.npr.org/2014/05/29/317127131/veterans-philoctetes-puts-modern-spin-on-ancient-greek-play (Accessed 17/1/2019).

Seigel, J. (2015). Theatre of War. *National Endowment for the Humanities Magazine*, 36 (2) www.neh.gov/humanities/2015/marchapril/feature/theater-war (Accessed 17/1/2019).

Settis, S. and Cameron, A. (2006). *The Future of the Classical*. Cambridge: Polity Press.

Shay, J. (1995). *Achilles in Vietnam: Combat Trauma and the Undoing of Character*. New York: Simon and Schuster.

Shay, J. (2003). *Odysseus in America: Combat Trauma and the Trials of Homecoming*. New York: Simon and Schuster.

Sherman, H. (2017). A Warrior Chorus. *Stage Directions Magazine*, May 24. http://stage-directions.com/current-issue/125-perspectives/9524-a-warrior-chorus.html. (Accessed 17/1/2019).

Sherman, N. (2015). *Afterwar: Healing the Moral Wounds of Our Soldiers*. Oxford: Oxford University Press.

Tritle, L.A. (2000). *From Melos to My Lai*. London and New York: Routledge.

Zusi, K. (2016). Greek Drama's Lessons for Veterans. *Yale School of Medicine Magazine*, Winter 2016. https://medicine.yale.edu/news/printarticle/greek-dramas-lessons-for-veterans.aspx (accessed 18/1/2019).

9

COMICS AND GRAPHIC MEDICINE AS A THIRD SPACE FOR THE HEALTH HUMANITIES

Susan M. Squier

Introduction

The retrospective view is a strange one for those of us who are university professors. We have been so trained to look forward; to estimate how many articles we can publish before tenure, to consider the chances that a wished-for grant will come through, to yearn for that sabbatical still five years away, to imagine what it will feel like when the book we are laboring over is finally in print, and even to anticipate retirement. To be asked to look back happens seldom. We may do so only when we compose a letter of recommendation, scanning our memory for the accomplishments of a valued graduate student, or when we have to undertake those deadly exercises the Dean requires: the annual "faculty activity report" linked to everything from merit raises to tenure turndowns.

Thanks to the invitation to contribute to this volume, however, I have recently been engaged in an act of retrospective assessment. I have been wondering when I turned to comics, and then to graphic medicine, in my research and teaching in the medical and health humanities. I have raided my file cabinet and retrieved some of the articles I have written in the field of medical and health humanities over the past 25 years. They have given me a picture of some of the social, cultural, and historical developments that led me to comics as I tried to grapple with some of the challenges of the medical and health humanities.

What I have found is that comics, and then graphic medicine, have served me as a third space in my scholarship and teaching.[1] While the concept of 'third space' will take on different meanings in the course of this brief essay, winding its way to the conclusion where I will offer a more formal definition, let's start with my personal, and even idiosyncratic, description: the third space is a zone where one can play with ideas not yet accessible to linear thinking, draw together concepts, communities, and practices conventionally kept separate, and enjoy the fireworks that result.

In 1990–1991, I was living in Melbourne, Australia on a Fulbright Scholarship to study reproductive technology (as we called it then). I was writing what would become *Babies in Bottles*, a study of the relations between twentieth-century literature, medical science, and culture (especially photography and film) in the development of reproductive technology (Squier, 1994). It seems a long time ago now, that era in which we argued, as feminists, that surrogacy exploited the bodies of working-class women and that the new technology of *in vitro* fertilization robbed women of agency, transferring it instead to doctors and medical institutions. Melbourne was a lively place to be if you were interested in reproductive innovation: surrogate motherhood had just emerged as an extremely controversial reproductive option, and the Deakin University IVF clinic of Dr. Alan Trounson was making waves for its risky policy of implanting as many as eight embryos. The newspapers were full of stories on these topics, so scanning the main Melbourne newspaper, *The Age*, was a standard part of my research.

On February 18, 1991, as the US Gulf War was being waged on live television, two cartoons appeared in *The Age* that caught my attention with their vivid treatment of the same visualization technologies I had been writing about. In the first, by cartoonist Michael Bean, a father and son are crouched in front of a TV, the father pointing at the image, while above them a caption reads "Television viewers marveled at the view from the tiny bullet camera as it entered an Iraqi stomach!" (Bean, 1991). In the other, by Peter Nicholson, a bomb with top-mounted camera speeds across the frame from left to right. The caption reads "A 'smart' bomb trying to work out the difference between a frightened Iraqi conscript and a frightened 80-year-old grandmother" (Nicholson, 1991). Seeing those cartoons kindled a connection between what I was currently writing about and what we were all watching, horribly, on our television news.

The cartoon of the father and son watching the bullet camera tunneling into an Iraqi stomach reminded me of the ways pregnant women were treated in reproductive technology, and I wrote an essay using those comics to think through the curious combination of intimacy and distance that linked the new reproductive technologies with the Gulf War:

> [W]e might extrapolate from an understanding of the function of the scopic embryo or foetus in IVF and surrogacy an understanding of the role of the video-image (be it of an Iraqi's stomach, a tank tower, or a bunker) in war. Just as the medical privileging of the image of the embryo or foetus functions to render the woman marginal, both as gestating body and as one who is pregnable, so the wartime emphasis on the video-image renders the targeted human body marginal. It is either too small or too far away to see, or (in the cartoon of the 'tiny bullet camera' in the Iraqi's intestine) it is too large, too close up.
>
> *(Squier, 1993: 11)*

By playing in the third space of comics I was able to formulate some of the connections between the world of medicine and the world of war. However, I would have to wait almost 25 years to find a thorough evaluation of how deeply entangling those connections really are—that is, until I read Jennifer Terry's brilliant analysis of the biomedicine–war nexus in *Attachments to War: Biomedical Logics and Violence in Twenty-First-Century America* (Terry, 2017). A challenge to inward-facing or internalist medical humanities, Terry's book demonstrates the vicious circle of attachment through which war both catalyzes and requires the techno–medical advances of contemporary treatment, rehabilitation, and prosthetics.

Over the next ten years, I wrote my next book, *Liminal Lives: Imagining the Human at the Frontiers of Biomedicine* (Squier, 2007), fueled by my sense that the human lifespan was being remade, and the human identity being reshaped, in literature and medicine in the era of biotechnology.[2] The arc of *Liminal Lives* stretched from the cultured cell to the ageing and dying individual, and once again comics helped me think about those subjects. I was particularly drawn to Ruben Bolling's brilliant comic *Bad Blastocyst*, arguing in the Coda that because it "enables us to enter, imaginatively, [a number of] complex, ambiguous debates" (Squier, 2004: 286), it provides an excellent teaching tool for addressing ethical issues ranging from capital punishment, abortion, disability studies, to animal experimentation (Bolling, 2004; Squier, 2007).[3]

Rereading that brief analysis of Bolling's nine-panel *Bad Blastocyst*, I am still convinced by my analysis. However, my naïveté as a comics scholar makes me cringe, especially at my description of comics as 'the most highly stigmatized fictional genre.' How times have changed since 2004—and how I have as well, thank goodness. Now I know that comics is not a genre, but a medium; that comics are (increasingly) not only fiction but also non-fiction and documentary; and that disciplinary and social narrowness has produced the stigma around comics. Although Fredric Wertham didn't help. In a lovely little footnote to the health humanities, psychiatrist Dr. Fredric Wertham launched a crusade against comics in 1948 when he spoke at a symposium on "The Psychopathology of Comics Books" sponsored by the American Association of Psychotherapy. Six years later, with his book *Seduction of the Innocent* (1954), Wertham catalyzed US Senate hearings that led to the voluntary adoption of the self-regulatory adoption of the Comics Code (Wertham, 1954; Hajdu, 2008). While I then read *Bad Blastocyst* mostly for its plot and themes, more recently I have focused on its innovative paneling and its attention to framing and perspective that subtly moves the reader from taking the perspective of the cleaning woman to assuming the point of view of the blastocyst (Squier, 2015). Even as a novice comics reader, however, I was happily able to appreciate the potential of a comic to express complex, ambiguous issues and thus to be pedagogically useful in discussions of medical ethics.

If that brief discussion in *Liminal Lives* was my first real foray into comics criticism, the next ten years gave me the chance to hone those skills as I thought my way through the changing relations between the medical humanities and a new arrival, the "health humanities." I had argued in *Liminal Lives* that the foundation of the human being—biological lifespan as well as embodied self—were under reconceptualization and reconstruction in the era of contemporary biomedicine. An interdisciplinary workshop organized by neurobiologist Gillian Einstein and philosopher Margrit Shildrick in 2006 created the opportunity to expand on those thoughts. Einstein and Shildrick bracingly challenged those of us who participated to examine women's health through a "postconventional" lens, that is to imagine women's health shaped by the converging impact of postmodern philosophy and contemporary biomedical technologies. What would it mean, they asked us, to imagine a human medicine attentive to issues of race, sex, class, ability, and age?

I wrote an essay prompted by that workshop, reflecting on the abilities of the medical humanities to grasp fully the complex, ambiguous, and difficult experience of illness (Squier, 2007; Squier, 2014). Reading two comics in the not-yet-christened genre of graphic medicine, Brian Fies's newly published Eisner award-winning *Mom's Cancer* and Harvey Pekar and Joyce Brabner's *Our Cancer Year*, I considered their very different views of cancer treatment, the first within a tightly defined clinical frame and the latter within a human rights and social justice framework (Fies, 2011; Pekar and Brabner, 1994). While Fies's comic did challenge the rigid distinctions patient and doctor and between illness and health, Brabner and Pekar's comic also plumbed the links between disease, illness, and broader sociopolitical threats to human health. Despite their differences, both comics honed the analytic skills of a reader interested in deciphering the tensions they contained between images and text—but where did that leave the term *medical* humanities, I wondered. Recalling Diane Price Herndl's crucial point that a problematic exclusivity structures both disability studies and the medical humanities, I maintained that:

> whatever label we choose, . . . a strategy of continuous reframing is essential if we want to do useful work . . . we can no longer afford to limit our scholarship to one perspective.

And we can no longer get away with defining our research fields as mutually exclusive, whether we define them as medical humanities, health humanities, or disability studies.

(Squier, 2007: 347)

The following year, I had the good fortune to present a lecture in honor of one of the most remarkable women in the field of medical humanities, Joanne Trautmann Banks, first professor in Medical Humanities at the Penn State College of Medicine and a founding editor of the journal *Literature and Medicine*. Once again, an awareness of the conflicting agendas of medical humanities and disability studies drew me to the third space of comics. But Jo Banks led me there. In her essay "Life as a Literary Laboratory," she foresaw the increasing importance of images in the field of literature and medicine. Recalling W.J.T. Mitchell's concept of the "imagetext," she wrote about finding it a helpful metaphor for her experience with her son Piers, who suffered from a rare form of epilepsy. She was "led to struggle for a new way to write about her son's experience" because she was increasingly interested in finding "a space where medical treatment could take a back seat to healing social encounters," and so she turned to the arts (Squier, 2008: 138–139). When I gave the first Jo Banks Memorial Lecture at the American Society for Bioethics and Humanities (ASBH) to an audience of philosophers, physicians, and medical humanists, I drew on comics as a third space in which to articulate Banks's powerful point: that we must leave behind both the exclusively medical approach *and* the narrowly conventional cultural archive as we move into the future of the health humanities.

Several years later, I was invited to write an essay in tribute to another senior scholar in the medical humanities, the distinguished Kathryn Montgomery. There, I recalled participating in the pathbreaking summer seminar on "Case History, Narrative, and the Construction of Objectivity" that Montgomery co-led at Northwestern University's Feinberg School of Medicine.[4] There I first encountered Ann Starr's brilliant art book, *Where Babies Come From: A Miracle Explained*, whose quirky drawings and wry text seemed to me "a lively example of graphic medicine almost avant la lettre" (Squier, 2013: 34). The seminar gave me a "renewed appreciation of the way attention to my own experience could loosen and deepen my own scholarly writing" (34). In addition to a raft of readings, we were treated to a range of interdisciplinary, hands-on, collaborative pedagogical techniques: from reader's theater and city walks, to improv theater, architectural tours, and charades.

This time, the medical and health humanities shaped my approach to teaching the doctoral seminars on comics and graphic narratives I was by then offering at Penn State. I included a "studio hour" in each three-hour class meeting, during which my students would experiment with the process of making comics. Moreover, channeling the Bruno Latour essay that had been my contribution to the reading list for Montgomery's seminar, I urged students to break away from stale critique toward concern, and select a topic related to medicine, illness, or disability (their own or that of a friend) not just for the four-page comics they created in studio, but for their final seminar paper as well. I found rare, passionate engagement both in my students' comics and also (to my surprise) in their final papers for that graphic medicine seminar, fortifying my conviction that the future of the health humanities lies with its junior scholars.

Comics also offers another valuable third space for both junior and senior scholars in the medical and health humanities: collaborative writing. When Thomas Couser invited me to contribute an essay to his journal *Life Writing*, I persuaded my junior colleague Krista Quesenberry to join me, and together we wrote what we called an experiment in epistolary criticism, "Life Writing and Graphic Narratives" (Quesenberry and Squier, 2016). Although Krista was in Pennsylvania and I was in Berlin on sabbatical, as we corresponded by email during the spring, summer, and fall of 2015, we found conceptual meeting ground in the visual and verbal spaces of Alison Bechdel's *Fun Home*, Justin Green's *Binky Brown Meets the Holy Virgin Mary* (Green, 1972), the illustrations for Charlotte Perkins Gilman's *The Yellow Wall-Paper*, Riva Lehrer's stunning portrait of Eli Clare, from her series "Circle Stories," Sarah Leavitt's graphic somatography *Tangles*, Ryan Pequin's *The Walk*, and James Kochalka's *The Cute Manifesto*. Looking at these works together we were able to consider some of the concerns that both comics and life-writing share: the role of gestural and graphic authentication, the use of counterpoint to manage conflicting perspectives, and the complexities that disrupt the expected pace, arc, and forward movement in a work that takes its form from life.

Comics scholar Amelia DeFalco credits Theresa Tesuan for the term "loiterature," referring to the kind of looping, recursive movement, a wandering in and out of the frame, back to the past and forward to the future, that is produced by the specific spatial affordances of comics—panels separated by blank spaces known as gutters (DeFalco, 2015). This retrospective essay on my experiences of culture, education, and the health humanities is more a work of loiterature than it is an objective history. And yet being prompted to engage in such loiterature has been a pleasure, because it has allowed me to pay tribute to the scholars, artists, and thinkers who have joined me in the fertile third space of comics, in the health humanities.

That brings me to the third space that is graphic medicine. Given its name by physician and cartoonist Ian Williams in 2007, this diverse and ever-growing group has hosted an annual international convention since 2010. There, cartoonists and scholars, patients, publishers, and people with disabilities, caregivers and family members, nurses, physicians, and librarians, all come together to present papers, share comics, offer workshops, and explore "the interaction of comics and healthcare," as the Graphic Medicine website puts it. (Graphic Medicine also hosts a virtual third space, www.graphicmedicine.org and also has its own book series of the same name at Penn State Press, which—full disclosure—I co-edit with Ian Williams.) The intent of these conferences, as of the scholarship that has emerged from them and around them, is to broaden and deepen our understanding of medicine, to reframe it to include the perspectives of disability studies and health, and to "scale up" the concept of health so it also applies to the microbial communities within and around us, to animals and plants, and indeed to the planet itself, challenged as it is by environmental pollution and climate change. Graphic Medicine is perhaps the best example of the formal definition of a third space that I promised at the beginning of this essay. As Edward W. Soja puts it, a third space is:

> a meeting point, a hybrid place, where one can move beyond existing borders . . . a place of the marginal women and men, where old connections can be disturbed and new ones emerge . . . a precondition to building a community of resistance to all forms of hegemonic power.
>
> *(Soja, 2008: 53)*

This retrospective look encourages me to take a prospective one as well: I hope graphic medicine will continue to serve as a welcoming third space for the growth of the health humanities. I will enjoy the fireworks that result.

Notes

1 I include both the terms "comics" and "graphic medicine" throughout this article because while I have been writing about comics since at least 1993, the term Graphic Medicine came on the scene in 2007, when Ian Williams MD, physician and cartoonist, coined it to refer to comics dealing with

medicine, illness, disability and caregiving, and I did not encounter the term until 2010, when I participated in the first international Comics and Medicine conference in London. https://nihre cord.nih.gov/newsletters/2018/05_04_2018/story1.htm A more extensive definition of Graphic Medicine, as well as a glimpse at the vibrant intellectual, artistic, therapeutic, and social world the field has created, can be found at www.graphicmedicine.org.

2 In an early chapter on organ donation in *Liminal Lives*, I used a cartoon *The Times* (London) set into an article addressing the global organ donor crisis to introduce a discussion of research into tissue culture. The cartoon pictures a man in an Argyle sweater swinging, pipe in mouth, from a light fixture. Below him, a woman grasping a newspaper with the headline "Pig Heart Transplants Unsafe" explains to the man beside her: "He opted for the Monkey Heart transplant instead."

3 Since then I have written about this comic several more times, particularly in my contribution to *Graphic Medicine Manifesto* (2015) and in *Epigenetic Landscapes* (2017). What a gem it is.

4 If my memory serves me right—and it has been more than 20 years—this seminar was co-led by Kathryn Montgomery Hunter, Tod Chambers, and Delese Wear. Apologies if I have misremembered.

References

Bean, M. 18 February 1991, *The Age*. Melbourne, Australia, p. 12.

Bolling, R. (2004). Bad Blastocyst. In: R. Bolling, *Thrilling Tom the Dancing Bug Stories: A Collection of the Weekly Comic Strip "Tom the Dancing Bug"*, Kansas City, MO: Andrews McMeel: 140.

DeFalco, A. (2015). Graphic Somatography: Life Writing, Comics, and the Ethics of Care. *Journal of Medical Humanities*, 37: 223–240.

Fies, B. (2011). *Mom's Cancer*, New York: Abrams.

Green, J. (1972). *Binky Brown Meets the Holy Virgin Mary*, San Francisco: Last Gasp.

Hajdu, D. (2008). *The Ten Cent Plague: The Great Comic-Book Scare and How It Changed America*, New York: Farrar: Straus & Giroux.

Nicholson, P. 18 February 1991, *The Age*. Melbourne, Australia, p. 13.

Pekar, H. and Brabner, J. (1994). *Our Cancer Year*, Philadelphia: Running Press.

Quesenberry, K. and Squier, S.M. (2016). Life Writing and Graphic Narratives. *Life Writing*, 13(1): 63–85.

Soja, E.W. (2008). Thirdspace: Towards a New Consciousness of Space and Spatiality. In: K. Ikas and G. Wagner, eds, *Communicating in the Third Space*, New York: Routledge: 49–61.

Squier, S.M. (1993). The [Impregnable] Mother of All Battles: War, Reproduction, and Visualization Technology. *Meridian*, 12(1): 3–9.

Squier, S.M. (1994). *Babies in Bottles: Twentieth-Century Visions of Reproductive Technology*, New Brunswick, NJ: Rutgers University Press.

Squier, S.M. (2007). Beyond Nescience: The Intersectional Insights of the Health Humanities. *Perspectives in Biology and Medicine*, 50(3): 334–347.

Squier, S.M. (2008). Literature and Medicine, Future Tense: Making it Graphic. *Literature and Medicine*, 27(2): 124–152.

Squier, S.M. (2013). Case Narrative and Objectivity: Chickens and Comics: My Story about Kathryn Montgomery. *Atrium*, 11: 32–35.

Squier, S.M. (2014). Comics in the Health Humanities: A New Approach to Sex and Gender Education. In: T. Jones, D. Wear, and L.D. Friedman, eds, *Health Humanities Reader*, New Brunswick, NJ: Rutgers University Press: 226–241.

Squier, S.M. (2015). The Uses of Graphic Medicine for Engaged Scholarship. In: M.K. Czerwiec, I. Williams, I., S.M. Squier, M.J. Green, K.R. Myers and S.T. Smith, eds, *Graphic Medicine Manifesto*, University Park: Penn State Press: 41–66.

Squier, S.M. (2017). *Liminal Lives: Imagining the Human at the Frontiers of Biomedicine*, Durham, NC: Duke University Press.

Starr, A. (1997). *Where Babies Come From: A Miracle Explained*, Wellesley, VT: Printed Matter Inc.

Terry, J. (2017). *Attachments to War: Biomedical Logics and Violence in Twenty-First-Century America*, Durham: Duke University Press.

Wertham, F. (1954). *Seduction of the Innocent*. New York: Reinhart.

10

MEDICINE WITHIN HEALTH HUMANITIES

Gail Allsopp

Introduction

Medicine is a multidisciplinary specialty. Increasingly, doctors work with a wide variety of practitioners within a multidisciplinary team. As a general practitioner this includes nurses, pharmacists, paramedics, and students, among others. But, importantly, at the center of our team is the patient and their family. When we think about creativity and health, we need to ensure every member of the team is involved, not only the "medics." For years, doctors talked of medical humanities as the relationship between medicine and the arts. This term originated in the United States in the 1960s (Evans and Greaves, 2010) and has grown from strength to strength. Why, though, do we limit creative approaches to health to medical humanities? Working as we increasingly do, in teams, we should no longer isolate our colleagues and our patients from our medicine–art interface, but instead celebrate the involvement of us all, together as a team. For this reason, medical humanities should not stand alone, but instead integrate itself within the inclusive umbrella of health humanities.

There are a variety of ways of using a creative approach within medicine, in health care, and with our teams. Many, as I describe below, we may do without thinking, without adding the label of medical or health humanities. Some activities we have observed others performing during our career and simply follow due to its success, some we take from our family lives, some develop spontaneously with the patient in front of you. The outcome is the same. There is joy when using creativity within our clinical practice and the evidence of benefit is overwhelming: not only for our patients and our team, but also for ourselves.

In this chapter I offer some reflections on the value of integrating a creative, humanities-based practice into patient care, the care of our colleagues, and of ourselves. This is based on my own reflective practice as a primary care physician. Whether you are a health professional or find yourself informally caring for others in a health setting, why not try some for yourself?

Creative practice with patients

If you have never knowingly used a creative approach with patients, start simply. During a consultation, use diagrams to explain a diagnosis, give written information to expand a consultation, or record consultations to allow the patient to listen again. These are all practical yet creative approaches that can be included under the "medical" or "health humanities" banner.

Build on each consultation by trying different or new techniques. Different approaches will elicit differing responses depending on the patient in front of you. Trial and error will allow you to develop your own style and toolbox of creative techniques. However, it is important to remember that creativity should always add to the consultation, not distract from the health issue presenting to you.

Children

Video

With an unwell child who is distressed due to illness, or is frightened of the doctor's office, consider using visual arts, such as video, to calm and distract. You might use your own computer screen, tablet, or smartphone, or ask the guardian to use theirs. Playing the child's favorite cartoon while you talk to the parents or try to stealthily examine the back of the child's chest can be a successful tactic as well.

Puppets

We do not need to have pre-prepared equipment or be a drama therapist to use puppetry to engage with a child. Be spontaneous: draw a face on the end of the throat spatula. One side happy, one side sad. Use the spatula to talk to the child. Allow the child to hold it and show you if they are happy or sad, or to talk to you "through" the puppet.

Or try blowing up a non-latex examination glove. Decorate it with a happy face, using the blown-up fingers as its hair. Allow the child to play with it as a "balloon" while you examine them. Anyone working with children knows distraction works, and these simple approaches cost little and have no infection control risk as we can dispose of them once our examination is complete.

Role-play

A seven-year-old patient who had been diagnosed with epilepsy required long-term medication. He refused, despite his mother trying every day, and his fits continued. Using role-play and imagination to explore his illness with him, the boy decided that inside his brain there was a battle occurring: a battle that needed a tank to win and restore the peace. Using visualization led by the mother, he accepted that the tank was out of petrol and needed refilling twice a day to keep the peace. The petrol? That was the carbamazepine that he had refused to take. The medicine that did not taste very nice, in his mind, became the petrol that the tank needed. Through visualization, he learnt that the only way to win the battle was to refuel the tank twice a day, so the child started to take his medication—a simple creative approach that cost nothing and made a meaningful difference to this boy, his epilepsy control, and his mother's happiness (as his carer).

Memory boxes

Used extensively in the hospice movement, pediatrics, and primary care, memory boxes come in many forms. Memory boxes generally involve the creation of a physical "box" of items (memories) that can be accessed in the longer term, once the relative or friend has died. Pictures, photographs, letters, trinkets, or jewelry belonging to the person are traditionally included. Taking it one step further to encourage the use of all of our senses to access memories is important, rather than relying on touch and sight alone. Including perfume or favorite creams so that the smell of a person (that sometimes can be lost through the passage of time) can be accessed. Making copies of their favorite music, or writing lists of their favorite foods (to include aural and taste sensations), can also benefit some relatives.

Encouraging all patients to create memory boxes, irrespective of their age, can be useful. They can be as important for a man married who loses his spouse of 50 years as they are for a child who loses a parent.

Adults

Visualization

A woman in her early forties who developed breast cancer asked for advice after a lengthy oncology appointment. Her breast cancer treatment was to include chemotherapy but she was too frightened of the potential side effects and had refused the treatment. After discussing the benefits and risks, we used visualization to try and look at the chemotherapy in a different way. She eventually decided she would have the treatment, but that every time they gave her chemotherapy, she would visualize a positive golden-colored concoction, full of goodness, flowing into her veins and throughout her body. This helped her complete the treatment as oncology had advised, while coping very well.

This type of visualization, using any variety of visual images that are meaningful for an individual patient, can be used with anyone undergoing chemotherapy or invasive treatment. It is essential to honestly discuss the positive and potential negatives of treatment. However, using guided visualization techniques can help with the anticipatory fear, prior to starting treatment, even if they then go on to have significant side effects during the treatment itself.

Laughter

Fitting contraceptive coils involves an intimate examination and many women are anxious during the procedure. Using gentle humor eases their anxiety, but more significant than that, when inserting the coil through the internal cervical os, there is often muscle spasm of the cervix. You can push hard, hurt the patient, and risk a false passage into the womb, or sit patiently and wait for the cervix to relax and open up. Anecdotally, I have found that telling jokes and making the women laugh speeds up the process of opening up the cervix. This may be distraction, endorphin release, or luck, but adding laughter to the procedure makes it easier for both the patient and the operator. Laughter is proven to release endorphins and may reduce pain in some circumstances (Dunbar et al., 2011). An unconventional creative approach perhaps, but one that works well.

Distraction

Operative procedures under local anesthetic, or even simple interventions such as taking blood, can be stressful for patients. To ease the stress and improve the patient experience creative approaches can be used. A choice of music to listen to while undergoing the treatment or using videos while you complete the procedure can help. This distraction is not limited to children, although is more often used with them. How many times have you sat in the dental chair and wished for something other than the sound of the drill to concentrate on? As adults, we need creative approaches and distraction just as much as our children do. It is easy to make simple changes in the clinical setting.

For example, a challenging procedure to fit a subcutaneous contraceptive implant into the arm of a 21-year-old girl with learning difficulties was requested. Looking for a creative approach to her care, discovering her love for the film *The Greatest Showman* and her passion for singing as loud as she could, at the top of her voice, the approach to inserting the implant became clear. The creative procedure went as follows:

- Using a local anesthetic cream to reduce any pain. Drawing a happy face on the dressing, to ensure she did not try and take it off. Convincing her the face was there to keep her arm pain-free and safe.
- Playing *The Greatest Showman* soundtrack as she first walked into a familiar room and throughout the procedure.
- While inserting the implant, encouraging her and everyone else in the room to sing along, as loud as they could.

By the time the first track had ended, the implant was inserted and a bandage firmly in place. The look on her mother's face said it all. Her daughter, who was usually so difficult in medical environments, had managed to have a local anesthetic procedure performed in primary care with a happy smile on her face throughout. Simply by using a creative approach to the procedure, capturing the creativity that was right for her, enabled success.

Environment

Why should only children's hospitals be bright and funky? As adults we still seek stimulation of art and theatre. We still have as many fears as children do, but are simply better at hiding them. Next time you walk into your consultation room, try and see it again for the first time. If you were anxious or unwell, would it be welcoming? Could you change anything? Simple creative changes like a poster on a ceiling to look at while lying down to be examined can help improve the patient experience.

In nursing homes

Increasingly, we are living longer. Our life expectancy is increasing, but not always the quality of that life. There is a large elderly population who live in nursing, care, or residential homes and the number over the age of 65 requiring care is expected to increase by 25% by 2025 (Guzman-Castillo et al., 2017); many of these individuals have dementia. Medical professionals are increasingly discouraged from prescribing sedating medication for this population, but instead to look at behavioral approaches to care and more creative approaches.

For example, art, music, and dance are increasingly being used to entertain, stimulate, and enhance the quality of the lives of this population—led not by therapists, but by the staff themselves. Nurseries are being set up in nursing homes across the United Kingdom to bring the old and young populations together for the benefit of both, using play to stimulate young and old minds alike. These are all creative and patient-centered approaches to care.

In death

We are all encouraged to talk to our own relatives and our patients when they are dying, with the belief that hearing is the last sense to leave us. As a general practitioner, when visiting patients in their last days of life, even if there is no family present and the patient is alone, there is usually a radio or TV playing in the background. However, it is important to think very carefully about this music, this "background" noise.

Imagine yourself lying drifting in and out of consciousness and you can hear your favorite band or style of music playing, comforting you. Imagine then a different scenario, that instead of *your* favorite music, it is the carer's or the family's favorite. How do you feel when someone of a different generation is playing their favorite artist, opera, or musical theatre? Do you like every type of music or does some irritate you? What about the volume of the music? Or do you prefer silence?

Using music to soothe and comfort is a standard creative approach in the last days and hours of life. However, we need to make sure it is the right music for that individual. This is something we must consider adding to our end-of-life discussions with patients. We ask about after-death plans, with many patients many choosing music for their own funerals, but it is equally important that we can choose the background music, or silence, to accompany our death in the clinical setting and in our own homes, to ensure that the aim of comforting is achieved, with no distress arising from the well-intentioned creativity.

In teaching

General practice is a "cradle to the grave" specialty, including patients of all ages. Indeed, Jaques' "seven ages of man" speech from Shakespeare's *As You Like It* (see Shakespeare, 1989) describes this variety perfectly:

> All the world's a stage,
> And all the men and women merely players;
> They have their exits and their entrances,
> And one man in his time plays many parts,
> His acts being seven ages . . .
> *(Act II, Sc. 7)*

This brief and poetic speech is freely available online, and can be used in many ways when teaching: with those considering a career in primary care to showcase the variety, or when thinking about continuity of care or lifelong relationships with patients, and the increasing and expanding aging population. Discussions surrounding dementia, disability, euthanasia, and death can all start from this one extract of Shakespeare. Using creativity in teaching enables a different approach to thinking and learning that, alongside standard health-care training, should be encouraged.

With our teams and for ourselves

We must never forget that, as caregivers, we also need healing, care, and support. I believe that the health humanities can give us that, especially in primary care, where clinicians can be isolated. The environment in which we work, the decoration, view, and noise level, will all affect how we feel. With the rapid turnover of patients (every ten minutes in the United Kingdom), and the increasing complexity of presentations, it is helpful between patients to create space for oneself. A moment of silence, a favorite picture, a poster on the wall to lose oneself in for a moment, or background music can all aid our resilience by clearing our mind to be ready for the next challenge, or the next patient encounter. Caring for the carer is as important as caring for the patient, and using creativity can help us as much as it can help our patients.

Conclusion

Medicine is both an art and a science. This chapter has given a brief overview of some ways in which we can use creativity within our practice, but doctors are not the only ones influencing patients. Our approach in medicine is increasingly multidisciplinary, just as our creativity should be.

As a primary care physician that regularly integrates creative practices into my health-care work, I see "health humanities" as an inclusive term, ensuring our patients and teams are all involved. Medical humanities, by contrast, is decidedly less so. It feels exclusive. It does not encourage nurses, paramedics, patients, or carers to be involved. The title sounds like a club that only the medical elite can belong to. There is a place for medical humanities, of course. Doctors will always want to work alongside other doctors, but since we are now all working in bigger and better multidisciplinary teams, it is essential that the whole of our team are included, feel invited, and want to belong. I therefore propose that the medical humanities remain as a strong and worthwhile discipline, but as a subheading under the bright, inclusive, and multidisciplinary umbrella of health humanities itself.

References

Dunbar, R.I., Baron, R., Frangou, A., Pearce, E., van Leeuwen, E.J., Stow, J., Partridge, G., MacDonald, I., Barra, V. and van Vugt, M. (2011). Social Laughter is Correlated with an Elevated Pain Threshold. Proceedings of the Royal Society. *Biological Sciences*, 279(1731): 1161–1167.

Evans, H. and Greaves, D. (2010). 10 Years of Medical Humanities: A Decade in the Life of a Journal and a Discipline. *Medical Humanities*, 36(2): 66–68.

Guzman-Castillo, M., Ahmadi-Abhari, S., Bandosz, P., Capewell, S., Steptoe, A., Singh-Manoux, A., Kivimaki, M., Shipley, M.J., Brunner, E.J. and O'Flaherty, M. (2017). Forecasted Trends in Disability and Life Expectancy in England and Wales up to 2025: A Modelling Study. *The Lancet Public Health*, 2(7): PE 307–E 313.

Shakespeare W. (1989). *The Illustrated Stratford Shakespeare*. 7th Edition. London: Chancellor Press: 224–225.

11

A HEALTH HUMANITIES SUBLIME

Bradley Lewis

Introduction

Mr. Ramsay, stumbling along a passage one dark morning, stretched his arms out, but Mrs. Ramsay having died rather suddenly the night before, his arms, though stretched out, remained empty.

Virginia Woolf, To the Lighthouse *(1927: 128)*

Joining with Mr. Ramsay through this passage in *To the Lighthouse*, we engage our finitude, and those of our loved ones, with the solace of aesthetic companionship. In short, we participate in what aesthetic theorists call "the sublime": an experiential response to overwhelming phenomena in art or nature that puts our worldly, everyday life in greater perspective and context. This chapter invites us to further explore the sublime as a conceptual touchstone for the emerging field of health humanities. As a field, health humanities shifts the focus of medical humanities from critical and/or narrative work to the companion work of construction and integration. Health humanities creates new ways of being with our suffering and our bodily and mental differences, by breaking down the segregation of "clinicians," "patients," and "caregivers" to build integrated spaces for mutual recovery and transformative cares of the self. The sublime is relevant to all these moves. Within this field it is a relatively unexplored resource for imagining and being with our morbidity and our mortality, and its usefulness cuts across health-care identity formation. Anyone can benefit from the transformative potentials of the sublime. To get a feel for how this is possible, let us work through some contemporary uses of the sublime.

Contemporary sublime

The "sublime" is an aesthetic term that dates back to the classical period and forward to current times (Lewis, 2018). We can get a synchronic slice of its contemporary use by look-ing at a recent Tate Modern wall description. The Tate tells us that, although the term is "much contested," the sublime denotes "an exalted state of mind, or an overwhelming response to art or nature that goes beyond everyday experience"; the sublime further expresses "formlessness, immensity, intense light or darkness, terror, solitude and silence," all of which can be overpowering and even traumatic (Tate Gallery, 2014). But, surprisingly, rather than overwhelm us or traumatize us, the sublime offers us "the solace of transcendence, an art in which one could lose oneself" (Tate Gallery, 2014). The sublime, then, is a two-step response to art or nature. In step one, the sublime overwhelms us. It brings us to a deep awareness of our vulnerability and our finitude. In step two, rather than leave us traumatized, it leaves us in state of deeper wisdom, peace, and contemplation.

Virginia Woolf's *To the Lighthouse* (1927) is a good place to begin an exploration of how the sublime has been mobilized by the arts of the past century. In a key scene, Mrs. Ramsay, the lead character, pauses at the end of the day to sit alone in the dark, quietly, and to let "life sink down for a moment" while she contemplates the lighthouse in the distance. She finds herself taken out of her attachments, away from "the fret, the hurry, the stir," "all the being and the doing," by the power of the regular, persistent, yet pitiless, remorseless long steady stroke of the lighthouse (62). Mrs. Ramsay's being is engulfed by this power, which reminds her, by the relentlessness of its sweep, that her existence in life is finite: "It will end, it will end," she realizes in a moment of clarity (63). She goes on to imagine her death in a kind of reverie, where the "stroke" of the lighthouse multiplies in meaning to become "her stroke," a deathly bursting of the "sealed vessels in her brain," and at the same time a loving stroke of "silver fingers" (65). As a sublime moment, however, the experience does not end in anguish or despair, but leaves her—and potentially the reader as well—in a deep feeling of "peace," "rest," "eternity," "delight," and "ecstasy" (62–65).

For Woolf, and writers of similar sensibility, the artistic sublime is an ethopoietic creation— that is, constructed by an author for a reader who makes an ethical choice to join with the author in embracing and co-constructing the experience. As D.T. O'Hara explains, the sublime for Woolf,

> is the work of reader or listener, the spectator, who projects his or her own receptivity (or 'echoing') into the visions of the creator and then assumes the position of, identifies with, the creator, in proud flight, hovering and soaring at will.
>
> *(O'Hara, 2015: 3)*

The ironic awareness of the constructed nature of the experience does not cancel out the consolation any more than awareness of the constructed nature of my apartment cancels out its protection from the rain and cold. The sublime, in this dance of perspectives, construction, and consolation, is a creative act inspired by active engagement with the imagination of great souls (as Longinus, the ancient Roman theorist of the sublime, might put it).

One can feel a similar ironic wink and a nod combined with the deepest of sublime art in blues guitarist Blind Willie Johnson's *Dark was the Night, Cold was the Ground* (1927). The ironic side comes out in the title, which quickly takes us to the first step of the sublime two-step, with its reference to death, burial, and crucifixion held at the same time in a kind of tongue and cheek. But, once the music begins, Johnson's playfulness is also deeply serious as he takes us into the heart of a sublime transformation. Johnson's *Dark was the Night, Cold was the Ground* follows on the legacy of slave songs that W.E.B. Du Bois calls, alternately, the "sorrow songs" and the "Jubilee songs"—sorrow because "the music of an unhappy people, of the children of disappointment: they tell of death and suffering"; jubilee because, at the same time, the songs represent an "unvoiced longing toward a truer world, of misty wanderings and hidden ways" (Du Bois, 1999: 157). Du Bois's perspective on this paradoxical combination can be seen as "the perfect metaphor the sublime" (Hubbard, 2003: 313), and Johnson's *Dark was the Night, Cold was the Ground*, a blues version of the sorrow song legacy, achieves an ethopoietic sublime consolation worthy of Ry Cooder's highest praise: "the most transcendent piece in all American music" (Obrecht, 2015: 111).

Eighty years later, Mark Doty's autographical poem, "Theory of the Sublime" (2006), brings out similar themes as Doty finds himself transported via "passage ways into the sublime" while visiting Gaudi's sublime and unfinished cathedral, the Sagrada Família. Through human "agency of metaphor" and the "made things" of art, the cathedral helped Doty create an experience of "wonder and fury" at the "strangeness and beauty of the world" and the "brevity of our tenure in it" (Doty, 2006: 16–17). Doty's memoir, *Heaven's Coast* (1997), articulates how such sublime passageways are not only aesthetic experiences, but also potentially deeply therapeutic. Doty tells the story of his grief after his lover, Wally, died from AIDS-related illness. During Wally's illness, Doty lived in dread and tension, with his life closing in around him, but after Wally died his "perception began to open again" and he found himself in some "vague lunar place, a winter shore lit only by starlight" in a kind of "porous state" in the mists of a "flux of change" (ix). Doty asks himself and the reader, "What is healing, but a shift in perspective?" and his memoir links the shifting perspective of grief with the shifting perspective of the sublime (ix). After Wally's death Doty spends his time recovering through long meditative walks along Provincetown beaches with his two dogs. But far from escaping the terror of impermanence and loss, the walks bring Doty face to face with the "cold dark deep and absolutely clear" reality of death and dying through a chain of encounters with mortally wounded seals stranded on the beach (22).

Doty, in his meditations, turns the seals into metaphors for sublime travelers "between worlds"—the material world of individual vulnerability (step one) and the oceanic world of fluid merger and peace (step two). In Doty's grieving, healing, sublime state of mind a wounded seal entering the water and a dying seal entering death become intertwined:

> A body that was wounded sits stranded, incapacitated. Gone into another element, that same being takes gorgeous, ready flight. I am filled, entirely, with the image of my wounded lover leaping from his body, blossoming into some welcoming other realm. Is it that I am in that porous state of grief, a heated psychic condition in which everything becomes metaphor?
>
> Or does the world consent, in some fashion, to offer me the particular image which imagination requires?
>
> *(Doty, 2006: 25)*

Consistent with the ironic sincerity of Woolf and Johnson, Doty keeps both questions, and therefore both elements—metaphor and the real world—alive. His metaphorical comparisons of seals above and below the water, of herons on the ground and in the air, with Wally's movement in and out of life is both sublime metaphor and consolation.

Doty knows that he is turning the seals into metaphor to help scaffold his healing transformation and that this does not really put him in control. "Make all the meaning you want, Death says, shape it how you will. Open the limits of your thinking or feeling, make room for me, accommodate how you will, nothing touches the plain truth of me" (36). For Doty, no matter how we respond, we are ultimately not able to dominate the other of death. "Hold your grief, release it, come to terms or don't—nothing touches the fact of the lifeless body" (36). And, yet, the creative aesthetic experience of the sublime two-step, from terror to consolation, and its link with healing and grief is no less meaningful for its limitations. When Doty comes back to this very same beach to scatter Wally's ashes, his mind returns to the consoling metaphors he inhabited there. Releasing the ashes,

I cried harder than I had for weeks, thinking of letting go this portion of the evidence of him. Whatever I think ashes are, the notion of flinging them into the blue and white emptiness of that place made me weep all the way from the depths of myself, sobbing from the bottom of my lungs, from some place inside the body light never reaches.

And out on the shore that day, the seals were swimming—the first I'd seen alive and unthreatened for weeks, and the last I would see that season. They were watching me and the dogs, floating there in their untouchable pack, beautiful faces looking back at me from the other world, which I was not allowed to reach.

(Doty, 2006: 36)

Lars von Trier's *Melancholia*

For a final example, Lars von Trier's film *Melancholia* (2011) develops the possible sublime intertwining of terror, consolation, and playful irony in a particularly imaginative way. The film begins with a preview of its ending—a rogue planet, "Melancholia," crashing into Earth to the sound of Wagner's prelude to *Tristan und Isolde*. In between, two sisters, Justine and Claire, go through alternating psychic crisis. In the first half of the film, Justine (played by Kirsten Dunst) descends into deep despair after her attempt at a normative marriage fails on the very night of the wedding. Justine revives in the second half of the film, paradoxically rebalanced and transformed by Melancholia's disruption of normative life. But her sister Claire (Charlotte Gainsbourg) goes in the opposite direction. Remarkably functional in everyday social life during the first half of the film, Claire becomes wracked by anxiety and terror as Melancholia approaches and life on earth is about to end. Von Trier seems to side with Justine and Wagner in this case, constructing the film such that the audience's affective response is less that of Claire's normative reaction and closer to Justine's sublime two-step—terror followed by consolation and peace (French and Shacklock, 2014). As film critic J. Hoberman put it, after leaving a Cannes screening, he felt not terror or melancholy but "light, rejuvenated and unconsciously happy" (Hoberman, 2011).

The sublime experience that von Trier gives us through the character of Justine is contrasted not only with Claire, but also with John, Claire's husband, and his attempt to control the situation and the experience through rational dominion. John feels the terror of the situation, but he transforms the experience through calm control. He pays close attention to scientific reports, he charts the course of Melancholia through telescopic observation, and he plans provisions and technological fixes. John feels himself superior in his reaction and adopts a condescendingly patriarchal relation to Claire and Justine. But when it turns out that Melancholia is too destructive for rational control, he is even worse off than Claire. His only "controlling" recourse at that point is to impulsively abandon his family and swallow a bottle of pills rather witness the apocalyptic denouement.

Justine, by contrast, uses her aesthetic understanding to bring consolation not only to herself, but to her family as well. With Claire and Claire's son, Leo, Justine helps her family create a "magic cave" in which they may seek shelter and solace as the end arrives. The magic cave, like von Trier's film, does not deny the limits of human control or the inevitability of human destruction. Rather it takes this knowledge into aesthetic creation of a sublime merger with the world beyond our temporary egos. As the rogue planet comes thundering into earth, the small family of characters and we, the viewers, are not alone. Through von Trier's creation we too have a magic cave in which we can hold hands together in our joint understanding of the human condition. As French and Schacklock point out in their analysis of the film's affective impact:

> At the peak of [its] visual and sonic assault the film cuts to black and the sound-track to silence, leaving the spectator with a transitory void characterized by the stopping of time and cessation of movement. It is a genuinely sublime moment of affective intensity that ... inevitably spills over into the spectator's life and reson-ates beyond the cinematic experience.
>
> *(French and Shacklock, 2014: 355)*

In the words of Jean-Luc Nancy and quoted by French and Shacklock, the sublime is "not so much what we're going back to as where we're coming from" (355).

The sublime as health humanities resource

These few examples provide a glimpse into the transformative power of the contemporary sublime. Looking to the specific case of health humanities, this capacity deserves greater con-sideration because human transformation is at the heart of healing: yet we have limited resources for human transformation. Other resources include medication, surgery, psychother-apy, mourning, and spiritual practice—but that list is noticeably short and some of those very methods have extensive side effects. This means that harnessing the sublime as a health humanities resource for self and mutual transformation is an invaluable theoretical and perhaps practical opportunity as well. Doing so adds to our limited list of transformative tools, and, fortuitously, its side effects are largely positive (it creates a more aesthetic world to live in).

To see an example of what happens when we do not do this kind of transformative work, it is instructive to compare *Melancholia* with Margaret Edson's *Wit* (1999). There is a deep similarity between John's reaction to the rogue planet and Dr. Kelekian's reaction to Professor Bearing's cancer. Kelekian responds to Bearing's stage IV ovarian cancer (which has a very low survival rate) with aggressive, rational control and experimental treatments. His biomedical attempt to dominate the cancer and its terror condescendingly dominates Bearing and her own aesthetically informed experience of death and dying (she is a scholar of John Donne, a seventeenth-century poet renowned for his meditations on mortality). When the treatment inevitably fails, Kelekian, like John in *Melancholia*, also has no resources left but panic and flight. Kelekian impulsively goes against the standards of care to order (in fact command) a morphine drip for Bearing. The drip is, in effect, an unconsented medical euthanasia in the face of Kelekian's inability to be with the realities of human vulnerability, impermanence, morbidity, and mortality.

But Kelekian's fear is not unusual in health-care settings. Indeed, it is hardly just clin-icians who must work through these kinds of reactions. By developing health humanities' understanding of sublime practices we might provide resources to help inoculate, treat, and palliate these kinds of understandably terrified reactions to our human vulnerabilities and finitude. Of course, a health humanities sublime will not resonate for everyone and it should not be our only resource. However, the arts of the sublime do have a power and potential to reach people in ways that the other resources do not; they show how powerful the arts can be in the service of human transformation. As a conceptual touchstone for health humanities, the sublime opens up a wealth of aesthetic resources that can be used as tools for life, illness, and death in the medical world and beyond. This realization is at the heart of emerging health humanities work.

References

Doty, M. (1997). *Heaven's Coast: A Memoir*. New York: Harper Collins.

Doty, M. (2006). "Theory of the Sublime" and "The Poet on the Poem." *American Poetry Review*, 35 (6): 16–17.

Du Bois, W.E.B. (1999). The Souls of Black Folk. In H.L. Gates and T.H. Oliver, eds, *The Souls of Black Folk: A Norton Critical Edition*. New York: W.W. Norton and Company: 1–167.

Edson, M. (1999). *Wit*. New York: Faber & Faber.

French, S and Shacklock, Z. (2014). "The Affective Sublime in Lars von Trier's *Melancholia* and Terrence Malick's." *The Tree of Life. New Review of Film and Television Studies*, 12 (4): 339–356.

Tate Gallery. (2014). Wall Text, *Transformed Visions: Abstraction and the Sublime*. London, UK: Tate Modern, London.

Hoberman, J. (2011, Nov 9). Not with a Whimper But a Bang: The End Times of *Melancholia*. *Village Voice*. Retrieved from www.villagevoice.com/2011/11/09/not-with-a-whimper-but-a-bang-the-end-times-of-melancholia/(Accessed 18/2/2019).

Hubbard, D. (2003). W.E.B. Du Bois and the invention of the sublime. In D. Hubbard, ed, *Souls of Black Folk One Hundred Years Later*. Minneapolis: University of Missouri Press: 298–321.

Johnson, Blind Willie. (1927). Dark Was the Night, Cold Was the Ground. *Dark was the night, Cold was the Ground*. Columbia Records, track 1.

Lewis, B. (2018). "A Medical Sublime". *Journal of Medical Humanities*. https://doi.org/10.1007/s10912-018-9536-y.

O'Hara, D. T. (2015). *Virginia Woolf and the Modern Sublime*. New York: Palgrave Macmillan.

Obrecht, J. (2015). *Early Blues*. St Paul: University of Minnesota Press.

von Trier, L. (2012). *Melancholia*. Magnolia Home Entertainment.

Woolf, V. (1927). *To the Lighthouse*. San Diego: Harcourt Brace & Company.

12

VISUALIZING WITHIN HEALTH-CARE PRACTICE

Colin Macduff

Introduction

The act of sense making is a central practice of health humanities. Writing in their foundational text in 2015, Crawford et al. draw on the work of Bruner (1990) and Stetler (2010) to advance the idea that meaning is dynamic and formed in situated action. Having worked as a nurse, health researcher, and educator for almost 40 years, this idea resonates with my own experiences. As a novice nurse in practice, meaning for me came primarily from situated interaction with those in need of health care and their families/friends and other colleagues involved in providing that care. Consideration of particular contexts and actions through the lens of wider knowledge from a range of disciplines developed over time, and helped build further understandings of what was going on for whom and why.

Thus the scholarship of others was and is vital in helping to create ongoing meaningful dialogue with practice experiences. This wider knowledge typically comes in the form of words and images, which can themselves influence ways of seeing, thinking, and acting. This is important for health-care provision because the three related practices of observation, imagination, and identification remain as crucial to high-quality nursing now as they were when highlighted by Florence Nightingale over 150 years ago (Macduff, 2017). Writing of nursing in her seminal 1860 text *Notes on Nursing*, Nightingale declares "there is nothing in the world, except perhaps education, so much the reverse of prosaic—or which requires so much power of throwing yourself into others' feelings which you have never felt" (Nightingale, 1860: 196). Good nursing requires not only observation and listening skills to try to apprehend at least some of what a person's feelings may be, but also a prospective act of imagination to seek to understand some of what this may mean for that person in context. This sense making requires more than the five senses, and this is particularly the case when nurses and other health-care professionals are dealing with aspects that are not necessarily directly visible or tangible (e.g., feelings of anxiety or the threat of invisible pathogens).

Accordingly, the role of imagination and what may influence it becomes a very relevant consideration for health-care practice and provision, and thereby for health humanities. As a full exploration of this is beyond the scope of this chapter, my particular focus here will be on how visual aspects of imagination may be relevant to health-care practice and research, within the broader domain of individual and collective visualization processes.

Individual and collective visualizing

According to *Oxford English Dictionary*, the term "imagination" stems from the Latin verb *imaginare*, to "picture to oneself," a visualizing aspect prominent in its formal definition as "the faculty or action of forming new ideas, or images or concepts of external objects not present to the senses" (Oxford English Dictionary, 2018). In layman's terms this aspect is known as *the mind's eye*, and Pearson et al.'s (2013) psychology-based review suggests that such image generation is built using the scaffolding of previously related, memorized perceptual information. Applied to health-care experiences, this raises the question of what influences the individual practitioner's (or patient's) mind's eye when envisaging a phenomenon. In turn this raises the linked matter of the relevance of externalized visual representations of the phenomenon produced to inform collective understandings and actions.

Visualizing the invisible

These questions have been a particular focus for my research in recent years. In my previous experiences as a nurse in clinical practice, I was usually aware at some level (conscious or liminally) of how relatively clean or dirty my hands were, even though no dirt might be visible. When later I was drawn into researching the efficacy of education to prevent and control health-care-associated infections (HAIs), I came to reflect on this in more depth. In discussions with other nursing colleagues it seemed that not everyone shared my internal gauge; one particularly respected colleague declared that nurses don't wash their hands when they don't see the dirt, because "seeing is believing." This led to my exploration of the extent to which practitioners actively envisage the invisible pathogens that cause HAIs and, in time, this became a foundational question within the Arts and Humanities Research Council (AHRC) and Scottish Funding Council-funded "Visualising the Invisible" (Visinvis) research study (Macduff et al., 2013).

While addressing this question through the lens of psychology may have been feasible, I was drawn more to the possibilities of combining health service research knowledge (nursing and microbiology) with approaches from the wider humanities, specifically art and design. In this way Sullivan's "Dimensions of Visualisation Framework" (from *Art Practice as Research*; Sullivan, 2005) informed our methods of elicitation, and our adaptation of his framework is summarized in Figure 12.1.

Starting from the right-hand panel, lower left quadrant, enlarged photographic images of a clinical setting were used to help us elicit 12 participants' perceptions of their role in context, pathogen risk points, and the extent to which pathogens were already envisioned *in situ* (left-hand, upper quadrant). Recorded dialogue continued during an activity where participants were asked to choose from a range of materials to create a representation of pathogens (right-hand, upper quadrant). This process built cumulative understandings of the conceptions of this mixed group (right-hand, lower quadrant), which comprised four nursing staff, five domestic services staff, two patient-focused public representatives, and one construction design management coordinator.

Data analysis showed that few participants reported actively visualizing pathogens in their mind's eye in clinical contexts. However, the study elicited mental images of pathogens from all participants, and all were able to create related models during the making activity. The attributes of these images and the models were manifold, covering aspects of dimension, color, texture, smell, emotion, and movement. Key referents included small animals and microbiological depictions.

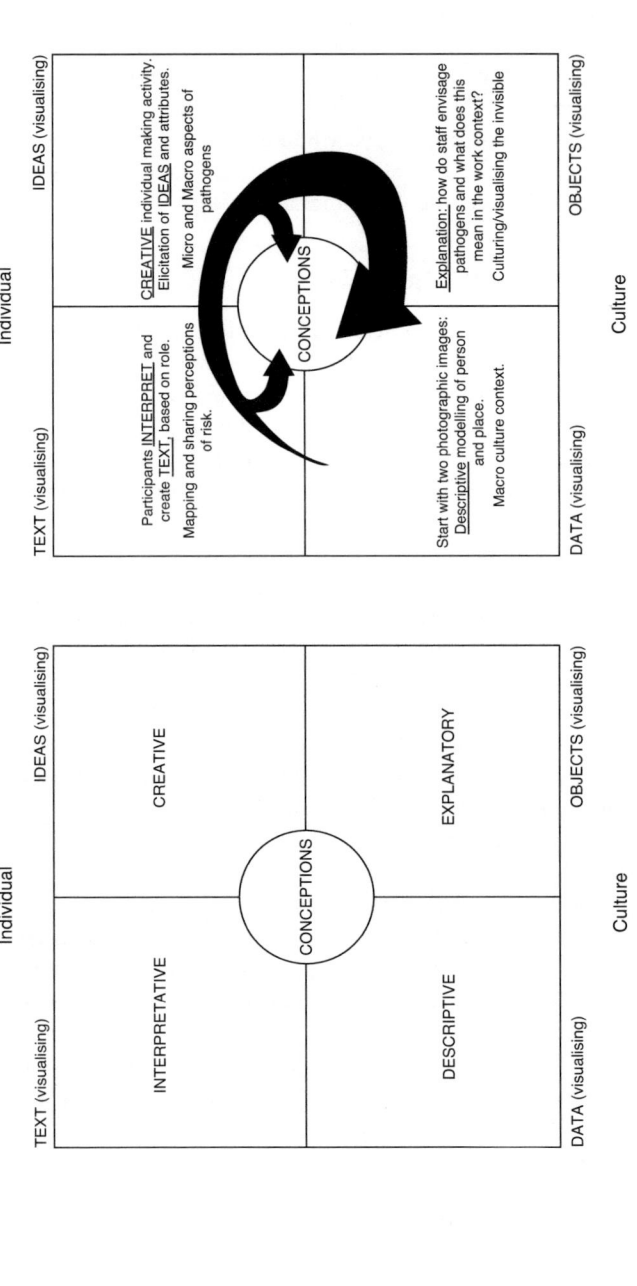

Figure 12.1 Study design based on dimensions of visualization
(adapted from Sullivan, 2005)

In this way some useful insights into individuals' envisagings, and what influenced these, were elicited. These findings, along with a related collaborative exploration of the meaningfulness of current ways of visually representing pathogens, then informed the design team members' development of a suite of three prototype digital visualizations, created to help health-care workers to visualize pathogens more dynamically in medical and surgical ward settings.

This suite of prototype visuals was then shown at a national health-care conference where they were reviewed and evaluated by almost 200 health-care professionals from varied backgrounds. For each prototype feedback was obtained regarding what these visuals could be used for, where they could best be deployed, and who would find this most meaningful and appropriate. All prototypes were seen to have substantive common strengths, but some nuanced differentiation of purpose and application was also usefully elicited (e.g., in relation to use in clinical or classroom environments).

To our knowledge this was the first study to explore internal and external aspects of visualization for HAIs in this way. However, the importance of internal images, in the form of mental models, has more recently been posited by leaders in the infection prevention and control field (Sax and Clack, 2015). Clearly, there is need and scope for further research.

VisionOn

Our own follow-up work, VisionOn (see Macdonald et al., 2017), has involved the development and evaluation of a prototype training tablet app for hospital staff, using interactive contextualized visuals rather than standard visualization of data via graphs, charts, and dashboards. To demonstrate different pathogen behavior, dynamic visualizations of norovirus (*Clostridium difficile*) and MRSA (methicillin-resistant *Staphylococcus aureus*) were developed in relation to location, survival, and transmission within a virtual hospital ward model using evidence-based microbiological and staff behavioral data. The three-stage iterative co-design and evaluation process involved a mixed sample of UK National Health Service (NHS) staff (doctors, nurses, and domestic services staff; $n = 150$).

Participants reported improved awareness and understanding of the pathogens responsible for HAI. They also gave feedback on the types of information relevant for different staff cohorts, and on which aspects of the visualizations worked well or were prone to cause misunderstandings, and provided suggestions for further development and improvement. Overall the tool appeared to offer staff a new perspective on these invisible pathogens by being able to "see" them newly contextualized in the virtual ward, thus making them seem more real.

As such the study suggests the possible value of a tool designed with active practitioner involvement to produce meaningful shared visualizations. In the process a number of conceptual and practical visualization challenges were identified, such as the tension between "realistic" visual rendering and the need to minimize the "clutter" of a typical ward environment so as to foreground key information (Macdonald et al., 2017). The VisionOn and Visinvis studies are also notable for including cleaning staff as key participants—crucial stakeholders that many studies, including those within health humanities (Crawford et al., 2015), tend to neglect. As we have noted previously (Macduff et al., 2013), the low status that society ascribes to domestic work makes cleaners almost as invisible as the pathogens that they work to control.

Other participatory approaches

Crawford et al. (2015) argue that "one important role of the arts and humanities in healthcare is to dramatically expand the scope of the social negotiations and verbal and visual narratives available as we make sense of health and illness" (6). Within the two linked research studies outlined above, it can be seen that combining arts and design approaches with those from nursing and microbiology can help to open up a topic. Importantly, this starts and continues by eliciting and incorporating the perspectives of health service workers themselves. One widely used approach that aspires to such inclusion is the "value stream mapping" aspect of Lean Kaizen quality improvement exercises, where a visual tool or template is typically used with staff to help generate collective visual representations of health-care delivery systems and processes. However, in my own experiences of being asked to take part in such exercises within clinical practice, scope for creativity and questioning was very much limited by the over-riding corporate agenda of achieving efficiencies. As such, the effect was, for me, a brief opening up followed by a swift shutting down. Less subject-ively, the overall evidence on staff satisfaction with this process (and its overall effectiveness for quality improvement) is at best mixed (Holden et al., 2015; Moraros et al., 2016; Nowak et al., 2017).

Within the context of collective visualization for practice improvement in infection pre-vention and control, it is important to note the potential value of the video-reflexive eth-nography approach as developed by Iedema and colleagues (Iedema et al., 2013, 2014). This involves the consensual filming of health service staff and patients in clinical contexts, which is then used by staff and patients as a basis for reflexive discussions around areas of practice that might be improved. Rather than focusing on the imagination and invisible phenomena such as pathogens, this recording and reflecting approach seeks to capture the complexity of visible clinical situations and highlight practices that have become unconscious and habitual. Importantly, this "exnovation" approach is designed to be appreciative in nature and to foster innovation from within by foregrounding "the ordinary, moment-to-moment unfold-ing of clinical work" (Iedema et al., 2013: 83). As such it seeks to open up thinking and dialogue about practice and systems, an intention that seems compatible with health human-ities perspectives on visualization.

Healthcare Associated Infection Visualisation and Ideation Research Network (HAIVAIRN)

A final example of how arts and humanities can contribute to the field of infection pre-vention and control/HAIs is manifest in the work of the Healthcare Associated Infection Visualisation and Ideation Research Network (HAIVAIRN). Through our experiences of developing the Visinvis and VisionOn studies as interdisciplinary projects, Alastair Macdon-ald and I became ever more conscious of the need to further expand and integrate research in the field by involving perspectives from other disciplines. Fortunately, this thinking was very much in line with the UK Research Councils, whose collaborative funding programs recognize that "wicked" issues such as antimicrobial resistance require combined expertise from across the academic spectrum. Nevertheless, on mentioning "visualization" and "health-care-associated infections" to members of the public and aca-demic colleagues, we found that the default mind's eye position tended to rest on the microscope's eyepiece.

Accordingly, the AHRC-funded HAIVAIRN project sought to address the question: *how can we better address the problem of HAIs through visualization-related ideation and applications?* This was an attempt to expand conceptions and the scope of verbal and visual narratives. The objectives were to:

- Coalesce a diverse range of national and international expertise around visualization-related ideas to address the prevention and control of HAIs, working from a foundation in arts and humanities.
- Explore and identify areas of research need and opportunity, articulating possible cross-disciplinary contributions through a series of workshop events.
- Create a set of visual mappings locating main priority themes for inquiry, promising subthemes, and related loci and foci for cross-disciplinary interactions.
- Generate a range of relevant researchable questions from this basis.
- Develop these as feasible cross-disciplinary proposals, and disseminate network activities to increase visibility and connectivity in this field.

The three workshop events brought together participants from design, nursing, health geography, human geography, microbiology, NHS domestic and support services management, psychology, health humanities, English literature, social policy, transport planning, anthropology, architecture, and sociology. The final report (Macdonald and Macduff, 2018) summarizes the collaborative processes and outputs achieved. The visual mapping of areas of research need and opportunity (Figure 12.2) shows the diversity of topics and methods generated by participants, and their contingent nature within an integrated schema.

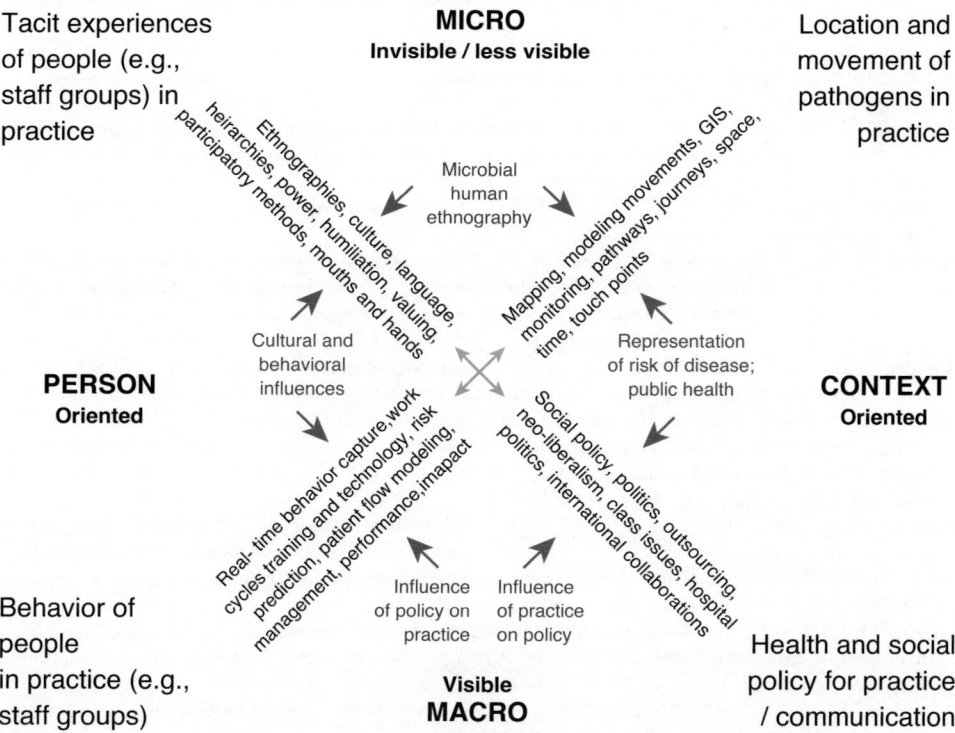

Areas of research need and opportunity for visualization approaches to HAIs (topics and methods)

Figure 12.2 The nature, location and interrelationship of the main topics and methods that HAIVAIRN participants saw as research needs and opportunities

During the lifetime of the project several members of the network developed ideas into funding bids, resulting in three new interdisciplinary research studies focusing on the related problem of antimicrobial resistance in the indoor and built environment. All of these three studies have visualization as a central element and are design led.

This brief chapter has sought to explore some relevant examples of individual and collective visualizing, ranging from internal imagined images to externalized representations. All seek to open up ways of seeing, thinking, and making sense that may help collaboratively address challenges in health-care practice. In this way the visual dimensions of health humanities can not only offer relevant processes, but also create designs, maps, windows, mirrors, and other artifacts to complement the magic of the microscope. In turn, these tools can help kindle the acts of imagination and breadth of vision that are needed for good quality care to flourish.

References

Bruner, J. (1990). *Acts of Meaning*. Cambridge, MA: Harvard University Press.

Crawford, P., Brown, B., Baker, C., Tischler, V. and Abrams, B. (2015). *Health Humanities*. Houndsmills: Palgrave Macmillan.

Holden, R., Eriksonn, A., Andreasson, J., Williamsson, A. and Dellve, L. (2015). Healthcare Workers' Perceptions of Lean: A Context-Sensitive Mixed Methods Study in Three Swedish Hospitals. *Applied Ergonomics*, 47: 181–192.

Iedema, R., Hor, S., Wyer, M., Gilbert, G., Jorm, C., Hooker, C. and O'Sullivan, M. (2014). An Innovative Approach to Strengthening Health Professionals' Infection Control and Limiting Hospital-Acquired Infection: Video-Reflexive Ethnography. *BMJ Innovations*, 1(4): 157–162.

Iedema, R., Mesman, J. and Carroll, K. (2013). *Visualising Healthcare Practice Improvement: Innovation from Within*. London: Radcliffe.

Macdonald, A. and Macduff, C. (2018). *HAIVAIRN: Report on the Healthcare Associated Infection Visualisation and Ideation Research Network*. Glasgow: The Glasgow School of Art. Available to download free at: http://radar.gsa.ac.uk/5642

Macdonald, A., Macduff, C., Loudon, D. and Wan, S. (2017). Evaluation of a Visual Tool Co-Developed for Training Hospital Staff on the Prevention and Control of the Spread of Healthcare Associated Infections. *Infection, Disease and Health*, 22(3): 105–116.

Macduff, C. (2017). A Brief Historical Review of Poetry's Place in Nursing. *Journal of Research in Nursing*, 22(6–7): 436–448.

Macduff, C., Wood, F., Hackett, C., Loudon, D., Macdonald, A., Dancer, S. and Karcher, A. (2013). Visualising the Invisible: Applying an Arts-Based Methodology to Explore How Healthcare Workers and Patient Representatives Envisage Pathogens in the Context of Healthcare Associated Infections. *Arts and Health: An International Journal for Research, Policy and Practice*, 6(2): 117–131.

Moraros, J., Lemstra, M. and Nwanko, C. (2016). Lean Interventions in Healthcare: Do They Actually Work? A Systematic Literature Review. *International Journal for Quality in Healthcare*, 28(2): 150–165.

Nightingale, F. (1860). *Notes on Nursing: What It Is and What It Is Not*. The Second Version – Library Standard Edition (July 1860). Reproduced in: Skretkowicz, V., ed., (2010). *Notes on Nursing: What It Is and What It Is Not* and *Notes on Nursing for the Labouring Classes*. Commemorative Edition with Historical Commentary: . ., . New York: Springer.

Nowak, M., Pfaff, H. and Karbach, U. (2017). Does Value Stream Mapping Affect the Structure, Process and Outcome Quality in Care Facilities? A Systematic Review. *Systematic Reviews*, 6(1): 170.

Oxford English Dictionaries (2018). https://en.oxforddictionaries.com/definition/imagination (Accessed 7/9/18).

Pearson, D., Deeprose, C., Wallace-Hadrill, S., Hayes, S. and Holmes, E. (2013). Assessing Mental Imagery in Clinical Psychology: A Review of Imagery Measures and a Guiding Famework. *Clinical Psychology Review*, 33: 1–23.

Sax, H. and Clack, L. (2015). Mental Models: A Basic Concept for Human Factors Design in Infection Prevention. *Journal of Hospital Infection*, 89(4): 335–339.

Stetler, R. (2010). Experienced Based, Body-Anchored Qualitative Research Interviewing. *Qualitative Health Research*, 2(6): 859–867.

Sullivan, G. (2005). *Art Practice as Research: Inquiry in the Visual Arts*. Thousand Oaks, CA: Sage.

13

HEALTH HUMANITIES AND THE CREATIVE DISCIPLINES

Victoria Tischler

Introduction

Creative practitioners, referred to as *creatives* in this chapter, include visual artists, musicians, theater directors, designers, writers, and poets. These practitioners regularly engage with health-care training and delivery, for example by participating in clinical educational programs enhancing the aesthetics and ambience in environments. This chapter considers what the health humanities have to offer creatives. I suggest that health humanities can play a greater role in the training and practice of creatives, offering individual opportunities as well as wider benefits to the community. The reciprocal benefits of creativity and health are considered historically, using visual arts and mental health as an example, and within the framework of co-creative practice.

Creative disciplines and health-care systems and research: uneasy bedfellows

Much has been written about what the arts bring to health care, including supporting well-being and enhancing quality of life for patients and staff (Arts Council England, 2016). The creative arts have even been considered a "shadow health service," helping to maintain good health as well as to address health problems (Crawford, 2018). However, the input of creatives and the arts that they offer are often instrumentalized, that is, considered a type of treatment much like a dose of medication. Such discourse is often framed in biomedical terms incorporating intervention, evidence, and standardized measurement, effectively reflecting the ongoing dominance of biomedicine in Western health care. A recent report identifies the "active ingredients" of arts programs in order to improve and better measure them (AESOP/BOP, 2018). This neglects the wider benefit of creative participation such as what psychologist Abraham Maslow referred to as *peak experience*, where artistic endeavor is associated with self-actualization, the highest form of human need fulfillment (Maslow, 1943).

More recently, it has been suggested that so-called "small-c creativity" can be beneficial by bringing arts and crafts into everyday activities (Bellass et al., 2018), and that "anti-perfectionism" may actually be key to happiness and fulfillment (Dolan, 2019). Beyond individual enhancement, the arts and humanities have demonstrated wider societal benefits including civic pride and social cohesion (e.g., Serota, 2018; Tischler, 2017).

The arts co-exist alongside a health-care context that has evolved into a highly technical and procedurally focused system; hence creative activities are often framed as "interventions." Historically, Western culture involves a tradition of health care that is doctor centered, with patients adopting a sick role. This positions doctors as authority figures at the pinnacle of the decision-making hierarchy within health-care systems, whereas patients are, by contrast, effectively passive recipients of care. While the sick role may be functional, assigning individuals exemption from their usual duties while they commit to help seeking and regaining full health (Parsons, 1951), it is increasingly recognized that optimal health care is delivered using a collaborative, negotiated model that is patient centered and multidisciplinary in approach. Such approaches are associated with improved health outcomes including patient satisfaction with health-care encounters and self-management (Rathert et al., 2013).

Within the health research environment, biomedical approaches also retain privilege. For instance, the results of randomized controlled trials are given "gold standard" status within hierarchies of evidence. Arts Council England's recent report (2018) acknowledged that such approaches are not sensitive to the nuance of arts activities that include process and transactional elements. This report also cites the motivations of creatives as a "sense of social justice or a desire to develop their practice through co-creation or simply a sense of adventure." Further, their satisfaction is derived from their facilitation of "a kind of epiphany or transformation for the individuals and groups they have been working with . . . and [contributing to or reshaping] their own artistic development" (66). This suggests clear motivation and benefits for creatives working in this realm.

In a wider context, the emphasis on health outcomes and the impact of arts on educational programs for health-care trainees (e.g., providing insights into the human condition, preparing students for narrative practice through patient stories, and improving visual acuity), reinforces the privileging of STEM (science, technology, engineering, and mathematics) subjects in society. However, this dominance of a scientific worldview has been challenged by an increased recognition of the critical role of the arts (Clarke, 2019), where the arts help to navigate uncertainty and ambiguity and to develop holistic consideration of the human condition. Simon Chaplin, Director of Culture, the Wellcome Trust, has acknowledged the importance of research "beyond the academy," including investigating a wider range of research methods that include scientific as well as "real world" perspectives (Arts Council England, 2018). Here the arts have a critical role to play within the development and delivery of services, as well as research.

Creativity and mental health: health care supporting artistic expression

A historical perspective helps to shape the multiple ways in which health might support creative development, amidst adverse circumstances, as in the case of artists with mental health problems. The exhibition "Art in the Asylum" (Djanogly Gallery, Nottingham, 2013) considered this by examining the origins of the use of art in mental health environments, both therapeutically and diagnostically. It also examined the crossover points where art by patients became considered art in its own right. Within this realm, we see numerous examples of creative development inspired by clinical or care contexts, often arising from collaboration with health-care professionals. These benefits included creative opportunities, privileged artistic status, and recovery potential.

W.A.F. Browne was asylum superintendent at the Crichton Royal Institution in Dumfries, Scotland from 1838 to 1857. He worked collaboratively with a patient named William Bartholomew (1819–1881), formerly an engraver and hat maker, before admission to the

Crichton. He was initially diagnosed with mania and later with delirium tremens (shaking usually attributable to alcohol withdrawal), but it was noted that after his admission to the asylum he began to read and draw. Browne was an early proponent of the moral treatment of patients in psychiatric settings, encouraging them to draw, paint, and act, also collecting their work and writing a scientific paper about "mad artists" in 1880.

Browne and Bartholomew worked on a series of large-scale portraits of patients (those incarcerated with Bartholomew) that depicted different types of conditions, including "idiocy" (learning disability), melancholia (depression) and *theomania extatica* (believing oneself to be God). These portraits were used by Browne when lecturing on "mental diseases" to medical and nursing students (Park, 2010); as Browne noted, "the species of alienation, diagnosed by the attendant physician, has been appended to each" (Park, 2010: 239). Although some of Bartholomew's other artistic output was noted by Browne to be "absurd and mythical" with "wild magnificence," it is likely that his portrait series provoked a more positive response, likely to have been beneficial to Bartholomew's status and treatment as an asylum patient. The collaboration represented an opportunity for a patient to showcase his artistic skills by providing technical expertise and personal insights, as well as creating an important visual teaching tool. This type of opportunity would have been a rarity at that time. Bartholomew's patient series is now housed at Edinburgh University Library.

A further example was the collaboration between British Surrealist artist Julian Trevelyan (1910–1988) and the Maudsley Hospital psychiatrists Eric Guttman and Walter Macclay. Alongside the clinicians and other psychiatric patients, Trevelyan took part in a series of mescaline experiments that sought to further understanding of visual hallucination. Surrealist artists such as Trevelyan were interested in psychical processes and such collaboration enabled them to gain insights into, for example, Freud's concept of the unconscious (Hogan, 2001) and influenced Trevelyan's later creative output.

Mary Barnes (1923–2001) was a patient at the psychiatrist R.D. (Ronnie) Laing's therapeutic community in East London during the 1960s. There she was encouraged to "go down" into her psychosis in order to recover. Her creative expression was encouraged by her psychiatrist Joseph Berke, who worked closely with Laing. Barnes used her experiences of psychosis and her relationships with Laing and Berke as creative material, often depicting them in her outputs (for example, "IT," which was composed of wild expressionist furies of oil paint that documented her psychotic rage, and the "Baby Bear" series featuring Berke). Barnes wrote definitively about the cathartic power of art and its ability to help create a new identity:

> Kingsley Hall saw the birth of my painting, in 1965. In a wild, breaking-down state … I was going down into the dark … I was going down, down into rage and despair, moaning, groaning, tearing and biting – to get out of a net, to escape from a murderous tangle … I was alive, at home, all inside my body.
>
> *(Barnes, 1970)*

After leaving Kingsley Hall Barnes lived and worked as an artist; her creative output helped define her as an artist rather than someone who experienced psychotic illness. She went on to co-write a book with Berke entitled *Two Accounts of a Journey Through Madness* (1971), detailing their often volatile relationship. In the past decade there have been two solo shows of her work in London: "Mary Barnes" at SPACE studios (2010–2011) and "Boo-Bah," Bow Arts, The Nunnery (2015).

New directions for co-creativity

Within arts and health discourse, critical consideration of current models of delivery, collaboration, and types of evidence are being negotiated. One concept gaining traction is *co-creativity*, a method of working collaboratively alongside diverse populations including those with cognitive impairments (for example, people with dementia). Co-creativity is characterized by shared decision making and ownership, reciprocity, and relationality (see Zeilig et al., 2018). Emergent findings indicate that this approach benefits all involved and that it promotes transdisciplinary processes, namely those that move beyond disciplinary boundaries, by enacting change in practice.

One such project explored co-creativity over 12 months in a series of four workshops, each focusing on a different art form: dance, visual art, theater, and music. The workshops shared leadership and decision making with all participants, including those with dementia and their partners. The sessions were found to generate novel artistic outputs, while developing and solidifying collaborative partnerships (Tischler et al., 2018). For creatives, the project inspired new work and new relationships, while strengthening others, as one said: "new ideas, creative partnerships, friendships and creative working practice have developed over this last year" (Tischler, 2019: 180).

There are an increasing number of roles for socially engaged artists, particularly those working in health and social care settings and for whom collaboration, activism, and community change is part of their practice. For those identifying as having lived experience of mental health problems, collaboration with the health sector can represent artistic opportunity, affirmation, and therapeutic benefits (Tischler, 2019). This is only achieved through bespoke and tailored support that enables full participation in collaborative projects. As an artist working with arts and health charity Daily Life Ltd. stated about her collaboration on a mental health–themed project: "I've grown so much this year. Just working with others and being a bit calmer and more measured" (180). Another refers to therapeutic benefits of these projects: "I was definitely feeling a bit angsty at the time and it just got out some catharsis."

Despite calls for more artists to work in health care, and potential benefits such as increased employment opportunities, creative stimulus, and job satisfaction, socially engaged roles are often undervalued and poorly remunerated (Artworks Evaluation Survey, 2014; Anderson, 2018). There are, however, socially engaged artists who are critically acclaimed, such as the architectural collective Assemble, whose work with communities won the lauded Turner Prize in 2015. The Co-Creative Change project was recently awarded £360 million by Arts Council England to form national and international networks that explore the role of artists and cultural organizations in co-creating change with local communities.

The Ben Uri Gallery and Museum provides an example of a cultural organization entirely reconfiguring itself to position it at the forefront of developments in arts and health. Founded in 1915 as a collection focused on the work of British and immigrant Jewish artists, it evolved to expand its remit to the individual, social, and political issues of identity and migration. With a substantive collection featuring work by artists including Marc Chagall, George Grosz, and David Bomberg, themes of war, religion, and identity feature prominently and provide powerful stimulus for therapeutic intervention. The collection has been featured in work on projects with asylum seekers, people with learning disabilities, and people living with dementia.

Beginning in 2019, the Ben Uri organization split its resources between two primary projects: research and exhibition of émigré art, and an arts and dementia research institute. This represents the first such initiative by a cultural organization to allocate equal resources between curatorial and art historical activity, and arts and health research. Although an altruistic motivation could underpin this decision, the move may also be viewed as a bold, strategic positioning of Ben Uri at the forefront of arts and health research and development. Ben Uri's position reflects the power of the health-care agenda, in this case the global public health priority of dementia to influence the strategic direction of a cultural arts organization.

Conclusion

The future for creatives with an interest in health appears bright. The health humanities offers increasing opportunities for collaboration, and for development of innovative research methodologies, and an enhanced role in the development and delivery of health care. While these are positive developments, co-creative approaches should be further implemented to ensure that creatives are fully valued and supported, recognized as equal collaborators with a unique and vital skill set. This will maximize opportunities for their own practice as well as benefiting health practices and systems and those cared for within them.

References

Aesop/BOP Consulting (2018). Active Ingredients. http://ae-sop.org/wp-content/uploads/2018/09/Active-Ingredients-Report-Sept-2018-Final-low-res.pdf (Accessed 18/2/2019).

Anderson (2018). Arts on Prescription? Try funding the artists first. 13 November, *The Guardian*, https://theguardian.com/commentisfree/2018/nov/13/matt-hancock-artists-health-secretary (Accessed 18/2/2019).

Art in the Asylum (2013). Creativity and the Evolution of Psychiatry, Djanogly gallery, Nottingham. https://vimeo.com/80921476 (Accessed 18/2/2019).

Arts Council England (2016). The Power of Art: Visual Arts: Evidence of Impact. Retrieved from https://artscouncil.org.uk/sites/default/files/download-file/power_of_art_visual_arts.pdf (Accessed 18/2/2019).

Arts Council England (2018). Arts and Culture in Health and Wellbeing and in the Criminal Justice System: A Summary of Evidence. Retrieved from https://artscouncil.org.uk/publication/arts-and-culture-health-and-wellbeing-and-criminal-justice-system-summary-evidence (Accessed 18/2/2019).

Artworks Evaluation Survey of Artists (2014). Paul Hamlyn Foundation. Retrieved from https://artworksalliance.org.uk/awa-resource/artworks-evaluation-survey-of-artists (Accessed 18/2/2019).

Barnes, M. (1970). Painting. *Motive Magazine* December. (Used with permission of Dr Joseph Berke, December 2019.)

Bellass, S., Balmer, S., May, V., Keady, J., Buse, C., Capstick, A., Burke, L., Bartlett, R. and Hodgson, J. (2018). Broadening the Debate on Creativity and Dementia: A Critical Approach. *Dementia*, doi: 10.1177/1471301218760906.

Clarke, M. (2019). STEM to STEAM: Policy and Practice. In: de la Garza A., Travis C. (eds), *The STEAM Revolution*. Springer, Cham.

Crawford, P. (2018). The Arts are a Shadow Health Service: Here's Why. Retrieved from http://theconversation.com/the-arts-are-a-shadow-health-service-heres-why-105610 (Accessed 18/2/2019).

Dolan, P. (2019). *Happy Ever After: Escaping the Myth of the Perfect Life*. London: Allen Lane.

Hogan, S. (2001). *Healing Arts*. London: Jessica Kingsley.

Maslow, A.H. (1943). A Theory of Human Motivation. *Psychological Review*, 50 (4): 370–396.

Park, M. (2010). *Art in Madness: Dr W A F Browne's Collection of Patient Art at Crichton Royal Institution*. Dumfries: Dumfries and Galloway Health Board.

Parsons, T. (1951). *The Social System*. New York: The Free Press.

Rathert, C., Wyrwich, M. D., and Boren, S. A. (2013). Patient-Centered Care and Outcomes: A Systematic Review of the Literature. *Medical Care Research and Review*, 70 (4): 351–379.

Serota, N. (2018). The Arts Must Reach More People If They Are to Help Our Divided Society. *The Guardian*, 11 Feb. https://theguardian.com/commentisfree/2018/feb/11/arts-council-reach-more-people-divided-society-city-of-culture-hull-nicholas-serota (Accessed 18/2/2019).

Tischler, V. (2017). 'It takes Me Into Another Dimension': An Evaluation of Mental Health-Themed Exhibitions in Outdoor Urban Areas. *Arts and Health: An International Journal for Research, Policy and Practice*, 10: 1–16.

Tischler, V. (2019). The Roving Diagnostic Unit: art, madness, fun and the potential for change. *Arts and Health: An International Journal for Research, Policy and Practice*, 11 (2): 174–182.

Tischler, V., Schneider, J., Morgner, C., Crawford, P., Dening, T., Brooker, D., Garabedian, C., Myers, T., Early, F., Shaughnessy, N., Innes, A., Duncan, K., Prashar, A., McDermott, O., Coaten, R., Eland, D. and Harvey, K. (2018). Stronger Together: Learning From an Interdisciplinary Dementia, Arts and Wellbeing Network (DA&WN). *Arts and Health: An International Journal for Research, Policy and Practice*, 11 (3): 272–277.

Zeilig, H., West, J. and van der Byl Williams, M. (2018). Co-Creativity: Possibilities for Using the Arts with People with a Dementia. *Quality in Ageing and Older Adults*, 19 (2): 135–145.

14

CO-DESIGN AS A DEMOCRATIZING FORCE

Alastair Macdonald

Introduction

Design is succinctly summarized as "a set of practices aimed at realizing a certain desirable future" (Storni, 2013: 51) and, as such, is predicated on the idea that the status quo can be improved. Immediately, a number of questions arise: Whose desirable future, and who should be involved in defining and deciding this? How to move toward an idea of an improved future that we have not yet had the opportunity to experience? This chapter sets out to provide an introductory overview of design's more recent practices and preoccupations, its contribution to the field of health care, and how these practices attempt to improve the health-care experience— for both those receiving it and those involved in its delivery— by helping realize some of the aspirations of the health humanities.

Design in the health-care setting

Within health care, design is a field advancing on a number of fronts; varied contributions are evidenced in Tsekleves and Cooper (2016). Robert and Macdonald (2017) characterize the health-care setting as follows:

> In terms of a service environment, several aspects of healthcare make it rather different from other sectors, not least its sheer scale, variety and complexity, as well as the (often) fragility, vulnerability and dependency of its clients. Healthcare organizations and services are also typically complex, hierarchical, and highly socio-technical settings. The dynamics within interdisciplinary healthcare teams are often as complex and hierarchical as those between teams and their patients.
>
> *(118)*

This immediately identifies a number of problematic issues within a largely biomedical paradigm that design, if it is to be involved, needs to acknowledge and address. The setting can be likened to a complex service ecosystem with a large cast of interacting players and agents: cohorts of individuals each with their differentiated roles, tasks, behaviors, and interactions;

the agents and mechanisms of threats to health care and treatment (such as infection); and the design of the environment and its positive or negative effects on recovery and well-being.

If a future is to be desirable, shared, and democratic—for patient, carer, and health-care provider alike—then all need to be involved in envisioning, creating, and realizing that future. Co-design, defined as "the meaningful involvement of end users in the design process" (Design Council, 2017), is now a common and well-established practice. Its roots lie in the 1970s Scandinavian "participatory design" (PD) movement, a phrase "often used as an umbrella term for participatory, co-creation and open design processes" (Chisholm, n.d.).

It is therefore worthwhile to differentiate design approaches that are merely consultative as distinct from truly meaningful participation. Savory (2010) provides a useful framework for incorporating patient and public involvement in translative health-care research, and both Arnstein and the New Economics Foundation (NEF) provide models representing the shifts in "people power." Arnstein's Ladder of Citizen Participation (1969) starts with "manipulation," and moves up through a number of stages including "consultation" and "partnership," eventually leading to "citizen control." In a simplified and more contemporary interpretation of this, NEF's Ladder of Engagement (2014) categorizes different types of approaches, progressively shifting from "doing to" (e.g., coercion), through "doing for," to "doing with" (i.e., co-production) at the top. Design's thrust is habitually toward the top end of this ladder.

A democratic space

Having declared the intent to co-design, and to bring together the relevant stakeholders to do so, how does one address the particularly problematic issues arising from health care and its setting (such as hierarchical roles) to create a space or forum removed from that setting? How might habituated behaviors and power dynamics in health-care settings be positively challenged by co-design? How can co-design in such spaces be practiced in democratic ways? Here, it is valuable to describe two approaches. One is the creation of a "publics," an open and neutral space, and the other an "infrastructuring," with materials and activities to enable co-design to take place within this space. Within this open space, the assembled team are "individuals bound by a common cause" (Le Dantec and DiSalvo, 2013: 243) that together create "a dynamic organization of individuals and groups formed by the desire to address an issue" (254). Turner (1969) coined the term "communitas," defined as a union of equal members. The designer does not have expertise in the clinical or care sense, nor is s/he a "virtuoso of experience" (Sanders, 2001); to enable "designing" to be carried out in a co-design approach by all stakeholders, the activities within this space need a degree of "infrastructuring" (Bjorgvinsson et al., 2010). The intention of such infrastructuring is "to capture particular views and ways of engaging when designing complex sustainable systems" (Seravalli and Eriksen, 2017: 246) and to allow for the designing of situations, activities, and materials to enable a "greater proportional symmetry" between the stakeholders involved (Strickfaden and Devlieger, 2011: 208). Examples might be materials such as visual stimulus cards, personas, storyboarding and narratives, design games, activities such as role-play, and enactment with paper mock-ups or functional prototypes to help reconceive and simulate a new hospital food management and nutrition monitoring system (Macdonald et al., 2012). Another example might be to reimagine how physical rehabilitation following stroke, using visualization techniques, could assist improved understanding and communication between therapist and patient (Loudon et al., 2014).

Building to think

These materials, along with the format and structure of these co-design sessions, not only invite contributions to ensure that all voices have a say; they also move beyond the *capture* of experience and insight to *embody* these voices in prototype and mock-up form—to help bring a degree of tangibility to ideas, whether these are for equipment, procedures, or services.

Sanders and Stappers discuss designers' ability to "make things that describe future objects" and cite how prototyping can play a number of roles, for example, to "allow the testing of a hypothesis" because prototyping "allows people to experience a situation that did not exist before" (2014: 6). It is worth stressing that in the inclusive co-design approach it is not the designer who is doing the designing. Rather, it is the stakeholders—enabled by the approaches, spaces, types of practice, and materials habitually used in design practice—who become actively involved in this collaborative venture.

In the context of using prototyping in policy making, Siodmok (2014) states, "to proto-type generates imperfect truths but with the right approach it also generates data about the future" and also "evidence of what works and, more importantly, what does not, can be very powerful." In the health-care setting, Coughlan et al. (2007) cite cases of the effective-ness of "rapid prototyping," discussing its value in such terms as "building to think," "giving permission to explore new behaviors ... in a nonthreatening, low-risk way" (9), as "learning tools" and "transitional objects ... that support a change from a current behaviour to a new behaviour" (10). Evidence-based design is very much about designing, making, prototyping, and testing with the intention of ultimately moving beyond research towards implementation. It involves thinking beyond the now, and toward the future.

Designerly and design-like

Until relatively recently, the design profession was hung up on the idea that it was the pro-fession to be doing all the designing. If one looks broadly at design since the mid-twentieth century one can see, comparable to the shifts in approach to engagement and participation outlined above, a paradigm shift from that of the consultant designer designing products *for* people to the late twentieth- and early twenty-first-century paradigm where the designer is collaborating much more *with* others. Increasingly, this work is further informed by interdis-ciplinary teams and the public, through what is much more widely understood and accepted as co-design today. This reflects the democratization of design activity, epitomized by the work of the Scandinavian PD movement, that is now more widely adopted and adapted. But what if this trajectory was taken to its logical conclusion? Could one have people designing without the need for designers at all? Is that possible? In fact, a form of this has already occurred using the experience-based co-design (EBCD) approach:

> [EBCD] is an approach that enables staff and patients (or other service users) to co-design services and/or care pathways, together in partnership. The approach is different to other service improvement techniques.
>
> *(Point of Care, 2018)*

Donetto et al. (2014) summarize a decade of EBCD's achievements in improving patient experiences, using the approach first piloted in a head and neck cancer service at a National Health Service hospital in England. This form of "designing" has been able to achieve what design has been unable to in terms of the consistent application, refinement, and uptake of the EBCD method in over 60 health-care organizations internationally. EBCD poses some interesting questions and challenges for design. Robert and Macdonald (2017) develop this discussion by differentiating "designerly" from "design-like" approaches and methods, highlighting the strengths, weaknesses, and the types of outcomes each approach tends to produce.

Co-design as anti-structure

Co-design practices and approaches, such as those described above, act to establish an "anti-structure" (Turner, 1969) capable of resisting and counteracting a hegemonic medicalized service paradigm. In its place, co-design provides opportunities to create an alternative space where no ideas are "off the table." This alternative space, and the types of materials, activities, and practices it involves, describes a shift "away from a technocratic view of innovation towards one that includes social innovation—innovation that arises out of social interactions ... and actions that arise from the constitutions of a public" (Le Dantec and DiSalvo, 2013: 247). The creation of that neutral and open space, supported—that is, infrastuctured—through appropriately inclusive materials and activities allows for a "plurality of voices, opinions and positions" (Strickfaden and Devlieger, 2011: 208) that assist thinking and building towards more appropriate future "solutions." These are the futures that are co-constructed and reconciled from the multiple narratives and desires of all those involved. As a consequence, such co-designed futures challenge epistemological privilege in conventional health-care knowledge and experience.

References

Arnstein, S. R. (1969). A Ladder of Citizen Participation. *Journal of the American Planning Association*, 35 (4): 216–224.

Björgvinsson, E., Ehn, P. and Hillgren, P. A. (2010). Participatory Design and Democratizing Innovation, in PDC '10: Proceedings of the 11th biennial participatory design. Conference, Sydney, Australia, 29 November – 3 December 2010. New York: ACM Press, 41–50.

Chisholm, J. n.d. What is co-design? Design for Europe: Available at http://designforeurope.eu/what-co-design (Accessed 23/11/2019).

Coughlan, P., Fulton Suri, J. and Canales, K. (2007). Prototypes as (design) tools for behavioral and organizational change: a design-based approach to help organizations change work behaviors. *Journal of Applied Behavioral Science*, 43(1): 122–134.

Design Council. (2017). *The A–Z of Co-Design*. Accessed 31 July 2018. Available at: www.designcouncil. org.uk/z-co-design (Accessed 18/2/2019).

Donetto, S., Tsianakas, V. and Robert, G. (2014). Using Experience-Based Co-Design to Improve the Quality of Healthcare: Mapping Where We Are Now and Establishing Future Directions. London: King's College London. Available at: www.kcl.ac.uk/nursing/research/nnru/publications/Reports/EBCD-Where-are-we-now-Report.pdf (Accessed 20/9/2018).

Le Dantec, C.A. and DiSalvo, C. (2013). Infrastructuring and the Formation of Publics in Participatory Design. *Social Studies of Science*, 43(2): 241–264.

Loudon, D., Taylor, A. and Macdonald, A.S. (2014). The Use of Qualitative Design Methods in the Design, Development and Evaluation of Virtual Technologies for Healthcare: Stroke Case Study. In: M. Ma, L.C. Jain and P. Anderson, eds, *Virtual and Augmented Reality in Healthcare 1*. Berlin Heidelberg: Springer-Verlag: 371–390.

Macdonald, A.S., Teal, G., Bamford, C. and Moynihan, P. J. (2012). Hospitalfoodie: An Inter-Professional Case Study of the Redesign of the Nutritional Management and Monitoring System for Vulnerable Older Hospital Patients. *Quality in Primary Care*, 20 (3): 169–177.

New Economics Foundation. (2014). Co-Production: Theory and Practice. [online] Available at: https://prezi.com/eitdkeaoly8t/co-production-theory-and-practice/?webgl=0 (Accessed 31/7/2018).

Point of Care. (2018). EBCD: Experience-Based Co-design Toolkit. Available at: www.pointofcarefoun dation.org.uk/resource/experience-based-co-design-ebcd-toolkit/(Accessed 31/7/2018).

Robert, G. and Macdonald, A. S. (2017). Co-design, organisational creativity and quality improvement in the healthcare sector: 'designerly' or 'design-like'? In: D. Sangiorgi and A. Prendiville, eds, *Designing for service*. London: Bloomsbury. 9: 117–130.

Sanders, E.B.-N. (2001). Virtuosos of the Experience Domain. [pdf] Maketools. Available at: www.make tools.com/articles-papers/VirtuososoftheExperienceDomain_Sanders_01.pdf (Accessed 31/7/2018).

Sanders, E. B.-N. and Stappers, P. J. (2014). Probes, Toolkits and Prototypes: Three Approaches to Making in Codesigning. *CoDesign: International Journal of CoCreation in Design and the Arts*, 10 (1): 5–14.

Savory, C. (2010). Patient and Public Involvement in Translative Healthcare Research. *Clinical Governance: An International Journal*, 15: 191–199.

Seravalli, A. and Eriksen, M. A. (2017). Beyond Collaborative Services: Service Design for Sharing and Collaboration as a Matter of Commons and Infrastructuring. In: D. Sangiorgi and A. Prendiville, eds, *Designing for Service*. London: Bloomsbury: 237–250.

Siodmok, A. (2014). Designer policies. [pdf] *RSA Journal* (4): 28–29. Available at: https://www.thersa. org/discover/publications-and-articles/journals/rsa-journal-issue-4-2014/ (Accessed 23/11/2019).

Storni, C. (2013). Design for Future Uses: Pluralism, Fetishism and Ignorance. Available at: www. nordes.org/opj/index.php/n13/article/viewFile/276/258 (Accessed 31/7/2018).

Strickfaden, M. and Devlieger, P. (2011). Empathy Through Accumulating Techné: Designing an Accessible Metro. *The Design Journal*, 14 (2): 207–230.

Tsekleves, E. and Cooper, R. (Eds) (2017). *Design for Health*. Abingdon: Routledge.

Turner, V. (1969). *The Ritual Process: Structure and Anti-Structure*. Cornell Paperbacks: Cornell University Press.

15

INDIGENOUS HEALTH HUMANITIES

Allison Crawford, Lisa Boivin and Lisa Richardson

Introduction

The image, *Sharing Bioethics*, by Dene artist and scholar Lisa Boivin (Figure 15.1), uses Boivin's image-based storytelling approach to both describe and make a space for holistic meaning making within two spheres: Western biomedicine and Dene medicine. In its story, Boivin imagines ways that these spheres might intersect, the tools of healing in Western medicine (such as the X-ray and stethoscope) coming into contact with the tools of Dene medicine: the medicine bundle, plants, and animals important for healing. This contact occurs through relationship with the two healers: their arms touch to create a third, shared space. This mutuality of touch allows interconnectedness without the obliteration of one space by another (more dominant) way of knowing (Crawford, 2018).

The *possibilities* in the points connecting the arms of each figure are fragile, perhaps even tentative, rather than firmly secured; small shifts may threaten the integrity of this new sphere of possibility. The image is part of a larger visual narrative by Boivin (2018) about the story of her family, particularly the story of her father's encounter with Canada's medical system as a young child with polio: enduring surgeries, forced hospitalization, and medical procedures throughout his life, often without informed consent. Boivin's father's experience exemplifies the colonial history of medicine. Through her storytelling, Boivin creates a new space for different knowledges to meet and to be in relationship, while simultaneously witnessing and documenting this colonial past that continues into the present. Through her images, the gaze that she turns on Western medicine is at once an invitation to explore the ways in which Indigenous and Western medicine can coexist, and a critique of biomedicine's colonial practices.

In a provocative 1998 essay, Warwick Anderson asked: where is the postcolonial history of medicine? (Anderson, 1998). He noted the absence within the history of medicine of accounts of the colonial encounter through medicine, and positioned the history of medicine as a means of engaging in the critical work of decolonization. Since then, academics in the history of medicine have begun to delineate the field, focusing mainly on the tropical South and medicine's role in shaping and sustaining the empires of imperialism (for example, Anderson, 2006; Vaughan, 1991). This is also an area that is beginning to be taken up in the larger domain of health humanities, utilizing narrative, as well as art by patients and providers from postcolonial cultures, including critical voices by postcolonial academics, and using frameworks drawn from postcolonial theory (see, for example, the work of DasGupta, 2006, 2017).

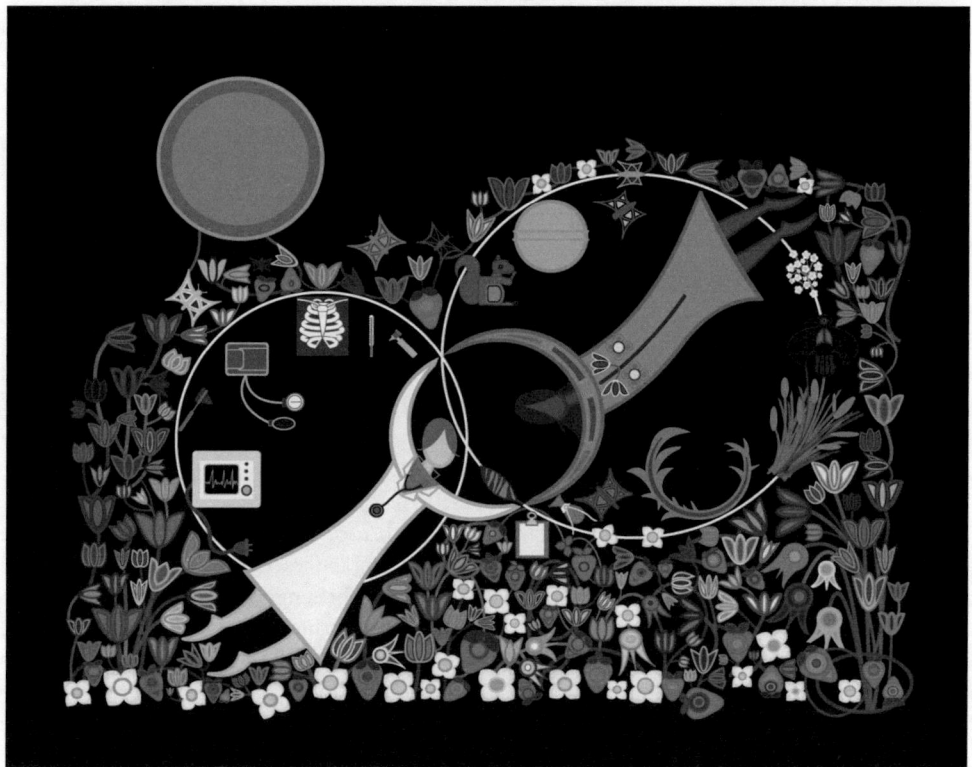

Figure 15.1 Sharing Bioethics, by Lisa Boivin

In this chapter we ask, where is the Indigenous history of medicine? What tools, perspectives, and critiques would an Indigenous health humanities offer? We draw upon new work in the areas of Indigenous life-writing, narrative, and art within health care, as well as critical writing about Indigenous knowledges and methodologies. We highlight the possibility of an Indigenous health humanities to create a culturally safe "third space" of relations within health care. However, we also delineate four areas for critique and further research within the Indigenous health humanities: (1) the arts not as separate from medicine, but *as* medicine; (2) art and story *as* knowledge and critique; (3) the specificity and diversity of "Indigenous" knowledges, and the languages, traditions, literatures, and arts of autonomous nations; and, (4) storytelling as a relational practice of being an ally reader/viewer/listener.

Indigenous history(ies) of medicine

If postcolonial approaches to the history of medicine have a fairly recent scholarly history, analysis of the colonial context and practices of Western medicine in Indigenous contexts is even more recent. In addition to his influential work on the colonial history of medicine in the Philippines (2006), Anderson explores issues of race, indigeneity, and medicine in Australia in *The Cultivation of Whiteness* (2005). He traces how white superiority was often constructed and reinforced through contrasts between white settlers and harsh, unfamiliar environments, and the racialized bodies of Indigenous others. Medical and scientific discourse, and research practices, were used to buttress the "naturalness" of these hierarchical comparisons.

Two important Canadian studies have investigated the role of racist attitudes as a cause of the health inequity for Indigenous peoples. Maureen Lux's (2001) *Medicine that Walks: Disease, Medicine, and Canadian Plains Native People*, 1880–1940, argues that government policies rooted in racist ideologies led to the steep decline of health in the reserve population of the prairies. In *Colonizing Bodies: Aboriginal Health and Healing in British Columbia*, Mary-Ellen Kelm (1998) argues that colonial attitudes, including the belief that Indigenous people in British Columbia were on the verge of extinction, justified government interventions as appropriate and necessary. Several important works extend these arguments, asserting that the health disparities that exist today for Indigenous peoples are not a result of inherent, racialized weakness, but were created by a number of political-economic factors resulting from early contact, including disease, starvation, loss of life, the reconfiguration of social groupings (ethnogenesis), and economic adversity. James Daschuk (2013) and Paul Kelton (2015) explore these colonial influences among Indigenous peoples in Western Canada and the Cherokee Nation, respectively. Waldram, Herring, and Kue Young (2006) similarly assert that political economy is the most appropriate interpretive lens to consider Indigenous health, taking into account biology, culture, history, and governmental policies and practices.

Indigenous scholars directly within the field of health care are also beginning to draw on (post)colonial critiques to address the ongoing colonial practices of health care (Allan and Smylie, 2015), challenge the framing of disease, and also challenge the capacity of Western medicine in turn to address this ongoing inequity.[1] One of the key questions raised in the discipline of medical history, particularly for historians of governmental and health policy, is if or how to intervene in current advocacy, policy making, and social action (Brandt, 2004). For Indigenous writers of history, the telling of the history of settler-colonialism is directly linked with a call for redress and action in the present.

Narrative medicine, postcolonial narrative medicine, and Indigenous narrative medicine

Awareness of the narrative dimensions of medicine has come largely from social scientists and anthropologists in the late 1980s, who drew attention to the ways that physicians communicated, taught, and practiced through stories (see, for example, Brody, 2003; Good, 1994; Kleinman, 1989). Kathryn Montgomery Hunter (1991) was one of the first to examine the narrative structure of medical knowledge using the tools of literary analysis, demonstrating that "the theory and methods of understanding that are traditional to the humanities are useful in understanding what it is that physicians do" (xiii). Physicians can be further understood as thinking, reasoning, and making decisions in narrative terms (Good and Delvecchio Good, 2000).

Rita Charon coined the term "narrative medicine" in 2000 to "refer to clinical practice fortified by narrative competence—the capacity to recognize, absorb, metabolize, interpret, and be moved by stories of illness. Simply, it is medicine practiced by someone who knows what to do with stories" (Charon, 2007: 1265). Elsewhere she specifies, "narrative medicine provides healthcare professionals with practical wisdom in comprehending what patients endure in illness and what they themselves undergo in the care of the sick" (Charon, 2018: vii). The phrase "narrative medicine came to me to signify a clinical practice informed by the theory and practice of reading, writing, telling, and receiving of stories" (viii).

In *The Practices and Practices of Narrative Medicine* (2017), Charon et al. voice their commitment through narrative medicine "to protest the social injustice of a global healthcare system that countenances tremendous health disparities and discriminatory policies and practices" (1) and later in the book list "action toward social justice" as one of six core principles for the field (172). However, despite the promise of narrative medicine and the enthusiastic embrace of it by many, one concern is that narrative medicine consistently focuses on canonical Western texts and narrative forms (Hooker and Noonan, 2011; Woods, 2011).

The reasons for failing to include cultural perspectives and narrative practices may be related to the centrality of close reading as a core technique of narrative medicine. Charon, in providing a history of this school of literary criticism—from its origins in Britain, through to the American New Critics of the 1950s—notes the sustained critique of close reading, including the charges of narrowly focusing on a small group of canonical texts, and, given the emphasis on text over context, the failure to "contextualize the work by time or space or person. Such matters as race, language, class, or gender are seen to not come in for the attention they require of the reader" (Charon et al., 2017: 162). Certainly, there is almost no reference to postcolonial criticism. While Charon acknowledges this critique, and also shows how more contemporary approaches to close reading are attuned to the emotional and moral consequences of reading (and therefore to the reader and the social beyond the text), she nevertheless continues to emphasize close reading, "a singular understanding of the transaction between this text and this reader" (164), rather than the larger sociality of texts.

There have been some attempts to use narrative medicine to begin this work. Sayantani DasGupta (2006, DasGupta et al., 2006), one of the founding members of the Columbia narrative medicine program, has described pedagogical approaches to narrative in several articles that suggest narrative can facilitate transcultural understanding. One of DasGupta's (2017) approaches adapts Melanie Tervalon and Jann Murray-Garcia's term "cultural humility" to the idea of narrative humility, "a sense of wonder and the understanding that some aspect of their stories will necessarily be unfamiliar or unknowable" (148). Instead of using narrative to render another culture "readable" by medicine, or to learn as many facts as we can about individual cultures, transcultural contact is an intersubjective exchange.

Additional features of postcolonial theory could contribute to narrative medicine's critical apparatus, but the literature exploring these possibilities is sparse.[2] Arthur Frank (2013) calls upon metaphoric associations, pronouncing colonization as central to the achievement of modern medicine itself: the colonization of the body by the technical. For those engaged in life-writing about their illness, he states, "those who work to express this voice are not only postmodern but, more specifically, postcolonial in their construction of self" (9). He relates the triumph of those who write illness narratives to another postcolonial critic, Gayatri Chakravorty Spivak, who "speaks of colonized people's efforts 'to see how the master texts need us in [their] construction ... without acknowledging that need'" (11). After Spivak, Frank provokes readers to consider, "What do the master texts of medicine need but not acknowledge?" (11).

Indigenous writing about narrative, illness, and medicine, and its intersection with settler-colonialism is also scant. There is life-writing about the lives of Indigenous physicians, such as Lori Arviso Alvord's autobiography (Alvord and Cohen, 2000), which specifically addresses how she incorporates traditional knowledge into her medical practice. Neal McLeod (Cree) (2007) examines family and community story as intergenerational forms of memory, whose unique narrative forms impart strength and resilience. An anthology of narratives, *Healing Histories: Stories from Canada's Indian Hospitals*, highlights the- care system (Meijer Drees, 2013); in that edited volume, Meijer Drees emphasizes the ability of narrative to preserve the voice of narrator, but more importantly she understands story as a means to confront the injustices and the subjective experiences of settler-colonialism.

In Inuit contexts there is very little writing on the overlap between narrative, illness, and medicine. In a 1991 article in the journal *Arctic Medical History*, Robin McGrath presages this field, writing about Inuit writing on illness (McGrath, 1991). McGrath addresses some of the stereotypes and romantic imagery through which Inuit are represented in popular imagination. She reports on the two Inuit periodicals—*Inuktitut Magazine* and *Northern Lights and Shadows*—that arose to entertain and provide a forum for Inuit patients at hospitals in the south. McGrath recognizes the lasting legacy of these health-care experiences for many Inuit, and looks toward narrative as part of "coming to terms" with this history and assisting other Inuit "who today are still suffering the trauma caused by the disease and its treatment" (31). Crawford (2018) looks to physician life-writing over the last hundred years to provide an account of the health care provided to Inuit in the Canadian Arctic, and of the importance of a critical, postcolonial reading of the narrative and discursive constructions of Inuit through these narratives and through health care itself.

A 2015 special issue of *Ars Medica: A Journal of Medicine, the Arts and Humanities*, edited by the authors of this chapter, arose out of an awareness of the need for Indigenous voices and perspectives in health care.[3] This elevation of critical and autonomous Indigenous voices into the field of health care can address the exclusion and marginalization of Indigenous perspectives from medicine and narrative medicine. Writing of Indigenous life-writing more broadly, Daniel Heath Justice (2008) does not eschew writing, noting in the words of Gloria Bird (Spokane) that writing "at its liberating best, it is a political act. Through writing we can undo the damaging stereotypes that are continually perpetuated about Native peoples. We can rewrite our history, and we can mobilize our future" (258).

However, Audra Simpson (Kanien'hehaka) (2014) is more circumspect; she labels the expectation of Indigenous peoples to tell their life stories "ethnographic entrapment," forcing Indigenous peoples into the position of what Rey Chow terms, "self-confessing subjects" (212). Ethnographic subjects "must live up to the ethnographic niche to which they have been assigned ... forced to display their ethnicity constantly as a form of confession that will set them free" (212). For Simpson, what will create liberation is not confessing truths and the recognition of humanity, but structural change. In her approach of "ethnographic refusal," recognition is instead sought from other Indigenous people, and other colonized people.

Simpson's alliance with other colonized peoples and her use of postcolonial theory is a strategy that is in turn problematized by other Indigenous writers. Emma LaRocque (Cree and Métis) (2016), who has also evolved what she calls a "resistance scholarship"—a "contrapuntal, anticolonial epistemology and pedagogy to highlight textual strategies of domination" (61) in mainstream Western narratives—resists incorporation into postcolonial studies. She cautions (72) that:

> the recent postcolonial emphasis on 'hybridity' (which is not to be confused with Métis Nation cultures), 'crossing boundaries,' or 'liminality' can serve to eclipse Aboriginal cultural knowledges, experiences (both national and individual) and what may be called the colonial experience ... no amount of disassembling 'the Native experience' to accommodate globalized postcolonial theories can undo this homegrown colonial burden.

This emerging field of Indigenous life-writing allows the possibility of new and critical perspectives on the health-care experiences of Indigenous peoples historically and into the present. Current debates in the field, and multiple critical perspectives, will continue to define the parameters and limitations of this field, and its possibilities for creating health equity and cultural safety for Indigenous peoples. The critiques of these approaches are important, as they will help to delineate methods for storytelling, reading, and witnessing. Here we highlight four areas where further research and dialogue are necessary.

1. Art and story as medicine

In Indigenous healing and medicine traditions, storytelling is itself medicine. In *Narrative Medicine: The Use of History and Story in the Healing Process* (Mehl-Madrona, 2007), for example, Lewis Mehl Madrona (Cherokee) writes about the centrality of story to Indigenous culture and of the healing power of stories. As with other aspects of cultural and ceremonial loss, loss of story is rooted in cultural genocide and attempts at assimilating Indigenous peoples into dominant culture. This understanding locates stories not just as a tool to critique health care, but as a primary means of reinstating cultural continuity, and of healing historical trauma and loss (Crawford, 2014).[4] Attempts to reduce narrative to a means of cross-cultural understanding, or as a commentary on Western medicine, minimizes and de-centers its intrinsic importance. Emma LaRoque (2016) also cautions against reading all Indigenous narrative as traumatic loss: "Not every Indigenous person is dislocated—many write and read literature securely from their cultural and epistemic home/lands" (70) As this field continues to emerge, all of these dialectical truths need to be held in tension. Ultimately, it is the knowledge keepers and storytellers of each community that will decide on the place of particular stories and their need for, and use as, medicine.

2. Art and story as knowledge and critique

Unlike contemporary Western traditions, story is not a lesser version of either reason or knowledge. Stories carry knowledge and teachings that go beyond providing a representation of Indigenous identities; they are able to carry instruction and teaching. These knowledges may offer useful critiques of health care, and the deployment of humanities in health care, but the knowledges contained in stories should not be reducible to these purposes. Again, the locus of that knowledge and the wisdom contained in stories resides within Elders, and knowledge keepers in a specific community. Linda Tuhiwai Smith (Māori) (2012), whose work on decolonizing methodologies has become a touchstone for many Indigenous scholars, is also cautious about adopting postcolonial frameworks. She equates being researched with being colonized, and forwards an alternative agenda for Indigenous research methods and practices that foregrounds social movement or action, community, tribe, and self-reflexivity or insider/outsider recognition, along with training Indigenous researchers. Tuhiwai Smith lists 25 Indigenous projects that these practices could be mobilized for, including six related to practices of life-writing: testimony; storytelling; remembering; reading; writing and theory making; and creating. Indigenous storytelling recognizes both that each individual story is powerful and that stories "contribute to a collective story in which every Indigenous person has a place," connecting past, future, land and people. She cites Margaret Kovach, who argues that because stories are connected to knowing, the story is both method and meaning, and therefore central to Indigenous research and knowledge methodologies.

One issue for Indigenous scholars and critics to contend with, within health humanities and other contexts, is how the knowledge and values of a story or artwork may be at odds with the system of values into which they are inserted. Elizabeth Cook-Lynn (Crow Creek

Sioux) (1998) also challenges the way Indigenous life-writing participates in Western traditions that uphold values antithetical to Indigenous values, such as privileging the solitary individual over the community. We need to continue to ask, *what are the values of health care, and the values of the humanities as applied to health care? How do we expect these stories to participate in this field, and is that aligned with their values?* As health humanities scholars we have to pay particular attention to the methods and practices we bring to reading stories, concepts that we often simply take for granted, such as point of view, narrative coherence, and closure.

3. Specificity, diversity, and sovereignty of Indigenous knowledges

This chapter, along with the term "Indigenous health humanities," threatens to collapse unique narrative and artistic traditions under a pan-Indigenous umbrella. Without critical reflexivity, attempts within the health humanities to understand "the" Indigenous voice may unwittingly perpetuate the colonial process of erasure of identity and sovereignty that health care has participated in. Marilyn Dumont (Cree-Métis) (1993: 45) writes of the ways that narrating the self in Western moulds is further constrained by expected forms of narration dictated by stereotypes that readers have of Indigenous peoples:

> If you are old, you are supposed to write legends … If you are young, you are expected to write stories of foster homes, street life and loss of culture; and if you are in the middle, you are supposed to write about alcoholism or residential school. And somehow throughout this, you are to infuse everything you write with symbols of the native world view, that is: the circle, mother earth, the number four or the trickster figure.

As we recognize the value of Indigenous stories and art, we must always locate and be aware of their rootedness in specific Nations, communities, languages, and land. Further, the medicine and knowledge carried within the story is also inseparable from the land that provides the story's context, and the language in which it is told.

4. Storytelling as relational: on being an ally reader/viewer/listener

Important to each of the three considerations above is awareness of the relationality of storytelling. The reader/viewer/listener is in relationship with the story and storyteller, and given the contextual (land, language, community) specificity of the story or art may be unable to (or be uninvited to) be in relation to the story. Some stories, just as some knowledges and practices, will be closed to the uninitiated. This resistance of story stands in direct opposition to attempts to subsume or subscribe stories, including under the banner of Western medicine or health humanities. The term "storywork" by Stó:lō scholar Jo-Ann Archibald (2008) includes the Indigenous protocols that attend storytelling and listening, and that invest these stories with their power, along with the relational work of stories.

Non-Indigenous readers/viewers/listeners in particular need to remain attuned to the work they need to do to be in relationship with a particular story or storyteller. *What does it mean to witness a story as an ally (rather than to consume it)? What are the responsibilities of an ally?*

The questions of how to stand in relation to a story or piece of art created by a First Nations, Inuit, Métis, or another Indigenous person, are critical and evolving. This very relationality requires at least the narrative humility described by DasGupta. Beyond that, as Glen Sean Coulthard (Dene) insists, such relationality must involve more than passive recognition. These stories demand action. In Canada, it has become a trope when discussing Indigenous peoples within institutional contexts—such as health care, education, and politics—to reference the importance of opportunities for reconciliation. The stories, art, and critical approaches that constitute the emerging field of Indigenous health humanities may offer opportunities for critical reflexivity within health care. However, in order for the Indigenous health humanities to engage in reconciliation it must be linked to the meaningful action of decolonizing health care and other social institutions.

Notes

1 Joseph Gone's work is exemplary, particularly Gone (2007).
2 New efforts in the larger field of health humanities are calling for greater interdisciplinary integration across the field. See, for example, Crawford et al. (2015) and Jones et al. (2014).
3 See http://ars-medica.ca/index.php/journal/issue/view/21/showToc.
4 Crawford (2014) has argued elsewhere, drawing on approaches to trauma studies in literary theory, that historical trauma can be understood as narrative. Nathanial Mohatt and his colleagues (2014) have extended this idea of the narrative structure of historical trauma to talk about the public dimensions of this narrative framework.

References

Allan, B., and Smylie, J. (2015). *First Peoples, Second Class Treatment: The Role of Racism in the Health and Wellbeing of Indigenous Peoples in Canada*. Toronto: Wellesley Institute. Available at: www.wellesleyin stitute.com/wp-content/uploads/2015/02/Summary-First-Peoples-Second-Class-Treatment-Final. pdf (Accessed 18/2/2019).

Alvord, L.A. and Cohen, E. (2000). *The Scalpel and the Silver Bear*. New York: Bantam Books.

Anderson, W. (1998). Where is the Postcolonial History of Medicine? Essay Review. *Bulletin of the History of Medicine*, 72(3): 522–530.

Anderson, W. (2005). The Cultivation of Whiteness: Science, Health and Racial Destiny in Australia. Carlton, Vic: Melbourne University Press.

Anderson, W. (2006). Colonial Pathologies: American Tropical Medicine, Race, and Hygiene in the Philippines. Durham: Duke University Press.

Archibald, J. (2008). Indigenous Storywork: Educating the Heart, Mind, Body, and Spirit. Vancouver: University of British Columbia Press.

Boivin, L. (2018). Image-Based Storytelling: A Visual Narrative of My Family's Story. *Canadian Medical Association Journal*, 190(37): E1112–E1113.

Brandt, A.M. (2004). From Analysis to Advocacy: Crossing Boundaries as a Historian of Health Policy. In F. Huisman and J.H. Warner, eds, *Locating Medical History: The Stories and Their Meanings*. Baltimore, MD: Johns Hopkins University Press: 469–484.

Brody, H. (2003). *Stories of Sickness*. 2nd ed. Oxford; New York: Oxford University Press.

Charon, R. (2007). What to Do with Stories: The Sciences of Narrative Medicine. *Canadian Family Physician*, 53(8): 1265–1267.

Charon, R. (2018). *Narrative Medicine: Honoring the Stories of Illness*. Oxford: Oxford University Press.

Charon, R., DasGupta, S., Hermann, N., Irvine, C., Marcus, E.R., Colon, E.R., Spencer, D. and Spiegel, M. (2017). *The Principles and Practice of Narrative Medicine*. New York: Oxford University Press.

Cook-Lynn, E. (1998). American Indian Intellectualism and the New Indian Story. In D.A. Mihesuah, ed, *Natives and Academics: Researching and Writing About American Indians*. Lincoln: University of Nebraska Press: 57–76.

Crawford, A. (2014). The Trauma Experienced by Generations Past Having an Effect in Their Descendants: Narrative and Historical Trauma Among Inuit in Nunavut, Canada. *Transcultural Psychiatry*, 51(3): 339–369.

Crawford, A. (2017). Where Sickness Comes From: Reading and Unsettling Medicine in the Canadian Arctic. Unpublished PhD thesis. University of Toronto.

Crawford, A. (2018). Dene and Western Medicine Meet in Image-Based Storytelling. *Canadian Medical Association Journal*, 190(36): E1085–E1086.

Crawford, P., Brown, B., Baker, C., Tischler, V. and Abrams, B. (2015). *Health Humanities*. New York: Palgrave Macmillan.

Daschuk, J.W. (2013). Clearing the Plains: Disease, Politics of Starvation, and the Loss of Aboriginal Life. Regina, SK: University of Regina Press.

DasGupta, S. (2006). How to Catch the Story But Not Fall down: Reading Our Way to More Culturally Appropriate Care. *Virtual Mentor*, 5: 315–318.

DasGupta, S. (2017). The Politics of Pedagogy: Cripping, Queering, and Un-Homing Health Humanities. In R. Charon, S. Dasgupta, N. Hermann, E.R. Marcus, E.R. Colon, D. Spencer and M. Spiegel, eds, *The Principles and Practice of Narrative Medicine*. New York: Oxford University Press: 137–156.

DasGupta, S., Meyer, D., Calero-Breckheimer, A., Costley, A.W. and Guillen, S. (2006). Teaching Cultural Competency Through Narrative Medicine: Intersections of Classroom and Community. *Teaching and Learning in Medicine*, 18(1): 14–17.

Dumont, M. (1993). Popular Images of Nativeness. In J.C. Armstrong, ed, *Looking at the Words of Our People: First Nations Analysis of Literature*. Penticton, BC: Theytus Books: 45–50.

Frank, A.W. (2013). *The Wounded Storyteller: Body, Illness, and Ethics*. Chicago: University of Chicago Press.

Gone, J.P. (2007). We Never Was Happy Living like a Whiteman : Mental Health Disparities and the Postcolonial Predicament in American Indian Communities. *American Journal of Community Psychology*, 40(3–4): 290–300.

Good, B. (1994). Medicine, Rationality, and Experience: An Anthropological Perspective. *The Lewis Henry Morgan Lectures 1990*. Cambridge; New York: Cambridge University Press.

Good, B. and Delvecchio Good, M.J. (2000). 'Fiction' and 'Historicity' in Doctors' Stories: Social and Narrative Dimensions of Learning Medicine. In C. Mattingly and L.C. Garro, eds, *Narrative and the Cultural Construction of Illness and Healing*. Berkeley: University of California Press: 50–69.

Hooker, C. and Noonan, E. (2011). Medical Humanities as Expressive of Western Culture. *Medical Humanities*, 37(2): 79–84.

Hunter, K.M. (1991). *Doctors' Stories: The Narrative Structure of Medical Knowledge*. Princeton, NJ: Princeton University Press.

Jones, T., Wear, D., Friedman, L.D. and Pachucki, K., eds, (2014). *Health Humanities Reader*. New Brunswick, NJ: Rutgers University Press.

Justice, D.H. (2008). No Indian Is an Island: On the Ethics of Teaching Indigenous Life Writing Texts. In M. Fuchs and C. Howes, eds, *Teaching Life-writing Texts*. New York: Modern Language Association of America: 252–259.

Kelm, M.E. (1998). Colonizing Bodies: Aboriginal Health and Healing in British Columbia, 1900–50. Vancouver, BC: UBC Press.

Kelton, P. (2015). Cherokee Medicine, Colonial Germs: An Indigenous Nation's Fight against Smallpox, 1518–1824. Norman: University of Oklahoma Press.

Kleinman, A. (1989). The Illness Narratives: Suffering, Healing, and the Human Condition. New York: Basic Books.

LaRoque, E. (2016). Teaching Aboriginal Literature: The Discourse of Margins and Mainstreams. In L. M. Morra and D. Reder, eds, *Learn, Teach, Challenge: Approaching Indigenous Literatures*. Waterloo, ON: Wilfrid Laurier University Press, Vol. 2016: 55–72.

Lux, M.K. (2001). Medicine That Walks: Disease, Medicine and Canadian Plains Native People, 1880–1940. Toronto; Buffalo: University of Toronto Press.

McGrath, R. (1991). Inuit Write about Illness: Standing on Thin Ice. *Arctic Medical Research*, 50(1): 30–36.

McLeod, N. (2007). Cree Narrative Memory: From Treaties to Contemporary Times. Saskatoon, SK: Purich.

Mehl-Madrona, L. (2007). Narrative Medicine: The Use of History and Story in the Healing Process. Rochester, VT: Bear and Company.

Meijer Drees, L. (2013). *Healing Histories: Stories from Canada's Indian Hospitals*. Edmonton: University of Alberta Press.

Mohatt, N.V., Thompson, A.B., Thai, N.D. and Tebes, J.K. (2014). Historical Trauma as Public Narrative: A Conceptual Review of How History Impacts Present-Day Health. *Social Science and Medicine*, 106: 128–136.

Simpson, A. and Smith, A., eds. (2014). *Theorizing Native Studies*. Durham, NC: Duke University Press.

Smith, L.T. (2012). Decolonizing Methodologies: Research and Indigenous Peoples. London: Zed Books.

Vaughan, M. (1991). *Curing Their Ills: Colonial Power and African Illness*. Stanford, Calif: Stanford University Press.

Waldram, J.B., Herring, A. and Kue Young, T. (2006). *Aboriginal Health in Canada: Historical, Cultural, and Epidemiological Perspectives*. 2nd ed. Toronto; Buffalo: University of Toronto Press.

Woods, A. (2011). The Limits of Narrative: Provocations for the Medical Humanities. *Medical Humanities*, 37(2): 73–78.

16

ACCESSIBILITY AND ADVOCACY IN HEALTH HUMANITIES

Susan Levy

Introduction

The landscape of health and social care is being transformed to address the growing complexity and multilayered nature of health. Within this evolving arena of practice, the arts are becoming increasingly visible and fundamental. Embedding access to the arts and humanities within the context of health and social care requires radical new perspectives, innovative ways of working, and the unsettling of established modes of professional practice. Health humanities is situated within this new landscape of health and social care and is exposing the logic of aligning a social lens alongside the prevailing medical paradigm within health. Practitioners have a key role in supporting the genesis of these new ways of working, namely, by advocating for the use of creative methodologies to enable patient narratives to be integral to patient care, and advocating for access to arts-based activities.

The use of the arts in the helping professions has a long history (Bartoli, 2013). Poetry, painting, creative writing, dance, music, and other art forms have been used as therapy, a form of communication, and a means of self-expression. The impact of involvement in the arts within health is situated at the nexus of where the arts and humanities connect with us at a human, social, and emotional level. This level of connection is contextualized in conceiving of art within health and social care as a process, an experience, and relationship (Dewey, 1934), where the "doing" of art leads to meaningful outcomes (Lloyd, 2015). Conceptualizing of art as an experience brings to the fore the importance of relationships, the patient–practitioner relationship, and the role of advocacy and access embedded within that relationship.

This chapter focuses on two key aspects that are essential to the successful integration of the arts into health—access and advocacy—and the role of practitioners in facilitating for both. First, advocacy and the patient voice are explored through the prism of the patient–practitioner relationship. The use of creative approaches is highlighted as a conduit to new ways of communicating and accessing the subjective worlds of patients. Second, the role of advocacy shifts to practitioners mediating and supporting access for patients to arts and humanities activities through social prescribing. The final section of the chapter addresses the need for caution in applying a creative discourse in practice.

Advocacy and accessing patients' voices

Health humanities connect the arts to the social dimensions of health and well-being, to empowering and giving voice to patients through positioning them at the nucleus of their care, which can be actualized through advocacy. As Garden (2015: 77) writes, the "health humanities are in essence a form of advocacy," and a means to represent the under-represented: to give voice to the unknown, to new perspectives that are personal and individual, to expose and make visible the complexity and intersectionality of patients' lives (Kumagai, 2008). For Squier (2007), health and social care practitioners can only know, and therefore represent, patients if they are able and willing to situate them within intersectional identities and their broader sociocultural context. An openness to listen and engage with new narratives, new knowledge, and new ways of seeing and experiencing the world is the foundation for making the social dimensions of people's lives relevant within health care and for enabling advocacy to flourish. This rich tapestry of narratives should be framed by a strengths-based approach (Saleeby, 2012) that celebrates and centers patients' capabilities alongside the differential impact that disability, illness, and health have on everyday lives.

Person-centered practice brings to the fore the voice, the experience, and the ambitions of patients within health care. Balancing the prevailing medical discourse alongside the narratives of patients, while a catalyst for change, is not unproblematic. The health and social care professions are turning to the arts and humanities to help expand the parameters of their understanding of patients' lives, and to see things from patients' perspectives. This paradigm shift requires extending the medical frame of vision to be inclusive of other knowledges and other voices (patients, service users, and carers), voices that for too long have been marginalized within health. The use of the arts and humanities in health and social care is beginning to unlock these voices. Access to the arts is opening innovative ways for patients to express themselves and to communicate with their practitioners. From using images to using their bodies, "the geography closest in" (Rich, 1986: 212), patients' lives are embodied through the arts. These developments are stimulating change and redefining the health and social care discourse (Crawford et al., 2015; Huss and Bos, 2018; Levy, 2018).

Let us consider what this might look like in practice, through a scenario of a health practitioner empowering their patients to advocate and (re)present themselves in their day-to-day life. The creative use of Photovoice (Capous-Desyllas and Bromfield, 2018) enables the practitioner to ask a patient, who would benefit from being more physically active, to take a photo of their daily walk or exercise. The photos provide an insight into the sociocultural aspects of the patient's life alongside their physical activity. The photos enable the patient to creatively (re)present themselves to their health practitioner and open a dialogue for reflective discussion. At the core of this simple and achievable example is a relationship between patient and practitioner: here, both have a voice and knowledge to contribute to identifying and achieving health outcomes. This scenario visualizes art as advocacy, enacted through practitioners integrating creative methodologies into the patient–practitioner relationship.

Creative approaches open a space for reimagining the relational dynamic that occurs between patients and practitioners (Atkinson et al., 2015). The emerging relationships that develop through this process are built on trust and are fluid, providing for reciprocal learning and unlearning, for knowing and unknowing. Advocacy emerges here through practitioners having the confidence, knowledge, and "permission" (Levy and Young, 2018) to work in new and innovative ways.

Social prescribing: advocating for access to the arts

Arts prescribing is a form of social prescribing that refers specifically to advocating for involvement in arts activities (Stickley and Eades, 2013; Stickley and Hui, 2012). Social prescribing involves health and social care practitioners working collaboratively with patients to identify and advocate for involvement in community-based activities, including the arts. (The generic term *social prescribing* is used in this chapter.) Social prescribing complements, and for some patients replaces, traditional medical interventions to enhance overall well-being and reduce hospital admissions, thus creating new possibilities for reimagining health prescribing. It is being used across the spectrum of medical and social dimensions of health, for conditions including Parkinson's (McGill et al., 2018), in mental health (Sapouna and Pamer, 2016), and in survivors of domestic violence (Gray and Schubert, 2010), through to patients who are marginalized and isolated (Loftus et al., 2017). It has been found to support the development of social capital (Bourdieu, 1986) and to address some of the underlying social determinants of health inequalities (Mani, 2017; Morton et al., 2015). Outcomes from prescribing involvement in arts-based activities coalesce around meaningful relationships, a sense of belonging, confidence, and overall well-being; "it is the quality of the human relationships and the atmosphere that is created by the service providers that was of most significance to the participants" (Stickley and Hui, 2012: 578).

The first UK survey of general practitioners' views on social prescribing and the use of arts in health care was launched in 2018 (Aesop, 2018). The findings reveal 66% of respondents in agreement that the arts could make a positive contribution to improving health and well-being. A key challenge and opportunity for general practitioners and other health professionals to translate this vision into reality is around access: access in relation to the availability of arts and humanities activities that are accessible (physically, socially, culturally. and economically); access to information about the availability of activities to signpost patients (Alliance-Scotland, 2016); and access to collaborative working between health, social care/social work and arts-based practitioners to share knowledge and co-produce meaningful outcomes. Throughout this chapter references to health care have intentionally been broadened to health and social care/social work. This is an acknowledgement of the need for collaborative working to achieve the ambitions of the arts contributing to health and well-being outcomes through social workers/social care practitioners facilitating access to community arts-based activities.

The following four points act as scaffolding to frame, guide, and support advocating for and mediating access to the arts as a conduit for transforming future health and social care:

1. *Knowledge-based advocacy*

    • Development of a comprehensive evidence base concerning the impact of the arts in health and social care, to support decision-making in advocating access to creative practices.

2. *Accessible arts*

    • Development of accessible, sustainable, and inclusive arts and humanities activities that can accommodate a diversity of health and social care needs.

3. *Accessible information*

    • Access for patients and health care and social care practitioners to relevant and current information on the availability and accessibility of arts and humanities-based activities.

4. *Integrated working*

- Effective collaborative working between patients and health-care, social care, and arts-based practitioners sharing different knowledges to co-produce health and well-being outcomes.

Creativity in policy and practice

The integration of arts and humanities into health and social care is occurring in parallel to a policy discourse around creativity. At a time of prevailing neoliberalism, austerity, and limited budgets, health and social care practitioners are tasked with being more innovative and creative in their practice. "The professional and the supported person should develop creative solutions to meet the outcomes identified in the support plan" (Scottish Government, 2013). Creative practice, if used uncritically, may achieve economic rationalization, but may fail to connect with the art, the emotional, relational, and affective aspects of creativity. As Negus and Pickering (2000: 260) have noted, creativity risks being a "dominant category, but a residual concept." Caution should thus be exercised in supporting greater access to creative practice that could inhibit "the articulation of crucial advocacy arguments" (Madden and Bloom, 2004:134; 2001) and enabling patients to (re)present themselves. The rationale for creativity in practice must retain a focus on advocating for and mediating access to activities that can stimulate aesthetic affect and change in patients' lives. Furthermore, the essence of creative freedom should not be stifled or suppressed through the assimilation of the arts into health care or the "ineffable character of arts ... lost in clinical service provision" (Broderick, 2011: 106). Strategic planning and policy development around the integration of arts into health care must be advocated through a united voice, that is, a voice that reflects and retains the unique attributes of each discipline: the arts, health care, and social care.

Conclusion

Health humanities offer a contemporary lens for advocating for change in the delivery and experience of health and social care. There is a natural synergy between health, social care, and the arts that practitioners can use as they integrate the social dimensions of health alongside or in place of traditional medical perspectives. The integration of the arts into health and social care practice has led to health narratives being diversified and inclusive of patient voices. These ambitions are being achieved through practitioners working more creatively, using arts-based methodologies in their practice to advocate for patients to (re)present themselves in context; and through social prescribing, advocating, and mediating access to arts and humanities activities. Further work is required to ensure these developments become sustainable, visible, and accessible; and that advocacy for the arts is sustained as a fundamental driver in the evolving landscape of health and social care.

References

Aesop (2018). *Aesop announces 'dramatic' results of a brand new survey of health professionals attitudes to the arts in social prescribing*, 23 July 2018, www.ae-sop.org/2018/07/23/aesop-announces-dramatic-results-of-a-brand-new-survey-of-health-professionals-attitudes-to-the-arts-role-in-social-prescribing/ (Accessed 18/2/2019).

Alliance-Scotland. (2016). *Developing a Culture of Health: The Role of Signposting and Social Prescribing in Improving Health and Wellbeing*. Edinburgh, Alliance-Scotland.

Atkinson, S., Evans, B., Woods, A. and Kearns, R. (2015). The 'Medical' and the 'Health' in a Critical Medical Humanities. *Journal of Medical Humanities*, 36: 71–81.

Bartoli, A. (2013). Creative Arts in the Professions: Contributions to Learning in Practice. *Journal of Practice Teaching and Learning*, 12(1): 3–5.

Bourdieu, P. (1986). *Distinction: A Social Critique of the Judgement of Taste*. London, Routledge and Kegan Paul.

Broderick, S. (2011). Arts Practices in Unreasonable Doubt? Reflections on Understandings of Arts Practices in Healthcare Contexts. *Arts and Health: An International Journal for Research, Policy and Practice*, 3(2): 95–109.

Capous-Desyllas, M. and Bromfield, N.F. (2018). Using an Arts-Informed Eclectic Approach to Photovoice Data Analysis. *International Journal of Qualitative Methods*, 17: 1–14.

Crawford, P., Brown, B., Baker, C. Tischler, V. and Abrams, B. (2015). *Health Humanities*. London, Palgrave Macmillan.

Dewey, J. (1934). *Art as Experience*. New York, Penguin.

Garden, R. (2015). Who Speaks For Whom? Health Humanities and the Ethics of Representation. *Medical Humanities*, 41: 77–80.

Gray, M. and Schubert, L. (2010). Turning Base Metal into Gold: Transmuting Art, Practice, Research and Experience into Knowledge. *British Journal of Social Work*, 40: 2308–2325.

Huss, E. and Bos, E. eds., (2018). *Art in Social Work Practice: Theory and Practice: International Perspectives*. London, Routledge.

Kumagai, A.K. (2008). A Conceptual Framework for the Use of Illness Narratives in Medical Education. *Academic Medicine*, 83(7): 653–658.

Levy, S. (2018). Recreating the Social Work Imagination: Embedding the Arts within Scottish Social Work. In: E. Huss and E. Bos, eds., *Art in Social Work Practice: Theory and Practice: International Perspectives*, London, Routledge: 44.

Levy, S. and Young, H. (2018). *The Ripple Effect: Relational Social Care through Art*. Dundee, University of Dundee. www.scribd.com/document/393964577/The-Ripple-Effect.

Lloyd, K. (2015). Being with, Across, Over and Through: Art's Caring Subjects, Ethics Debates and Encounters. In: A. Dimitrakaki and K. Lloyd, eds., *Economy, Art, Production and the Subject in the 21st Century*, Liverpool, Liverpool University Press: 140–157.

Loftus, A.M., McCauley, F. and McCarron, M.O. (2017). Impact of Social Prescribing on General Practice Workload and Polypharmacy. *Public Health*, 148: 96–101.

Madden, C. and Bloom, T. (2001). Advocating Creativity. *Cultural Policy*, 7(3): 409–436.

Madden, C. and Bloom, T. (2004). Creativity, Health and Arts Advocacy. *International Journal of Cultural Policy*, 10(2): 133–156.

Mani, G. (2017). Social Prescribing for Healthy Aging: Sustaining Social Capital in India. *Family Medicine and Community Health*, 5(3): 208–210.

McGill, A., Houston, S. and Lee, R.Y.W. (2018). The Effects of a Ballet-Based Dance Intervention on Gait Variability and Balance Confidence on People with Parkinson's. *Arts and Health: An International Journal for Research and Practice*, 11(2): 133–146.

Morton, L., Ferguson, M. and Baty, F. (2015). Improving Wellbeing and Self-efficacy by Social Prescription. *Public Health*, 129: 286–289.

Negus, K. and Pickering, M. (2000). Creativity and Cultural Production. *International Journal of Cultural Policy*, 6(2): 259–282.

Rich, A. (1986). *Blood, Bread, and Poetry: Selected Prose, 1079–1985*. New York, Norton and Co.

Saleeby, D. ed., (2012). *The Strengths Perspective in Social Work Practice*. 6th ed. Boston, Pearson Education.

Sapouna, L. and Pamer, E. (2016). The Transformative Potential of the Arts in Mental Health Recovery: An Irish Research Project. *Arts and Health: An International Journal for Research and Practice*, 8(1): 1–12.

Scottish Government (2013). *Statutory guidance to accompany the social care (Self-Directed Support) (Scotland) Act 2013* www.gov.scot/publications/statutory-guidance-accompany-social-care-self-directed-support-scotland-act-2013/#res446933 (Accessed 18/2/2019).

Squier, S.M. (2007). Beyond Nescience: The Intersectional Insights of the Health Humanities. *Perspectives in Biological Medicine*, 50(3): 334–347.

Stickley, T. and Eades, M. (2013). Arts on Prescription: A Qualitative Outcomes Study. *Public Health*, 127: 727–734.

Stickley, T. and Hui, A. (2012). Social Prescribing through Arts on Prescription in a UK City: Participants' Perspectives (1). *Public Health*, 126: 574–579.

17

THE ROLE OF THE IMAGINATION IN THE PRACTICES OF THE HEALTH HUMANITIES

Marina Tsaplina and Raymond Barfield

Introduction

Whoever you are, no matter how lonely,
the world offers itself to your imagination,
calls to you like the wild geese, harsh and exciting –
over and over announcing your place
in the family of things.

> *(Mary Oliver, "Wild Geese")*

We are still reluctant to admit that the poetic imagination sets the bounds for human thought. At the heart of philosophy's quarrel with poetry is the fear that the imagination goes all the way down.

> *(Rorty, 2016: 3)*

Health-care practices are rapidly changing under the forces of economic realities, corporate transformation of institutions, and advances in artificial intelligence. In the next decade these structural forces, if left un-reimagined, will alter the landscape of medical education, practice, and economics, and increase the risk of exacerbating dehumanization in health care. The threat is substantial, but because highly developed communication skills are required for decision making in these ever more complicated health-care settings, there will be new opportunities, and urgent need, for deeper integration of the arts and humanities into the pedagogies and practices of health care.

The trust implicit in the virtuous practice of medicine demands that clinicians learn to reach beyond their own assumptions in order to hear and be affected by the details of the unfamiliar worlds of patients. Bruno Latour described this as developing "an articulate body ... holding to a dynamic definition of the body as 'learning to be affected'" (Latour, 2004: 209). This demands acknowledging the vulnerability and variation of human bodies, including the clinician's own (Mol, 2011; Butler, 2014; Charon, 2016; Dasgupta, 2008), and training clinician imaginations to perceive the way structural foundations of health (Metzl and Hansen, 2014) and biopolitical power (Washington, 2010; Casper and Moore, 2009; Clare, 2017) shape embodied lives. The details of a patient's world are revealed through the stories they tell through multiple material languages. Without curiosity and respect for these stories, medical technology can become an act of assault rather than an act of healing. Likewise, people who are seeking health care must learn to listen to the stories of their own bodies and be shown that these testimonies (Woods, 2012; Frank, 2013) will be received by their health-care team.

The act of telling and listening to stories of any kind depends upon the imagination, that dimension of the body–mind capable of arranging and rearranging elements of an as yet unknown, or only partially known, emerging life-world. Defining *imagination* is itself a creative task that evokes the dynamism of imagination as a living act of the mind, resisting completion and finality. Definitions of the imagination are placeholders, important for discussion but inclining toward a stasis that is foreign to the very function of imagination. This is demonstrated by noticing what is shared and what is different in the following definitions, made 150 years apart:

> Imagination: The power to recombine the materials furnished by experience or memory, for the accomplishment of an elevated purpose; the power of conceiving and expressing the ideal.
>
> *(Webster and Porter, 1895: 730)*

> [The act of imagination poses a puzzle] between the *transcendent* uses of imagination, which enable one to escape from or look beyond the world as it is, and the *instructive* uses of imagination, which enable one to learn about the world as it is ... the two uses differ not in kind, but in degree—specifically, the degree of constraint on imaginings.
>
> *(Liao and Gendler, 2019)*

Both of these definitions illuminate the place of imagination in rich articulations of the meaning of *health*, such as this one:

> Imagine health as the capacity to acknowledge and artistically mobilize *memory* and *hope* as ongoing features of the unique qualities of being human ... The journey of health requires a capacity to create meaning from a chaotic past while bringing forward the image of a hoped-for future.
>
> *(Lederach and Lederach, 2010: 202)*

However we define imagination (see also Kind and Kung, 2016), when clinicians begin to talk about purpose and meaning in the life of an individual, they have stopped using the methods of science, and have started using a kind of imaginative work more closely associated with the humanities and the arts. This chapter will address the role of imagination in cooperative medical decision making and will discuss approaches to fostering imaginative nimbleness, richness, and maturity. It will provide a frame for understanding the central role of imagination in health-care practices that facilitate care as an embodied, relational process as opposed to a transactional product (Mol, 2011; Montori, 2017), and it will draw on the humanities and the arts as our best reservoir of insight into the content and concrete practices of the imagination.

Storytelling between and beyond words

One comment by physician William Osler has been passed down in medical education for over a century because of how deeply it resonates with so many in medicine: "It is much more important to know what sort of patient has a disease than to know which disease a patient has." For patients, storytelling in the hospital is literally a matter of life and death. If illness stories are not at the center of clinical encounters, all sorts of terrible things can happen. In whatever ways modern health care changes, beauty and suffering still meet in the arena of storytelling. Storytelling makes use of every aspect of imagination because it reaches into every aspect of human meaning.

In order for clinicians to receive and discern the full story of a person, they must employ a dimension of imaginative reach that has been called *sociological imagination* (Mills, 2000 [1959]). The concept of sociological imagination acknowledges the ways an individual's biography and health emerge from historical processes that occur within larger social and economic contexts, strengthening structural competency (Metzl and Hansen, 2014; Tsevat et al., 2015). Such imaginative reach allows our perceptions to move past a narrow focus on individualized biological function, and to open into the multidimensional lived experiences of human beings embedded in histories.

Unfortunately, modern medicine often lacks the imaginative capacity to receive such stories and to be changed by them. How clinicians imagine human worth and dignity holds great consequence (Schoen, 2005; Urwin, 2019). Patient communities are constantly searching for the languages that may articulate their lives. The difficulty of giving an account of one's self in the middle of the often-disorienting experience of illness or disability is profound, because both illness and structural violence (Farmer et al., 2006) may tear through and fracture the self. These fractures are re-created through institutions, policies, procedures, and violations enacted along historically gendered, racialized, and normative body lines. Ordinary language can be rendered incoherent, leaving people with little more than a checklist of events recounted in a way that further numbs us to our experience of the unspeakable. Certain kinds of suffering seem to demand silence, suffering that would only be accentuated were we to attempt to speak—especially when the language that is our way of saying what is most important is rendered invalid by an institution or a practice. Great pain and violence can tear apart our familiar languages. In such cases, "when experiences become unrepresentable and conventional language insufficient, voice beyond words needs a new language" (Lederach, 2011: 189).

Two stories of imagination in suffering, care, and healing

Story #1

The increased morphine doses had no effect on reducing the pain of the old man who was dying from cancer. The nights of screaming remained uncountable. Begging, again, for an enema, he was told he just had three in the past several days. The author of this article leaned over the hospital bed and whispered "Papa, the enema won't help. It's the cancer." These words suddenly seemed to create an understanding in him that before was unreachable. "The ... cancer?," he repeated, and immediately exclaimed "Then pull it out!" The nurse in the room who had previously administered the morphine raised his hands and, half-laughing in helplessness, said to the daughter, "I'm sorry, I can't do that, that's not possible." Her rational, atheist, dogmatic father was screaming in pain for his cancer to be pulled out from him on what was to be the last night of his life, and with nothing left to offer, she began to pull. Not touching her father but doing the gesture of pulling to help her own belief in the reality of the imaginative act, she told him how awful that substance was, how disgusting it was. "Papa, I'm pulling it out. Is it helping?" "Yes! Yes! Keep pulling!," he yelled. She told him that it was so painful and strong and horrible that she barely had enough strength to pull it all out, but that she will be strong enough. After minutes, or centuries, she said, "I have pulled it all out, Papa. Do you feel better?" "Yes," he said, "yes . . ." And soon after, he fell asleep.

Story #2

The doctor had known exactly what to say to her at the beginning, when "cure" was still possible. But as the patient grew sicker from side effects of the bone marrow transplant—the only thing that remained in his doctor-toolbox—the doctor became mute. He became mute, except when he was endlessly disturbing the silence with chatter about changes in laboratories and X-rays and dialysis schedules. He did not know what to do with her mortality other than to listen to her heart with his stethoscope and say things about the next experimental medicine he would try. He did not know what to do when he asked where it hurt, and she answered, "It hurts everywhere." One night he was at home and his phone rang: "She died, and they are asking for you." What could he possibly say to the family? She was only 12 years old. Why did he feel so much failure? Why did he feel relief? Why would they be asking for him to come to the bedside, when he had failed to cure her? He drove into the hospital, listening to a song by Jeffrey Foucault, "Stripping Cane." When he walked into the room, and saw her on the bed, her mother came over to him and hugged him and said, "Thank you." Thank you? People in the room were laughing and telling stories. They invited him to be human. They invited him to grow his imagination about what the practice of medicine means. He accepted the invitation.

Imagination is a practice

The imaginations of health-care providers need to be trained to be able to reimagine the metaphors (Bleakley, 2017), and thus the contours, of medical practice. If clinicians are trained to perceive, and to discern, the nuances of embodied experience, they may begin to hear in their patients' testimonies one of the main points of metaphor: the achievement of intimacy (Cohen, 1978). The maker of the metaphor offers a concealed invitation that the listener deliberately, and with intentional effort, interprets and accepts. Such an exchange acknowledges and is even constitutive of community.

Imagination is the force that allows the mind to become aware of reality that exists at the margin of the mind's current experience, expanding what is available to rational thought, to feeling, and to the language we use to express thought and feeling. Reality will always be larger than our language, which means that imaginative leaps will always be required for discovery. The elasticity of the imagination allows our minds to create schemas of reality and to adapt to reality, as our schemas grow. Languages of various sorts—words, painting, music, dance, drama—are the grappling hooks that imagination uses to ascend, to climb, to discover, and cultivate articulate, affected bodies. Francis Bacon (1561–1626) said the excellent question is half of wisdom. We might add (and Bacon would likely agree) that the source of the excellent question is the imagination.

The imagination is the origin of any hypothesis that leads to discovery, because the imagination first glimpses the discoverable law, extending the mind's reach into new territory, and shining light into areas that are as yet dark to our understanding. When points of information appear in the world, the imagination apprehends the invisible connections that make a whole from the pieces. The imagination and the power of rationality are always working in tandem when genuine insight into reality is at hand. In the great artist, just as in the great scientist, rationality must be developed along with imagination's power to reach toward the unfamiliar and the unknown, and to contribute to new articulations of reality. All great discovery depends upon this. Knowledge grows in this way. If only one of these forces is developed, the result is bad art and bad science. Trouble comes when our philosophical frames dogmatically truncate the reach of imagination. Philosophy is fundamentally the ability to see the world, increasing our awareness of reality in a way that depends on our commitments. But these commitments depend upon the capacity of our imaginations, the ability of our minds to reach past what we take as already known within our lived experience (Barfield, 2017).

As discovery involves meaningful connections we have not seen before, artistic practice and inquiry constitutes a substantive research practice that may yield knowledge, a form of questioning that progresses through the formation and reformation of reality, and our responses to it. Art renders the familiar world strange and through this process inspires revelation, allowing for a tired reality to once again be seen with wonder. A successful artistic work is testimony to a shaping-through-questioning of reality, forging new connections among the infinite dots of information that were once unconnected, or reconnecting existing patterns in striking ways. For this reason, there is no end to the meanings of aesthetic experiences. Works of art have a claim on us, not simply because they are significant in themselves, but because they are capable of transforming our matrix of meanings and associations, and by doing so they may change our entire horizon of understanding (Cunningham et al., 2007). This is broadly true of human experience in the world, and it is certainly true of human experience within the strange world of health care that encounters us when we are at the limits of our fragility and strength.

The label of "patient" or of "clinician" does not describe the entirety of the person's involved in a clinical encounter. But if the urgent, human work that occurs in the arena of medical practice is to be careful and kind, the work of the imagination is necessary to bridge the permanent gap (Barabino and Assal, 2009) between the world of a person who is a patient for a time, and the world of a person who is a clinician for a time.

The strangeness of disembodied medicine

One astonishing aspect of the current crisis in medicine is that its practices are strangely disembodied. Numbers, laboratory values, radiographic images, and reports are often valued as the primary accounts—the primary *articulations* (Latour, 2004)—of the reality of the body. These "objects of medicine" presuppose forms of imagination, perception, and activity (Good, 1994), and are generated through specific medical practices and technologies (Mol, 2002). Medicine's articulations of the body are held to be true, objective, and primary, while the multiple articulations of the lived body by patients—who hold their own sets of material language practices—are seen as secondary and merely "subjective." Yet what if we follow the great proposal of Bruno Latour while not immediately disturbing medicine's hierarchy of reality that is divided along the objective/subjective divide? What if we supplement it with practices, frameworks, and pedagogies that can hold the multiple, multiplying, and contrasting articulations of bodies-in-illness for both health-care providers and patients alike? Doing so might lead to the formation of new ways of seeing the human being within medicine. In fact, it might lead to the recovery of embodiment in health care.

The body is the ground of our history, retaining memory, trauma, imagination, and desire. Illness can fracture this body, and through such fractures surprising aspects of the self often emerge. A fractured self may be healed in the domains of breath, thought, feeling, imagination, and history. The fractures can be reintegrated, even if the physical condition does not leave. This is why a cure may not necessarily heal, and healing does not depend on a cure.

Embodiment requires the integration of all of these dimensions in the human being (Tsaplina et al., 2018), and is indispensable to an embodied practice of health care. This echoes ancient Chinese wisdom that holds that we are not born fully human, but rather only become so as we cultivate ourselves and our relations with others (Kleinman, 2009). This integration also depends on recognizing that the physical and metaphysical are interwoven and inseparable (Nancy,1999). This can lead to conclusions that go against the grain of medicine's standard account of the body, but this is to be expected. Medicine emphasizes biological materiality, to the exclusion of what might be called *poetic materiality*—a way of accounting for how the imagination wraps around and shapes our experience of physical structures and even the physical structures themselves across personal, social, historic, and biopolitical planes.

This active, interchanging relationship between the observer and the observed is supported by the evolving views of cognitive scientists, who now widely accept that human cognition emerges not from observing a static object and environment that is separate from the self, but rather from a dynamic interaction and co-creation between the perceiver and the environment.

> Organisms do not passively receive information from their environments, which they then translate into internal representations. Natural cognitive systems ... participate in the generation of meaning through their bodies and action, often engaging in transformational and not merely informational interactions: they enact a world.
>
> *(Paolo et al., 2014: 39; Varela et al., 2016)*

"Enactivism" posits that observers actively shape the worlds they perceive: an *enacted* world cannot be described from a third-person perspective. This insight is one that resonates deeply with Eastern understandings of consciousness in the practices of meditation and mindfulness, as mindfulness is always a mindfulness *of* something, cultivating a steady awareness of the deep interrelationality of all matter and beings (Ricard and Singer, 2018). Such a view can lead to radically different ways of framing even the most technologically advanced parts of medicine.

Care as a relational embodied process

Medical education will not prepare clinicians for great practice in this most human of arenas unless it learns to cultivate an understanding about care as something neither idealized nor transactional: that is, as not antithetical to technological advancement, or conceivable as a "transactional product" that can be packaged into an efficient set of procedures with a factory-like beginning, middle, and end. Rather, care is a process rooted in daily practices that attempt to respond and attune to the changing needs of unpredictable body–minds. "The logic of care starts out from the fleshiness and fragility of life" (Mol, 2011: 13). The response of care is also a deeply imaginative act.

When a clinician walks into a room, meets a family, closes the door, and engages in the partnership that occurs in the ideal practice of health care, everyone in the room becomes vulnerable in a way that would not have occurred apart from that circumstance. This originates in the vulnerability of the patient's body, whether or not this is acknowledged by the patient, family, and clinician. This vulnerability creates an imbalance of need, which in turn creates an imbalance of power. The intrinsic fragility of this relationship, brought about in part by the power imbalance, is mitigated only when the vulnerability of the clinician's own body is acknowledged by both the clinician and the patient. Acknowledging this shared vulnerability and mutual interdependence can reduce the potential for violence toward patients that is made possible when one person has power over another (Shapiro, 2018). It can also reduce the isolation clinicians experience when they are placed outside the sphere of human vulnerability by being assigned a role that demands that they never make a mistake, never show weakness, and never fail to solve a problem, cure an illness, or fix something that is broken. "Care is goal-driven, but it is irreducible to the outcome ... it acknowledges that bodies with disease are unpredictable" (Mol, 2011: 23).

If medical education wants to meet the pragmatic challenges the future holds, while also giving students a deeper view of what the body is, what illness is, and what a person is, it must incorporate practices from the arts and the humanities into its pedagogy. These are where human wisdom related to embodied experience is stored. There is no other way to nurture imaginative inquiry. Artistic inquiry is a research practice that asks questions and makes discoveries through making, giving form to the imagination through forming and reforming the patterns of our perceptions of reality, researching and playing with the relationship between the human being and our world. It is through rigorous and reflective practice that theoretical knowledges and lived experiences can be embodied, made meaningful, and thus contribute to the generation of new understandings (Barbour, 2006).

Embodied artistic inquiry helps clinicians gain *articulated bodies* (Latour, 2004), that is, bodies that have learned to be affected (Despret, 2004). It gives form and voice even to questions whose answers can never be complete, but whose asking is indispensable to being authentically human. Imaginative inquiry tempers the place of control held by technological innovation and biomedicine, by reminding us to be reverent toward the integrity of living things whose transient, but beautiful, forms express poetic materiality. The language of imagination is sometimes strange to our ears, until we have moved deep into the ways the humanities and the arts illuminate health-care practices. But medicine also, and quite often, asks patients to accept language and concepts that are unfamiliar and strange: it is fair to ask clinicians to return the favor of remaining open, curious, and willing to learn something new.

References

Barabino, B. and Assal, J.-P. (2009). Art Beyond Therapy: When Patients and Healthcare Providers Share the Limelight. *DiabetesVoice*, 54(Special Issue): 36–39.

Barbour, K. (2006). Embodied Engagement in Arts Research. *International Journal of the Arts in Society*, 1(2): 85–91.

Barfield, R. (2017). *Wager: Beauty, Suffering, and Being in the World*, Eugene, OR: Cascade Books.

Bleakley, A. (2017). *Thinking with Metaphors in Medicine: The State of the Art*. Abingdon, Oxon: Routledge.

Butler, J. (2014). *Vulnerability and Resistance*. https://profession.mla.org/vulnerability-and-resistance/ (Accessed 8/12/2019).

Casper, M.J. and Moore, L.J. (2009). *Missing Bodies: The Politics of Visibility*. New York: New York University Press.

Charon, R. (2016). The Shock of Attention. *Enthymema*, 16: 6–17.

Clare, E. (2017). *Brilliant Imperfection: Grappling with Cure*. Durham: Duke University Press.

Cohen, T. (1978). Metaphor and the Cultivation of Intimacy. *Critical Inquiry*, 5(1): 3–12.

Cunningham, C., Candler, P.M. and Davey, N. (2007). Doubled Reflection: Gadamer, Aesthetics and the Question of Spiritual Experience. In: C. Cunningham and P.M. Candler, eds, *Transcendence and Phenomenology*. London: SCM Press: 151–173.

Dasgupta, S. (2008). Narrative Humility. *Lancet*, 371(9617): 980–981.

Despret, V. (2004). The Body We Care For: Figures of Anthropo-Zoo-Genesis. *Body & Society*, 10(2–3): 111–134.

Farmer, P.E., Nizeye, B., Stulac, S. and Keshavjee, S. (2006). Structural Violence and Clinical Medicine. *PLoS medicine*, 3(10): e449.

Frank, A. (2013). *The Wounded Storyteller: Body, Illness, and Ethics*, Chicago, IL: University of Chicago Press.

Good, B.J. (1994). How Medicine Constructs Its Objects. In: B.J. Good, ed, Medicine, Rationality, and Experience: An Anthropological Perspective. Cambridge: Cambridge University Press: 68.

Kind, A. and Kung, P. (2016). *Knowledge Through Imagination*. Oxford: Oxford University Press.

Kleinman, A. (2009). Caregiving: The Odyssey of Becoming More Human. *The Lancet*, 373(9660): 292–293.

Latour, B. (2004). How to Talk About the Body? The Normative Dimension of Science Studies. *Body & Society*, 10(2–3): 205–229.

Lederach, J.P. and Lederach, A.J. (2010). The Resonating Echo of Social Healing. In: J.P. Lederach and A.J. Lederach, eds, *When Blood and Bones Cry Out: Journeys Through the Soundscape of Healing and Reconciliation*. New York, NY: Oxford University Press: 197–224.

Liao, S.-yi and Gendler, T. (2019). Imagination. *Stanford Encyclopedia of Philosophy*. Available at: https://plato.stanford.edu/entries/imagination/ (Accessed 29/1/2019).

Metzl, J.M. and Hansen, H. (2014). Structural Competency: Theorizing a New Medical Engagement with Stigma and Inequality. *Social Science and Medicine*, 103: 126–133.

Mills, C.W. (2000). *The Sociological Imagination*. New York, NY: Oxford University Press.

Mol, A., and Duke University Press. (2002). *The Body Multiple: Ontology in Medical Practice*. Durham, NC: Duke University Press.

Mol, A. (2011). *The Logic of Care: Health and the Problem of Patient Choice*. London: Routledge.

Montori, V.M. (2017). *Why We Revolt: A Patient Revolution for Careful and Kind Care*. Rochester, MN: The Patient Revolution.

Nancy, J.-L. (1999). L'Intrus. Available at: www.maxvanmanen.com/files/2014/10/Nancy-LIntrus.pdf (Accessed 19/2/2019).

Oliver, M. (1986). Wild Geese. In: M. Oliver, *Dream Work*. Boston: Atlantic Monthly Press.

Paolo, E., Rhohde, M. and Jaegher, H. (2014). Horizons for the Enactive Mind: Values, Social Interaction, and Play. In: S. Stewart, O. Gapenne and E.A. Di Paolo, eds, *Enaction: Toward a New Paradigm for Cognitive Science*. Cambridge, MA: MIT Press: 33–88.

Ricard, M. and Singer, W. (2018). *Beyond the Self: Conversations Between Buddhism and Neuroscience*. Cambridge, MA: MIT Press.

Rorty, R. (2016). *Philosophy as Poetry*. Charlottesville: University of Virginia Press.

Schoen, J. (2005). *Choice & Coercion: Birth Control, Sterilization, and Abortion in Public Health and Welfare*. Chapel Hill: University of North Carolina Press.

Shapiro, J. (2018). "Violence" in Medicine: Necessary and Unnecessary, Intentional and Unintentional. *Philosophy, Ethics, and Humanities in Medicine*, 13(1). doi:10.1186/s13010-018-0059-y.

Tsaplina, M., Odendahl-James, J. and Bend, T. (2018). Attending to the Illusion of life: Reimagining Medicine Through the Art of Puppetry Practice. *Puppetry International*, 44(Puppetry Social Action/Social Justice special issue): 16–19.

Tsevat, R.K., Sinha, A.A., Gutierrez, K.J. and DasGupta, S. (2015). Bringing Home the Health Humanities: Narrative Humility, Structural Competency, and Engaged Pedagogy. *Academic Medicine*, 90(11): 1462–1465.

Urwin, R. (2019, May 12). Doctors Are Warned That Learning Disability or Down's Syndrome Is No Reason Not to Resuscitate a Patient. Retrieved from www.thetimes.co.uk/article/doctors-warned-that-learning-disabilities-or-downs-no-reason-not-to-resuscitate-patients-62jfwqxht

Varela, F.J., Thompson, E. and Rosch, E. (2016). *The Embodied Mind Cognitive Science and Human Experience.* Cambridge, MA: MIT Press.

Washington, H. A. (2010). *Medical Apartheid The Dark History of Medical Experimentation on Black Americans from Colonial Times to the Present.* Paradise, CA: Paw Prints.

Webster, N. and Porter, N. (1895). Imagination. In: *Webster's International Dictionary of the English Language; Being the Authentic Edition of Webster's Unabridged Dictionary, Comprising the Issues of 1864, 1879, and 1884,* Springfield, MA: G. and G. Merriam: 730.

Woods, A. (2012). Rethinking "Patient Testimony" in the Medical Humanities: The Case of *Schizophrenia Bulletin*'s First Person Accounts. *Journal of Literature and Science,* 6(1): 38–54.

18

INVENTING EDWARD JENNER

Historicizing anti-vaccination

Travis Chi Wing Lau

Introduction

Mary Wortley Montagu's importation of Turkish variolation in 1818 marked one of the earliest attempts in English culture to prevent smallpox epidemics, which continued to claim upwards of 400,000 lives each year in the eighteenth century. Medical professionals believed that variolation—the process of deliberately infecting an individual with smallpox material taken from an infected or recently variolated person to produce a mild case—protected the inoculated for life after inducing a mild case of smallpox and, as a kind of "natural infection," would less likely be fatal. Yet frequently cases of variolation became full-blown outbreaks of smallpox, which scarred or even killed those who consented to the lancet. In many cases, the inoculated still contracted bouts of smallpox. By the 1760s medical men like John Fewster, Benjamin Jesty, and Peter Plett were considering the use of cowpox as a smallpox substitute in inoculation procedures. Edward Jenner's experiments in 1796 were meant to intervene in this culture of inoculation inconsistently and dangerously performed. Yet, ultimately, Jenner's sights were on something grander: the elimination of smallpox entirely. His efforts would popularize a practice that would lead to over 100,000 vaccinations by the turn of the century and, ultimately, the first and only instance of an epidemic disease being eradicated on a global scale.

Yet vaccination's success story has obscured the history of the late eighteenth-century culture wars that led to the very invention of "the Jennerian technique" as a nationalized medical procedure. It would also be these culture wars waged between Jenner and his detractors that would transform his public image from country doctor to medical hero. Edward Jenner was not the first person to discover vaccination, but he was the first to recognize its potential to galvanize an English public that could rally behind the practice's symbolic and biological value. His strategic collaborations with men of letters, physicians, and politicians helped to consolidate a narrative of salvific vaccination that claimed to preserve the English national body from the dangers of revolutionary fervor and fevers coming from France and the colonies: the immunizing of individual citizen's bodies contributed to the collective protection of the body politic and the affirmation of a healthy national body. How did Jenner dispel insecurities about vaccination's dangers while simultaneously selling its novelty and supposedly inherent Englishness? This chapter examines the understudied archive of propaganda from this pamphlet war to trace how insecurities about vaccination were imagined by figures on both sides of the debate. I argue that the rhetoric from these documents still underpins contemporary anti-vaccination movements resistant to scientific and political claims of vaccination's undeniable necessity. The politicization of preventative medicine through the circulation and reproduction of Jennerian—as well as anti-Jennerian—propaganda reveals the vast extent to which vaccination became a battleground over what constituted personal, public, and political security.

Jenner's (re)invention

Before Edward Jenner embarked on his public campaigns for vaccination, he began as an apprentice to both an apothecary and a surgeon. While this garnered Jenner practical experience that may have set him apart from other physicians, such hands-on training was still understood to be a "long way from being abstract and bookish[;] it emphasizes practice, not medical theory" (Jordanova, 2000: 87). Surgeons and apothecaries, seen as a rank below their more learned counterparts, steadily aimed to reform their image as lesser medical men. Jenner was deeply aware of these stereotypes surrounding the "lower" orders of eighteenth-century medicine and sought to revise them in his vaccination campaigns by intentionally blurring the already shifting professional boundaries of medicine. The ideal vaccinator, Jenner imagined, would be a triple threat: (1) he conducted himself as a learned physician with practical knowledge of the body; (2) he knew, through repeated experiment and refinement, the technical details of his own procedure, from managing calf lymph to preparing the vaccine doses; and (3) he skillfully wielded the vaccination lancet.

Although Jenner would ultimately be known for his vaccination practices, it was his passion for natural history that first garnered him acclaim in scientific circles. In 1788 Jenner published a paper on the behavior of fledgling cuckoos, which put him in good favor with members of the Royal Society. His election as a Fellow in 1789 gave him enough standing to obtain a medical degree from St. Andrew's University in Scotland by 1792. His professionalization, however unconventional, allowed Jenner to credibly establish a general practice in his home town of Berkeley, in Gloucestershire, and later to act as a consultant for wealthy patients at Cheltenham spa. Jenner's enmeshment in spa culture, which involved patrons visiting health resorts like Bath to drink and bathe in waters, also enabled him to advertise vaccination as a form of practical preventative therapy in a market primarily dominated by physicians offering advice for daily living. The turning point for Jenner's acceptance into higher society, particularly among more professional medical circles, was his tutelage for two years under Scottish surgeon John Hunter at St. George's Hospital in London. Through John Hunter, he met the other esteemed Hunter brother, William, and connected with other metropolitan men of science like Joseph Banks, who would become a crucial patron of his vaccination agenda. Attention to Jenner's biography presents an entirely different narrative of vaccine's triumph than one of individualistic heroism. Jenner's early career depended heavily on these networks for legitimacy and patronage in the form of Parliamentary grants for the foundation of the Royal Jennerian Society, whose sole purpose was spreading the gospel of vaccination nationwide. Part of Jenner's success involved convincing the English elite to invest prominently into public health, thereby cultivating an interdependence between science and society at large. Vaccination catalyzed a paradigm shift in the way governments viewed their populaces: as a national body composed of individual citizen's bodies in need of immune protection.

Prior to Jenner's turn to cowpox, Mary Wortley Montagu had followed her husband to Constantinople upon his appointment as Ambassador to the Ottoman Empire in 1716. There, she witnessed smallpox variolation in which live smallpox fluid was taken from a blister and introduced by scratching into the skin of an uninfected person—what she would term "engraftment" in her famous letter to Sarah Chiswell in 1717. The use of fluid from smallpox pustules as a prophylactic had been well recorded in accounts by travelers in the East, but Montagu's public inoculation of her children and the 1721 Royal Experiment ensured its continued circulation (and debate) within English high society. While variolation struggled to gain traction, Scottish and Welsh folk practices of "buying the pox," which involved purchasing an encounter between an infected child and a healthy child or purchasing smallpox matter taken from the infected child to be "ingrafted" onto the healthy child, flourished. Early inoculation culture inaugurated a fluid economy of smallpox lymph that could be bought, sold, and trafficked from one locale and body to the next. Some parents, having heard rumors of failed procedures or severe side effects, expressed deep apprehension about exposing their children to potential harm even though it was supposedly for their own good, especially because so many children were left "pock-fretted" or "pock-holed" by the encounter. In many cases, the inoculated developed more aggressive cases of smallpox that proved fatal or were easily communicated to others if quarantine procedures were not in place. Similarly, the violence of scratching the skin and inserting infectious matter from smallpox pustules into the body of the person being inoculated also seemed to some, particularly the religious, a violation of bodily sanctity. Despite private decisions to inoculate individuals, variolation "involved either bringing the disease into the community pre-emptively or exposing the community by remaining susceptible" (Bennett, 2008: 502).

In Daniel Defoe's *Journal of the Plague Year* (1721), citizens who deliberately expose themselves to the plague are portrayed as fanatical and crazed; by the middle of the century, however, early inoculators rationalized variolation as a benevolent preventative measure, changing public perception of what it meant to choose exposure to an infectious disease. The early history of vaccination involved persistent attempts on behalf of inoculators and local governments to manage health insecurity by destigmatizing the practice of inoculation. The persistent dangers of arm-to-arm procedures and technical inconsistencies prompted physicians like Robert Sutton to consider new inoculation regimens (pre- and post-procedure) that would increase safety and success. Sutton began experimenting with variolation in 1757 after a botched attempt at inoculating his own son. By 1762 he had developed and marketed a secret "new method of inoculating for small-pox," which was so successful that it developed into an entire industry of variolation clinics and convalescence houses with over 300,000 people in just over a decade. It took until 1796 for Sutton's eldest son, Daniel, to reveal in their publication, *The Inoculator*, that the famous Suttonian method consisted of shallow scratching, using the matter from only those with mild cases of smallpox, and a regimen of bloodletting and sequestering. Montagu and Sutton contributed to the developing technologies and the market for inoculation in the period, but more importantly, they helped to universalize the idea of smallpox as an affliction that could *affect* all English people but not necessarily kill them. The inoculated often bore small pock marks from their cases of smallpox and scars at their inoculation sites, but both physical indications of encounter with the disease were being slowly rewritten as symbols of a commitment to bodily well-being, community health, and heroic survival. Inoculation's increasing popularity "actualized a new visual ambience" in that more living people were seen with evidence of the pox; inoculators in local communities "moderated the visceral fear of the disease and help to initiate a specific practice of bodily exhibitionism" (Kerr, 2013: 132–33). Instead of a death sentence, safely contracting the pox through proper inoculation (and the accompanying scar) became a badge of honor that indicated one's commitment to their health and that of the community.

In the summer of 1798 Jenner articulated in writing what he had long observed of milkmaids and their ruddy complexions: their vocational exposure to cowpox altered their constitutions, rendering them immune to smallpox. By the time Jenner published his pamphlet, *An Inquiry into the Causes and Effects of the Variolae Vaccinae*, Montagu's variolation procedure was well-known to the English public, but Jenner's procedure drew support for its accessibility and increased safety in comparison to variolation. Jenner's key claim, that cowpox (*vaccinia*) could be a viable, convenient substitute for live smallpox in inoculation procedures, allowed him to conclude that "the person who has been thus affected is for ever after *secure* from the infection of the Small Pox" (Jenner, 1978, orig. 1798; my emphasis). Jenner's interest in natural history helped him theorize that a disease in horses known as "the Grease" was frequently communicated to cows via farmers who handled both. Milkmaids milking the cows would touch the nipples and udders, where the pox tended to manifest, and would contract painful bouts of cowpox that would render them immune to future smallpox infection. Jenner documented this phenomenon in his collection of case histories that proved the efficacy of his "Jennerian technique."

In Case XVI, Jenner describes milkmaid Sarah Nelmes's poxed hand and arm:

> Sarah Nelmes, a dairymaid at a Farmer's near this place, was infected with the Cow Pox from her master's cows in May, 1796. She received the infection on a part of the hand which had been previously in a slight degree injured from a scratch from a thorn. A large pustulous sore and the usual symptoms accompanying the disease were produced in consequence. The pustule was so expressive of the true character of the Cow Pox, as it commonly appears upon the hand, that I have given a representation of it in the annexed plate."
>
> *(Jenner, 1978, orig. 1798: 31)*

Depending on how useful a case was for the explication of his technique, Jenner would include visual illustrations of both naturally occurring smallpox cases, which were useful for harvesting viable vaccination material, and the results of his procedure. These images typically depict a close-up rendering of the subject's wrist, arm, or hand with smallpox pustules or scars. Reinforcing the shift in the visual understanding of smallpox brought on by earlier inoculators, Jenner's images, which seem detached from any specific, identifiable body, emphasize the recognizable nature of ideal cowpox cases for the purposes of vaccination. Nelmes's symptoms speak for themselves and for his method, for the pustules on her hand and wrist are "expressive of the true character of the Cow Pox." Jenner's deliberate inclusion of the accompanying plates models what viable cowpox looked like and gave an empirical basis to what some dismissed as mere folk tales. In addition, these images provided examples for other practitioners to replicate and circulate.

Furthermore, the treatise represents cowpox as a desirable, even useful blemish on the human form. For Jenner, Nelmes's case is both ordinary and exemplary: the case history is full of cases similar to Nelmes's, but her idealized bodily manifestation of cowpox, primed for use in vaccination, speaks the truth of *vaccinia*'s efficacy as that which can be repurposed from nature for human defense. This promise is then verified by the subsequent Case XVII, featuring James Phipps, whom Jenner inoculated with the lymph from Nelmes:

The more accurately to observe the progress of the infection, I selected a healthy boy, about eight years old, for the purpose of inoculation for the Cow Pox. The matter was taken from a sore on the hand of a dairymaid, who was infected by her master's cows, and it was inserted, on the 14th of May, 1796, into the arm of the boy by means of two superficial incisions, barely penetrating the cutis, each about half an inch long.

In order to ascertain whether the boy, after feeling so slight an affection of the system from the Cow-pox virus, was secure from the contagion of the Small-pox, he was inoculated the 1st of July following with variolous matter, immediately taken from a pustule. Several slight punctures and incisions were made on both his arms, and the matter was carefully inserted, but no disease followed. The same appearances were observable on the arms as we commonly see when a patient has had variolous matter applied, after having either the Cow-pox or the Small-pox. Several months afterwards, he was again inoculated with variolous matter, but no sensible effect was produced in the constitution.

(Jenner, 1978, orig. 1798: 32–34)

Phipps's youth, Jenner implies, leads to a successful procedure with extremely limited side effects and "security from the contagion of" not only cowpox, but also smallpox. Over the course of the volume follows a narrative pattern of lymph being harvested for the vaccination of another. This circulating lymph produces a fluid link among the vaccinated bodies included in the *Inquiry* and creates a community of those treated by Jenner. Vaccination (and, ultimately, herd immunity) is thus fundamentally a practice of interdependence against contagion: an individual's infection benefits another, and the collective benefits from the acts of individuals.

Jenner puts vaccination in terms of English identity and citizenship: in this practice, *English* bodies preserve each other. *Vaccinia*'s origins still remain in debate; Jenner, however, entitles the pamphlet with a regional descriptor: he explicitly indicates that *variolae vaccinae* is a "disease discovered in some of the western counties of England, particularly Gloucestershire." To identify cowpox as an endemic disease allows Jenner to argue further for its viability as a replacement for smallpox vaccinations precisely because it is locally sourced and does not need to be imported from abroad. In fact, he makes the case that England now has a highly valuable medical export that can then be used for the good of the empire. What could, then, be read as repetitive medical reportage—case after case of vaccination success—is actually less an "inquiry" than a refrain: the cowpoxed body of the English country laborer, whose "constitution [is] in a state of perfect security from the infection of the Small-pox," (Jenner, 1978, orig. 1798: 67) is a source of protection from epidemic disease. It is this utopic promise of "perfect security" and how that security might be achieved and ensured that ultimately became the center of the vaccination propaganda wars.

While Jenner proffered "perfect security" with his "Jennerian technique," his detractors in turn highlighted its many failures to secure anything at all: *could the future of England be in the literally poxed hands of a milkmaid, and should such rural bodies, so often in proximity to animal bodies, be used for the preservation of national health?* The strategic repackaging of Jenner's technique as a nationalistic innovation and the virulent backlash it inspired reveal the stakes of what health security should constitute for citizens, as well as to what extent the state could achieve and justify that security during the increasingly insecure late eighteenth-century revolutionary period.

Jenner's pastoral security

Tim Fulford and Debbie Lee have characterized the Jennerian propaganda campaign as one "designed to convince the socially powerful that Britain would benefit from the healing power of nature ... and make his pastoral medicine seem socially and politically conservative as they sought public approval in a Britain dominated by war with revolutionary France" (Fulford and Lee, 2004: 202). I contend that this refashioning of pastoral medicine within conservative terms was linked to a much broader reconceptualization and politicizing of preventative medicine. Part of the challenge of publicizing and universalizing vaccination was to ensure that it was of benefit to citizens on every rung of the social ladder. Jenner's calls for vaccination departed from the methods of physicians who tended to profit from treatment and cure rather than from preventative practice. Since George Cheyne's *The English Malady* and William Buchan's *Domestic Medicine*, prevention had been a concern of English physicians, but one still primarily addressed in terms of lifestyle management, particularly regarding excessive aristocratic consumption of food and drink. While the consistent moderation of intake was understood as an active means of preserving health, vaccination took this theory one step further: resistance to or security from contagious disease could be intentionally "ingrafted" into the body by the lancet.

In 1803, Jenner wrote to T. Cobb, one of his London-based patients whom he had likely met at Cheltenham, proclaiming,

> my opinion is, that the Metropolis is the very Focus of Infection, and that destroying the Disease here will be essential in lessening its calamities in the Country. We hope soon to see Societies form'd throughout the Empire for the Extermination of the Smallpox.
>
> *(Jenner, 1983; orig. 1803: 20)*

As he suggests throughout his correspondence from the 1780s through to the beginning of the nineteenth century, Jenner's intent was never to confine vaccination to the countryside, but to directly target the metropolitan epicenters of the disease by normalizing vaccination as common practice and by establishing proxy societies that could spread vaccination throughout the British empire. This benevolent rather than profiteering agenda enhanced Jenner's professional image against accusations of quackery. Jenner spoke of vaccination as communal effort, encouraged reproduction of his methods, assisted in the procurement of lymph for other practitioners, and frequently responded to feedback on his procedure from colleagues in the metropole and beyond. As opposed to developing an entire inoculation industry out of a secretive regimen, as the Suttonian method had done, Jenner imagined a nationwide public health network of vaccination societies that could bank and disseminate cowpox lymph for vaccination, educate, and provide vaccine services. Jenner's model of preventative medicine was unique both temporally and spatially: (1) to be "perfectly secure" from smallpox demanded prevention well in advance of infection rather than treatment or cure after the fact, and (2) this security would need to be taken up on local and national levels as a concern of the *entire English population*.

Jenner's most influential supporters were those most eager to frame vaccination "as a benign symbol of the natural powers of healing" emerging from England's countryside (Shuttleton, 2007: 187). One of the most prominent of Jenner's supporters was Robert Bloomfield, a London shoemaker and farmer whose autobiographical poem "The Farmer's Boy" (1800) and collection *Rural Tales, Ballads and Songs* (1802) launched him into the public scene as a rural poet intimately acquainted with and outspoken about the experience of England's laboring classes. Bloomfield himself had lost family to smallpox and felt a personal investment in furthering the vaccination cause in his family's name and for his children's future: "I have, in my own, insured the lives of four children by Vaccine Inoculation, who, I trust, are destined to look back upon the Small-pox as the scourge of days gone by" (Bloomfield, 1804). Bloomfield evidently shared Jenner's belief in an English future without what Jenner called "the speckled monster" throughout his campaigns.

Bloomfield's pro-vaccination poem, "Good Tidings; or News from the Farm" (1804), begins with a dedication to Jenner and the members of the Royal Jennerian Society and a brief "Advertisement":

> I have employed my thoughts on the importance of Dr. JENNER's discovery, and the downfall of the Small-pox, it has generally and almost unexceptionably appeared a subject of little promise; peculiarly unfit indeed for poetry. My method of treating it has endeared it to myself, for it indulges in domestic anecdote.
>
> *(Bloomfield, 1804)*

Since "The Farmer's Boy," Bloomfield had employed "domestic anecdote" as a form that conveyed pastoral experience otherwise unavailable to metropolitan readers. In this poem, vaccination becomes a topic worthy of being cast within the rustic, autobiographical style for which Bloomfield became known. "Good Tidings" opens with the archetypal figure of the farm boy, a symbol of rural innocence, but

> where the reader of a pastoral poem expects to be presented with a rural idyll, Bloomfield confronts them with this emblematic tale of the misery caused by a contagion which pointedly emanates from the towns and destroys any hopes of domestic rural happiness.
>
> *(Shuttleton, 2007: 196)*

The poem's opening gambit refuses what pastoral poetry so often aestheticizes: the simplicity and peace of rustic life. Instead, the consequence of leaving contagion unchecked moving from town to town can only be disaster and disability.

Drawing from his own experience witnessing smallpox epidemics ravaging the English countryside, Bloomfield represents the young boy's social isolation and misery as a result of his illness, and his mother's guilt at being unable to nurse him back to full health:

> My boy was healthy, and my rest was sound
> When last year's corn was green upon the ground:
> From yonder town infection found its way;
> Around me putrid dead and dying lay,
> I trembled for his fate: but all my care
> avail'd not, for he breath'd the tainted air;
> Sickness ensu'd—in terror and dismay
> I nurs'd him in my arms both night and day,
> When his soft skin from head to foot became
> One swelling purple sore, unfit to name:
> Hour after hour, when all was still beside,
> When the pale night-light in its socket died,

126

Alone I sat; the thought still sooths my heart,
That surely I perform'd a mother's part,
Watching with such anxiety and pain
Till he might smile and look on me again;
But that was not to be—ask no more:
Go keep small-pox and blindness from your door!
(Bloomfield, 1804: 14–15)

Bloomfield dramatizes the pathos of health insecurity: in the span of under five lines, the boy moves from "healthy" to "sickness." The mobile "infection" from "yonder town" entirely undermines the "mother's part," however diligently "perform'd." To recall Jenner's "security" (from the Latin *securitas*, meaning to be free from cares), Bloomfield suggests that despite the mother's "care," "anxiety and pain," she can do nothing to stop the marring of her child's eyes and his disfigurement: he becomes almost an unrecognizable "swelling purple sore, unfit to name." The child, as a symbol of English futurity, is reduced entirely to one abject smallpox pustule, not even dignified with a name. The speaker's injunction to "go keep small-pox and blindness from your door" echoes the call for nationwide preventative medicine from township to city. The speaker supports by name Jenner and his allies who aim "to spread a saving conquest round the earth,/till ev'ry land shall bow the grateful knee" (Bloomfield, 1804: 15). The panacea from the countryside becomes the key to the "saving conquest" of an entire world affected by smallpox.

Bloomfield's mythologizing of Jenner translates the revolutionary nature of Jenner's technique into accessible terms:

Dear must that moment be when first the mind,
Ranging the paths of science unconfin'd,
Strikes a new light; when, obvious to the sense,
Springs the fresh spark of brilliant intelligence.
So felt the towering soul of Montagu,
Her sex's glory, and her country's too;
Who gave the spotted plague one deadly blow,
and bade its mitigated poison flow
With half its terrors; yet, with loathing still,
We hous'd a visitant with pow'r to kill.
Then when the healthful blood, though often tried,
Foil'd the keen lancet by the Severn side,
Resisting, uncontaminated still,
The purple pest and unremitting skill;
When the plain truth tradition seem'd to know,
And simply pointed to the harmless Cow,
Doubt and distrust to reason might appeal
But when hope triumph'd, what did Jenner feel!
(Bloomfield, 1804: 18)

Bloomfield links Jenner to the longer history of inoculation exemplified by Montagu (also represented as a hero), "who gave the spotted plague one deadly blow." Fulford and Lee, as well as Michael Bennett, have noted the prevalence of military metaphors in pro-vaccination discourse, arguing that "portraying vaccination as a holy war ensured that Jenner's medicine appeared to the public as a cause for national pride" against foreign (read: French) conta-gions (Bennett, 2008: 502; Fulford and Lee, 2004: 218). Bloomfield recasts vaccination as a humanitarian enterprise:

> Where even hope itself could scarcely rise
> To scan the vast, inestimable prize?
> Perhaps supreme, alone, triumphant stood
> The great, the conscious power of doing good,
> The power to will, and wishes to embrace
> Th'emancipation of the human race;
> A joy that must all mortal praise outlive,
> A wealth that grateful nations cannot give.
> (Bloomfield, 1804: 17–18)

Bloomfield frames this war against "the purple pest" as one of Enlightenment rationality ("strikes a new light," "springs the fresh spark of intelligence") and one of benevolence and humanitarian generosity ("The great, conscious power of doing good," "th'emancipation of the human race"). Refuting anti-vaccination arguments that suggested vaccination was tanta-mount to irrational self-harm or even suicide, Bloomfield insists that it is "ranging the paths of science unconfin'd"—that is, vaccination is not merely folk medicine but scientifically sound medical practice, one that has made sense of what "plain truth tradition seem'd to know" by "simply point[ing] to the harmless Cow." Rural figures like the blind boy and the "harmless cow," already heroized and made mascots for the pro-vaccination cause by Jenner's associate, the Quaker physician John Coakley Lettsom, in his *Observations on the Cow-Pock* (1801), find themselves in the heroic company of Jenner and Montagu. Bound together within the poem's heroic couplets, their "glory" becomes "the country's too" as their labor benefits their communities and the British nation.

For most of the poem, Bloomfield devotes his verses to lionizing Jenner as an English medical hero in the battle against epidemic disease. But the practice of vaccination itself begs poetic transformation: the speaker enacts the poem's own vaccination procedure by converting what was earlier an "infection" into florality:

> Forth sped the truth immediate from his hand,
> and confirmations sprung in ev'ry land;
> In ev'ry land, on beauty's lily arm,
> On infant softness, like magic charm,
> Appear'd the gift that conquers as it goes;
> The dairy's boast, the simple, saving *Rose!*
> (Bloomfield, 1804: 19)

Originally titled "The Vaccine Rose," "Good Tidings" alludes to the botanical origins of inoculation as a grafting of a bud or scion into a tree to preserve it from illness. Fulford and Lee read this as Bloomfield's transformation of "the blister raised in the vaccinated arm into a symbol of natural beauty and fertility" (Fulford and Lee, 2004: 215). As Jenner did in his *Inquiry,* Bloomfield aestheticizes the sites of cowpox eruption on English arms. In contrast to the hideous purple smallpox pustule that engulfs the entire being of the blind boy, the pustule at the vaccination site blossoms as a "simple, saving Rose." Bloomfield stages Jen-ner's appropriation of one of nature's "simple gifts" for the purpose of enabling healthy

English bodies to flower. Bloomfield's pro-vaccination poem welcomes and models inter-corporeal mixture (of rural and urban, of animal and human, of young and old) as part of the process of attaining a blissful security characterized by the "good tidings" of pastoral beauty and industrious good health. Yet this magical thinking would be precisely the target of ire and mockery by Jenner's critics.

Revealing Jenner's insecurity

Confident as Jenner was in his *Inquiry*, his letters to fellow medical men suggest constant concerns about the proper execution of vaccination and the management of lymph. In a 1798 letter to Edward Bevan, a surgeon at Stoke upon Trent, Jenner insists caution be used "in the selection of your matter—Much confusion may arise from its being used when par-tially decomposed by putrefaction, as in that case a disease would arise which would not give security from the contagion of smallpox" (Jenner, 1983; orig. 1803: 9). Brief notes like this abound in Jenner's correspondence and underscore that the judicious selection of matter and its proper transportation and preparation proved to be far more difficult than Jenner suggests. Like variolation before it, vaccination too risked being improperly performed, pos-sibly to fatal consequences for the vaccinated. In the *Inquiry*, Jenner overstates the frequency of cowpox cases in Gloucestershire. Cowpox was endemically rare and required vaccinators to arrange for safe transport of cowpox lymph from distant locations. These constraints required the development of a vaccination infrastructure more elaborate than Jenner himself imagined.

As Andrea Rusnock outlines in her study of the material history of vaccination, cowpox lymph was transported in three different ways: "in a dried state, in a fluid state, and by vac-cinated individuals" (Rusnock, 2009: 24). The dry threads were convenient for mailing by post but had a high rate of failure due to damage or loss in transit, which then prompted attempts to preserve the lymph in a liquid form on the lancet itself. This aqueous solution, sometimes incorrectly prepared, rusted the lancet and ruined the solution or required extremely expensive lancets of superior metals hardly accessible to middle- and working-class patients. Heat and other environmental factors also made cowpox lymph exceedingly difficult to transport over great distances or to more remote locations in the colonies. Lymph samples were sometimes faked and led to vaccine injuries and even death. Until techniques were developed in the mid-nineteenth century for harvesting lymph from cows directly, arm–to–arm transfer was still the primary means of maintaining a steady supply of lymph. For vaccinators, this arm–to–arm method ensured a chain of infection for the vaccin-ation of larger populations. Yet cowpox was fragile and often died out in the process, sever-ing this vital chain. Despite Jenner's intent to eliminate the problems brought on by variolation, the continued reliance on arm–to–arm transfer and unstable technologies meant that vaccination remained precarious. Without clear guidelines for determining and insuring vaccine contents, vaccinators and their patients would often have had to trust the lymph suppliers. Many physicians remained unsure if their sources harvested lymph from the right cases of cowpox or if the lymph was indeed lymph at all. Insecurities about vaccination materials attached easily to ongoing anxieties about the appropriateness and efficacy of injecting animal fluids into human bodies.

James Gillray's 1802 "The Cow-Pock or the wonderful Effects of the New Inocula-tions!" famously caricatured the vaccination clinic by depicting it as a sensationalized theater of inappropriate social and bodily mixture, where Jenner's "patients" quite literally turn into cows after being vaccinated. At the center of this orgy of bodies sprouting hooves and horns is Jenner, depicted as the stereotype of the quack physician (skinny, sinister, and unsympathetic), as he punctures a female laborer with an exaggeratedly large, dagger-like lancet. Directly targeting Jenner's credibility as a gentleman-doctor, the satirical print dramatizes the violence of the vaccination procedure as one that involves intentional trauma to the body. This scene's tension is also deeply gendered: the act of vaccination is represented as a disturbing encounter between male physician and vulnerable female patient whose fear is written upon her face—a face which, we are to infer, will soon to be transformed into a bovine likeness, like those of the other bodies around her. As a political cartoon, Gillray's print also plays upon post-revolutionary anxieties about working-class laborers as themselves beastly bearers of contagion and social discord. Gillray directly counters pro-vaccination claims for the value of the Jennerian technique: its novelty, its safety, and its benefit to collective health. Rather than ushering in the new, vaccination only seems to bring out these laborers' inherent bestiality or hasten their inevitable transformation into mindless, unsophisticated animals from which they were little different to begin with. Most powerfully, the image gothicizes the fluid connection established among the vaccinated: the bodies crammed densely into the frame are connected by their chain of infection from a procedure meant to offer them and Britain protection. The Jennerian network, meant to spread the gospel and the security of vaccination, seems here to proliferate physical and ideological corruption instead.

This fear that bovine vaccine serum would cause "Cow-Mania" had already been suggested by Jenner's outspoken opponent, Dr. Benjamin Moseley, who claimed that "in the year 1798 the Cow Pox Inoculation Mania seized the people of England *en masse*" (Moseley, 1800: 183). Moseley's rhetoric built upon this language of "seizure" and "mania" to represent vaccination as Jenner's quackery infecting English minds with its false promises and bad science. His mudslinging took the form of alarmist reports that vaccinated patients were developing a scrofulous bestial disease that compelled women, like Pasiphaë from classical mythology, to copulate with bulls and ultimately give birth to minotaurs. The transference of what Moseley mockingly termed a "*quadrupedan* sympathy" that would result in the unwholesome production of a race of cow–human hybrids was not the only consequence of injecting human bodies with the essence of cows (Moseley, 1800: 183; original emphasis). Moseley's moralistic strategy also relied on connecting 'Cow-Mania' with syphilis as a disease of sin, excess, and deviant sexuality. David Shuttleton notes how Moseley's neologism for cowpox lymph, the "*Lues Bovilla*, a bestial humour," "is an etymological adaptation of *Lues Venerea* (i.e., syphilis) deliberately designed to counter Jenner's term *Variolae Vaccinae* and foster the implication that cow-pox implants a bestial form of syphilis" (Shuttleton, 2007: 184). Moseley's inflammatory rhetoric drew skeptical resistance to the security Bloomfield argued that Jennerian vaccination would bring to the English public: "What misery may be brought on a family after many years of imaginary security!" (Moseley, 1800: 184).

Moseley partnered with William Rowley to give a number of public lectures on the injustices and pseudoscience underlying vaccination. Resident physician to the Marylebone Infirmary and member of the Royal College of Physicians, Rowley became widely known after publishing his polemic *Cow-Pox Inoculation No Security Against Small-Pox Infection* (1805). Rowley describes his treatise as a necessary corrective to "many medical errors," and as needed "to establish demonstrative truths in the theory and practice of the art" through a collection of 504 documented cases of vaccination injury, seventy-five of which led to death (Rowley, 1805: v). These injuries primarily take the form of what Rowley variously calls "*cow-pox mange, evil, blotches, ulcers, and mortification*" and "filthy *beastly disease*," which he claims will dissuade any rational person from supporting "universal vaccination" (Rowley, 1805: viii; original emphasis). The deception of vaccination, then, is in its false promise of full "security" from smallpox that ultimately proves to be but "temporary security" and one "not definable" (Rowley, 1805: xi).

While Bloomfield worked to connect Jenner to his variolating predecessors in his poetic account of vaccination, Rowley deliberately denies Jenner's connection to the "Suttons, Dimsdales, Jones, Dr. Archer and many others," whom he holds in high esteem for practicing legitimate medicine. Rowley's model of immunity excludes the possibility of interspecies immunity based on Levitican injunctions against human–beast contact:

> The Small Pox is a visitation from God, and originates in man; but the Cow Pox is produced by presumptuous, impious man: the former heaven ordained; the latter is, perhaps a daring and profane violation of our holy religion.
>
> *(Rowley, 1805: 8)*

Smallpox variolation, he declares, is safer by virtue of the fact that smallpox happens naturally *in humans* and the smallpox lymph used to produce an immune response is extracted *from humans*. Vaccination, on the other hand, is a contrived solution made out of the constitutions of beasts, which are not compatible with human ones. If vaccination's effectiveness against smallpox is only tested during cases of exposure, Rowley believes, many supposed success cases are in fact failures waiting to reveal themselves in time, often when it is too late to intervene. "Why leave a certainty for an uncertainty?," Rowley asks his readers (Rowley, 1805: 4). Pro-vaccination advocates, consumed by "visionary conceits, irrational projects, and obstinate perseverance in error, united to uncontrolled arrogance," have produced more insecurity, rather than the security they promised (Rowley, 1805: 1).

In contrast to Bloomfield's idealized blind boy, Rowley invokes the pathetic figure of the "innocent infant" forcibly vaccinated against her will or without her knowledge:

> Parents, affectionate, unsuspicious parents, from the plausible pretensions and indefatigable activity, rash over-heated boastings, and extravagant promises of the vaccinators, were induced credulously to sacrifice their innocent infants to this new shrine, this new altar of probability.—They left a reality for an experiment, a known *good* for a probable *evil*.
>
> *(Rowley, 1805: 5–6; original emphasis)*

In place of rationality and sound judgment, "pretension" and "rash over-heated boastings" fool parents into "sacrificing" their infants to vaccination likened to a cult. Rowley cleverly recasts the language of mathematics and science ("probability," "experiment") as part of the duplicitous project of the vaccination cause. Here, variolation's certain protection far outweighs the experimental evils of vaccination. In Rowley's judgment, the hubris of Jenner and his co-conspirators has led to a nationwide mania, producing deluded vaccine supporters and a silent epidemic of vaccine-injured children suppressed by vaccinators wanting to protect their cause.

Drawing upon the same lurid visual vocabulary seen in Gillray's print, Rowley's pamphlet included two hand-colored engraved plates of "The Cowpoxed Ox-Faced Boy" and the "Cowpoxed Mangey Girl." Featuring a close-up of the boy's face and an exposed female body, these plates were frequently used for their shock factor at Rowley's public lectures. By drawing attention to the boy's swollen face and the girl's body covered in bloody abscesses, Rowley decried vaccination's transgression of religious taboos and claimed that transgression led to the children's physical marring. Rowley's logic echoes medieval and early modern reproductive theories of maternal imprinting in which illicit behavior or external stimuli could affect the physical form of even an unborn child. The misguided parents, cajoled into allowing bestiality in the form of medicine, were being punished through their children's deformities. Rowley devotes the concluding section of his treatise to the spectacular public exhibition of these two vaccine-injured children:

> The scene was truly affecting and distressing to humanity. The first case brought into the lecture-room, was case 26, *Joules*, the *cow-poxed, ox-faced boy*, who likewise, has a terribly diseased elbow-joint. Marianne Lewis, case 88, was the second who was covered with Cow-Pox blotches, like a leopard. The indentations were shewn in these two cases, and they were compared and viewed by all the gentlemen present, with the print so well and faithfully executed by the ingenious Mr. Pugh and Mr. Anniss. The exactitude of the drawings were acknowledged by all.
>
> After these, a load of children, brought in a cart from Sleaford-street, Battersea-fields, &c. appeared; amongst whom were the six surviving children of eight, two having *died* of Small Pox after vaccination. The *indentations* in the arms were all seen and acknowledged, and they all now have the Cow-Pox mange. Cases 50 to 57.
>
> When these had been viewed, a very great number of other cases followed, all mentioned in the book, where Small Pox had happened after vaccination. The *indentations* or scars in their arms were examined and proved by all present, nearly 100 auditors, to be incontrovertible facts.
>
> (Rowley, 1806: 126–27; original emphasis)

In his recreation of this "scene truly affecting and distressing to humanity," Rowley details what reads like a freak show, a form of entertainment involving the exhibition of extraordinary bodies that would become increasingly popular throughout the nineteenth century. Like Jenner's strategy of repetition in his case histories, Rowley uses a sentimental narrative of child disfigurement to enhance what has been primarily a book of tables documenting vaccine injury. While the quantity of cases he has collected into a single volume serves to prove Rowley's point, these concluding paragraphs of narrative description put faces to those cases.

Conclusion

With the rise of teaching hospitals over the course of the eighteenth and nineteenth centuries (as Michel Foucault has described), the medical theater was often an exclusive space where medical knowledge was shared among a professional community of male physicians. As readers, we are given access to this space and can virtually witness this public reading of the children's bodies as "incontrovertible facts" of vaccine danger. The children, reduced to their case numbers and held up as exemplary manifestations of vaccination injury, are displayed to the audience of gentlemen and are reproduced in drawings, which reappear in Rowley's publication among others. Aside from their names and symptoms, we are given no other information about the children. The children are not quoted or given any opportunity to voice their subjective experience of vaccine injury. Alongside the cartloads of unnamed children bearing all degrees of cowpox "evils," they become sentimental proof of the severity of vaccination injury. Unsurprisingly, the child would become the most frequently invoked figure in nineteenth-century anti-vaccination movements.

The vaccination culture wars reveal how both pro- and anti-vaccinators envisioned an English population whose health could be threatened and also managed by state interventions. Anti-vaccinators refused the wishful thinking of Jenner's vaccination agenda, which they saw as a futile endeavor to preserve health that only led to further corruption of English health and to the undermining of social and religious hierarchies. Yet both sides deployed vivid, if contrasting, imaginaries of health insecurity, Moseley and Rowley's nightmarish vision of "Cow Mania" spreading unchecked against Jenner and Bloomfield's fantasy of idyllic bliss. Attention to the transits between medicine and literature during the eighteenth and nineteenth centuries reveals that vaccination's preventative function has never been purely a biological issue. Resurgences in practices like "chicken pox parties" or deliberate refusals of childhood vaccine schedules by concerned parents are hardly new; rather, they redeploy centuries-old arguments and metaphors against what anti-vaccinators believed was the overreach and violence of medicine increasingly aligned with state power. Movements against vaccination draw on long-standing anxieties about bodily permeability and autonomy now exaggerated in a post-9/11 world of proliferating risks. These same risks underpin pro-vaccination strategies to insist upon the absolute necessity of vaccination as a public health practice aimed at protecting some of the most vulnerable members of the population. This historical tension between how pro- and anti-vaccinators imagined health insecurity and its management continues to animate current debates over vaccination, which cannot be reducible to purely its science.

References

Bennett, M. (2008). Jenner's Ladies: Women and Vaccination against Smallpox in Early Nineteenth-Century Britain. *History*, 93(4): 497–513.

Bloomfield, R. (1804). *Good Tidings; or, News from the Farm*. London: Parnassian Press, for Vernor and Hood, 31, Poultry; Longman and Rees, Paternoster Row.

Fulford, T. and Lee, D. (2004). The Beast Within: Vaccination, Romanticism, and the Jenneration of Disease. In D. Lee, P. Kitson and T. Fulford, eds., *Literature, Science, and Exploration in the Romantic Era: Bodies of Knowledge*. Cambridge: Cambridge University Press: 198–227.

Jenner, E. (1978; 1798). *An Inquiry into the Causes and Effects of the Variolae Vaccinae: A Disease Discovered in Some of the Western Counties of England, Particularly Gloucestershire, and Known by the Name of the Cow Pox*. Special ed. Birmingham: Classics of Medicine Library.

Jenner, E. (1983; 1803). To T. Cobb, Esq., Banbury, Oxfordshire, 8 March 1803. In G. Miller., ed., *Letters of Edward Jenner and Other Documents Concerning the Early History of Vaccination*. Baltimore: Johns Hopkins University Press: 20.

Jordanova, L. (2000). *Defining Features: Scientific and Medical Portraits, 1660–2000*. London: Reaktion Books.

Kerr, M. (2013). "An Alteration in the Human Countenance": Inoculation, Vaccination, and the Face of Smallpox in the Age of Jenner. In J. Reinarz and K. Siena, eds., *A Medical History of Skin*. London: Pickering Chatto: 129–146.

Moseley, B. (1800). *Medical Tracts*. London: John Nichols, Red-Lion Passage, Fleet Street, For T. Cadell and W. Davies, Strand.

Rowley, W. (1806). *Cow-Pox Inoculation No Security Against Small-Pox Infection*. London: Printed, for the Author, by J. Barfield, Wardour-Street; and sold by J. Harris, Corner of Ludgate-Hill; J Murray, Left-Street.

Rusnock, A. (2009). Catching Cowpox: The Early Spread of Smallpox Vaccination, 1798–1810. *Bulletin of the History of Medicine*, 83(1): 17–36.

Shuttleton, D. (2007). *Smallpox and the Literary Imagination, 1660–1820*. Cambridge: Cambridge University Press.

19

SELLING THE DE-PHARMACEUTICALIZATION OF INSOMNIA

Semiotics, drug advertising, and the social life of Belsomra

Lorenzo Servitje

Introduction

"Big pharma" has become something of an easy target in the wake of trends like the increased attention to drug companies' legislative lobbying, pricing, and marketing in the United States and global markets elsewhere. Innumerable parodies of pharmaceutical advertisements on syndicated television shows like *Saturday Night Live* and digital media platforms like YouTube speak to the running joke that drugs have inched their way into so many dimensions of our lives (Dumit, 2012). The desire for pharmaceuticals is no longer limited to the elimination of sickness and disease but now encompasses the infinite reduction of medical risk and the asymptotic ideal of being "better than well" (Elliot, 2003).

There is a general cultural recognition of the increased jurisdiction of medicine, a process medical sociologists termed "medicalization" in the 1970s, which has attracted a vast scholarship (e.g., Conrad, 1992; Rose, 2007; Zola, 1972).[1] The increased scope of pharmaceutical intervention, "pharmaceuticalization," is a specific engine of medicalization, characterized by using medication to treat both conventionally accepted medical problems and those formerly outside the control and rule of medicine, along with also being agents of enhancement (see Abraham, 2010; Bell and Figert, 2012; Conrad, 2005).[2] Joe Dumit has described the economic logics that underlie the processes of pharmaceuticalization as "surplus health"—the increased volume of drugs consumed in terms of numbers of patients and duration of treatment. Surplus health defines the research, development, and consumption of drugs in the United States by co-producing a threshold of diseases and their diagnosis (Dumit, 2012). In the face of public awareness, condemnation of, and seemingly complacence with an ideology of surplus health, how might we interpret the continued pressures applied by the pharmaceutical industry on patients and medical practitioners? How do drug companies market their products to a culture that is becoming contemptuous of its marketing practices? In this chapter, I suggest that integrating the work of medical sociologists and science and technology scholars on pharmaceutical culture with the humanistic lenses of semiotic close reading and cultural studies can help us make sense of this phenomenon, specifically in terms of insomnia. Belsomra, Merck and Co's novel sleeping medication approved by the US Food and Drug Administration (FDA) in 2014, is an especially productive object of inquiry in this vein.

Belsomra works differently than the previous generation of soporifics, including benzodi-azepines such as Halcion (triazolam), Restoril (temazepam), and Ativan (lorazepam), and their closely related cousins, the "Z-drugs," such as Ambien (zolpidem), Lunesta (eszopiclone), and Sonata (zalepon), all of which act on GABA receptors.[3] Belsomra is the first FDA-approved member of a new class of therapeutic agents (orexin antagonists) for the treatment of insomnia. However, the pharmacology of its mechanism of action is not the central focus of this paper; rather, it is how that mechanism of action is discursively mobilized to mitigate the stigma surrounding sleeping medication and incorporate Belsomra within the commodified culture of wellness. A well-circulated and memorable 2015 advertisement for the drug, "Cats and Dogs" (Belsomra, 2015), capitalizes on apprehensions individuals might feel about considering treating insomnia with a "sleeping pill."

Understanding this process entails following one dimension of Belsomra's "social life." A drug's "social life" encompasses the biography of a material substance that produces physiological responses, including how it moves between different actors, settings, and attributes various forms of value, revealing the social and performative effects, along with the way that it "confirm[s] sickness, and demonstrate[s] the character and intentions of those who administer them" (Whyte et al., 2002; 15).[4] In focusing on the cultural work of Belsomra's marketing, this chapter shows how interdisciplinary inquiry yields insight into the broader context of so many prescriber–patient interactions: the commodification of health and wellness, returning to normal functioning, and self-improvement. Looking to direct-to-consumer advertising (DTCA)—the use of television, digital, or print media to advertise prescription medication to (potential) patients directly rather than medical professionals—reveals some of the ideological underpinnings in medical discourse that shape how people define themselves as productive, responsible, and healthy. In what follows, I will briefly summarize the broader contexts of DTCA and the sociological understandings of sleep and soporifics to frame my close reading of the 2015 Belsomra advertisement.[5] I will con-clude by addressing responses to the advert by the public, media, and Merck, and discuss how health humanistic work can have a productive impact when unraveling the social life of a drug by examining its cultural production.

DTCA: semiotics, economics, and the de-pharmaceuticalization of sleeplessness

DTCA, like any advertisements, rely on cultural mythologies and ideologies, represented through visual, narrative, textual, or auditory signs. By *sign* I mean a relationship between two elements: a signified—a mental concept—and a signifier—the form that concept takes. Signs can be anything from written words like *Belsomra*, to images and icons, to material objects. We are all on the same page when we hear the word "stethoscope," which repre-sents the idea behind a device that mediates acoustic sounds of the cardiovascular and respiratory systems from one body into the ears of another. But beyond their strict definition (denotation), signs also carry associative meanings that are culturally determined (connota-tion). For instance, the stethoscope can be an icon or synecdoche of a medical professional without ever being used. It could, at once, connote doctor–patient contact, and proximity and closeness (a doctor putting their hands on a patient and listening to one's body, in contrast to staying trained on a laptop); on the other hand, the stethoscope could connote distance, objectification (a doctor mediating contact between a patient and themselves, making the patient only a body to be professionally interpreted). Signs, whether material objects, or visual or textual representations work though metaphors, symbols, metonymies, in turn, existing in relation to larger constellations of other signs.

DTCA capitalizes on the negative connotations surrounding disease by imbuing a drug with positive connotations. That is, they do not really sell the drug itself; rather they commodify the lifestyle, identity, or idea the drug represents: an active sex life and masculinity (erectile disfunction drugs), productivity (anti-narcoleptics and stimulants), control over secondary sex characteristics or reproduction (hormones), "responsible" mitigation of risk (anti-hyperlipidemics and antihypertensives), etc. While these are not monolithic determining desires or subjectivities, advertisements for drugs like these naturalize associations between a disease, cultural value, myth, or ideology, and posit a drug as the remediation for any deficiency or misalignment between the viewer and whatever the advertisement suggests is normal or desirable (Dumit, 2012: 60).

In an effort to maximize new consumers, these ads often introduce the possibility or risk of disease in individuals who might not manifest symptoms. Phrases like "these might be signs of a serious condition" or "you could possibly be suffering from ..." are precisely constructed in their grammar to stay within the threshold of legally allowable claims (DTCA cannot diagnose any condition) while deploying the possibility of pathology; phrases like these convert *modalization* (the conceptual space between probability and necessity) into *mobilization* (action on the part of the individual to talk to their doctor) (Dumit, 2012: 60). To understand how this works in a drug like Belsomra, we need to have a basic understanding of the history and regulations surrounding DTCA.[6]

Belsomra's advertisement works off of a set of expected conventions, rhetorical shorthands, and rules. Part of the reason so many of these product claim ads feel the same is that they all have the same end (i.e., direct consumers to request the drug in the clinical encounter), yet are limited in what they can say, have to say, show, and claim. While there is a long history of drug advertisements going back to the nineteenth century, drug advertisements as they exist in American culture today began to focus on patients in the 1970s with the advent of the patient rights and the consumer health movement of the 1980s. During this period, the public began to demand more information and more of a role in medical decision making. Pharmaceutical companies where quick to abide. DTCA began to take shape in the early 1980s, with the first two televised advertisements airing in 1981. But, due to the amount of information they were forced to disclose about side effects, they were expensive to air. This changed in 1997 when an FDA ruling allowed them to substitute shorter statements and refer patients to more information (Greene and Herzberg, 2010). As blockbusters like Viagra, Lipitor, and Ambien emerged on the scene, companies diverted more money into DTCA. From 1997 to 2016, drug companies increased the amount of money spent on marketing from $2.1 billion (11% of total spending) to $9.6 billion (32% of total spending). During the same period the number of occurrences of advertisements rose from 79,000 (72,000 of which were television commercials) in 1997 to 4.6 million (663,000 television commercials) in 2017 (Schwartz and Woloshin, 2019).[7] Currently, marketing prescription drugs directly to patients is only allowed in the United States and New Zealand.

Despite changes in media consumption—from broadcast television to streaming, from print media to digital—DTCA shows no signs of abating. In 2011, it was estimated that, on average, US citizens were exposed to nine direct-to-consumer ads per day (Klara et al., 2018). As of 2016 the number of ads that appeared to consumers increased by 65% from

2014 (Kaufman, 2017). The amount of money spent on these advertisements speaks to the prevalence of these narratives, images, and texts that navigate the gray boundaries of allowable representations. Moreover, while there are currently and have been regulations over DTCA, they still provide much room for pharmaceutical companies to work with. The FDA requires that companies submit all promotional materials to its Office of Prescription Drug Promotion but, due to the volume, the Office does not review every advertisement (Klara et al., 2018: 651).

The marketing regulations that pharmaceutical companies contend with pertain mostly to the kind and amount of information provided, along with the scope of claims they can make about their product's use. DTCA broadcast ads must provide a "fair balance" of risk and efficacy information; they must communicate "major risks" in audio format, as long as the ad also provides a source to access FDA-approved labeling of the drug. The FDA restricts companies from promoting drugs for off-label (not officially designated diagnosis) use, although drug companies have challenged these restrictions under the First Amendment and the FDA has allowed some off-label advertising to physicians. Despite these, among other, regulations, oversight by the FDA remains limited (Klara et al., 2018: 662). One study that analyzed DTCA ads aired between January 2015 and July 2016 concluded that even in the face of these regulations many ads are misleading and, in a select few cases, are demonstrably false. "Overall," the authors contend, "few ads were fully compliant with FDA guidelines for DTC advertising and the quality of information presented in the broadcast DTC ads for prescription drugs was low" (Klara et al., 2018: 657). It is important to clarify that it is not just a matter of providing information per se. Compelling marketers to make visible and balance information does not get at the root of the problem. Even if the information is accurate, their presentation so often "involves the use of evocative imagery and language that (subtly or otherwise) convey narratives and themes that move beyond facts to appeal to universals such as the dread of sickness and desire to be better" (Doran, 2016: 334). This is precisely the kind of analysis humanistic inquiry affords, all the more when it incorporates quantitative and qualitative research to evidence interpretative readings.

Despite increased spending on DTCA and the ability of marketers to skirt regulation, the specific epoch Belsomra emerged from was not the most conducive to selling sleeping medication. Although finance research suggests growth in the market for the pharmacological treatment of insomnia (Markets and Markets, 2017), some quantitative population health studies have shown a decline in the number of prescriptions for it (e.g., Moloney et al., 2019). One explanation for the decrease in using medication in a multi-billion dollar market for the "sleep-industrial complex" and prescription drugs in general is the possibility that sleep is being "de-pharmaceuticalized," the social process whereby individuals are turning less to medication and more toward lifestyle changes and other products—in the case of insomnia, these include sleep tracking, sleep hygiene, and treatments such as cognitive behavioral therapy (CBT), and sleep "coaching" (Gabe et al., 2017: 49).[8] Qualitative studies using focus groups have found that numerous patients with insomnia who have and have not taken soporifics view them irresolutely. The drugs are frequently characterized as "unnatural" interventions and not "real sleep"; and they are often associated with addiction and lack of control (Gabe et al., 2016). Constructed ideas of "naturalness and normality" often lead patients to forego or limit the use of sleep medication—even in the cases where they asked for it (Moloney et al., 2019: 341). Gabe concludes that the (de)pharmaceuticalization of sleep is in a "state of flux": while sedative hypnotics continue to be commonplace, they are "rarely embraced unquestionably" (Gabe et al., 2016: 641–642). Instead, individuals were ambivalent and reflexive in their thinking about these medications, expressing "moral repertoires" associated with the use of sedative hypnotics: how the drugs are understood and negotiated in everyday life; how they play a role in presenting oneself as a moral being; and how they are based on a relatively coherent system of meaning for evaluating and defining behaviors, events, and other phenomenon. Gabe et al. (2016: 632) taxonomized these repertoires into the following: "the deserving patient," "the responsible user," "the compliant patient," "the addict," and the "noble non-user." The views reflecting the rejection, hesitancy, or qualification in these repertoires have been associated with the numerous negative portrayals in the media about sedative hypnotics specifically. Some of these representations, which are discussed below, have been linked with the decrease in prescription of Z-drugs (Moloney et al., 2019).[9] As a whole, much of the sociological literature on sleep and medicine recurrently cites oppositional trends and discourse with respect to soporifics. It is, then, in the face of contradictory messages—idealizing productivity and improving health, exerting better living through control (chemical or not), needing more sleep, needing to avoid sleeping pills—and in the face of DTCA's affordances and restrictions that Merck had to make Belsomra desirable.

Beslomra's delicate balancing act

What is so interesting about Merck's advertisement "Cats and Dogs" is the way it negotiates these challenges and contradictions, working to expand market reach and destigmatize the use of sleeping medication. If we were to distill the cultural negotiations Belsomra's marketing performs down to a single conceptual metaphor, it would perhaps be best represented by "medicine is equipoise." The advertisement's visual, auditory, narrative, and textual signs suggest that the drug reconciles the proposed binaries of *sleep* and *wake* into harmonious coexistence. I use the term *coexistence* here not merely as rhetorical flourish but to follow the advertisement's casting of distinct animals as signifiers for sleep and wake. The animal characters not only appeal to a wide audience (more than half of American families have pets); they also represent the idiomatic understanding of cat/dog as an opposition, as in the simile "they fight like cats and dogs." Upon closer analysis, however, it becomes clear that the ad presents this seemingly dichotomy only to upend it—the ad posits that the relationship between sleep and wake is not oppositional but rather dyadic. This conceptual recasting of the relationship between these two states structures how Merck positions Belsomra's mechanism of action as a new kind of sleeping medication, one that is not really a "sleeping medication" at all.

The rhetorical construction of Belsomra as the non-sleeping-pill sleeping pill begins with a halcyon exposition. Framed in a medium shot, we see a woman reading in bed with a white cat figure, before the next scene cuts within the first second to a medium close-up of the cat. "Ah, Sleep," the sonorous narrator opens, "*remember when* it *used* to welcome you as a friend" (emphasis added), as the cat stretches to reveal it literally embodies the word *sleep*. The cat is serene; it gracefully expands its flexible body to show its silken fur. Sleep-cat allows itself to be affectionately embraced by the woman. Everything about this figure is soporific. The smooth CGI tail evokes a feeling of cool, silk sheets. Sleep-cat is the perfect size for hugging, mimicking the space of a small pillow or stuffed animal to let the arms remain passively flexed in a common sleeping position. The composition of the scene, with the woman's gaze directed to the gracefully hypnotic swaying tail, makes it easy to miss the male partner already in deep repose. While the male partner's presence is subtle, it contributes to the fanciful ideal of pre-insomnia life as normal, ordered. Everyone and everything is in their right place, right rhythm. The fact that the narrator begins in the interrogative mood introduces the assumption to the viewer that they, indeed, have seen more restful nights in the past. From the very beginning, the ad interpellates all viewers as disordered sleepers.

The tranquillity does not last. A quick fade to black marks the intrusion of conflict: "But then, it became more elusive," the voice continues, as the change in perspective places the viewer under the bed; we can see the woman search for her ensconcing pet in the middle of the night. Having captured the viewer's attention with this complication, the narrator continues to stoke curiosity—"But why?" As the woman searches through her house, the camera cuts to the attic where the canine-shaped "wake" contraposes sleep-cat (Figure 19.1). Sleep-cat becomes skittish and aloof in the face of wake-dog's emboldened approach. The shift in setting to the attic is significant to the interaction between these figures. Unlike the bedroom, which is tidy and elegant in its simplicity, the attic is, in comparison, disordered. Boxes on the floor, a blanket tossed on a chair. Some of the floorboards are lifted. This frames how the antagonism between sleep-cat and wake-dog serve two specific, related—yet seemingly contradictory—functions: first, representing the conflict between sleep and wakefulness as abnormal, a disorder, when we compare the bedroom with the attic; second, suggesting that the setting and arrangement of this scene is normal, given that it is not at all uncommon to have an attic that looks unkempt and less well maintained when compared with the rooms below. The implication is that it is in fact normal to struggle with this disorder; it is normal to "lose" sleep, but not because it has fled on its own, rather because it has been driven away by its opposing state, wakefulness. But there is a solution.

Belsomra: the reconciling agent that at once, puts sleep and wake back into balance, and makes sense of the paradoxical normal abnormality of the sleeplessness it treats. The proposed pharmaceutical solution's mechanism of action and introduction thematically follow the way the drug is presented on screen. The attic scene cuts to Belsomra's icon, set in a white background, featuring the standard generic name in parenthesis, along with dosage and other mandated information. We are informed that "Belsomra is a prescription medication for adults who have trouble falling or staying asleep," as the logo dissolves back into the diegetic world of the advertisement. Meanwhile, the woman leads wake-dog down from the attic to the bedroom. Here, it is easy to miss the distinctive, contrasting editing techniques of these two sections of the narrative. The transition from the attic conflict to the Belsomra graphics is a hard, abrupt cut. While the entire proposition of the drug and its

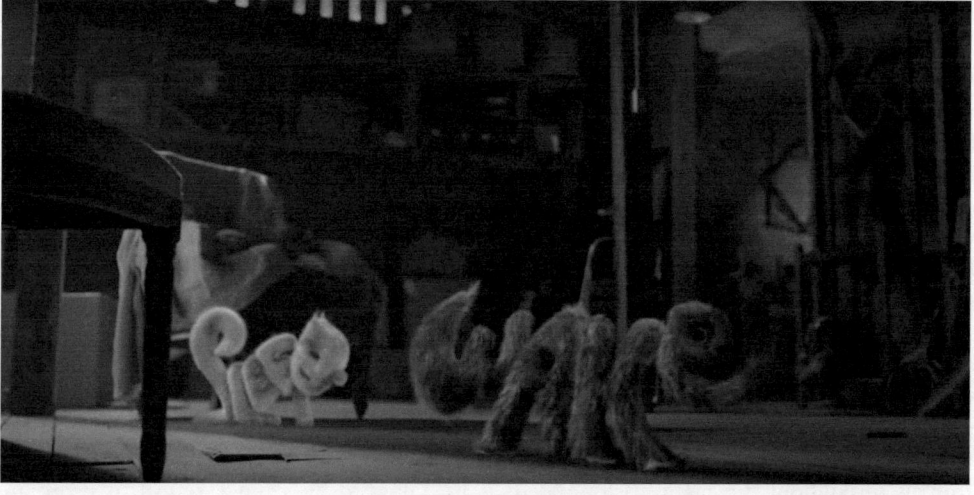

Figure 19.1 "When you have insomnia, it may affect the wake-neurotransmitters in your brain." (0:17)

ad is balance and continuity, no one wants their insomnia to go away gradually. Concomitantly, the resolution the drug catalyzes is immediate. By opposing insomnia, Belsomra ends it. At the same time, however, Merck is careful not to attach any aggressive connotations to the drug, less it be read as a "knock-out drug," one that has too rapid of an onset and is incapacitating. Everything thus far has been framed in a way that distinguishes Belsomra from benzodiazepine and Z-drug sedative hypnotics, and even more so from their barbiturate precursors. In contrast to the cut from the attic to the Belsomra graphics, the transition from Belsomra graphics to the woman leading wake-dog down to the bedroom flows in a measured dissolve. The mood is placid; the resolution for insomnia as a disorder might be quick, but the actual effect it produces is a gradual easement into "natural" sleep. The climax does not feel like one, because the burden of insomnia has been deescalated, sublimated into a tameable, measured balancing act of modulating neurotransmitters.

The use of editing to represent at once the smooth flow of the drug's tempering effects while also highlighting the strength of its intervention follows the representational forms of and resolution between wake-dog and sleep-cat's conflict. After the logo, the focus turns to address wakefulness specifically, following an explanation of the drug's mechanism of action. The woman lovingly pats wake-dog, as the figure gladly follows her direction. "Belsomra is thought to help turn down wake messages by targeting and inhibiting the action of orexin," the voiceover informs, "a neurotransmitter that plays a central role in sending wake messages." The woman crawls into bed, followed by sleep-cat's reappearance as it jumps on the bed and once again allows her to gently embrace its body. Unlike "sleeping pills" in all their pejorative connotations (i.e. sedative hypnotics), "Only Belsomra works this way."

The focus on training wake-dog rather than sleep-cat does not just mirror Belsomra's pharmacology; it makes an argument in favor of controlling insomnia not by inducing or forcing sleep, but by disciplining wakefulness. This is a cognitively dissonant logic that posits an assertive, willful control of a natural process while still holding "natural" sleep as an ideal. In other words, it reflects the need to impose order over a biological and/or socially determined disorder, while also holding in contempt pharmacologically induced control, as this can represent "unnatural interference with a natural state" (Gabe et al., 2017: 45). This resistance is tied to an espousal of "a moral strength to not relying on artificial props—a form of pharmaceutical Calvinism" (Gabe et al., 2016: 638).[10] The contradiction is obfuscated in the ad. The connotations of natural sleep and self-control obfuscate the reality that the pharmaceutical is what allows one to conduct sleep and wakefulness. In the next scene, wake-dog has, indeed, awoken, from his Belsomra-branded bed. Front paws on the bed, tail wagging, the dog playfully seeks the woman's attention. The woman, who is resting peacefully with sleep-cat by her pillow, wakes up. Her eyes open and momentarily flutter before she rolls over to the opposite side of the bed, ignoring both the dog and the urge to wake completely. Sleep-cat, likewise, lifts its head ever so slightly only to fall back asleep, aloof to the dog's attempted interruption. Paying no heed to wake-dog's attention-seeking behavior follows commonly applied pet-training techniques. Belsomra's method does not restrain, deride, or punish wake-dog. Wakefulness, then, is not actively suppressed; it is disciplined.

The very fact that the woman wakes up, even just momentarily, contributes to the overall argument of the ad. If Belsomra is being advertised as a medication that treats insomnia, why, then, would Merck include any kind of sleep disruption? Clearly, the interaction symbolically represents a negligible momentary awakening; and it is, in fact, this momentary awakening that further normalizes the medically induced sleep effects of Belsomra. Minor nocturnal arousals throughout the night, as long as they are followed by a quick return to sleep, are normal (Reading, 2013: 2). Belsomra appears to effect balanced, natural sleep, along with its normal imperfections, its standard disruptions. Moreover, by including a normal disruption, Merck detaches the unnatural, knock-out sedation associated with "sleeping pills." Belsomra navigates the tightrope balance, if not dialectical, form of de-pharmaceuticalization.

In step with the formal and thematic use of balance to make the drug seem less like a drug, toward the end of the ad the narrative action combined with sound ameliorates potential objections to the medication's side effects. Part of the backlash against pharmaceuticalization, particularly of sleep, is not just the connotation of unnatural sleep but also the side effects. Ambien has had a notably sordid history in the news media with respect to hypnosedative-induced complex behaviors, such as sleepwalking, eating, driving, and sex. A number of celebrities have very recently pointed to Ambien—or, the "Devil's Aspirin"—as the cause of strange and dangerous behaviors that resulted in embarrassment, public backlash, and in some cases criminal charges (Gabbatt, 2018). In "Cats and Dogs," the FDA-mandated declaration of common side effects include these behaviors, relayed during the falling action. The woman, accompanied by wake-dog, appears active and social—meeting with a friend outside her house (who is escorted by her own wake-dog), exercising, and then simply enjoying a newspaper in her backyard. Concurrently, viewers are informed that one should not drive or operate heavy machinery while taking Belsomra, that "walking, eating, driving or engaging in other activities while asleep without remembering it the next day have been reported." "Abnormal behaviors may include aggressiveness, confusion, agitation, or hallucinations," the voice over continues, adding that "the temporary inability to move while falling asleep or waking up and temporary leg weakness have also been reported," a symptom of sleep paralysis.

These side effects are certainly alarming, but understanding how they are commonly perceived from a psychological as well as literary-cultural perspective puts into question how this convention, a requirement by the FDA, has less informative power than one might assume. One writer from the *Huffington Post* comically points out, "The ad makers are hoping you won't notice this dark turn, since the terrifying effects they describe are recited over a backdrop of soothing music" (Gregoire, 2015). While this account is certainly accurate, the catalysts for distraction and dismissal are a bit more complex than "soothing music." First, the narratorial voice changes from a man to a woman; this narrator has a softer, less resonant voice compared with the other narrator; with the classical music soundtrack, her message is ever so slightly muted. Without a doubt, just the reduction in volume downplays the message —the list of side effects. Second, and as a visual adjunctive to the voice-over change, is what the woman does while the narrator describes sleep paralysis: she is walking in exercise clothes, from the left to the right side of the screen with wake-dog; when the narrator moves to "temporary leg weakness," we are once again inside the house, but we see the woman walking up the stairs, leading wake-dog into the bedroom. Her movement, the ability to walk at a brisk pace for exercise, and the strength to ascend stairs with ease together contrapose the kinesthetic impairment that a patient might experience while taking the drug.

Finally, given that explicit recitation of side effects is an FDA mandate for pharmaceutical companies, I would argue that this concerning list of side effects can often work more as a trope in the DTCA genre, and less as useful information.[11] That is, however dramatic and serious the side effects might be, many viewers will be so used to the convention, that they do not consider the elements in the list in the most substantive way. One might argue otherwise, pointing to the innumerable jokes, parodies, and direct references to side effects. These references are so idiomatic, so commonplace, and so voluminous in American culture, however, that these very qualities facilitate indifference. (It is particularly telling, that the popular website *TV-Tropes* includes an entry for "Side Effects May Include …").[12] Compounding this is the documented psychological dimension: the recitation of side effects produces an "argument dilution effect," where, in the case of DTCA, "the practice of listing both severe and frequent but minor side effects paradoxically plays down the risk factors in assessing the suitability of the drug and in turn increases its attractiveness" (Sivanathan and Kakkar, 2017: 797).[13] In other words, the DTCA genre, through the very requirement of listing side effects, actually affords a paratactical overload. This barrage of possibilities can nullify whatever informative value presenting them to viewers might have.

Having faced the hurdle—or met the generic convention—of compulsory side effect divulgence, the ad imparts closure by returning to the bedroom. Wake-dog walks itself to the dog bed without direction from the woman, as sleep-cat allows itself to be gently lifted into her arms, the way it used to. The ad cuts to the final scene where the woman is resting serenely, hugging sleep-cat as the camera zooms out revealing the entirety of the bed, which now includes the woman's male partner with equal weight in the frame—"Ah, sleep." Although the man was partially visible early on, his fuller inclusion at the end doubles-down on the ad's thematic balancing: two sides of the bed are occupied by each respective person, composing an even domestic partnership, mirroring the complementary states of sleeping and waking. The medical problem having been resolved, the ad re-intro-duces normativity, a common structure in many pharmaceutical advertisements, not unique to Belsomra. The logo becomes visible once again, superimposed upon the image of the sleeping couple. Concluding with a brand name's logo is another generic convention, but certainly a rhetorically significant one in this case. The Belsomra logo imposes a lasting impression not only aesthetically, but also semiotically.

The logo—three sinusoidal-like waves above the *Belsomra* text—evokes the rhythm of sleep and wakefulness, along with the merger of the two in a third wave that represents their conciliation, something not unlike a normal circadian rhythm of a person's day-to-day life. While this icon as graph does not exactly match up to the complexity of a sleep cycle graphed through an EEG, it does capture the concept. The graph icon could very likely resonate with individuals that use sleep-tracking devices, a key feature of more recent smart watches and fitness wearables, which further encourage control over the impossible ideal of perfect sleep, a pathology that one group of researcher's term "orthosomnia" (Baron et al., 2017: 351). The associative connection with digital sleep hygiene-tracking technologies fur-ther obscures Belsomra's pharmacological essence, and likely makes it an appealing option even for "noble non-users."

The use of waves as a visual sign, moreover, corresponds to the advertisement's use of music. The advertisement's score is a waltz, specifically a Chopin-romantic waltz. The sig-nificance of this specific kind of music for this specific kind of dance follows the logic of balance, harmony, and rhythm established above. In a waltz, each partner's step mirrors the others, which conceptually might also be understood as a kind of cycle, following the graphical wave form. The ad's use of different instruments and how their notes are syn-chronized with events on the screen contributes to this rhetoric. Throughout most of the ad, there is a notable contrast between legato melody (notes that are strung together smoothly without interruption) and the staccato accompaniment (short, punctuated notes that are detached from the others). This contrast at once indicates a tension (insomnia) but also the normal ebb and flow of the sleep–wake cycle that might include abrupt inflections, such as the normal interruptions to sleep. Therefore, the dialectic of normal minor abnor-mality and of sleep and wake neurotransmitters is reinforced by auditory means, comple-menting the visual and narrative thematics. Ultimately, the suggestion is that it is potentially normal to have insomnia, but that with Belsomra one can return to ideal—but not too perfect—sleep. In the last few seconds of the ad, viewers are presented with an auditory closure by way of a shift from minor to major keys using flutes, a typical way to signify resolution in a classical composition.[14] Belsomra is the solution to this conflict, just as it is to the ambivalence surrounding soporifics.

The afterlife of cats and dogs

While "Cats and Dogs" is by no means dated, it only lasted a short time in circulation. This did not, however, stop it from receiving a significant amount of attention. A short survey of tweets mentioning or hashtagging "Belsomra" reveals two prominent critiques: first, the concerning side effects, which as noted above, while seemingly distressing, are not often a determining factor in turning people away from a drug. Second, many viewers commenting on social media found the ad to be "creepy," often joking that sleep-cat and wake-dog ironically materialize Belsomra's possible hallucinatory side effect (Gregoire, 2015). Merck discontinued the ad and produced a replacement. The replacement, "Distractions," does not feature sleep-cat and wake-dog and does not thematically or formally convey the metaphor of medicine as balance in the same figurative dimensions the way "Cats and Dogs" does.[15] That said, it is still operating on the broader wave of de-pharmaceuticalization by way of invoking sleep hygiene. Using another female protagonist, the ad visually narrates common techniques associated with habits and environmental modifications that are conducive to falling and staying asleep. In the "Distractions" ad, a woman begins by turning off her television, which displays credits of some unknown program. The credits signal a sense of an ending. The listing function of the credits gesture towards the idea of a checklist, appropriate for elements of a sleep hygiene protocol: she proceeds to turn off the light, shut down her phone, and close her window.

And yet, "Despite all of the things you do to get a good night's sleep," we are told, "it can feel as if they get … undone, while you lie there, restless." As if by some insomnio-genic poltergeist, all of the disciplined elements of sleep hygiene are literally undone: the window shade comes up, and light enters; the TV turns on, *in medias res*, to a lion roaring. Cue the solution:

> Maybe you should talk to your doctor about Belsomra. Belsomra is an FDA sleep aid that works *differently* because it targets and inhibits the action of orexin, a neurotransmitter that is believed to play a central role in keeping you awake.
>
> *(emphasis added)*

The fading to black transitions a sequence of scenes showing a woman resting peacefully—including a brief, normal interruption, not unlike the one in "Cats and Dogs"—before she awakens to a strip of sunlight from the window cast perfectly across her eyes. She opens her windows to a new, refreshing day. "So, if you are looking to get more sleep, keep doing the things that help but also talk to your doctor about Belsomra." The paradoxical message is that if you are trying not to use sleeping pills for insomnia, because you want natural control over sleep, Belsomra can help as part of a balanced, responsible program. It works on the same broader logic of equipoise, as pharmacological intervention under the guise of de-pharmaceuticalization.

Accounting for the language in Merck's change in marketing strategy provides an important consideration for health humanities researchers and practitioners. Doug Black, US marketing leader for insomnia at Merck, commented that the "original ad did tremendously well," saying that

[it] had served its purpose. We were a very late entrant to the market, and at the time, the team felt we needed to break through. What we've learned since then as we've listened to our consumers, is that to reach a broader audience, we needed to find a more empathetic message.

(Bulik, 2017)

Despite Black's affirmation of listening to consumers, it is unclear how the new ad is anymore "empathetic" than the previous one. If we define empathy as the affinity for another's circumstances and related feelings, it remains uncertain that the "Cats and Dogs" effected any to begin with, beyond simply using simile to represent what insomnia "can feel *like*." This is perhaps a poignant reminder, especially given the history of empathy's role as a justification and imperative in medical humanities (not without contention) (Garden, 2007) that incorporating a humanistic lens towards health and medicine requires nuance, or it risks facile appropriation by interested stakeholders and the propagation of a one-dimensional deployment.

This chapter has not been an attempt to demonize Belsomra or the use of soporifics, or to question insomnia as a diagnosis. Rather, it has sought to demystify what subtends the "good sleep" Belsomra's etymology promises. Bound within Belsomra's harmonizing logic are an amalgam of opposing forces and contradictions that scale from the molecular to the social to the ideological. At the pharmacological level, Belsomra works by inhibiting orexin, and consequently suppress the wake process in an individual body. In relation to other individual bodies, insomniatic or not, it promotes ordered participation in the social. If, as Wolf-Meyer suggests, sleep operates as a matter of responsibility to meet work and societal demands, then it consequently "binds individuals to institutions ... and when disordered sleep disrupts the interactions medicine intervenes to reorder the everyday" (Wolf-Meyer, 2012: 3). At the ideological level, what organizes and ideationally fuels so much of the social, Belsomra reflects a culture that at once warns that "lack of sleep may kill you" while also espousing "sleep[ing] when you're dead" (Barbee et al., 2018: 6). Belsomra manifests the commodification of "natural" wellness while also living better through chemistry. Furthermore, the drug and its marketing lend themselves to a medicalized model where a complaint like insomnia is at once "common" and "abnormal" (Conrad, 2005: 6). If Belsomra's core logic is equipoise, it does, indeed, perform quite the balancing act.

As this extended analysis of DTCA demonstrates, interdisciplinary semiotic readings of pharmaceutical advertisements are productive starting points for considering the cultural dimensions of a drug's social life: how it is linked to lifestyles, attitudes, and "attractive imaginaries," how it is working in the world, and how that aligns—or does not—with its intended uses (Hardon and Sanabria, 2017: 122). It gives us a way to interpret the relationship between a drug's biological, societal, and cultural effects. Engaging with this form of semiotic reading defamiliarizes the genre, moving us from tired denunciation and facile parody to a more nuanced understanding of DTCA's aesthetics, rhetoric, and logics.

Without pressing the need to immediately instrumentalize this specific reading and method for use in the clinic, we should be mindful of the fact that thinking through how these advertisements work provides a unique opportunity in the proverbially increasingly vexed relationships between prescribers and patients. Accounting for the rhetorical complexity of the advertisements, the influence of DTCA on prescribing practices, and the role pharmaceuticals can play in identity formation (moral repertoires in the case of sedative hypnotics), suggests both participants in a clinical interaction might benefit from asking each other about DTCA. In the vein of narrative medicine and pathography, listening and discussing what strikes a patient to request a particular drug, rather than chastising or rejecting them under the auspices of medical authority, creates an opportunity to build trust and can potentially yield clinically relevant information pertaining to illness and sickness rather than just disease (Kleinman, 1988). It can, moreover, educate both patient and practitioner. In the case of the patient, prescribers can explain what the drug advertisement glosses over and the difficulties and challenges of assessing risks and benefits. Patients can articulate signs and symptoms of disease, along with the lived, narrative experience of illness, and collaboratively contemplate the cultural scripts that advertisements could cater to. This mode of exchange has the potential to reduce the pressure prescribers often feel when requested to prescribe a specific drug and the condescension patients often face when they posit whatever version of lay pharmacological expertise they might present. To get here, however, we begin with capacious contextualization paired with sustained interrogation of a single text, rather than judgment. Perhaps, then, we could be better served by asking not if Belsomra—or DTCA more broadly—is right for us, but rather *how* and *why* its representations might seem to be.

Notes

1 This term was expanded to "biomedicalization" to delimit its transformations post-1985. See: Clarke, A., Shim, J.K., Marno, L., Fosket, J.R. and Fishman, J.R (2003) Biomedicalization: Technoscientific Transformations of Health, Illness, and U.S. Biomedicine. *American Sociological Review*, 68(2), 161–194.

2 Pharmaceuticalization, moreover, distinctly considers the use of medications for lifestyle, recreation, and enhancement—certainly gray rubrics—and access to them from outside licit medical channels (the internet and black market.) See Gabe et al. (2017).

3 In the simplest terms, GABA (gamma-aminobutyric acid) is a neurotransmitter that plays an inhibitory role in the nervous system. A GABA-agonist potentiates this system. An exception to the drugs named above is Rozerem, which is a melatonin receptor agonist. Z-drugs are technically referred of as non-benzodiazepine sedative-hypnotics.

4 Following Appadurai's anthropological work on commodities and material items, Whyte, Geest, and Hardon trace the lives of drugs specifically in terms of "their production and marketing, their prescription, their distribution through intertwined formal and informal channels, and their deaths through one or another form of consumption, and finally their lives after death in the form of efficacy in modifying bodies" (Whyte et al.,2002: 13–14).

5 Because there are a number of different classes of medications (e.g. tranquilizers, sedatives, sedative-hypnotics), I use *soporific* here as the broadest term for an agent that induces sleep.

6 For more details on the history of DTCA, see Greene and Herzberg (2010) and Schwartz and Woloshin (2019).

7 1997 figure reported in 2016 dollar equivalent.

8 On the sleep industrial complex, see Mooallem, J. (2007) The Sleep-Industrial Complex. *New York Times*, November 18. https://www.nytimes.com/2007/11/18/health/18iht-18sleept.8377935.html. Accessed November 28, 2019.

9 Here, Moloney references Gabe et al.'s (2017) study.
    On a taxonomy of common this kind of figurative language, see Scott et al. (2004: 23).

10 Although Gabe et al. (2017) draw data from a sampling of the UK's population, there is quantitative and qualitative evidence of at the very least resistance to or reluctant acceptance of medicalization, if not a more concentrated process of de-pharmaceuticalization in the United States. See Moloney et al. (2019: 5).
    On pharmacological Calvinism, see Conrad (2005) *The Medicalization of Society: On the Transformation of Human Conditions into Treatable Disorders*. Baltimore: Johns Hopkins University Press: 106. The term was first coined in Klerman, G. (1972) Psychotropic Hedonism vs. Pharmacological Calvinism. *Hastings Center Report*, 2(4): 1–3.

11 Indeed, if we are thinking paratextually, side effect warnings are part of drugs as consumable objects. Because the FDA requires that prescription drugs are dispensed with package inserts, whether we read them or not, drugs have a textual, media component. In fact, the very fact that

we are so quick to throw away the 40-page, 1000-line document that includes everything from chemical structure, pharmacokinetics, and clinical trial information on top of side.

12 See "Side-Effects Include …," *TVtropes*. Accessed July 30, 2019. https://tvtropes.org/pmwiki/pmwiki.php/Main/SideEffectsInclude.

13 The authors understand the dilution effect as an "effect [that] occurs whereby those who assess the mixed set of diagnostic and non-diagnostic information arrive at less extreme predictions in comparison with those who assessed only diagnostic information. That is, the nondiagnostic information—information of little value and consequence for outcome prediction—dilutes the value and importance of the diagnostic information in our prognostication" (797).

14 I am indebted to my colleagues Suzanne Edwards and Mark and Alyssa Volker that were generous in sharing their extensive knowledge of musicology to substantiate this reading.

15 See Belsomra, "Distractions," Television advertisement, 2017. Accessed July 30, 2019. https://www.ispot.tv/ad/wKsO/belsomra-distractions.

Acknowledgements

This chapter would not have been possible without the insight and research on the financial aspects of DTCA provided by Shaelyn Heft. The help with the musicological reading is grounded in the invaluable specifics and information offered by Suzanne Edwards, Mark Volker, and Alyssa Volker. I would also like to thank Gillian Andrews for her suggestions and edits on the chapter as a whole.

References

Abraham, J. (2010). Pharmaceuticalization of Society in Context: Theoretical, Empirical and Health Dimensions. *Sociology*, 44(4): 603–622.

Barbee, H., Moloney, M.E. and Konrad, T.R. (2018). Selling Slumber: American Neoliberalism and the Medicalization of Sleeplessness. *Sociology Compass*, 12(10), doi:10.1111/soc4.12622

Baron, K. G., Abbott, S., Jao, N., Manalo, N., & Mullen, R. (2017). Orthosomnia: Are Some Patients Taking the Quantified Self Too Far? *Journal of Clinical Sleep Medicine*, 13(2): 351–354.

Bell, S.E. and Figert, A.E. (2012). Medicalization and Pharmaceuticalization at the Intersections: Looking Backward, Sideways and Forward. *Social Sciences and Medicine*, 75(5): 778–783.

Belsomra. (2015). Cats and Dogs. *Television advertisement*. Accessed 30 July, 2019. www.ispot.tv/ad/7UYo/belsomra-cats-and-dogs

Bulik, B.S. (2017). Goodbye to Belsomra's Furry Mascots. Merck's Focusing on Sleepless Patients Instead. *Fierce Pharma*. October 9 2017. Accessed July 30, 2019. www.fiercepharma.com/marketing/good-bye-sleep-cat-and-wake-dog-merck-s-belsomra-new-marketing-direction-built-patient

Conrad, P. (1992). Medicalization and Social Control. *Annual Review of Sociology*, 18: 209–232.

Conrad, P. (2005). The Shifting Engines of Medicalization. *Journal of Health and Social Behavior*, 46(1): 3–14.

Doran, E. (2016). Trouble Spots in Online Direct-to-Consumer Prescription Drug Promotion: Teaching Drug Marketers How to Inform Better or Spin Better? Comment on "Trouble Spots in Online Direct-to-Consumer Prescription Drug Promotion: A Content Analysis of FDA Warning Letters". *International Journal of Health Policy Management*, 5(5): 334.

Dumit, J. (2012). *Drugs for Life: How Pharmaceutical Companies Define Our Health*. Durham: Duke University Press.

Elliot, C. (2003). *Better Than Well: American Medicine Meets the American Dream*. New York: Norton.

Gabbatt, A. (2018). "The Devil's Aspirin": Why Do So Many Celebrities Blame Ambien? *The Guardian*, August 17 2018. Accessed July 30, 2019. www.theguardian.com/technology/2018/aug/17/ambien-elon-musk-roseanne-celebrities-blame-sedative-behaviour

Gabe, J., Coveney, C.M. and Williams, S.J. (2016). Prescriptions and Proscriptions: Moralising Sleep Medicines. *Sociology of Health and Illness*, 38(4): 628–639.

Gabe, J., Williams, S.J. and Coveney, C.M. (2017). Prescription Hypnotics in the News: A Study of UK Audiences. *Social Science and Medicine*, 174: 43–52.

Garden, R. (2007). The Problem of Empathy: Medicine and the Humanities. *New Literary History*, 38(3): 551–567.

Greene, J. and Herzberg, D. (2010). Hidden in Plain Sight: Marketing Prescription Drugs to Consumers in the Twentieth Century. *American Journal of Public Health*, 100(5): 793–803.

Gregoire, C. (2015). This Sleeping Pill Commercial is Absolutely Terrifying. *Huffpost*, 17 September. Accessed July 30, 2019. www.huffpost.com/entry/belsomra-commercial_n_55f83fcbe4b00e2cd5e7fd50

Hardon, A. and Sanabria, E. (2017). Fluid Drugs: Revisiting the Anthropology of Pharmaceuticals. *Annual Review of Anthropology*, 46(1): 122.

Kaufman, J. (2017). Think You're Seeing More Drug Ads on TV? You Are, and Here's Why. *New York Times*, 24 December. Accessed July 30, 2019. www.nytimes.com/2017/12/24/business/media/prescription-drugs-advertising-tv.html.

Klara, K., Kim, J. and Ross, J.S. (2018). Direct-to-Consumer Broadcast Advertisements for Pharmaceuticals: Off-Label Promotion and Adherence to FDA Guidelines. *Journal of General of Internal Medicine*, 33(5): 651–658.

Kleinman, A. (1988). *The Illness Narratives: Suffering, Healing, and the Human Condition*. New York: Basic Books.

Markets and Markets. (2017) 8 *U.S. Insomnia Market by Non-Pharmacological Therapy (CBTI, Hypnotherapy), Prescription Sleep Aids (Benzodiazepines, Non-Benzodiazepines (Zaleplon), Orexin Antagonist) and OTC Treatment (Antihistamine, Melatonin, Valerian Root) - Forecasts to 2021*. Online: Accessed August 16, 2019. www.researchandmarkets.com/research/jgq9qr/u_s_insomnia

Moloney, M.E., Ciciurkaite, G. and Brown, R.L. (2019). The Medicalization of Sleeplessness: Results of U.S. Office Visit Outcomes, 2008–2015. *SSM Population Health*, August 8: 100388. doi:10.1016/j.ssmph.2019.100388

Reading, P. (2013). *ABC of Sleep Medicine*. Oxford: John Wiley and Sons.

Rose, N. (2007). Beyond Medicalization. *Lancet*, 369(9562): 700–702.

Schwartz, L.M. and Woloshin, S. (2019). Medical Marketing in the United States, 1997–2016. *JAMA*, 321(1): 80–96.

Scott, T., Stanford, N. and Thompson, D.R. (2004). Killing Me Softly: Myth in Pharmaceutical Advertising. *British Medical Journal*, 329: 1484–1488.

Sivanathan, N. and Kakkar, H. (2017). The Unintended Consequences of Argument Dilution in Direct-to-Consumer Drug Advertisements. *Nature Human Behaviour*, 1(11): 797–802.

Whyte, S.R. et al. (2002). *Social Lives of Medicines*. New York: Cambridge University Press.

Wolf-Meyer, M. (2012). *Slumbering Masses: Sleep, Medicine, and Modern American Life*. Minneapolis: University of Minnesota Press.

Zola, I. (1972). Medicine as an Institution of Social Control. *Sociological Review*, 20(4): 487–504.

20

THE PROBLEM WITH "BURNOUT"

Neoliberalization, biomedicine, and other soul mates

Shane Neilson

Introduction

Because the number of Canadian medical doctors with PhDs in the humanities is small, I feel justified in starting off this article with two anecdotes intended to validate the need for more dual-trained physicians as the discipline of medicine drifts further into gospelized clinical practice guidelines. The first anecdote comes from what I call biomedicine's "trenches." In the summer of 2018, I met with a cohort of first-year students at one of Ontario's medical schools as part of a careers talk over the lunch hour. Before discussing the value of a scholarly humanities deployed within the discipline of medicine, I took stock of my audience. "How many of you here have degrees in the humanities or social sciences?"

No hands raised. I realized I was asking the question the wrong way around. "How many, then, have degrees in the sciences?" A majority of hands shot up. But some *didn't* go up, and I wondered what background those people had. Perhaps I had misphrased my original question? "For those who didn't raise their hand, tell me: what training do you have?"

The remainder of the room had engineering, business, health sciences, and information technology degrees, some of them qualified at the Master's level. No one had training or experience in anything else. Alarmed, I asked the group, "Do you know what biomedicine is?" No one knew, or admitted to knowing.

Although this anecdote is true, it is a bit cooked in terms of context. In truth, I was already well aware that the game had been lost, long ago—this audience merely confirmed an established fact. They were the biomedical epistemology in embodied form, or at least the fleshly results of it, the epistemology's desired outcome.[1] The students had subscribed to the plan without even knowing what it was, electing to follow a well-demarcated path that led to acceptance into medical school. Their silence was a testimonial to the power of the epistemology: they didn't know what it was that they subscribed to, but they did what they were implicitly told anyway. What better master to serve in the years before application than the same master?

My second anecdote comes from the humanities job-search trenches. During that same summer I lunched with the medical students, I interviewed for a job in disability studies. I talked about my work critiquing the discipline of medicine, thinking this aspect of unique appeal, a distinguishing factor among applicants. I shared with the hiring committee a vision of renovating the medical school (part of the larger campus family) with humanities methodologies. At one point, a frustrated committee member said, "But you're talking so much about medicine. Our students in disability studies don't go on to become doctors. They don't care so much about medicine. What would *you* do for *our* students?"

Like the first anecdote, this reaction is also familiar to me. I had known of the "two solitudes" problem of the humanities and medicine, but I never had a clearer articulation of disaffection towards medicine been offered so boldly and baldly to my face before. Reacting to such irritation, I confess my mind turned to the defensive. *Isn't it easy to live in one's cloistered, factional little world?*, I thought. But rather than giving voice to that reaction, I responded by saying, "Having a medical doctor who is trained to be a collaborative critic of medicine, and who self-identifies as disabled, as one of your professors of disability studies … wouldn't be of interest to your students?" I followed this by repeating aloud a version of the first anecdote, and then added:

> But there is a version of the same phenomenon happening in the humanities, and you've just shown that. Don't you think a revolution would happen in the discipline of medicine if disability studies students were *encouraged* to become physicians? What might change in care practices as a result?

I encountered a different silence after that provocation, one that struck me as either jealous resentment (humanities faculties often eye medical faculties with justifiable frustration in terms of funding disparities) or the understandable conversational gap that occurs when an interviewee sinks his own ship. Either way, trying to interpret the symmetrical silences in both anecdotes over a year later, I am struck by how comfortable (speaking generally) two traditions of knowledge production are at ignoring or avoiding one another when they very much need one another.

With this relative lack of critique from within medicine in mind, my article will suggest that the concept of "burnout" is misframed by medicine because it is conceived of by medicine itself. I will move from a discussion of what medicine thinks burnout is, and why this definition's biomedical and neoliberal rhetorical sponsors are a problem, to ask this question: if what medicine values as reflected in its admissions processes is consistent, self-sacrificing dominance with respect to the management of data, then how can a course correction ever be achieved? My inquiry is informed by the field of the philosophies of medicine (biomedicine and neoliberalization of care), literary studies (Vincent Lam's *Bloodletting and Miraculous Cures* and various publications by the Canadian Medical Association), and a field interview to provide some real-world coordinates for my arguments. Along the way, I hope to enact the value of critique from the inside.

Survey says: neoliberal rhetoric and the Canadian Medical Association National Physician Health Survey

On October 10, 2018, the Canadian Medical Association (CMA) published the *CMA National Physician Health Survey* (NPHS), a document that was widely reported on in broader Canadian media. For example, the *Toronto Star*'s headline read "Canadian doctors are suffering from burnout at an 'alarming' rate." Although the crisis-hawking headline isn't wrong, there is so much to critique about the NPHS's concept of "burnout" that the headline isn't quite right, either. But to be fair, what newspaper features headlines like "Canadian doctors are suffering from crushing biomedical and neoliberal imperatives?"

One need not move beyond the first page of the NPHS to understand the rhetorical basis of the plight physicians are in. In that first graph, biomedicine appears immediately: "Our goals were to generate an up-to-date and relevant baseline dataset for use by other organizations, researchers, educators and stakeholders and to use this dataset to inform and advance physician health initiatives" (Canadian Medical Association, 2018: 1). Like all reasonable people, I am all for quantifying a problem to get a sense of size and scope, and I trust that, like me, the readers of this article will be "alarmed" by the "burnout" on offer. I also hope that readers appreciate irony. Shouldn't we be discomfited by the NPHS's unwitting adherence to the same body-rendered-into-data transformation—the project of biomedicine—that necessitated its very existence? If an epistemology does not know the *meaning* of its ass from its head, but has exact weights and measurements attesting to the *numerical* difference, then how can such an epistemology be used to help physicians get better? How is an initiative designed to quantify how sick physicians are, operating as it does out of the very force that is making physicians sick, supposed to help physicians?

Although neither are defined in the discussion section of the NPHS (tellingly, one must skip to the appendix), "resiliency" and "burnout" are mentioned often and have numerical values attached attesting to their burden in the profession. As one might expect, the equation goes more or less like this: low-resiliency physicians = high likelihood of burnout. Yet the appendix's definition of "burnout" is worth reviewing, for it suggests the existential problem at work when rendering affective/spiritual states in quantitative terms:

> The two-item Maslach Burnout Inventory (MBI 2 . . .) was used to measure burn-out. This scale has been deemed reliable and valid in physician populations . . . The MBI 2 is recommended as an appropriate alternative to the full MBI-22 for large-scale and multifaceted national surveys where space is an important . . . The two questions assess emotional exhaustion ("I feel burned out from my work") and depersonalization ("I have become more callous towards people since I took this job"), which are indicators of burnout. Responses are measured on a scale ranging from 0 ("never") to 6 ("everyday"). To be classified as burned out, an individual must experience high levels of emotional exhaustion and/or depersonalization. High levels on these subscales are defined as occurring at least weekly.
>
> (Canadian Medical Association, 2018: 27)

According to the tool, emotional exhaustion and depersonalization are the components of "burnout," which seems reasonable enough on the face of things. Who would disagree that doctors who become less caring over time, and who are exhausted in emotional terms, are not burned out? My problem with this definition is not on the plane of scientific validation—I'm sure biomedicine did its job—but rather on the *discourse* of burnout, on what burnout *means* in the context of this survey. If, as the NPHS maintains, burnout—a metaphor suggesting consumed husks, exhausted resources, immolated futures, fiery hellacious negativity—is a cause of "alarm," then what can be done by and for a discipline given over wholly to biomedicine? How can we care for our "burnouts" and is it even possible to change things from within? Is the alarm bell truly pulled by biomedicine for the good of the discipline, or is it ringing an alarm bell cynically, so that its "physician workforce"—a term shot through the NPHS—can continue to be good, functioning care drones? Can we trust biomedicine to take care of our souls?

Based on the NPHS's rhetoric, I argue that the aforementioned "alarm" is pulled with significant ambiguity: "We believe that strengthening the health and wellness of the physician workforce is a shared responsibility. Individual physicians must take steps to maintain their personal health and wellness, while system-level initiatives involving numerous institutions, organizations and communities are also necessary" (Canadian Medical Association, 2018: 2). Admittedly, the "belief" just transcribed identifies "system-level" responsibilities, which seems responsible enough at first glance. Not everything is dumped onto poor, burned-out individuals and their capacity to adapt or to take care of themselves. On second glance, one notes the hierarchy established by sequence. The individual is called to account first, and the "system" is mentioned second; moreover, what system and prevailing conditions are we even talking about?

My argument—not a novel one, but one still worth making—is that the "belief" of the NPHS is, ultimately, authored by the philosophy of neoliberalism. Neoliberalism's encouragement of resiliency as something to be cultivated at the level of the individual in order to compensate for its curtailment of the welfare state compromises the good intentions of the NPHS.

Let me define what I mean by the oft-invoked, but confusingly polysemous, term "neoliberalism." For this article, neoliberalism denotes a cluster of changes to monetary policy by Western governments beginning in the 1970s but accelerating to the present. These changes reflect "a general orientation towards a strongly market-based approach, which emphasises deregulation, minimalisation of the State, privatisation, and the emergence of individual responsibility" (Sakellariou and Rotarou, 2019: 2). The rise of neoliberal monetary policy in the latter part of the twentieth century has largely meant the dismantling (or "privatizing") of the welfare state. In the introduction to a special issue of *Social Science in Medicine* concerning the role of civil society in health-care system reform, Giarelli et al. (2014: 160) write, "Across the world public provision of healthcare is being rolled back or precluded in favor of free market principles associated with global neoliberalism." Canada has not been spared the curtailments inherent to doctrines of efficiency, for as Toba Bryant (2009: 203) argues, "[t]he rise of neoliberalism has influenced welfare state policies in Canada." As the philosophy increased its hold on governments in the twenty-first century, neoliberalism now poses an overt philosophical threat to socialized medicine, for as Sakellariou and Rotarou (2019: 1) state, neoliberalism emphasizes the "free market rather than the right to health."

With this context in mind, the NPHS can be interpreted as a document that adopts neoliberal rhetoric (e.g., referring to the "physician workforce" repeatedly). The basic premise of the document is that doctors are important because of the work that they do, not because they have intrinsic value as people, and this constitutes a real problem for biomedicine's burnouts. Isn't it hard to get better if one identifies as a job and not a human being? Why not call the physician burnout problem what it is: a self-selecting and economically remunerative (but spiritually destroying) form of exploitation? "Burnout" strikes me as a misnomer for what physicians are suffering, as individuals and as a collectivity, for we feel the inevitable strain of a system that *imposes* the coping strategy of depersonalization. The system offloads its impossibility to its "workforce." The terms of our practice are set according to a rhetoric of efficiency, productivity, and volume. "Burnout" can hardly be called an unintended outcome of this system, but rather a *byproduct* of the industrialization of care as well as a consequence of cuts to the socialized health-care system.[2] "Burnout" in this sense is not emotional exhaustion and depersonalization but an understandable, and possibly even desired, result of monetary policy changes (to wring the most efficiency out of a system, one must break a few eggs). To place, as the NPHS does, the individual alongside the twin giant-tyrants of biomedicine and neoliberalism (the NPHS's "systemic factors") in the context of burnout is to assign numbers to a problem based on the systematization of individual reportage, but the exact dimensions of all individuals surveyed is two. We are crushed as flat as a pancake under the boots of the giants.

Dissecting biomedicine's "study techniques": burnout as destiny

Perhaps we should begin at the beginning, and not with the NPHS's contemporaneous numbers. Let's talk about what it means to practice medicine. As mentioned in my first anecdote, the "burnout" problem begins long before entry into medical school; it is foretold in the processes of becoming a doctor, which follow an accepted, predetermined path. This path is mapped by Giller-winning physician-writer Vincent Lam in "How to Get into Medical School, Part One," the first short story in his *Bloodletting and Miraculous Cures*, in which strategies of work are already laid down in the pre-med stage:

> For self-identified "med school keeners" (the label was inherently self-designated even for those who publicly denied it), study tables were the monks' cells of exam time. Adherents arrived early in the morning and sat silently except for whispered exchanges. There was a desperate devotion to the impending sacrament and judgement of the exam. The faithful departed late at night, and returned upon the library's opening.
>
> *(Lam, 2006: 9)*

The remainder of the story contrasts two personalities, those of Ming and Fitzgerald, two prospective medical students, who have quite different study methods. Ming focuses on data, trivia—on digestible, testable, regurgitatable fact—where Fitzgerald focuses instead on comprehension:

> Sometimes, Fitzgerald closed his eyes and mouthed words while he memorized. Ming pretended to look out the window, allowed herself to briefly watch the half-image of his reflection speaking silently. She could see that he was immersed in the material, that he was trying to get inside it. She admired this, and longed for Fitzgerald because of it. Ming had decided to be occupied primarily with the facts in her textbooks, and less with comprehension. Ionic channels were not a wonderful riddle to her, as she knew they were to Fitzgerald. They were simply a means to an end, that end being a perfect set of grades and a medical school admission letter. Hers was the more common attitude in the life sciences faculty, and so Ming regarded Fitzgerald as being pure and noble, if strategically unwise.
>
> *(Lam, 2006: 9–10)*

Ming, of course, achieves the kind of marks that will eventually gain her early admittance to medical school, but Fitzgerald performs in a mediocre fashion. Ming attributes her success to her "study techniques" (Lam, 2006: 10) that involve rote memorization, obsessive note taking, and a systematic approach to processing the information she is expected to distribute back to her examiners. (Any medical person reading this must be nodding their head; the acuity of the description is hard to read.) In the story, Ming is eventually accepted into medical school, and Fitzgerald is not, although he does get accepted a year later, only after he alters his "study techniques" ("dissected" by Ming as a gesture of help) to more closely align with those of Ming.

This short story has what I would call a rich admissions discourse, replete as it is with "study techniques," interview strategy, and MCAT folklore. Perhaps the chief deficit in how to get into medical school dramatized by the story is the incredible gap between knowing what it takes to get into medical school (Ming is expert, and Fitzgerald, albeit with less successful study techniques, is no mere acolyte) and what it means to be a doctor. At one point, Ming and Fitzgerald share a meal as a break between study sessions, and they:

> talked about their need to become physicians. Others were not genuine, they agreed, and transparently wanted to become doctors for money and prestige. Ming and Fitzgerald wanted medicine for the right reasons, they told each other: service, humanity, giving. Because their motivations were clean, they were certain they deserved it more than those among them. They did not ask why they wanted to serve, be humane, or to give. They simply felt like the right motivations, and being correctly motivated should improve their chances of success. This was enough, and these sentiments felt easy and immune from questioning. If forced to reflect, both Ming and Fitzgerald would have had to admit that these convictions were, at their core, somewhat improvised.
>
> *(Lam, 2006: 10)*

The path to medicine is clear, but the apprehension of what medicine *is*, what it is like practicing medicine, is missing. Only a vague desire to help people is sketched by Lam as motivation, and I cannot say that it was any different for me as a prospective medical student, so I do not view the characters of Ming and Fitzgerald with scorn, but rather with a wincing acknowledgement that incites me to ask this question: if the path to medicine— subscription to monastic self-discipline to achieve academic dominance—is clear, but the meaning of what being a doctor is not, then biomedicine has tilted the table against the humanities early, and that the table is titled because biomedicine *prefers* certain kinds of disciples. This point is hit home when Ming reviews Fitzgerald's biochemistry exam, for which he receives a mediocre grade. In the passage that follows, Ming tries to find places where more marks should have been given:

> "I can't find marks, but you understand this stuff. You're losing marks on detail. The Krebs cycle—you know it better than I do. The problem is the way you study and write." She said this not only to be kind, but because she found his answers elegant and insightful. Ming's own responses were always factually complete in point form, convenient to check off for a perfect score.
>
> *(Lam, 2006: 15)*

Fitzgerald writes epically idiosyncratic answers replete with self-made diagrams; Ming recapitulates, taxonomizes, differentiates—and tries to tailor her answer to what is expected to be the answer. Fitzgerald takes philosophy as his "humanities elective"[3]—a single one of these requisite for many medical schools—and he is "top of the class" (Lam, 2006: 17) with a mark of "seventy-one." On hearing how he performed, Ming tells Fitz that he needs to "strategize [his] electives" (Lam, 2006: 17). The narrator tells us that her elective was "introductory psychology, a course that fulfilled its reputation of providing an easy A+" (Lam, 2006: 17). Humanities scholars reading this piece, feel free to emit a groan of recognition.

In a sense, the story is a simple fable of how two different systems of knowledge production lead to two different fates. Biomedicine rewards Ming, its true disciple, and it eventually rewards its convert, Fitzgerald. The story is not about what it means to be a doctor, and how could it be? The story is titled the way it is for a reason. Yet I argue that without instilling an understanding of what being a doctor is for the "med school keeners," without conveying somehow what being a doctor *means*[4] in the face of ritualized consumption of data, then burnout is not only a predictable outcome for physicians, it is an *intended* one—as I will argue next, using another of Lam's stories.

The duet of Jill and Chen: emergency departments are ground zero for neoliberal health policy

To close the loop on the implicit prophecy of "How To Get Into Medical School, Part One," Lam's *book* ends with "Before Light," a short story about burnout. In this tale, Dr. Chen—introduced as a medical student earlier on in the book—is now a full-fledged attending physician in the emergency department at "Toronto Southern." Also earlier in the book, Chen lives through the SARS crisis, contracting the illness himself, and performs a resuscitation on his alcoholic friend Fitzgerald (at the time of "Before Light" also a medical doctor, although the contribution of medicine to his addiction is not directly provided), but Chen is never presented as cynical, exhausted, or at odds with his profession ... until "Before Light."

The bona fides of Chen's burnout as defined by the NPHS are omnipresent in the story. Chen is emotionally exhausted. He loses patience at work when others place frivolous demands on his time (Lam, 2006: 322), he publicly intimidates a consultant who condescends to him (Lam, 2006: 331), he rationalizes his aggressive driving patterns because of his sacrifice to the discipline of medicine (Lam, 2006: 311), and there is a section in the story's middle in which Chen depersonalizes at great length:

> Stretcher rolls in, trundles across the floor ... It feels like those films of men on the moon who jump and take a forever leap, who launch a gold ball that disappears against the black sky while the narrator says, *All skies would be black without our oxygenated atmosphere. Beep beep beep.* The guy has a shit blood pressure. His skin is the white on white blue webbing lines of death. This is also my nightmare of war; the enemy invisible, shots in the dark, everyone rushing, confused, but in one tiny panicked place all is such calm because the end is near or the end is far, but there is no way to know. Somewhere there is a truce. Nurses and medics shout to grab this, hand me that, push it here, get the blue box ... Once, I saw Neil Armstrong with a soundtrack to Erik Satie's piano *Gymnopedies*—the astronauts suspended on delicate melody. Like that, floating, I call the orders, touch the patient, feel his belly, put my stethoscope on his side. I shine light in his eyes, they squeeze reflexively: dreamy, unreal. I say, "Atropine point eight." Each small move is accentuated. I say something, call out an order, and someone begins to do it, like my own golf ball hurtling away.
>
> *(Lam, 2006: 326–327)*

In the story, the various behaviors of Chen are not narrated as coping techniques, but this is in fact what they are, developed because of the relative impossibility of the expectations placed upon him. He must stay awake and spend himself at a complex, gruelling, technically demanding, and high-risk workplace in order to fulfill his role as a physician in the hospital. The story does not didactically point out the impossibility of working in this space and remaining well (it is not the job of fiction to tell) but rather dramatizes that impossibility through the character of Chen, who elsewhere in the book is depicted as a caring, compassionate, competent doctor. The reader sees the point Chen has reached, from diligent student to fraught physician, and draws their own conclusions.

Chen is, at the least, likely to seriously injure himself or die, as reflected in the final few pages of the story, where he is depicted comically slapping his own face and screaming nonsense aloud in order to stay awake on the drive home. He does not quite manage to completely stay awake, although no disaster ensues. After making it home, he falls asleep in the car park and awakens only when the caretaker knocks on his window, saying, "Morning, sir. I was knocking for awhile, getting worried, about to call the ambulance" (Lam, 2006: 336). That Chen is at risk is, I trust, apparent; but is he at risk because of himself, his failure to "have the stronger mind" as the story will develop, or is his failure to be well the result of the "system-level" factors vaguely referenced by the NPHS? Is Chen "at risk" because of biomedical and neoliberal philosophies that demand the impossible from him?

Linda Duxbury, professor at Carleton University's Sprott School of Business, delivered a keynote speech at the Canadian Conference on Physician Leadership 2019 that was reported on in the *Canadian Medical Association Journal*. Duxbury argues that "the health care system takes advantage of the willingness of physicians to work excessive hours and sometimes provide their time for free." Because "[h]ospitals have people who give a damn working for them ... the system survives" (Rich, 2019). The costs to individuals that constitute the medical profession are obvious, even obvious *to* them; but if what can be done about those offloaded costs must involve increased investment, then how can such investment be achieved when the rhetorics—"efficiency," etc.—are so stacked against change? For who doesn't want to be efficient, resilient, adaptable?

To get a better sense of the applicability of this idea in the real world, I interviewed Dr. Diana Toubassi, a family physician who works out of Toronto Western (this hospital being the likely stand-in for Lam's "Toronto Southern." Dr. Toubassi is a diminutive woman with a sprightly sense of humour and an air of conspiratorial hilarity, which made interviewing her about burnout intriguing. The whole interview confirms many of the contentions and themes within this article, but I will focus on verification of Chen's work process.

In response to a question about her work satisfaction, Dr. Toubassi admits that she is "struggling with the [low] frequency" of making a meaningful connection with her patients "and whether it's happening often enough to justify the pain and suffering associated with a career in medicine." When I follow up on this point and ask if the issue is one of workload, Diana responds:

> It's not so much workload as work *process*. I think I struggle with the amount—the lack of time we have to spend with each individual patient and the rush to push each individual patient through. I also struggle with whether the majority of the patients I'm seeing truly need to be seen *medically* and how much what they're looking for from me was potentially being provided by people like clergy or extended family in previous generations. I think a lot of patients are also looking for something from their doctor that is hard to give in a ten-minute visit where you're dealing with a sore throat.

Dr. Toubassi then sketches in the impossibility of her typical day:

> [Y]esterday I was 13 or 14 patients into the clinic. I had a green trainee with me who hadn't done any clinical rotations yet. We were running behind and I felt like

we were drowning in patients. I had her go and see a newborn baby that was there for their first visit. Mom was clearly overwhelmed and tearful already. Baby was jaundiced and not gaining weight. At the same time, I was seeing an elderly woman in her 80s who had recently been discharged from hospital. She hadn't been recovering well from home and had brought with her a written list of 8 issues that she wanted me to deal with in the ten minutes that we had together. I took pause for a moment, and I thought about how I was going to be the best person that I could be for both of these people at the same time, knowing that I also had to be at an important meeting ten minutes later. While I was seeing this elderly lady and my medical student was seeing the newborn baby, the nurse knocked on my door and said that the person who didn't show at 9 this morning made a mistake with their appointment time and she's here to see you and she needs a renewal of her medication and can you still see her? You have moments like that and you know there is just no human way, no way, that I can be at three places in the same time and give these three patients what they need from me today. It's just not possible. Or it's not possible for me to do that and still be intact enough with me to proceed with my day in a reasonable manner.

I'll bring Dr. Toubassi back in the next section, but for now let me ask the following questions: what is the place of terminology like efficiency and adaptability in this context? How long can we sustain unsustainable impossibility? No doctor can be present in "three places at the same time" but this is what the system requires in order to function.

The various threads I am trying to draw together—neoliberalization of the socialized system, burnout, internalization, and compensation for the system's inadequacies—is nicely dramatized by Lam in a scene that involves the interaction of Chen and a nurse, Jill, who work together concerning Mr. Santorini, a man having a heart attack. Mr. Santorini is in denial, and Chen, who is tried to convince Mr. Santorini in various ways under a literal time pressure (Chen repeatedly thinks "time is muscle" [Lam, 2006: 317]), resorts to a neo-liberal rationale in order to mobilize Mr. Santorini's consent:

> "Sir," I say. Do you pay your taxes?
> I fix my gaze on him, to take his attention away from Jill's new jab in his arm.
> Of course. I have a slick accountant, but sure, I—
> I come close to his face. I look straight and unblinking into his eyes. 'Do you know why you pay your taxes?" The drug in the vial is now dissolved. I draw up the clear liquid, a little more than the exact dose.
> I have to, otherwise—
> "You pay your taxes so that I can be here at midnight after having spent many years in school, and so that I can tell you without a shadow of a doubt that your heart is in the process of infracting and we need to use your tax dollars to do something about it." I say it nicely—like I would sell a used Hyundai if I were a car salesman.
>
> *(Lam, 2006: 318)*

Mr. Santorini, who rejects all of Chen's other reasoning up to that point, including biomedical reasoning in which Chen interprets test results to prove, unequivocally, that a myocardial infarction is progressing, is ultimately won over with Chen's economic rationale. Adding to the satire of the scene is that Chen sells himself the same script; he too subscribes to the same economic rationale for working his shift. He is there "at midnight after having spent many years in school." This same logic is recapitulated a little later in the scene:

> We have the state of the art, the best, the latest. This is the Cadillac, Mr. Santorini. This is recombinant thrombolytic. It was a breakthrough twenty years ago, and it's been refined since then, and it's superb ... I want the best for you, because you are an upstanding citizen, a taxpayer, and a rollerblader. You owe it to yourself, and I owe it to you.
>
> *(Lam, 2006: 319)*

In this instance, biomedicine is given its due, but is comically subordinated ("a rollerblader") within larger neoliberal frameworks of citizenship and taxes. Not only is biomedicine subordinated here by the one who calls its tune, but Chen acknowledges himself as so subordinated when he says "I owe it to you."

The scene is demonstrative in another sense. Chen's nurse, Jill, is a useful foil for Chen's silent, dutiful, and passive-aggressive compensatory efforts to support the system. While trying to get an IV on Mr. Santorini, a seriously ill man who should receive the attention of at least a couple of nurses, Jill voices her frustration with a health-care system that is underfunded and underresourced. While taking care of Mr. Santorini in front of Chen, she shouts out in the emergency department, "Lenny! Where is Lenny! These damn agency nurses, why can't this hospital staff the place properly? You know, Dr. Chen, this place is so screwed up" (Lam, 2006: 316). That a major Toronto hospital in this fictional universe requires "agency nurses" in order to maintain staffing complements speaks volumes about hiring practices, benefits, conditions of work, and consistency of care under the regime of neoliberalism; that, later in the story, the department's shown to not have enough equipment to start an IV, says more on the same score; but more germane to the topic of burnout and this article is Chen's response to Jill: "I stand out of Mr. Santorini's field of vision and hold a finger to my lips at Jill. She giggles. This seems very funny to her" (Lam, 2006: 316).

This duet is repeated a little later in the scene:

> The line doesn't run. She says, "It's blown. This is pathetic. Am I alone?" She says louder, "What does it take to get some help in here?"
>
> I stand again where Mr. Santorini can't see me. I wave my hands, bare my teeth, and mouth *stop it!* at Jill, who laughs.
>
> *(Lam, 2006: 317)*

The contrast between personalities is illustrative. Jill voices her frustrations about the care environment aloud, directly in front of the patient: which is honest, to say the least. Chen, on the other hand, whose job is to make everything work despite the prevailing limitations, who must reach into himself in order to compensate for systemic inadequacy, tries to passive-aggressively silence Jill for speaking the truth. Although a discussion of relative work cultures between nursing and medicine might result in a useful analysis (nurses are unionized, and therefore more inclined to "grieve" problems), this little drama within the larger story serves to emphasize Chen's self-entrapment: having internalized the workings of biomedicine and neoliberalism, having accepted the impossibility of the expectations he must meet, he agrees to keep the pantomime alive while borrowing against himself. Jill can say what she's thinking, but Chen can only come at problems sideways—and that's why he's the doctor. Based on the contract struck before even becoming a physician, he "owes" it to people like Mr. Santorini.

"The stronger mind": resiliency and individual capacity

"First Light" has another, related problem dramatized within, that of "resiliency." In Philippe Bourbeau's "A Genealogy of Resilience," a recent article that admirably maps out all the interesting turns the term has adopted over the past 50 years in various discourses, the medical/health context of the term is summarized as follows: "For the past two decades, psychologists and social workers have sought to fully detach the concept of resilience from the 'blaming the victim' problem that comes with understanding resilience as a personal trait" (Bourbeau, 2018: 30). In an editorial also summarizing various trends regarding resilience in health care, Carmel Mary Martin explains the common definition of resilience: "In medicine and health care, interest has typically focussed on psychological resilience as a mindset in the face of chronic disease and major life stressors" (Martin, 2019a: 1319). Using this logic, it is clearly unfair to blame Chen for not having the "resilience" to be able to withstand a toxic system, even when supplied with the techniques that neoliberalism so prides itself on.

"First Light," a story about the spiritual corrosions of burnout, starts with Chen trying to fall asleep, but he cannot. He clockwatches, making things worse. He has an exact count on the number of minutes he's been trying to fall asleep—"I've been lying here for seventeen minutes" (Lam, 2006: 307)—and even has subdivided that time in terms of position: "nine minutes on my left, then eight on my right" (Lam, 2006: 307). As Lam's first-person monologue informs us, Chen feels:

> sad and cheated. I resent my overnight shift in the emergency department, which starts at 23:30. I can never sleep before this late shift ... I hate my job ... I despise it. I have to get out of this. I can't do this forever.
>
> *(Lam, 2006: 307)*

After more close attention paid to Chen's sleeplessness and his consciousness of same, including a failed breath experiment, he explains:

> In medical school, they once brought a relaxation specialist to our class. She guided a hundred and seventy-seven students, all sitting in the tall and echo-filled lecture hall, through an exercise. We visualized looseness spreading from our toes, to our ankles, to our knees, to our bellies, as tension flowed out of our skin.
>
> *(Lam, 2006: 308)*

This is significant, for it's the only pedagogical instance of self-care narrated by Lam in the novel, the only time Lam depicts the institution of medicine demonstrating awareness and compassion to its future "workforce." Yet the technique is, at bottom, part of the larger culture of "resilience" advocated by neoliberalism itself, in which time-limited interventions are provided to individuals so that they can learn techniques of self-regulation.[5]

Chen's failure to master this efficiently delivered technique (in a big hall, with an entire year's cohort of medical students) seems to be less his own personal failure and more a matter the unreconcilable pedagogies of restorative self-care and neoliberal resiliency:

> I couldn't get past my ankles. My toes felt too big to relax. My feet ached. I couldn't make my ankles go limp. I asked myself whether the stronger minds were those who were able to allow the relaxation to take them over, to submit to the

slackness of their bodies, or those like myself whose knees and necks continued to fidget and fight. Then I became irritated with myself—*why did it matter who had the stronger mind?*

(Lam, 2006: 309)

Chen cannot succeed at this task because he compares himself with others in a competitive fashion. Noting that others in the hall have fallen asleep, he wonders what's wrong with himself, why he can't do as the other students do. He tries to understand his own inadequacy using a logic of strength, of competence, of a paradox of dominance and submission, of dedication and focus embodied in Ming's "study techniques." Ultimately, he feels worse about himself for resorting to these strategies. Chen's failure is simple: he needs to be able to relax, but he can't, and that he can't is partly the fault of the prevailing philosophies that rule him (biomedicine: know everything; neoliberalism: all is outcome, all is bang for buck). Chen doesn't know how to relax using the technique, and it is possibly not the way he can relax because he has been rhetorically positioned to be both omniscient and omnicompetent according to an underlying propulsive force of anxiety. The resiliency-based technique he has been tasked with will not work because it conceptualizes relaxation as a thought-switch being flipped, as a ritual to follow, as something to *do*, and Chen has core disciplinary knowledge that the mastery of technique is paramount. He needs to master something he cannot master, and this is an existential problem. His problem (also medicine's problem) is much bigger than that which can be dealt with in an hour's mass relaxation session. As Chen asks, why does it matter who has the stronger mind? It doesn't, for if one wants to recover or relax, then mastery of a technique is not a productive stance for all. But in the discipline of medicine, knowledge and mastery are strength, are the keys to the kingdom.

As former residency director of Toronto Western's family medicine program, Dr. Toubassi is familiar with this kind of approach to the problem of burnout:

[W]e incorporate wellness into our curriculum is by saying to residents, twice a year, "You can do and do yoga this morning and we are excusing you from clinical activity. Go do yoga." To me, that's an absurd approach to fostering wellness. That's one thing. We talk a good game, but things don't substantially change in terms of what we're actually teaching our residents. We don't approach it as a skill that is the way we approach everything else that we teach them, not as a body of knowledge. We just say, "The way that we're giving you wellness is by giving you less time to be in the hospital." To me, that's not the answer. The answer is more, "How do we teach you to be well even though you're here? How do we teach you to derive meaning so that the difficult parts of your job are maybe more bearable to you? That's where narrative comes in for me, because it's a skill set, it's a way to allow our trainees to conceptualize themselves and their experiences, and to share that with their peers in a way that will allow them to maintain their wellness going forward.

Yoga is something the individual can do, is a "skill." Alas, the NPHS's concept of resilience—unlike that of more contemporary research in the social sciences—remains rooted in individual capacity:

The two-item Connor-Davidson Resilience Scale (CD-RISC 2...) was used to measure resilience. The CD-RISC 2 includes two questions pertaining to adaptability and the ability to bounce back from hardships. Responses are measured on a scale ranging from 0 ("not true at all") to 4 ("true nearly all of the time"), for a maximum score of 8. The mean resilience score in the general population is 6.91 … Given this positive skew, scores were coded into two categories: low resilience (score 0–5) and high resilience (score 6–8).

(Canadian Medical Association, 2018: 27)

Thus "resilience" is "adaptability"—a term frequently used in neoliberal discourses that concern national economies—and the "ability to bounce back." But what if the system is itself the hardship, the chronic stressor? What does one "bounce back" to, when one is bouncing away from?

Full circle: in lieu of a "fix for a generation"

To solve a problem, one must first know that there is a problem. Then, one must refine the problem as a concept, understand all of its implications. Coincidently or subsequently, one must change how the problem is understood so that the problem can be shown to be inadequately understood. At some point, two paths emerge: (1) implementation of change, or (2) acquiescing to intractability. Also at some point, redefining the problem ceases to be useful.

From this day of May 6, 2019, a day I picked up the most recent issue of *CMAJ* from my mailbox, I think the profession is pretty much at (2). Consider the following items taken from this issue:

- Dr. Sam Campbell, a professor of Emergency Medicine at Dalhousie University—the same specialty as Vincent Lam and his fictional character, Dr. Chen—writes in "It Is The System That Is 'Failing To Cope,' Not The Emergency Department", our system is one "where the demand for services exceeds the availability of resources to supply them" (Campbell, 2019: E401). He adds that he and his colleagues "daily witness the suffering of patients who arrive for emergency care but are denied it because emergency resources are being redirected to counter the failure of other, unrelated parts of the system"(13).
- In "How Should We Act on the Social Determinants of Health," Trevor Drummer states the obvious by concluding, "If we emphasize the role of structural forces and societal dynamics in the social determinants of health, we find an opportunity to tackle the causes of the causes of health inequities. But, there are challenges to overcome before they can be properly addressed" (1242).
- Finally, the news article "Promises To Change Working Culture of Medicine Still Mostly Lip Service" (Glauser, 2019) functions as the capping entry to a trilogy.

The news is that this is news? The news is that more investment is required to fix a system that cannot meet the needs of providers and patients? I would like to conclude with something snappy, bring William Carlos Williams to the fore here, suggest that the meaning inherent to being a physician is somehow connectable to his great poem "Asphodel, that greeny flower". I could make the connection, but in truth, what change would that connection make? I could no more convince my fellow physicians to read poetry than I could come up with the trillions of dollars in perpetuity required to deliver on Paul Martin's laughably doomed promise of a "fix for a generation" (Martin, 2019b) for health care.

The problem is vast, and medicine is not technically eating its young, for the pre-med students are pre-consumed. One solution will strike many as bizarre, perhaps even ridiculous: what if the institution of medicine hired humanities scholars and employed them throughout the curriculum such that biomedicine met its match? Bear with me here. Just yesterday, I walked a young woman through what she might do when suffering a panic attack. Before progressive muscle relaxation and before deep breathing exercises, I encourage her to take the first step of naming the feeling in order to reduce its power, to put it on notice: "I am feeling anxiety." I then provide the second step, of validation: "I am feeling anxiety and it is okay." The third step is one of exploding the eternity of the feeling, disrupting its chronology: "I am feeling anxiety now. I've felt it before, and I got through it. I'll feel it again, it's inevitable." Humanities scholars can enact this kind of metaphor curriculum-wide with regards to burnout and biomedicine, giving permission to name the thing that both keeps the system functioning but makes the system corrosive to its subjects.

Notes

1 In this instance, and in the rest of the chapter, I define the "biomedical epistemology"—usually shortened to just "biomedicine"—as the idea that all human physiology and consciousness can be known and modified via laboratory experimentation because it is material. As Nikolas Rose (2007: 4) writes: "It is now at the molecular level that human life is understood, at the molecular level that its processes can be anatomized, and at the molecular level that life can be engineered." Rose adds (and I agree) that according to this basic orientation of science to humanity, "it seems ... there is nothing mystical or incomprehensible about our vitality—anything and everything appears, in principle, to be intelligible, and hence to be open to calculated interventions in the service of our desires."

2 A list of these cuts can be found in "Update: Mounting Healthcare Cuts" from the Ontario Health Coalition. To get a sense of the neoliberal flavor of the government's discourse, see Health Minister Christine Ford quest for "efficiencies" in the following CBC News Online article: "What we are looking at is improving patient efficiency. We are restructuring the system in many respects, moving people into different positions within that structure, because the way things are operating within the LHIN structure, it's not working right now. And providers are operating in silos. We want to break down those silos" (Draaisma, 2019).

3 If faculties of medicine require a "humanities elective" from their students, what does this really mean? For one thing, it predicts the present: the humanities within the institution of medicine is not considered central or essential, but is conceived of as a value-added or ancillary commodity. Trying to change this is hard because medicine knows what it wants and the table is tilted from the beginning. The humanities can be said to "have a place" but are also "put in their place" at the same time.

4 One of the ways to do this is to have dual-trained scholars collaborating with humanities faculties to show that medicine has another life.

5 As explained by Bennett et al. (2018: 1342), "personal skills training, and complementary, mind-body (e.g., mindfulness, meditation) interventions to mitigate stress perception have shown promising results in allowing individuals to recover following the PTE and to develop new coping skills."

References

Bennett, J.M., Rohleder, N. and Sturmberg, J.P. (2018). Biopsychosocial Approach to Understanding Resilience: Stress Habituation and Where to Intervene. *Journal of Evaluation in Clinical Practice*, 24: 1330–1346.

Bourbeau, P. (2018). A Genealogy of Resistance. *International Political Sociology*, 12: 19–35.

Boyle, T. (2018). Canadian Doctors are Suffering from Burnout at an 'Alarming' Rate, Survey Finds. *Toronto Star*, A3: 10 October.

Bryant, T. (2009). *An Introduction to Health Policy*. Toronto: Canadian Scholars Press.

Campbell, S. (2019). It Is The System That Is 'Failing To Cope,' Not The Emergency Department. *Canadian Medical Association Journal*, 191(14): E401.

Canadian Medical Association. (2018). *CMA National Physician Health Survey: A National Snapshot.* Ottawa: Canadian Medical Association.

Draaisma, M. (2019). Ontario Minister Says Cutting Jobs is Not the Intent of New Health-Care Legislation. *CBC News Online* 27 Feb.

Drummer, T. (2018). How Should We Act on the Social Determinants of Health. *Canadian Medical Association Journal.*190(42): E1241–E1242.

Giarelli, G., Annandale, E. and Ruzza, C. (2014). Introduction: The Role of Civil Society in Healthcare Systems Reforms. *Social Science and Medicine,* 123: 160–167.

Glauser, W. (2019). Promises To Change Working Culture of Medicine Still Mostly Lip Service. *Canadian Medical Association Journal,* 191(15): E432–E433.

Lam, V. (2006). *Bloodletting and Miraculous Cures.* Toronto: Doubleday.

Martin, C.M. (2019a). Resilience and Health Care: A Dynamic Adaptive Perspective. *Journal of Evaluation in Clinical Practice,* 24: 1319–1322.

Martin, P. (2019b). Moving Canada Forward: The Paul Martin Plan for Getting Things Done. *POLTEXT.* Web. Accessed 5 May 2019.

Rich, P. (2019). Health Care System Takes Advantage of Doctors' Work Ethic. *CMAJ News.* Web. Accessed 30 April 2019.

Rose, N. (2007). *The Politics of Life Itself: Biomedicine, Power, and Subjectivity in the Twenty-First Century.* Princeton: Princeton University Press.

Sakellariou, D. and Rotarou, E.S. (2019). The Effects of Neoliberal Policies on Access to Healthcare for People with Disabilities. *International Journal for Equity in Health,* 16(1): 1.

21
MEDICAL POETICS
Representing global health humanities and the case of 心

Lan A. Li

Introduction

"Dying is very easy," said Liao Jialun.

I crouched next to her wheelchair as she crushed open a *hetao* 核桃, literally translated as a "peach pit." The walnut's thick shell split down the middle and exposed a soft meaty interior. Liao often said that she was not afraid of dying, even though it was the season for dying. Winters in Tongzhou dropped below freezing and Liao took numerous precautions.[1] She draped a perennial polyester blanket over her lap, layered wool sweaters on top of cotton thermals, checked the weather reports every hour, and never left the apartment.

Many things could kill: pneumonia, diarrhea, fever, broken bones, common colds. But Liao would not die of hypothermia. She was more concerned about preserving her *xin* 心. "Nurturing life requires happiness,[2] requires adjusting your *xin* 心. To truly accomplish this is not easy." She added,

> 我目前做很很有进步。我不计较个人得失不是怕人家给我提意见。不过有时候心情还是不行。我目前这个状况就必须要这么做。要不然就一条路- 气死。
>
> Recently, I've made some improvements. I don't fuss over what I've gained or lost; I'm not afraid of what other people think. But sometimes my attitude falters. In my current condition I have to be this way. Or else, there is only one path: to die of anger.

Liao dug out the walnut meat. She popped the woody fruit into her mouth and slowly chewed with her remaining teeth. At 87 years old, she was good at living. Her "current condition" meant long hours sitting in the dark with the TV on and the sound off. She napped, read messages from relatives on WeChat, and listened to guided qigong techniques on tape. When she listened, she craned her neck to hear what she could and relied on her memory to fill in the rest. Liao had lived this way for ten years in Tongzhou. She was committed to this version of life.

Global pitfalls

This chapter uses Liao's *xin* 心 as one version of a "global" health humanities, but it does not take "global" at face value. The paradox of "global" is that it suggests a view from everywhere and nowhere. It is at once omniscient and placeless. One cannot be comprehensive about everything always. Of course, this impulse is not new: "global" histories are remnants of "world" histories that often inflect teleological time with dusty narratives of ancient civilizations in Egypt, Mesopotamia, and China to which we draw a direct line. Traditional temporalities construct binaries that separate present from past, here from there, East from West.

Shallow dives into discourses of "global" health stand in contrast to microhistories, cultural histories, and material histories. Still, historians have collectively tried to use the microscopic, cultural, and material to articulate new varieties of "global." Numerous scholars have harnessed the movement of people and their possessions to take "global" out of the abstract (e.g., Gómez, 2017; Wils et al., 2017; Worton and Tagoe, 2004).

They often focus on transnational encounters in the time of young nations to thoughtfully offer accounts of colonial and postcolonial population health from infertility to infectious diseases (see Marsh and Ronner, 1996; Peckham, 2016). Social and political imperatives offer many points of entry. Yet there remains more to the world of health humanities.

The world looks slightly different from the perspective of *xin* 心. As a noun and a verb, *xin* 心 could mean thinking and/or thoughts, feeling and/or heart, cognition and/or brain. How scholars arrive at these interpretations depend on their modes of inquiry.[3] When I use *xin* 心 as a way into "global" health humanities, I aim to do three things. First, I use *xin* 心 to join different intellectual genealogies in history, literature, and religion—already inherently transdisciplinary fields.[4] Second, I untie *xin* 心 from orientalist narratives of health and healing. I do not claim that *xin* 心 belongs to "Chinese" medicine, but instead include it in histories of health, embodiment, and the imagination. Third, I draw on my work as a filmmaker to address the practical concerns of moving between the health humanities and the digital humanities. Having turned Liao's *xin* 心 into a short film, I take seriously narrative as a form of representation. And having used edited interviews and podcasts as tools for working through questions about *xin* 心, I appreciate the role of conversation in creativity. In other words, I understand discourse as a skill that is central to reconfiguring the amorphous and overwhelming scope of the "global" health humanities. Sometimes we just need to talk through our ideas.

Each of these aims deal with translation at different levels: rendering embodied experiences into words, foreign events into familiar encounters, social concerns into personal struggles. These struggles are not new for scholars of semiotics and science studies (e.g., Callon, 1984; Liu, 2000). Politics get in the way of making unknown encounters knowable. Epistemic standards get in the way of establishing truth claims. The limits of language get in the way of expression.

Meanwhile, *xin* 心 requires a different kind of translation that is often absent in histories of public health. This makes sense: pronouncements of improving one's *xin* 心 did not neutralize infectious viruses; common understandings of *xin* 心 did not eliminate childhood polio. But *xin* 心 can open up a realm of private health. Although Liao Jialun's encounter with her *xin* 心 is not exactly Roy Porter's view of history from "below," nor is it a standard of Arthur Kleinman's "illness narrative," it is a chance for me to use the medical anthropologist's method of inquiry to excavate cosmologies of health and raise conceptual questions

(Kleinman, 1989; Porter, 1985). Like Bharat Venkat's telling of tuberculosis in India after anti-biotics, I take Liao's vignette to retell the case of *xin* 心 in the form of medical poetics. In other words, the poetics of *xin* 心 means working different cosmologies of the body into everyday language to cross genres of academic writing.

心 on the mind[5]

Knowing the caveats of translation, I use Liao's 心 to ask: what does 心 look like? As a thing and an action, Liao's 心 occupies multiple dimensions. When Liao sat in front of the TV, she worked on her 心. When Liao woke up from a nap, she worked on her 心. When Liao felt slighted by her daughter, she worked on her 心. When Liao shuffled from her seat to her wheelchair, she worked on her 心.

Those already familiar with 心 recognize Liao's constant vigilance. Laboring over 心 could be Daoist, or Confucian, or Buddhist in practice. The character 心, pronounced *kokoro* in Japanese and *sin* in Korean, had many functions. As sinologist Jana Benická recounted, 心's high-level and low-level attributes involved various forms of cognition and personhood (Benická, 2006). It formed attention and attitudes. It channeled care and feeling. It reflected intellect and ideas. It manifested sincerity and interest. It represented a kind of essence and spirit. 心 served the need to think and feel, and contained impulses for thinking and feeling. It gave these compulsions shape and direction. It became a kind of "home," in On-cho Ng's words, to "volition, sentiments, and intellect" (Ng, 1999: 89). More than that, 心 could be built and rebuilt. 心 was not limitless, although it was full of possibility. At 87, Liao's 心 remained agile and responsive as long as she was willing to openly shape and reshape it. Liao may not need to know how her 心 looked because she already knew how it felt. As long as she did not allow her emotions to dominate, her 心 would be fine. 心 as an anatomical and physiological object grounded her body and motivated her to measure up to better ways of being.[6] 心 bridged her idiosyncratic and idealized self.

Sinologists often define 心 in terms of what it is not: it is not merely rational, not merely romantic, not merely the beating heart. Elisa Sabattini has firmly denounced the common and "atrocious" translation of 心 as "heart–mind" because it is the heart and the mind, but it is not only the heart and the mind (Sabattini, 2015). "Heart–mind" misguides the reader to place 心 in an oversimplified Cartesian hierarchy, Sabattini asserts. I agree. This is part of the struggle of translation. For instance, historian Mark Csikszentmihalyi takes 心 as a state of mind when dealing with premodern texts. For instance, he translates *zhongxin* 中心 as the "inner mind" (Csikszentmihalyi, 2004: 71). Csikszentmihalyi's take on exercising virtue sound a lot like "states" that one can enter and leave. But 心 is *not* not a state, although occasionally it can function a lot like a state. Of Nancy Shephard Hughes and Margaret Lock's famous three bodies (the body-self, the social body, and the body politic), 心 can look a lot like a body politic (Scheper-Hughes and Lock, 1987). Some texts overtly describe 心 as a ruler and a ruler as the 心, both flanked by subordinates. Numerous prints and reprints of classical descriptions of 心 introduce the senses as occupying an "office" where the superior "controls" for the "benefit" of the entire "government" (Geaney, 2002: 17–18). The individual body-self of a ruler, an inherently social body, is the heart of the body politic. Elisa Sabattini translates "上下一心" (literally "up, down, one *xin*") as "superiors and inferiors share one heart" or "unanimity between superiors and inferiors," knowing that there is more to this phrase (Sabattini, 2015: 66).

Discussions of 心 can get messy. It is an object, an area, a site. It is a thing in motion. 心 could be in the chest, conspiring with the heart or the lungs, but if you opened the chest to see the heart and lungs, you would not find the 心.[7] Unlike the ears, 心 is not a useless sense organ. More like the imagination, 心 needs attention, exercise, and practice.

The organ 心 thus folds into many metaphors. At this stage, ideas of metaphorization require clarification. Those who subscribe to Aristotelian notions of metaphor take it as a transfer of names and, unlike analogy, as a way of knowing (Aristotle, 2013: 43–44). This kind of definition does not entirely apply to something like 心. As literary scholar Pauline Yu has argued, seemingly metaphorical images in classical Chinese poetry can invoke multiple references. Moonlight and white rabbits refer to minor gods, even though these references do not necessarily deviate from ordinary speech (Yu, 1981). They appeared in poetry, but were not poetic devices. According to Yu, classical poetry did not distinguish between the lyrical and empirical because it assumed that its readers shared a common language of reality. Poetry assumed a shared intersubjectivity. For instance, if you were like the seventeenth-century writer Liu Rushi 柳如是 (1618–1664) and shared some variation of her subject identity, her economic position, her province affiliation, her in-court relationships, her education, her musical preference—what sociologists might anachronistically call "demographics data" and what historians of science might say determined "commensurability"—then, perhaps, you might experience what she experienced. One would assume.

In effect, 心 is hard to define despite our use of metaphors because metaphors are hard to define. They are both cultural objects, both fixed and flexible, and they both travel with some difficulty. In this case, I find Alexander Wragge-Morley's definition of metaphors in early modern European history of science most helpful: it is an inherently affective category meant to induce pleasure, but does not generate knowledge (Wragge-Morley, 2020).[8] Metaphors do not tell you anything useful. They are not empirical; they do not make meaning.[9]

If we use this definition, 心 is almost a metaphor.

Tree–brain–branches

So, what *does* 心 look like? Although you, the reader, may not always know where to find it, you might already know what it looks like not because of what it does, but because of how it appears on the page. You have seen 心 because it looks like 心—three splashes over a gentle curve. Without any reference to sound or pronunciation, 心 shows you the organ on its own. It is both a character and an image. As Wragge-Morley put it, 心 is a case where "the physical organ of thought is expressed in the idea of thought."[10] This is unlike the Latin *cogitare*, the English *cogitate*, and the French *cognition* that address thinking and feeling without any reference to the organ(s) responsible for thinking and feeling.

心 did not always look this way. In earlier variations, one version featured a long branch that stretched from the top of the image to the bottom. Three arms reached out, two on the left, one on the right, each thick, stout, stunted. It stood upright as if to face the viewer. In another variation, these branches curved. They converged at the center to form the shape of a vessel. It resembled something like Poseidon's trident, only softer and with three grooves instead of two. Or perhaps it looked nothing like a spear. With an additional gap at the center, this version looked more like pot for steaming with one cavern at the center flanked by compartments on either side. The trunk hung from the base of the vessel and curled like a tail.

From studying these early cup–vase–spear–tree-like versions of 心, classicist Guangming Li has suggested a third meaning: the brain.[11] This is not to say that early anatomical illustrations from the tenth and thirteenth centuries and famous charts like the *mingtang tu* did not account for the brain; they did.[12] Only what appeared inside the head was an inscription that roughly read: "The ocean of Yin bone marrow penetrates all the way down."[13] In other words, the most Yin of the bone marrow moved from the head through the spine and down the back. The solid brain did not matter as much as the elements that guided and guarded it. The head was a cavern. Inside was fluid.

The physical appearance of 心 resembled the physical brain, in addition to the fluid thingy-ness of thinking/feeling/knowing/being/discerning. But the character as the brain, or at least the space of the brain that moved bone marrow down the back, did not make any reference to flesh. Compared with its compatriots, 心 had no meat. Often listed as one of the *wuzang* 五臟, or "five viscera," or "five orbs," or "five storehouses," depending on your translation, 心 was at the center.[14] And 心 was different from the others.

In other words, not all organs were made of flesh, even though the character for organ, *zang* 臟, featured the flesh radical 月. For instance, the same flesh radical appeared in four of the five viscera/orbs/storehouses: spleen 脾, kidney 腎, stomach 胃, and liver 肝.[15] Each of these were explicitly associated with flesh. That is, except for 心. Even the contemporary character for "brain" or *nao* 腦 featured 月—a direct reference to fleshiness. But *nao* 腦 was a fairly new name for an old body part. Historically, *nao* 腦 referred to a shell. It was etymologically connected to fruits like walnuts, almonds, and pistachios where *nao* 腦 identified nuts by their outer casings and not by their edible interiors. Similarly, *nao* 腦 as "brain" may have referred to a hard exterior more than a soft interior.

Like most aspects of physiology, the effects of 心 remained unseen, depending on what you were looking for. Invisible things had material effects. They mattered because they registered movement in the world. For instance, Qi 氣, which animated 心, looked like wind over rice. Literally, the compound character 氣 featured the character/image/word of wind over the character/image/word for rice. 氣 was an analogy for Qi, but it did not represent Qi. It showed the implications of a material thing. Another variation of Qi came in the form of 炁, which offered a more explicit vision of Qi. With 炁, Qi came in the form of "nothing" over "water," or alternatively, "nothing" over "flame." Like 心, Qi/chi/氣/炁 moved across phases. It could be the effects of wind, water, or fire. However frustratingly formless, its visible effects made it fundamentally material, effective, embodied.

The embodied reality and ontological ambiguity of 心 challenged many medical writers in the nineteenth century. For instance, readers of neuroscience including Benjamin Hobson (1819–1873) and Tang Zonghai (1851–1908) often lamented how classical texts overlooked the brain (Lei, 2014). This, they thought, mirrored a fatal ignorance that would cripple the feudalistic, pre-modern, archaic, obsolete, backward, incorrigible, stagnant, floundering, incompetent Qing empire. In the final decades of the Qing, scholars of Chinese classical medical texts looked to Japan to borrow new ideas of the body and supplement for their insufficiencies.[16]

And yet, 心 remained a useful object for desiring/discerning/deliberating. While some translators tried to alter the look and feel of characters, their process of translation for things like 氣/炁 got lost in partial metaphors and analogies. For instance, as historian Sean Lei has described in his excellent article, the nineteenth-century Scottish missionary Benjamin Hobson directly linked the character of Qi to steam and the steam engine (Lei, 2012). Like steam, Qi as 氣 and as 汽 (notice the drops of water) did a tremendous amount of work. They could change phases and move among different organs, from the bladder to the triple burner/*sanjiao* to the kidneys, just as compressed vapor did when it pulled up and down the giant pistons of an engine. Qi, like steam, was powerful.

Digital diaries

Despite discursive debates, 心 was not so mysterious. Medical humanities scholars have long appreciated the multiplicity of things. Bio-socio-medico-techno entities are anything but singular despite naming practices, which historians, anthropologists, and literary scholars have meaningfully disassembled. Annemarie Mol's ethnography did this with atherosclerosis (Mol, 2003). Jeremy Greene's institutional history did this with hypertension (Greene, 2008).

Liao Jialun's 心 was multiple and knowable in is multiplicity. She could track how it changed over time. "[W]hen I can't think through a problem or I'm slightly unhappy, I think about it, and in a second, it's over," she said. Adjusting her 心 came as a form of problem solving. "Before I would get angry, extremely angry, frustrated for the entire day," she added, "Not anymore ..." As she reflected on her anger management, units of time stretched and compressed. Frustrations could last for an entire day, or they could vanish at an instant. As she reconsidered her "current condition" she added:

觉得人生很有滋味。大家对我都挺好。有时候想起来觉得挺有意思的。
I feel like there is still meaning to life. People are kind to me. It's really interesting when you think about it.

This made Liao good at living, or at least good enough despite other limitations. And as we spoke, I tried to understand and potentially mitigate the scope of those limitations.

I first started filming Liao in 2016. She sat for hours at a time in her shaded solarium, which never saw any sun and always felt five degrees colder than the rest of the apartment that she shared with her daughter and son-in-law. I spent many long mornings and after-noons following her schedule, and my camera focused on the details of her life then. This was a technique that I often used when filming patients or socially vulnerable individuals. In previous projects, patients sometimes wanted to be anonymized after I had completed the first round of edits. Instead of blurring faces, which I consider a kind of violent erasure of identity, I included a careful selection of their belongings. Viewers have no way to see beyond the frame, but only focus on the textures on screen. Like classic cinéma vérité, the camera took you where your eyes could not go so that the face became less important in the context of the film.[17] In this case, I focused on Liao's hands, her eyes, her crushing of walnuts.

Liao did not like seeing herself on film. "You and your camera," she would say, vaguely amused. "There is nothing to film with this old lady." When I showed her some of the raw footage, she scoffed. "Look, how fat," she jeered. "A giant fatty." Still, it amazed her to see her home and her hands from my point of view. "Play it again," she sometimes asked. And I did.

Liao knew that she was privileged to be close to family. She knew that she was lucky that most of her relatives had survived the violence of the 1970s, the famines of the 1960s, the revolutions of the 1950s, the civil wars of the 1940s, and the military coups of the 1930s. She was born in 1928, "the same year Coca-Cola was invented," she would say.[18] Her mother had been the favorite wife of the mayor of Pujiang County in Sichuan. "My father was a large man," Liao remembered. "He was so fat that I could stuff a ping pong ball in his belly button." He died from a heart attack when she was eight.

I recognized in Liao a resilience that I did not possess. The glowing light of the CCTV news closed in every morning. Liao had been a teacher, choir director, librarian, and political prisoner. In the 1960s, she directed a two-hour performance of *Dong Fang Hong* ("The East is Red") in Tiananmen Square. In the early 1980s, she was an unofficial artistic ambassador when she traveled to Bloomington, Vancouver, and Los Angeles.

Now, she worked on her 心. As I kneeled next to her wheelchair and watched her crush open walnuts, I wanted to highlight the things that she liked about herself and her home. I played with depth of focus to catch the half hour of sunlight that reflected from the neighboring buildings and barely illuminated her balcony. I walked to her husband's old work desk on the opposite side of the apartment and focused on how the direct sunlight raked his old paint brushes. They sat unused and surrounded by a cluster of houseplants. I focused on how the purple shield leaves glowed in the afternoon and grew brighter at the edges.

One day, Liao decided to take stock of her husband's paintings. With the help of her older granddaughter, she gathered dozens of lightly stacked rolls and unfurled them one by one. I looked at Liao's eyes and hands. She knew how to handle the thin sheets of mulberry paper. Although some of the unmounted folios frayed at the edges, they never tore at her touch. When she came across one of her favorite paintings, she said, "The birds look so real. It's if they're going to fly off the page." This was her highest form of praise.

Later in the day, I took out my pocket-sized Sony recorder and sat next to Liao. I asked about her day and tried to minimize my intrusion of recording devices.

"Dying is very easy," she said. "Recently, I've made some improvements ..."

Our conversation sometimes returned to her childhood, to her days as a choir director, to her thoughts about the anchorman's new haircut ("Does *he* think he looks good?"), her music preferences, her grandson's work, the anchorwoman's new outfit ("Does *she* think she looks good?").

Before leaving Tongzhou, I showed Liao the rough cuts of our conversation—clips of the glowing purple plant, the paint brushes, the spokes on her wheelchair, the portraits of butterflies and sparrows. She nodded approvingly, "Good, as long as this is useful for your research." I later screened the same clip for Rishi Goyal's students in the Medicine, Literature, and Society major at Columbia.[19] He noticed that even though Liao had difficulty walking, she cared more about the dexterity of her hands than the strength of her legs. I played Liao's film in my own class and explained how I separated filming the video and recording the interview. I wanted to be less obvious in the room to deliver a narrative about 心 and aging that was both intimate and familiar. The film itself was placeless because I did not tell my students that Liao lived one hour outside of Beijing, which could be useful context for a different conversation. But they saw what I wanted them to see in Liao's home. The specificity of location mattered, only it mattered at different degrees. I tracked how Liao's image traveled, not to universalize experiences of 心, but instead to initiate conversations about the tree–brain–cup–organ responsible for contemplation, cogitation, and contentment.

Endings and beginnings

My appeal to medical poetics is at its early stages. Anthropologists and socially minded filmmakers have told a number of important and troubling stories in the health humanities, including Judith Helfand, Chris Walley, and Penelope Jagessar Chaffer, to name a few. Still, more stories can be told through voices, languages, and cosmologies without bizarre orientalist inflections.[20]

As scholars of the humanities, we use lots of conceptual tools to assess human data. My tools include microphones, cameras, battery packs, miscellaneous adapters, and editing software that shape how I move in the world and how I understand the ethical implications of my work. I identify as a historian, but recognize the writer's attention to narrative form and the anthropologists' attention to social theory. As an editor, I see my value in collaborative projects to refashion narratives of "global" health humanities. Like Shigehisa Kuriyama's emphasis on styles of writing and presentation, I join the digital and medical humanities as an exercise in ethics and aesthetics.[21]

Most academic conferences feature screens, projectors, and sound systems, which automatically render text-based scholars into visual storytellers. Already, we have an abundance of resources to make the most of high and low technologies, such as Scott McCloud's guide to comics and Edward Tufte's workshops on visual storytelling (McCloud and Martin, 2014; Tufte, 2006). Although historians do not need to become professional artists and filmmakers, scholars can reconfigure genres of presentation and writing to extend the reach of the humanities.

Joining methods in history, science studies, anthropology, literature, and film has allowed me to articulate the multiplicity of 心 with the help of Liao Jialun. Because 心 can be described as a way of being, an anatomical organ, and a physiological response, it travels more easily than other things—more easily than, for instance, theories of meridian paths that guide needling and heating practices, or acupuncture-moxabustion, which I explore elsewhere.[22] In all of this, 心 remains somewhat straightforward despite the challenges of translation and comparison.[23] And because of its ubiquity, we can generate new perspectives of a familiar object famous for its ambiguity.

Notes

1 Liao lived in the district of Tongzhou, one-hour east of Beijing's city center.
2 Many scholars translate the process of *yangsheng* 養生 as "nurturing life." To understand the longer history of *yangsheng* 養生, Kevin Buckelew has shown how the verb *yang* 養 evolved from fifth-century Buddhist texts in the common practice of "nurturing the embryo." Indeed, different versions of *yangsheng* 養生looked different under different circumstances; for instance, historian Ruth Rogaski has demonstrated how *yangsheng* 養生 took on new implications in the early twentieth century in public health discourse. But at all times, *yang* 養 invoked numerous ritualized, choreographed, and discursive processes. Anthropologist Judith Farquhar and philosopher Qicheng Zhang have further illuminated on the varieties of *yangsheng* 養生 and its sustained relevance in Beijing at the turn of the twenty-first century. See: Rogaski, R. (2014). *Hygienic Modernity: Meanings of Health and Disease in Treaty-Port China*. Reprint edition. Berkeley: University of California Press; Buckelew, K. (2018). Pregnant Metaphor: Embryology, Embodiment, and the Ends of Figurative Imagery in Chinese Buddhism. *Harvard Journal of Asiatic Studies*, 78(2): 381; Farquhar, J. and Zhang, Q. (2012). *Ten Thousand Things: Nurturing Life in Contemporary Beijing*. York: Zone Books.
3 Later in the article, I will argue for different version of *xin* 心. For instance, literary scholars place it in the chest and in the mind. Medical scholars place it in the lungs and in the heart. And if we look at the character itself, it offers yet another pictographic clue of potentially invoking the brain.
4 These kinds of deep temporal cuts are especially necessary for historians of medicine in East Asia because of physicians and institutions that support the persistence of classical texts that are printed and reprinted. See, for example, excellent collections of long medical histories such as: Hinrichs, T. J. and Barnes, L.L. (2012). *Chinese Medicine and Healing: An Illustrated History*. Cambridge, MA.; London: Belknap; Lo, V. and Barrett, P. (2018). *Imagining Chinese Medicine*. Leiden: Brill. Certainly, "Chinese" medicine is by no means homogenous. See Scheid, V. (2002). *Chinese Medicine in Contemporary China: Plurality and Synthesis*. Durham, NC: Duke University Press Books.
5 For the remainder of the chapter, I will no longer include the Romanization of 心 as *xin* to appreciate its multiplicity of meanings and pronunciations.

6 Or what Caroline Bynum would distinguish as "a" body, "the" body, and "Liao's" body. Each of these types of bodies invoke different aspects of the individual and the ideal. See Bynum, C. (1995). Why All the Fuss about the Body? A Medievalist's Perspective. *Critical Inquiry*, 22(1): 1–33.

7 Michael Carr has offered an analysis of the relationship between organs and issues of the 心 in the *Shijing* 詩經, often known as *The Book of Songs*. See Carr, M. (1983). Sidelights of Xin "Heart, Mind" In the *Shijing*." In *Proceedings of the 31st CISHAAN*, 824–25. Tokyo and Kyoto.

8 Wragge-Morley grounds his definition in early modern European history of science where most natural philosophers considered metaphors with great suspicion, but relied on them regardless. For more on the aesthetics of science, see Wragge-Morley, A. (2020). *Aesthetic Science: Representing Nature in the Royal Society of London, 1650–1720*. Chicago: University of Chicago Press.

9 On varieties of metaphorical treatment in the early modern English context, see Wragge-Morley, A. (2012). Vividness in English Natural History and Anatomy, 1650–1700. *Notes and Records of the Royal Society of London*, 66(4): 341–356.

10 For the full podcast episode with Alex Wragge-Morley and our interview with Dr. Guangming Li, see our episode "Multiple Organs: 心 as Heart-Mind-Brain" at https://cargocollective.com/mind-metaphors/THINKING-ORGANS.

11 More on this possibility in "Multiple Organs: 心 as Heart-Mind-Brain" at https://cargocollective.com/mind-metaphors/THINKING-ORGANS.

12 For a catalogue of *mingtang tu* reproductions into the twentieth century, see Huang, L. (2003). *Zhongguo Zhenjiu Shi Tujian [Atlases of Chinese Acupuncture Moxabustion History]*. Vol. 1. Qingdao: Qingdao Publishing: 79–86.

13 This is a rough translation, the original reads: 髓海至陰之在通尾骶. The *suihai* 髓海 or "bone marrow sea" is one of the "four seas" listed in the *Huangdi neijing lingshu hailun pian* 33. The others include *xuehai* 血海, *qihai* 气海, and *shuigu zhihai* 水穀之海, or very roughly the sea of Blood, Qi, and Water/Millet each found very roughly in the meridians, chest, and abdomen.

14 Medical historians Vivienne Lo and Catherine Despeux translate *wuzang* 五臟 as "five viscera." For a discussion of the translation of *wuzang* 五臟, see Major, J.S., Queen, S.A., Meyer, A.S. and Roth, H.D. (2010) (with additional contributions by Michael Puett, and Judson Murray), eds. *The Huainanzi*. New York: Columbia University Press: 900.

15 Even the characters for invisible meridian paths in the body known as *jingmai* 經脈 and *jingluo* 經絡 made references to some kind of fleshy network of things. For a discussion about the materiality of *mai/mo/*脈, see Kuriyama, S. (2002). *The Expressiveness of the Body and the Divergence of Greek and Chinese Medicine*. New York: Zone Books: 229–230.

16 This was the case with naming nerves as *shenjing* 神經, which scholars borrowed from the Japanese *shinkei* that was coined in the eighteenth century. See Shapiro, H. (2003). How Different Are Western and Chinese Medicine? The Case of Nerves. In: H. Selin, ed., *Medicine Across Cultures: History and Practice of Medicine in Non-Western Cultures*. Dordrecht: Springer Netherlands: 351–372.

17 For more on the history and techniques of cinéma verité Barnouw, E. (1993). *Documentary: A History of the Non-Fiction Film*. 2nd revised edition. New York: Oxford University Press: 253–256.

18 Coke was not invented in 1928, but it was the year that Coke was first trademarked in China. Nevertheless, Coke was Liao's favorite drink. Her son-in law often stocked dozens of mini Coke bottles in her mini refrigerator.

19 The link to the short film can be found here: http://lan-a-li.com/on-aging.

20 Some thoughtful examples include Shireen Hamza's podcast *Ventricles*: https://src.hds.harvard.edu/ventricles and Ahmed Ragab's *Cosmologics* http://cosmologicsmagazine.com/.

21 While Kant has written at length about the aesthetics of ethics, I follow landscape architect Ron Henderson's concern for the ethics of aesthetics.

22 I use the case of body maps to compare the movement of medical theories and clinical practice. More on this in the introduction to my forthcoming book, *Intimate Cartographies: Body Maps and the Assembly of Medical Imagination*.

23 For instance, Caroline Bynum has elegantly explored issues of universality and formal comparisons, which preoccupy art historians. See: Bynum, C. (1995) Why All the Fuss about the Body? A Medievalist's Perspective. *Critical Inquiry*, 22(1): 1–33.

References

Aristotle. (2013). *Poetics*, trans. Anthony Kenny. Oxford: Oxford University Press.

Benická, J. (2006). Xin as a "Qualitatively Equal" Co-Constituent of Phenomena in Chinese Mahayana Buddhism: Some Remarks on Its Interpretations by Using the Terms of Western Philosophical Discourse. *Monumenta Serica*, 54: 185–194.

Callon, M. (1984). Some Elements of a Sociology of Translation: Domestication of the Scallops and the Fishermen of St Brieuc Bay. *The Sociological Review*, 32: 196–233.

Csikszentmihalyi, M. (2004). *Material Virtue: Ethics and the Body in Early China*. Leiden: Brill.

Geaney, J. (2002). *On the Epistemology of the Senses in Early Chinese Thought*. Honolulu: University of Hawai'i Press.

Gómez, P.F. (2017). *The Experiential Caribbean: Creating Knowledge and Healing in the Early Modern Atlantic*. Chapel Hill: University of North Carolina Press.

Greene, J.A. (2008). *Prescribing by Numbers: Drugs and the Definition of Disease*. Baltimore: Johns Hopkins University Press.

Lei, S. H-l. (2012). Qi-Transformation and the Steam Engine The Incorporation of Western Anatomy and Re-Conceptualisation of the Body in Nineteenth-Century Chinese Medicine. *Asian Medicine*, 7 (2): 319–357.

Kleinman, A. (1989). *The Illness Narratives: Suffering, Healing, and the Human Condition*. Reprint edition. New York: Basic Books.

Lei, S.H-L. (2014). *Neither Donkey nor Horse: Medicine in the Struggle over China's Modernity*. Reprint edition. Chicago: University of Chicago Press.

Liu, L.H., ed. (2000). *Tokens of Exchange: The Problem of Translation in Global Circulations*. Durham, NC: Duke University Press Books.

Marsh, M.S. and Ronner, W. (1996). *Empty Cradle: Infertility in America From Colonial Times to the Present*. Baltimore: Johns Hopkins University Press.

McCloud, S. and Martin, M. (2014). *Understanding Comics: The Invisible Art*. New York, NY: William Morrow.

Mol, A. (2003). *The Body Multiple: Ontology in Medical Practice*. Durham: Duke University Press.

Ng, O-c. (1999). An Early Qing Critique of the Philosophy of Mind-Heart (Xin): The Confucian Quest for Doctrinal Purity and the Doxic Role of Chan Buddhism. *Journal of Chinese Philosophy*, 26 (1): 89–120.

Peckham, R. (2016). *Epidemics in Modern Asia*. Cambridge, United Kingdom: Cambridge University Press.

Porter, R. (1985). The Patient's View: Doing Medical History from Below. *Theory and Society*, 14(2): 175–198.

Sabattini, E. (2015). The Physiology of 'Xin' (Heart) in Chinese Political Argumentation: The Western Han Dynasty and the Pre-Imperial Legacy. *Frontiers of Philosophy in China*, 10(1): 58–74.

Scheper-Hughes, N. and Lock, M.M. (1987). The Mindful Body: A Prolegomenon to Future Work in Medical Anthropology. *Medical Anthropology Quarterly*, 1(1): 6–41.

Tufte, E.R. (2006). *Beautiful Evidence*. Third Printing edition. Cheshire, Conn: Graphics Pr.

Wils, K., de Bont, R. and Au, S., eds. (2017). *Bodies Beyond Borders: Moving Anatomies, 1750–1950*. Leuven, Belgium: Leuven University Press.

Worton, M. and Wilson, T., eds. (2004) *National Healths: Gender, Sexuality and Health in a Cross-Cultural Context*. London: Routledge.

Wragge-Morley, A (2020). *Aesthetic Science: Representing Nature in the Royal Society of London, 1650–1720*. Chicago: University of Chicago Press.

Yu, P. (1981). Metaphor and Chinese Poetry. *Chinese Literature: Essays, Articles, Reviews (CLEAR)*, 3(2): 205–224.

22

CREATIVE ARTS ADULT COMMUNITY LEARNING

Lydia Lewis

Introduction

Adult community learning (ACL) is non-formal learning with people in community settings. Often encompassing an element of social action, ACL is sometimes targeted at socioeconomically disadvantaged communities and other groups including people with long-term health conditions, people experiencing mental health issues, and informal carers. ACL is largely provided by local authorities and the voluntary and community (third) sector. Women tend to be over-represented among participants in ACL and there is also relatively high participation among older people (Lewis, 2019).

Although ACL across a range of subjects and activities has been shown to be beneficial for mental health and well-being, creative arts subjects—including visual arts, crafting, and creative writing—are often considered to be particularly beneficial in this regard. There is now a body of research which demonstrates that participation in the arts and creativity is associated with enhanced well-being and quality of life, better general health, and improved community health (DH Mental Health Division, 2010). Creative arts have been a key tenet of "social prescribing" initiatives across the United Kingdom, which link people experiencing mental health issues with sources of support in their local area, with evidence of these leading to "improved self-esteem, feelings of empowerment and improved quality of life" (Robotham et al., 2011: 12). Creative activities are also often advocated as being beneficial for "active aging" for older adults, producing benefits for physical health and social and psychological well-being (e.g., Cohen, 2006).

The idea that there are distinctive features of creative arts learning that mean it is particularly suited to meeting mental health and well-being aims has supported maintenance of creative arts in the ACL curriculum in the United Kingdom while other subjects such as social sciences have shrunk (Lewis et al., 2016). However, critics have argued that creative arts ACL should be seen as having value in its own right and should not have to be justified on the grounds of serving other agendas such as mental health and well-being (e.g., Meyer, 2008). This agenda, it is suggested, risks foreshadowing the core educational purpose and aims of ACL, refocusing it towards the creation of social spaces and psychosocial goals such as raising self-esteem and, thereby, depoliticizing the provision and changing its liberating nature (Caldwell, 2013; Ecclestone, 2004; Thompson, 2007). Indeed, some authors have suggested that creative arts provision for mental health and well-being is serving to placate, as opposed to "empower," participants, to divert attention from the social structural inequalities and injustice underpinning mental health issues, and to contain people's distress (see Mirza, 2006). Furthermore, "It should not be assumed that involvement in creative arts ... is automatically beneficial to mental health" (Lewis et al., 2016: 258). Indeed, a range of potential disbenefits of taking part in ACL may also be identified (see Lewis, 2019). While acknowledging these points, the aim of this chapter is to review research evidence, in light of the above policy debates, in response to two questions: (1) does creative arts ACL have particular benefits for mental health and well-being in comparison to other kinds of learning?, and (2) what are the (distinctive) processes through which creative arts ACL produces mental health and well-being benefits? A short discussion of mental health and well-being outcomes for ACL in creative arts subjects compared with other kinds of learning is provided first. An overview of the generative effects of creative arts ACL for a range of processes related to mental health and well-being follows. As this chapter draws on research about the generation of mutuality (forms of reciprocity and sharing between people) through creative arts ACL (Lewis et al., 2016), the discussion focused on the relational processes involved, although some more individualistic ones such as absorption and relaxation are also encompassed. In conclusion, implications for creative arts ACL provision in the context of the mental health and well-being agenda are considered.

ACL in the creative arts compared with other kinds of learning

Some studies have compared ACL in creative arts with other subjects. For example, a UK study that used data from the English Longitudinal Study of Ageing (ELSA) (Jenkins, 2011), found that for adults over 50 years, particularly women, while creative subjects such as music and arts were associated with improvements in well-being over time, formal courses were not, and gym/exercise classes were only associated with improvements in quality of life for adults over 70 and those who were widowed. Jenkins tentatively attributes these findings to the intrinsic enjoyment of the creative arts subjects as a motivator for learning and to the opportunities for socializing that this ACL offered. He concludes that the findings "suggest that, for older adults, it is the sometimes disparaged 'leisure courses' rather than narrowly vocational courses that are most likely to sustain and enhance wellbeing over time" (414).

Reynolds (2010: 136), in a study of older women's visual art-making as a leisure activity, asks, "Do cultural and creative occupations have a distinctive role to play in maintaining well-being in later life?" She cites a survey of 400 relatively young retirees which found that, as a leisure domain, cultural activities were most strongly associated with life satisfaction scores (Nimrod, 2007). She also cites Cohen (2006) who found that older people averaging 79 years of age who volunteered for a cultural program showed better maintenance of health, morale, and weekly activities compared with those who volunteered for a "usual activity" group. It is noted that in this latter study, participants' motives for volunteering for the different groups need to be considered, as they were not randomly assigned. Nevertheless, Reynolds (2010: 137) concludes that "the evidence reviewed suggests that high investment, effortful and self-expressive leisure activities are associated with subjective well-being in later life."

Mirroring the above findings, in a qualitative study involving 124 adults with a wide range of learning experiences, Hammond (2004a: 55) found that courses leading to vocational qualifications that were competence-based "led to few health and social capital benefits." She suggests it may be the complexity of the relationships that make it hard to identify positive health impacts from competence-based education. However, she also argues that "subjects and teaching styles that encourage reflection, creativity and self-expression are particularly important in relation to developing self-understanding and independent thinking," as well as a clearer sense of identity (55)—psychosocial qualities that mediate the effects of learning on health-related outcomes such as "improved well-being, increased efficacy, protection and recovery from mental health difficulties, and more effective coping" (Hammond, 2004b: 553). She reports how, in accounts of learning that led to these learning outcomes, "The creative arts—art, crafts, drama, dance, opera, singing, and creative writing—were mentioned because they opened people up, enabling them to re-evaluate issues, express their feelings, and grow as people," although other subjects that encouraged reflection, such as anthropology and counselling, were also found to be "effective in terms of growth" (Hammond, 2004b: 561).

Other studies do not report differences in mental health and well-being–related outcomes between adult learning in creative activities compared to others. For example, in a study of two lifelong learning programs for adults over 50 years of age in the USA that included classes in singing, art, and current affairs at an adult education center, and history, political science, and biology in a university setting, and used a measure of state-related affect, Simone. and Cesena (2010: 433) report "an immediate benefit in mood" for students regardless of program, class type, or location. The authors conclude that "adults who choose to engage in lifelong learning find the experience to be uplifting" (433).

In the context of ACL that is targeted for mental health recovery, provision across a range of subjects has been found to be beneficial. For example, in one study of mental health ACL, benefits are reported across a range of courses including numeracy and literacy and "self-help for life," which encompassed multiple subjects including social sciences, philosophy, and psychology (Lewis, 2014). In this research, recovery was supported through the development of resources, including cultural capital (knowledge and learning) and social capital (social connection, relationships, and social support), and the personal recognition afforded by the humanistic learning environment. These facets, in turn, served to enhance people's agency, or self-determination, which was found to be a key recovery process. Similarly, in a report dealing specifically with developing confidence and self-esteem through ACL, Eldred et al. (2004: 31) describe these mental health and well-being–related benefits across a wide range of contexts and subjects, including vocational and life skills, community development, personal development, drama, arts, and culture: "A common strand running through this diversity was that almost all the learners experienced successful learning and their confidence increased."

Some authors suggest that it is the act of engaging in adult learning or leisure activities, rather than the actual activities or the content of the learning involved, that can promote the shifts in subjectivity and identity work associated with mental health recovery. For example, leisure activities may help women to challenge depression through enabling them to experience feelings of enjoyment and a different sense of self as a result of making time for themself (Fullagar, 2008; see also Sagan, 2007). Such shifts in subjectivity may involve coming to see oneself as creative (in the case of creative activities), "actively embodied" (in the case of health and fitness–related activities), or part of a friendship group (in the case of social activities) (Fullagar, 2008). Others highlight the qualities of the tutor and the learning environment created, and the pedagogical ethos as crucial factors (e.g., Lewis, 2014).

Overall, then, the literature suggests that there may be mental health and well-being–related benefits associated with a range of adult learning activities where these encourage reflection and re-evaluation of experiences and ideas, self-expression and self-growth.,

Enjoyment and social connection are also important themes. For mental health recovery more specifically, enhancement of self-identity, and expansion of agency are additional key processes. However, the research also suggests that creative subjects can have particular generative effects for a range of processes relating to mental health and well-being outcomes. Some of these are explored in more detail in the next section.

The processes through which creative arts ACL produces mental health and well-being benefits

A recent review of ACL, mental health and well-being describes how the mental health and well-being–related benefits from ACL include the intrinsic benefits of learning something new and developing a new skill or interest, course participation giving people time for themselves to do something enjoyable and something to look forward to, providing an external focus, and enhancing people's personal identities. They also include social aspects such as gaining friendships.

This section examines why creative arts may be considered particularly effective for generating these benefits through ACL, with a particular focus on ideas of relationality and mutuality. It shows how the reasons involved include creative arts "being viewed as non-threatening, accessible subjects, and the fact that they provide particular opportunities for participatory practice, sharing experiences, building social support and mutual help among adult learners" (Lewis, 2019: 11). The section also considers some of the more distinctive mental health and well-being–related factors associated with creative arts ACL, including absorption and relaxation, a theme that is discussed first. Research findings concerning self-expression, communication and understanding of self and others, including in relation to "empowerment," are then expounded. The subsequent subsection takes up the theme of enduring interest, enjoyment, and social connection and support. Lastly, identity work, social contribution, and reciprocity are discussed.

Absorption, relaxation, and "being present"

There is a range of research that describes how the health-related benefits of adult learning include providing a focus, distraction from anxieties, and psychological displacement activity, for example in the face of bereavement or other kinds of loss, and how this function of adult learning is "important in promoting wellbeing, mental health and positive coping mechanisms" (Aldridge and Lavender, 2000; Hammond, 2004a: 51; Harding et al., 2013; Robotham et al., 2011). Research also suggests that creative arts subjects are particularly good for generating these kinds of psychological benefits, and for helping to rebalance or "re-center" oneself in the face of emotional stress or turmoil, as, in comparison to other kinds of learning, they more readily create "moments of 'flow', of complete and utter absorption" in the activity (Field, 2009: 187).

For example, in a qualitative study of creative arts activities and mental health and well-being involving five ACL groups and two targeted participatory arts organizations in England (Lewis et al., 2016), the theme of absorption was particularly strong in the accounts of members of a jewelry-making group attended by, mainly older, women. Both the group members and the facilitators also undertook the craft work at home and reflected on how they found the practice absorbing and relaxing, enabling them to "switch off" from their worries due to the concentration required. For example, one commented, "I find it's a way of me shutting all my problems behind me," and another said, "It just takes your mind off absolutely everything. I do get lost in it and everything; you don't think about anything else because you're concentrating so hard on that" (148). Informal care work was one important context in which the practice was found to have these benefits, providing "a good escape."

Qualities of the craft work which meant it was found to be absorbing and relaxing included "it's something to do with my hands and keeps me occupied, my mind occupied all the while" (148), the technical challenges involved, the intricacy of the beading work, and the scope offered by the craft practice. On this point, another participant reflected:

> I feel, myself, as if, I just get me stuff out and that's it, and I'm in a world of me own, you know, thinking, "Oh, can I do this," or," can I do that? "and… it's nice and quiet, you know
>
> *(p. 148)*

These findings mirror the research of Reynolds (2000) on women's needlecraft in the context of depression. In a similar way to the participants above, she notes how needlecraft can result in psychological calming and mind relaxation due to it requiring complete concentration, meaning that no intrusive, worrying thoughts can occur. Furthermore, as illustrated by the above quotation, "during craft activity a fresh and controllable world may be created," providing a relaxing antidote to life's stresses and responsibilities (Reynolds, 2000: 110).

Similar findings were reported in ACL art groups in Lewis et al.'s (2016) study. In a mainstream painting and drawing course, one participant reflected on the sessions: "It's not like watching TV or something … you're really focused on what you're doing and I think that's why the time goes by so quickly" (147). Another who was a full-time informal carer described how the art work provided a psychological break for her as "once you get doing something and you're concentrating on that, that's it, that's all you think about, really, is the work" (147). In an art group that was targeted for mental health recovery, one participant described the art-making as therapeutic in providing a "distraction" from her anxieties. The tutor on this course commented too that the meditative nature of the art work meant it provided respite from distressing thoughts and this was important in helping people to deal with mental health issues.

Lewis et al. (2016) also report findings from ACL creative writing groups. In one poetry group hosted in a mental health arts organization, participants described how the initiative was helpful to them in providing an external, constructive focus and how being mentally engaged and "present" with others at group meetings helped to relieve anxiety rooted in past troubles:

> Mental health is a kind of area which one can't really cure, you know, because it is something within the history of person … But poetry time relieves that tension, or art can, because it in involves you for that certain time, for two hours here everybody is working so that brings that kind of … you know, the tension has gone and you are here.
>
> *(p. 146)*

The above participants' comments indicate the therapeutic value of shared engagement in creativity in the face of mental health issues in focusing the mind and bringing one into the present moment. Related findings regarding the subjective benefits of creative community spaces in providing a shift in consciousness have been reported elsewhere (Fullagar, 2008; Fullagar and O'Brien, 2014) and are further discussed below.

Self-expression, communication, and understanding of self and others

Creative arts are often advocated for mental health and well-being because they enable self-expression, exploration, and understanding of the self, and a means of communicating with others, helping to address the "gap between the inner reality of feeling and the available ways of communicating what we feel" (Milner, 1950: 131 in Sagan, 2007: 316). Reynolds (2000: 108, citing Read Johnson, 1998) describes how, in the context of "depression," from a psychodynamic perspective, the tendency to self-punish and turn anger inwards may be released through verbal or art-based means. Where negative feelings are highly threatening and repressed, art work may provide a safer, more oblique means of exploration than verbal therapy (Dekker, 1996), perhaps through use of metaphor. Art work may also present a "container" for expressed emotions (Schaverien, 1989) as well as a way of accessing hidden inner knowledge and strength (Lipson Lawrence, 2008).

Similarly in the case of creative writing, difficult personal experiences and emotions can be explored indirectly and the practice can also be used to provide (relatively) non-threatening ways to explore and provoke a discussion of taboo subjects. For example, in the context of mental health targeted provision, poetry can allow for safe expression of distressing experiences, giving people "access to feelings and permission to process them" and "a means of redirecting and reshaping them" (Gillispie, 2003: 106; Lewis et al., 2016). In this context, creative writing groups can also be helpful in enabling people to identify with the feelings of others and to share experiences, for example through "open[ing] up discussion of what it means to be 'depressed'," something which participants can find affirming and empowering (Wertheimer, 1997: 39; see also Lewis et al., 2016).

Sagan (2007, 2008) in an English study of a literacy/creative writing group at a mental health day center, describes how participants felt the activity to be beneficial in helping to make their thoughts concrete. She also conveys the affinity and empathy within the group, with "the combination of joint discussion of personal themes with the challenge of writing about these appear[ing] to bind the group to itself in a private and intimate way not shared by other social groupings and cliques at the centre" (Sagan, 2007: 318). However, taking a psychoanalytic perspective, she also argues that, in the context of mental health recovery, writing about oneself can produce feelings of loneliness due to this engendering a shifting sense of self. Noting how the course offered a form of "containment within which new subject positions could be taken up and new identities explored" (Sagan, 2007: 317), she suggests that loneliness is part of the reparation processes involved in recovery as one's self-identity becomes refashioned.

Other research demonstrates the value of creative activities for facilitating communication and understanding between individuals who are differently placed, for example in terms of age or experiences of mental health issues (Lewis et al., 2016), and between workers, informal carers, and clients in care settings. For example, Gottlieb-Tanaka et al. (2003) report on a creative expression program that combined different domains of creativity into one activity in a Canadian residential setting for older people with dementia. They argue that creativity can be "a tool for communication between seniors and caregivers when verbal communication is failing" and that this can enhance a sense of control for this group as well as "bring joy, friendship and a sense of belonging," thereby improving quality of life (127; see also Bungay et al., 2019). At a deeper level, shared creative practice can help break down inter-personal barriers between workers and clients in organizational care settings through enabling people to move beyond their respective roles and status to appreciate their shared humanity, thereby supporting "relational wellbeing" (Crawford et al., 2018).

Lipson Lawrence (2008) discusses affective learning through the arts. She suggests that through our emotional reactions to the arts, and reflecting on these, we can "deepen our understanding of self, others and the world around us" (76), and emphasizes how the arts can promote "transformative learning in the context of emotionally laden issues" (68). A painting, a poem, or a dance can stir up emotion as it touches something deep inside us. Perhaps we connect to a personal experience of our own, or we tap into empathic connections with issues of universal concern. Learning can therefore take place "through the affective experiences of creating art and in encountering art created by others," with the witnessing of art having the potential to expand our worldview through "taking us to new places and allowing us to enter into the lifeworld of another" (Lipson Lawrence, 2008: 74, 75). In this manner, she asserts, the arts can help us envision alternative realities for the future, and can be powerful agents of personal, collective and community transformation and healing.

ACL that aims to be transformative may have an explicitly political dimension, involving consciousness-raising and informed action in the Freirean tradition (Freire, 1996)—learning that "transform[s] understanding from the personal to the social" (Caldwell, 2013: 41). For example, Austin (1999: 259, citing Ruddock and Worral, 1997) describes creative writing classes in South Yorkshire that were used to "challenge the pattern of disempowerment which is rife amongst people with mental health difficulties," through covering basic educational needs as well as "encouraging personal expression of opinion and group membership" and enabling examination of the oppressive aspects of people's lives "through classes designed specifically to move people forward."

Pettit (2010: 33) describes how there is a tradition of "creative and embodied learning emerging from popular theatre, storytelling and art" which can be very useful for "learning about power and developing capacities to be strategic with it—particularly when engaging with forms of power that are internalised and embodied." A particularly well known example is "Theatre of the oppressed," developed by the Brazilian theater practitioner Augusto Boal. Lipson Lawrence (2008) notes how such popular theater projects can work to generate both affective and embodied knowing as well as personal and collective transformation through "restorying lives."

In one popular theater mental health initiative for women, reported by Novitsky (2014), involvement helped the women generate insight into the factors affecting their own mental health and that of their children, as well as strategies for action. Another, reported by Noble (2005), involved development and performance of a play depicting experiences of people with multiple psychiatric diagnoses as a collaborative endeavor with counsellors, who also took part in the performance (called *Shaken: Not Disturbed … with a Twist!*). The popular theater piece, described as an exercise in transgressive and liberatory learning and "collective knowledge creation and action" (52), illustrated lives on the social margins and aimed to challenge social perceptions surrounding mental illness. The project involved reconfiguring "rituals of power" in the participants' lives "into new rites of personal power for themselves"—a process called "recodification," and to educate the audience, which included health-care workers, about such "nonvisible" lives (49).

Enduring interest, enjoyment, and social connection and support

Adult learning as a leisure activity may be defined as "serious leisure" that requires effort and commitment to learn the required knowledge and skills (Stebbins, 1982), with the creative arts being a central tenet of this (DH Mental Health Division, 2010). Studies demonstrate how leisure can generate social support and coping and stress-buffering effects

(Fullagar, 2008, citing Caldwell, 2005; Craike and Coleman, 2005). However, opportunities for leisure and enjoyment may be culturally or structurally denied to certain segments of society such as women, those experiencing long-term mental health issues and informal carers (Fullagar and O'Brien, 2014; Pieris and Craik, 2004). Populations focused on in studies of the benefits of leisure have therefore included these groups as well as older people, for whom leisure is often considered important in providing physical, social, and mental stimulation for "healthy aging."

In the UK context, in the report on Learn2b, a targeted ACL program for people with mild to moderate depression and anxiety, which included creative expression (Robotham et al., 2011), one participant described regaining her interest in art and learning to enjoy it as part of her recovery, while several women taking part in creative writing groups felt the activity was beneficial in providing something interesting and enjoyable to focus on and making time for oneself, aside from work and caring responsibilities. This was seen to help in terms of "getting back in touch" with or "refinding" oneself. One participant also commented on the value of undertaking creative activities in connection with others: "I have found new people to write, sing and make music with" (33).

The above findings support other research that has shown the value of women's creative practices for challenging depression in the context of informal caring through providing space for oneself, enjoyment, and temporary escape from responsibilities (e.g., Fullagar, 2008; Fullagar and O'Brien, 2014; Lewis et al., 2016; Reynolds, 2000). Fullagar (2008) suggests that this is an important aspect of recovery because enjoyment is often lacking in the lives of women experiencing depression, and women often have a harsh and punitive relation to the self. (Re)finding enjoyment, she argues, can help women to develop self-compassion and a more playful self-relation.

Similar findings are reported by Reynolds (2010) in a UK study of the contribution of visual art-making, including painting, pottery, textiles, card-making, weaving, lace-making, and other arts and crafts, as a leisure activity to support older women's well-being. Describing her findings in terms of "colour and communion," she tells of how the women enjoyed the sensuality of the art-making, the playful experimentation it allowed, developing new skills, and the challenges and fresh ambitions it generated, as well as the way in which it "promoted feelings of connectedness with the wider physical and social worlds" (138), beyond the home and immediate family. She also describes how "some created their own groups of like-minded friends, with art-making activities providing the mutual focus of their meetings together" (141) and how outside the group meetings, the art-making activities additionally supported family relationships through providing a shared activity.

Reflecting these findings, Gauntlett (2011) suggests three definitive motivations for making and everyday creativity: "pleasure and an enhanced sense of self as creative agent; feeling alive in the world through the ability to do things as an active participant engaged in dialogue with a community; and recognition by like-minded people." These themes also resonate in a Canadian study of a community-based lifelong learning program for older adults. Observing five different classes (calligraphy, sewing, Chinese poetry, folkdance, and fitness) and interviewing 15 members (10 women and five men), Narushima (2008) identified three main health-related outcomes of the learning: "(1) the effects of enduring interest, (2) classrooms as social support networks, and (3) the awareness of the right to learn" (673). She describes how "these learning effects are closely inter-related, working as a single, synergetic health-enhancing mechanism" (687).

Narushima reports on the value of "learning something interesting together with others" and how the adult learning helped reinforce perceived control—"an important means to sustain an independent and functioning life in old age" (683). As Reynolds (2000: 112) notes, temporary experiences of autonomy, choice, and control, which were also reported by the women undertaking needlecraft in her study, "may be particularly valued when personal decision-making or control are limited in other facets of life" and are helpful to countering depression. Furthermore, such experiences may be translated into other areas of people's lives, thereby contributing to agency enhancement (Lewis et al., 2016).

The space provided by taking part in creative arts ACL and engagement in the creative activities can also be helpful in allowing people to reappraise problems in their lives and to find constructive responses to these (Fancourt et al., 2019). The generation of social connection and support through ACL spaces is additionally helpful in this regard. Narushima (2008: 688) describes the contribution of adult learning to generating "informal mutual support networks," with both instrumental and emotional supports found to buffer the impacts of health problems in older age. One of her key findings related to the lowering of social hierarchies through the craft activities and how this sense of equality deriving from the pursuit of a common interest contributed to a classroom affinity and mutual care. She quotes one participant, Betty:

> We are together. We don't care whether other people are younger or from different backgrounds. Here everyone is the same. We all like sewing. We learn, talk, laugh together. We share patterns and tools. When the semester is over, everyone hugs each other and says good-bye for a while.
>
> *(684)*

Narushima (2008) also expounds the way in which the seniors in her study all contributed to the learning environment:

> "I think this program helps me stay healthy. Because I ENJOY. The enjoyment is the best medicine." As this participant's words drive home, each individual senior's interests, pleasure and determination to keep learning and be healthy while facing all the challenges of later life, positively influences other classmates and the atmosphere of the classroom. The comfortable learning environment with an experienced engaging instructor, friendly classmates, a sense of community and other mutual supports motivates seniors to remain in a single course. This in turn reinforces each individual's interest, life satisfaction, self-efficacy, and self-management—all important intermediate factors for psychosocial well-being and effective coping in later life.
>
> *(687)*

These extracts illustrate how, in ACL contexts, creative activities such as sewing constitute a kind of participatory practice which can produce a feeling of "togetherness" and, as elaborated next, provides opportunities for various other kinds of sharing and reciprocity. Under such circumstances ACL can become a collective endeavor in which individuals in a group grow together, in connection with one another, and interactively with the development of the group as a whole (Lewis et al., 2016; McDowell, 1998) through a kind of "incorporation of the collective into the individual" (Edwards, 2007: 259). Establishing ethos and building the group, including through mobilizing and sharing resources, are therefore important to achieving both educational and health-related aims, with the tutor playing a key role in these respects (Lewis, 2014).

In studies of arts participation for people experiencing severe and enduring mental health issues mental health-related benefits are similarly often described in terms of social inclusion and mutual support. Reflecting the studies described above, enjoyment, interest, and the creation of a stable, non-threatening environment in which participants can start to experience a sense of control over their lives and enhanced agency are strong themes (e.g., Lewis et al., 2016). These themes are illuminated well by Horghagen et al. (2014) in a Norwegian ethnographic study of craft activities in community-based mental health centers called "meeting places" for people with long-lasting mental illness. They describe how guided craft groups, encompassing textiles, woodwork, paintings, and glasswork and ceramics, promoted social participation for the nine women and three men taking part, with importance attached to staff participation in the activities as well. The benefits of the craft work included its low threshold for participation and its cultural familiarity and ordinariness within the Norwegian context, which provided mechanisms for participation and social interaction in the form of "small talk," while also meaning participants were able to shape identities as "artisans." Doing the crafts together facilitated social interaction as "having crafts such as knitting in their hands made it easier for participants to socialize and move in and out of conversations" (148). They also note how the communal craft work enabled social inclusion as participants felt part of a group, even if they were just sitting together with people undertaking crafts. Participation was therefore "enabled by the fact that there were no defined demands for the level of engagement" (150).

Crafting is described by Horghagen et al. as helpful in providing stability, routine, predictability, and control with the familiarity of both the group and crafting activity giving participants "a network of relational safety and support" (149) and a base for achievement in other domains. The habitual craft work seemed to generate strong connections between participants and facilitated peer support as, "while crafting, participants shared knowledge, experiences ... served as role models for each other ... and advised one another" (149). Both aspects of their participation—the craft work and the support—helped group members to manage their daily lives. Furthermore, the activities promoted joy and self-respect, and this helped free participants from the constraints of "mental illness." The learning experiences enabled participants to become "gradually more active in decision-making regarding how to organize craft production," while "the feedback received and given by participants ... strengthened their self-confidence in their [self-]management skills" (150–151). The dynamic interrelationship between the act of doing crafts and the social relations in the group is thus emphasized in this study, with the "socially interactive and collaborative craft production" seen as producing a transactional space for recovery (151).

Identity work, social contribution and reciprocity

Moody and Phinney (2012: 62) point out that, for older people, involvement in "serious leisure," such as arts programs, can contribute to social inclusion through "offer[ing] entry into a unique social world, providing for participants a sense of belonging and collective identity." As noted in the previous discussion of Horghagen et al.'s (2014) study, identity work through involvement in creative arts initiatives can also be an important part of social inclusion and recovery for those experiencing long-term, debilitating mental health issues. Studies of mental health participatory arts organizations have shown that, for many participants, belonging to a community of artists provides not only a valued social role but also an identity as an artist, which can be important to recovery in displacing negative identities associated with mental illness (e.g., Lewis and Spandler, 2019).

Research into creative arts ACL and mental health and well-being in both mental health–targeted and mainstream settings show how this adult learning can generate personal and social recognition, and hence be a source of identity work, for participants, not only because the shared practice involves undertaking creative work together with others, but also because it may involve the sharing of skills, materials, and creative outputs. Studies often mention a sense of pride, achievement, and satisfaction from creating and sharing tangible creative outputs as important psychosocial outcomes from the adult learning (e.g., Fisher and Specht, 1999; Hammond, 2004a, 2004b; HEA, 1999; Lewis et al., 2016), with these being linked to the wider outcomes of enhanced sense of meaning, fulfilment, and purpose that are often described in relation to involvement in the creative arts (DH Mental Health Division, 2010).

"Appraisal support" (Heany and Israel, 2002) is thus important in this context. For instance, Reynolds (2010) describes how, for older women engaged in visual art-making, "praise from fellow artists (whether amateurs or professionals) was experienced as offering a specific and potent source of validation" that "strengthened a positive self-image, as well as motivation to continue" (141). She also describes how the creative activity was important to the older women's subjective experiences surrounding having a role and "feeling useful" when previous work or family roles were reduced or no longer occupied. In this context, the creative practice helped to preserve reciprocity and equal status in relationships, "based on mutual interests and care-giving, rather than age or dependency . . ., shared topics of conversation and the exchange of skills and materials" (Reynolds, 2010: 140–141). This helped the women to maintain a valued identity, and to resist the stereotypes and exclusions often experienced in later life. Discussing a qualitative study of older people's art-making by Howie et al. (2002), Reynolds (2010) also describes how creative activities can serve a kind of identity work through providing

> a means of 'crafting the self', through for example, expressing continuities of self in past, present and future projects, maintaining family traditions, engaging in self-reflection, gaining affirmative responses from others, and acquiring a valued identity as an artist.
>
> *(Reynolds, 2010: 137)*

Elsewhere, Reynolds (1997: 12; 2000: 107, 111) describes needlework as offering "validation of the self" and a way of "preserving or regaining a satisfactory sense of self" for women who had acquired a disability or chronic illness in adulthood, and, for women experiencing depression, as "providing themselves and others with evidence of a healthy, achieving self." In the latter context, she argues that "craft products confirm an alternative self (extending work/family roles)" and "craft skills may contribute to valued roles and sources of status (e.g., charity work, teaching skills to others)" (Reynolds, 2000: 111). Public recognition of needlework products, she reflects, "enhanced feelings of accomplishment, and increased the person's sense of occupying a valued place in her social network" (Reynolds, 2000: 111).

The literature on mental health recovery includes other examples of how producing creative items can provide a way of giving back to family members or helpers and how this can help regain reciprocal qualities for personal relationships (e.g., Carlton, 2006). In addition, research in the context of care homes for the elderly shows how shared creative activities involving residents, relatives, and staff can help (re)generate this reciprocity through producing shared enjoyment, a shared experience and interest, and a common purpose (e.g.,

Bungay et al., 2019). The shared activities can also enable staff appreciation of residents' abilities and the value of arts participation for residents (Bungay et al., 2019; Gottlieb-Tanaka et al., 2003).

As Reynolds' research also shows, then, the generation of friendship through creative arts ACL can be another important source of reciprocity that can benefit well-being and mental health recovery. This may be through helping rebalance an over-emphasis on being the (dependent) recipient of care, or on giving to/caring for others—something particularly relevant to challenging women's depression given the cultural context of their family and working lives (Fullagar, 2008; Fullagar and O'Brien, 2014). In the former context, Halperin and Boz-Mizrahi (2009) report on the Israel Amitim program, which involved leisure activities, including classes in music, art, and dance for service users, volunteers, and staff in a mental health community center. They describe how participants valued the opportunity for personal development as contributors in social interaction and to experience "true friendship and a long-lasting relationship" (155), and a reduction in stigmatizing attitudes among the community center workers involved.

Lastly, as Reynolds' research indicates, creative arts ACL can provide particular opportunities for social contribution because it lends itself to collaborative approaches to learning, including shared learning between tutors and adult learners and intergenerational learning. In addition, it provides opportunities for wider social contribution, and for social and political engagement, for example through exhibiting art work, giving performances, or facilitating participatory arts events. These opportunities can be particularly valued when people are experiencing diminished social roles, for example due to older age or mental health issues. For example, reflecting on helping facilitate a jewelry-making session with a group of "young mums," one member of the jewelry-making group in Lewis et al.'s (2016) study commented, "I went home thinking, 'Well, I've done something worth it this afternoon'" (189; see also Lewis and Spandler, 2019; Moody and Phinney, 2012). Moody and Phinney (2012: 62) argue that "experiences of reciprocity within a community are important to the health and well-being of older adults" and "being able to contribute to a community in a meaningful way may make it easier for seniors to accept help and support from the community in a reciprocal manner."

Conclusion

Research on ACL and mental health and well-being has focused on mental health targeted provision and provision for older people. In these contexts it has demonstrated mental health and well-being–related benefits from various ACL curriculum areas. It suggests that these benefits are associated with the nature of the adult learning in terms of providing opportunities for personal growth. However, research also suggests that creative arts ACL is particularly amenable to generating a range of interconnected psychosocial processes which promote well-being and mental health recovery. In relational terms, mutuality, including understanding of self and others and reciprocity at interpersonal and social levels, is important to these processes (Lewis, 2019; see also Torronen et al., 2018).

The literature also suggests that the psychosocial processes associated with ACL benefits for mental health and well-being "appear to be similar across the whole dimension of psychological health, from despair and depression to flourishing" (Hammond, 2004b: 565). Yet these processes and, in particular, their combining to support an expansion of agency are particularly applicable to understanding ACL in the context of mental health recovery (Lewis, 2014; Lewis et al., 2016). In addition, as Sagan's (2007, 2008) research highlights, there may be more pain associated with adult learning in this context, compared with mainstream provision or that which aims towards promoting well-being. This is because recovery may involve revisiting difficult or traumatic experiences, coming to terms with loss of various kinds, and reparation processes including reconfiguring one's sense of self (Sagan, 2008).

As noted by way of introduction, there may also be "disbenefits" associated with creative arts ACL. For example, while the provision may generate group solidarity and a sense of community for most participants, some may experience attempts to take part as exclusionary, particularly if they do not fit the social profile of the group (Lewis et al., 2016). And while creative arts involvement can be a welcome break for women with caring responsibilities, pressure to take part in such activities can be another burden on carers (Rizk et al., 2011) in the context of "restricted" lives (Twigg, 1994).

In terms of the social critique set out in the introduction to this chapter, in so far as some creative arts ACL may help people cope with stress rather than to understand, and potentially challenge, the conditions of their lives which are producing this, it could be described as having placating effects. However, in the context of mental health issues in particular, there is a legitimate function for adult learning in providing a constructive external focus and distraction from worrying or intrusive thoughts. Moreover, the creative arts provide opportunities for "holistic learning" across cognitive, affective, somatic, and spiritual domains (Lipson Lawrence, 2008). They "embody life" (Goldberg, 2001), working in a reflective manner to help us understand the world around us and to contextualize our experience, and in a constructive manner to help us shape our social worlds. In ACL, while some of this learning may be an overt part of the creative arts curriculum, some of the educational processes involved which are agency-enhancing are implicit, taking place through the interactions and experience of the learning environment. As such, as Belzer (2004: 5) points out, "even when curriculum is not explicitly focused on topics related to social justice, equity and other issues of social change, it is implicitly taking a critical stance on power relationships inside and outside the classroom."

In addition, in the context of mental health or well-being issues, creative arts ACL can often be a first step for adults returning to education, potentially leading to participation in other areas of learning as well, and involvement in creative arts ACL is not exclusive to participation in other kinds of adult learning. Indeed, it is important to maintain a wide ACL curriculum, which includes creative arts, social sciences, and other subjects, to expand opportunities for learning across a range of areas, including in the context of mental health targeted provision and provision for older people (Hammond, 2004b; Kang and Russ, 2009; Lewis, 2014, 2019).

As the arts and creativity provide opportunities for broad-ranging and "holistic" learning, as described above, they should be viewed as an important element of wider curricula for ACL programming for mental health and well-being. But the degree to which this ACL provision supports the development of agency is likely to be dependent on the nature of the provision, the approach taken, and the knowledge and skills of the adult learning practitioners involved. In particular, whether or not there is a liberatory or "empowering" pedagogical approach that is informed by an understanding of power relations and their role in relation to mental health is likely to be pivotal (Lewis, 2014). Creative arts ACL for mental health recovery therefore needs to be focused on the creative arts education, while encompassing concern with the implicit educational, psychosocial, and affective processes involved. Crucially, the learning should help to open up different ways of thinking for adults and expand opportunities to view personal experiences through a wide social and political lens (Lewis, 2014; Lewis et al., 2016). Democratic principles and collaborative methods that actively involve adult learners in shaping the learning and the learning context (Austin, 1999; Belzer, 2004), together with reflective practice, can further ensure that such a broadening of knowledge and perspective includes everyone involved in the learning process and, potentially, members of the wider community as well.

Acknowledgements

This chapter draws on a literature review and research funded by an AHRC/RCUK Connected Communities large grant, no. AH/K003364/1.

References

Aldridge, F., and Lavender, P. (2000). *The Impact of Learning on Health*. Leicester: NIACE.

Austin, T. (1999). The Role of Education in the Lives of People with Mental Health Difficulties. In: C. Newnes, G. Holmes and C. Dunn, eds, *This is Madness: A Critical Look at Psychiatry and the Future of Mental Health Services*. Ross-on-Wye: PCCS Books: 253–262.

Belzer, A. (2004). Blundering Toward Critical Pedagogy: True Tales From the Adult Literacy Classroom. *New Directions for Adult and Continuing Education*, 102: 5–13.

Bungay, H., Munn-Giddings, C., Wilson, C. and Daddswell, A. (2019). *Creative Journeys. The Role of Participatory Arts in Promoting Social Relationships for Older People in Care Home Settings*. Cambridge: Anglia Ruskin University.

Caldwell, L. (2005). Leisure and Health: Why Is Leisure Therapeutic? *British Journal of Guidance and Counselling*, 33(1): 7–26.

Caldwell, P. (2013). Recreating Social Purpose Adult Education. *Adults Learning*, 25(4): 39–41.

Carlton, T. (2006). *Journeys of Recovery: Stories of hope and recovery from long-term mental health problems*. Glasgow: Scottish Recovery Network.

Cohen, G. D. (2006). *The Creativity and Aging Study: The Impact of Professionally Conducted Cultural Programs on Older Adults*. Retrieved from: www.nea.gov/resources/accessibility/Cna-Rep4-30-06.pdf (Accessed 1/8/2019).

Craike, M. and Coleman, D. (2005). Buffering effects of leisure self-determination on the mental health of older adults. *Leisure/Loisir*, 29(2): 301–328.

Crawford, P., Hogan, S., Wilson, M., Williamon, A., Manning, N., Brown, B. and Lewis, L. (2018). *Creative Practice as Mutual Recovery. Research Programme Final Report*. University of Nottingham, UK. April. Available: www.healthhumanities.org/creative_practice_mutual_recovery/.

Dekker, M. (1996). Why Oblique and Why Jung? In: J. Pearson, ed, *Discovering the Self Through Drama and Movement*. London, Jessica Kingsley Publishers: 39–45.

DH Mental Health Division. (2010). *Confident Communities, Brighter Futures, A Framework for Developing Wellbeing*. London: Department of Health.

Ecclestone, K. (2004). Developing Self-esteem and Emotional Well-being: Inclusion or Intrusion? *Adults Learning*, 16(3): 11–13.

Edwards, A. (2007). Working Collaboratively to Build Resilience: A CHAT Approach. *Social Policy and Society*, 6(2): 255–264.

Eldred, J., Ward, J., Dutton, Y and Snowdon, K. (2004). *Catching Confidence*. Leicester: NIACE.

Fancourt, D., Garnett, C., Spiro, N., West, R. and Mullensiefen, D. (2019). How Do Artistic Creative Activities Regulate Our Emotions? Validation of the Emotion Regulation Strategies for Artistic Creative Activities Scale (ERS-ACA). *PLoS ONE*, 14(2): e0211362.

Field, J. (2009). Good for your soul? Adult learning and mental well-being. *International Journal of Lifelong Education*, 28(2): 175–191.

Fisher, B. J., and Specht, D. (1999). Successful aging and creativity in later life. *Journal of Aging Studies*, 13: 457–472.

Freire, P. (1996). *Pedagogy of the Oppressed*. Trans. Myra Bergman Ramos. London: Penguin Books.

Fullagar, S. (2008). Leisure Practices as Counter-Depressants: Emotion-Work and Emotion-Play within Women's Recovery from Depression. *Leisure Sciences*, 30: 35–52.

Fullagar, S. and O'Brien, W. (2014). Social Recovery and the Move Beyond Deficit Models of Depression: A Feminist Analysis of Mid-Life Women's Self-Care Practices. *Social Science and Medicine*, 117: 116–124.

Gauntlett, D. (2011). *Making is Connecting*. Keynote presentation (abstract), Crafting Communities Connected Communities workshop. Available: http://connectingcraftcommunities.wordpress.com/workshop/1-crafting-communities/1-audio/(Accessed 1/8/2019).

Gillispie, C. (2003). Poetry Therapy Techniques Applied to a Recreation/Adult Education Group for the Mentally Ill. *Journal of Poetry Therapy*, 16(2): 97–106.

Goldberg, M. (2001). *Arts and Learning*. New York: Addison Wesley Longman.

Gottlieb-Tanaka, D., Small, J. and Yassi, A. (2003). A Program of Creative Expression Activities for Seniors with Dementia. *Dementia: The International Journal of Social Research and Practice*, 2(1): 127–133.

Halperin, G. and Boz-Mizrahi, T. (2009). The Amitim Program: An Innovative Program for the Social Rehabilitation of People with Mental Illness in the Community. *Israel Journal of Psychiatry and Related Sciences*, 46(2): 149–156.

Hammond, C. (2004a). The Impacts of Learning on Well-Being, Mental Health and Effective Coping. In: T. Schuller, J. Preston, C. Hammond, A. Brassett-Grundy and J. Bynner, eds, *The Benefits of Learning. The Impact of Education on Health, Family Life and Social Capital*. London: Routledge: 37–56.

Hammond, C. (2004b). Impacts of Lifelong Learning Upon Emotional Resilience, Psychological and Mental Health: Fieldwork Evidence. *Oxford Review of Education*, 30(4): 551–568.

Harding, C. Simon, A., Evans, L., Joyce, L., Stockley R. and Peters, M. (2013). *Community Learning Learner Survey Report*. BIS Research paper no. 108. London: BIS.

HEA (Health Education Authority) (1999). *Art for health: a review of good practice in community based arts projects and interventions which impact on health and wellbeing*. London: HEA.

Heany, C. A. and Israel, B. A. (2002). Social Networks and Social Support. In: K. Glanz, B. Rimer, and F. Lewis, eds, *Health Behaviour and Health Education: Theory, Research, and Practice*. San Francisco: Jossey-Bass: 185–209.

Horghagen, S., Fostvedt, B. and Alsaker, S. (2014). Craft Activities in Groups at Meeting Places: Supporting Mental Health Users' Everyday Occupations. *Scandinavian Journal of Occupational Therapy*, 21: 145–152.

Howie, L., Coulter, M., and Feldman, S. (2004). Crafting the self: Older persons' narratives of occupational identity. *American Journal of Occupational Therapy*, 58: 446–454.

Jenkins, A. (2011). Participation in Learning and Wellbeing Among Older Adults. *International Journal of Lifelong Education*, 30(3): 403–420.

Kang, M. and Russ, R. (2009). Activities That Promote Wellness for Older Adults in Rural Communities. *Journal of Extension*, 47(5): 1–5.

Lewis, L. (2014). Responding to the Mental Health and Wellbeing Agenda in Adult Community Learning. *Journal of Research in Post-Compulsory Education*, 19(4): 357–377.

Lewis, L. (2019). Adult Community Learning, Wellbeing and Mental Health Recovery. In: R. Papa and D. Matheson, eds, *Handbook on Promoting Social Justice in Education*. New York:, Springer: (in press).1–33.

Lewis, L. and Spandler, H. (2019). Breaking Down Boundaries? Exploring Shared Art-Making in an Open Studio Mental Health Setting. *Journal of Applied Arts and Health*, 10(1): 9–23.

Lewis, L., Spandler, H., Tew, J. and Ecclestone, K. (with Croft, H.) (2016). *Mutuality, Wellbeing and Mental Health Recovery: Exploring the Roles of Creative Arts Adult Community Learning and Participatory Arts Initiatives, Final Research Report*. University of Wolverhampton, April.

Lipson Lawrence, R. (2008). Powerful Feelings: Exploring the Affective Domain of Informal and Arts-Based Learning. *New Directions for Adult and Continuing Education*, 120: 65–77.

McDowell A. (1998). Creative Writing: How is it Viewed by Adults with Learning Disabilities? *British Journal of Therapy and Rehabilitation*, 5(9): 465–467.

Meyer, S. (2008). Truth, Beauty and the Meaning of Life. *Adults Learning*, 19(8): 7. www.learningandwork.org.uk/resource/adults-learning/

Milner, M. (1950). *On Not Being Able to Paint*. Oxford: Heinemann.

Mirza, M. (2006). The Arts as Painkiller. In: M. Mirza, ed, *Culture Vultures: Is UK Arts Policy Damaging the Arts?* London, Policy Exchange: 93–110.

Moody, E. and Phinney, A. (2012). A Community-Engaged Art Program for Older People: Fostering Social Inclusion. *Canadian Journal on Aging*, 31(1): 55–64.

Narushima, M. (2008). More Than Nickels and Dimes: The Health Benefits of a Community-Based Lifelong Learning Programme for Older Adults. *International Journal of Lifelong Education*, 27(6): 673–692.

Nimrod, G. (2007). Retirees' Leisure: Activities, Benefits, and their Contribution to Life Satisfaction. *Leisure Studies*, 26(1): 65–80.

Noble, S. (2005). Mental illness through popular theatre: Performing (in)sanely. *New Directions for Adult and Continuing Education*, 107: 45–53.

Novitsky, J. (2014). *Community Learning and Health, CLIF Impact Project*. Leicester: NIACE.

Pettit, J. (2010). Multiple Faces of Power and Learning. *IDS Bulletin*, 41(3): 25–35.

Pieris, Y. and Craik C. (2004). Factors Enabling and Hindering Participation in Leisure for People with Mental Health Problems. *British Journal of Occupational Therapy*, 67(6): 240–247.

Read Johnson, D. (1998). On the Therapeutic Action of the Creative Arts Therapies: The Psycho-dynamic Model. *The Arts in Psychotherapy*, 25(2): 85–99.

Reynolds, F. (1997). Coping with Chronic Illness and Disability Through Creative Needlecraft. *British Journal of Occupational Therapy*, 60(8): 352–356.

Reynolds, F. (2000). Managing Depression Through Needlecraft Creative Activities, A Qualitative Study. *The Arts in Psychotherapy*, 27(2): 107–114.

Reynolds, F. (2010). 'Colour and Communion': Exploring the Influences of Visual Art-Making as a Leisure Activity on Older Women's Subjective Well-Being. *Journal of Aging Studies*, 24: 135–143.

Rizk, S., Pizur-Barnekow, K. and Darragh, A. (2011). Leisure and Social Participation and Health-Related Quality of Life in Caregivers of Children with Autism. *OTJR: Occupation, Participation and Health*, 31(4): 164–171.

Robotham, D., Morgan, K. and James, K. (2011). *Learning for Life; Adult Learning, Mental Health and Well-Being*. London: Mental Health Foundation.

Ruddock, H. and Worral, I. (1997). *An Outline of a Current Project in Creative Writing and Literacy for People Experiencing Mental Health Difficulties*. Rotherham: Dearne Valley College.

Sagan, O. (2007). An Interplay of Learning, Creativity and Narrative Biography in a Mental Health Setting: Bertie's Story. *Journal of Social Work Practice*, 21(3): 311–321.

Sagan, O. (2008). The Loneliness of the Long-Anxious Learner: Mental Illness, Narrative Biography and Learning to Write. *Psychodynamic Practice*, 14(1): 43–58.

Schaverien, J. (1989). The Picture Within the Frame. In: A. Gilroy and T. Dalley, eds, *Pictures at an Exhibition: Selected Essays on Art and Art Therapy*. London: Routledge: 147–155.

Simone. P. and Cesena, J. (2010). Student Demographics, Satisfaction and Cognitive Demand in Two Lifelong Learning Programs. *Educational Gerontology*, 36: 425–434.

Stebbins, R.A. (1982). Serious Leisure: A Conceptual Statement. *Pacific Sociological Review*, 25: 251–272.

Thompson, J. (2007). *More Words in Edgeways. Rediscovering Adult Education*. Leicester: NIACE.

Torronen, M., Munn-Giddings, C. and Tarkiainen, L., eds. (2018). *Reciprocal Relationships and Well-being: Implications for Social Work and Social Policy*. London: Routledge.

Twigg, J. (1994). *CARERS Perceived: Policy and Practice in Informal Care*. Buckinghamshire: OU Press.

Wertheimer, A. (1997). *Images of Possibility. Creating Learning Opportunities for Adults with Mental Health Difficulties*. Leicester: NIACE.

23

WHAT ZOMBIES CAN TELL US ABOUT CONTEMPORARY HEALTH CARE

Steven Schlozman

Introduction

Whenever I am asked to write about zombies (let alone zombies and health care) I take solace in the writings of John Donne. I admit that this is a bit of a ruse, and a narcissistic one at that. In referencing Donne, I am hoping that this potentially obscure allusion will help to establish my credentials as a rather erudite and clever fellow despite my putative expertise in a topic as silly as zombies. But there is another, more, shall we say, *biting* reason for my beginning this chapter by citing the metaphysics of a seventeenth-century poet. That reason leads me to write about John Donne and his take on the lowly flea.

Donne wrote a great poem about fleas. In fact, the least creative thing about the poem is the name of the poem itself. He called it *The Flea* (Donne, 1663). For all intents and purposes, and certainly at first glance, the poem appears to be exactly and only about a flea. It is on the surface a heartfelt love song to the blood-sucking proclivities of this particularly bothersome arthropod. But is that all that his poem is about?

Of course not. Donne was a metaphysicist. As such, he delighted in comparing two or more seemingly incomparable concepts. To paraphrase Freud's descriptions of the ever-present cigar, the flea isn't only a flea. The flea serves as a potent metaphor for love and for lust.

Donne chose to use the actions of the flea—the unbridled lust for blood and flesh—as a perfect, if somewhat off-putting, analogy for the throws of romance and eroticism. Although his reasons for engaging in this poetic sleight of hand are beyond the scope of this chapter (now is a good time to remember that this is a chapter about zombies), I can turn to his analogy as perhaps the only metaphor that readers will find even more grotesque than the thesis of this essay: namely, that one can compare with equal fervency the zombie story and the story of health care. In other words, if Donne can write about blood-sucking bugs and erotic desire, then any piece of writing that draws together zombie films and the trials and tribulations of modern health care ought to be a walk in the park. Still, experience has taught me that, even with such careful introductions, I must begin any chapter about zombies by issuing a series of disclaimers. First of all, the cinematic zombie that first stumbled across our movie screens with 1968's *Night of the Living Dead* are not now, nor have they ever been, real. As a physician, I feel compelled to issue this caveat. And second, as with all works of lasting art, the popularity of the zombie trope tells us that zombie stories are perceived by many as surprisingly revealing and profound. Because health care is also incredibly profound, it stands to reason that we can draw from the profundities of zombie films and apply what we learn to the profound challenges facing health and wellness today.

Thank you, Mr. Donne. You have provided cover for my thesis. Zombies, despite the fact that they can barely walk, can through analyses of their stories tell us some pretty important things about health. But to do this, we need to establish the rules.

First, we will focus primarily on two of the greatest zombie films ever made: *Night of the Living Dead* (Romero, 1968) and *Dawn of the Dead* (Romero, 1978). Both films were written and directed by the late George A. Romero, and both are regarded as masterpieces within and outside of the horror world. Although it is true that there are true zombies—the spell-ridden individuals of Caribbean and West African tradition—these zombies will not be our focus. We will stick to Romero's films because they map uncomfortably well onto the plagues of modern health care.

Second, after a summary of the films themselves (and the compulsory spoiler alerts that each summary necessitates), we will move to a Donne-like discussion of the comparisons that these themes afford in an honest and somewhat painful discussion of health care.

Finally, we will end this chapter by tying these ideas together. At the end of the day (and many zombie films are in fact literally about the end of *all* days), despite all of their grunting, zombies have lots to say.

Night of the living dead

Night of the Living Dead was Romero's first film. It was a low-budget but brilliantly prognostic horror flick that changed, almost overnight, the nature of scary movies. After Romero's first masterpiece, there was no going back to larks like *I Married a Teenage Werewolf*.

In *Night of the Living Dead*, western Pennsylvania and later the entire United States finds itself in the grips of what appears to be the early stages of an epidemic. Dead people are rising from their graves as mindless and uncoordinated flesh eaters. Romero in fact first called his film *Night of the Flesh Eaters*, until it occurred to him and his collaborators that *Night of the Living Dead* had an oxymoronic symmetry that was itself reflective of the film's central message. The dead cannot be living. One concept cancels the other. But if the dead are indeed alive but can barely even walk, then they ought to be pretty easy to defeat. How resourceful can a stumbling dead person be?

Nevertheless, the remaining humans in this first ever, modern zombie tale allow their prejudices and ignorance to overwhelm whatever chances they have of surviving. The white woman mistrusts the black man almost more than she mistrusts the largely Caucasian ghouls outside the windows of the house in which they both take refuge. The father who is hiding with his family in the basement uses his perceived and perhaps rationalized sense that his only responsibility is to his family alone and locks himself below the house when he finds himself unexpectedly in the company of other survivors. As such, he is powerless to stop the death of his wife at the hand of his infected daughter. At the end of the film, most devastating of all, the Black protagonist, after having dutifully helped others as best he could and at the same time making it through the night, is shot in the head and tossed onto a pile of burning bodies. We get the feeling that his blackness makes him not worth the risk of making sure he is not infected. After all, we are treated to the point of view of the man who shoots him. We see that the protagonist is acting with intention—with clear human intention—but he is shot nonetheless.

The film is therefore entirely devastating, but not just for its ending. We leave the movie with the sinking feeling that all of the mishaps could have been avoided. The zombies can barely move, after all. They are terrified and easily held at bay by fire. Put a fence around these zombies and the problem is solved. Then we can learn about them. We can save the ones that are not too sick, and humanely treat the ones we cannot. We have done exactly that with stray dogs for centuries. Why can't we do it with humans in *Night of the Living Dead*?

One might ask the same question of modern health care. To be clear, I am not suggesting that health care has led us to treat those who suffer in the same manner in which we treat stray animals. But I am noting that any viewing of *Night of the Living Dead* is ripe with "what ifs" and "whys" that are highly pertinent to the provisions of ensuring health in today's complicated world.

What if the characters in *Night of the Living Dead* had decided to work together rather than to bicker unproductively? *Why* didn't the characters take what seemed to be some obvious steps towards making their circumstances better? All of this conjecture leads to one particularly vexing inquiry: *how could the poor souls of Night of the Living Dead fail to predict their unfortunate outcome?*

These very questions have been asked again and again about today's state of health. Could we have foreseen the depersonalization, indeed the "zombification," of modern health delivery? With the advent of technology, did it not stand to reason that we would drift apart from one another, clinician from patient, human from human, and in the process lose that which we have always held most precious to being well—the connections we feel with each other. Zombies are deeply impersonal, and being sick and providing care for the sick has become in many ways equally forlorn.

As Elgin et al. (2015) note, nurses began asking this question some time ago. Back in 1988, economists wondered whether giving patients more say in their care would improve patient satisfaction (Beisecker, 1988). Given that satisfaction continues to plummet, it seems that the transformation of the patient purely into consumer yielded the same lack of cooperative problem solving that plagued the sole humans walled off in the house in Romero's first film. We humans, in the absence of mindful regulation, have a tendency to become self-interested. We create different standards for ourselves than we do for our neighbors. This is what happens with the frightened father in the basement in *Night of the Living Dead*.

With Romero's first film, we can ask if the displacement that fiction offers reveals where our health care may have gone off track. If we feel under attack by something that we do not understand, the rules of civility are quickly forgotten, and health care certainly feels too big to totally grasp. We therefore search for principles we understand to make sense of how the delivery and receiving of decent health got so muddled and complicated. This led many to consider the rules of abject and unbridled consumerism, and these concepts were exactly the focus of Romero's next zombie tale.

Dawn of the dead

Dawn of the Dead leaves the Cold War paranoia of the late 1960s and brings instead the seemingly unstoppable zombie pandemic into the consumer-frenzied world of the late 1970s and 1980s.

When the movie begins, zombies are everywhere. Social order has broken down entirely. The opening scene features a newsroom in comical disarray, and then cuts abruptly to a housing project in the Northeast United States where the military are preparing to rid the high-rise apartments of an unclear number of zombie inhabitants.

191

This sets the scene for the sense of entitlement that wealth brings to chaotic circumstances. One of the soldiers preparing to attack the housing project is incensed that the impoverished and now likely infected residents of the low-income residences have any residences at all. "How the hell come we stick these low-life bastards in these big-ass hotels anyway," he asks. "Shit, man! This is better than I got" (Romero, 1978).

In other words, the residents of the hotel are dehumanized even before we know for certain whether they are infected. They are expendable because they lack the resources to pay for their safety. That in and of itself feels highly relevant to the consumerist health-care themes of the 1980s. Those who are deserving of care are those who can pay for care. This was a fundamental driving principle that was present throughout the world, but perhaps voiced most of all in the United States—that is, that the free market is the overarching and by far the most success-ridden way for our society to function. Economists such as Milton Friedman famously wrote that there

> is one and only one social responsibility of business – to use its resources and engage in activities designed to increase its profits so long as it stays within the rules of the game, which is to say, engages in open and free competition without deception or fraud.
>
> *(Friedman, 1992)*

Although Friedman first wrote these words in 1962, many have interpreted this statement as an endorsement of the reality that businesses, including the businesses of health care, will and should provide most of all for those who can afford it. This was certainly an emerging and sometimes dominant health-care philosophy of the 1980s that has persisted to this day.

It is no surprise, therefore, that our protagonists in *Dawn of the Dead* find safe harbor in a shopping mall. What better example of consumerist principles than a gargantuan edifice, quite literally a church where we place upon altars all the stuff we can buy. And, for a while, the protagonists are safe and even happy. They are at the top of the consumer pyramid. The hordes who cannot pay—in this case, the zombies—are kept outside the mall in a Dickensian scene where they are forced to watch what others have without being able to have any of it at all. Those on the inside enjoy hot coffee, fresh food, fur coats, and even an ice skating rink.

Soon, however, the impersonal nature of the mall becomes a nidus for dangerous boredom. Stuff, after all, is just stuff. A fur coat has no purpose in a mall. Outside of the larger world, all of the goods that the mall has to offer serve no real purpose. Just as in to *Night of the Living Dead*, the humans turn on one another. They are not satisfied by having stuff without the meaning that stuff affords. They even seem to welcome the ruffians who break into the mall to wage chaos. At least now they can meaningfully interact. The zombies, it seems, are an afterthought. They just want to get inside the mall, and they are relatively easily avoided.

It is not much of a reach to connect these themes to the crises of technology in modern health and wellness. We have, by all accounts, plenty of stuff. We have machines that can take photos by Bluetooth as they pass through the digestive tract of a patient. We have thousand-dollar drugs that miraculously prolong life. We have a treatment for every ailment and some might lament that we sell hope the way Apple sells computers. If you have the dollars, some argue, then we can give you, even without care, the hope you so desperately crave (Burki, 2014).

Except we are and always have been social creatures. All humans bring meaning to one another, regardless of their monetary value (Krauss, 2005). If we thought that meaning-making was measurable only as a function of wealth, then we would eschew the meaning that teachers, social workers, public servants, and all manner of arguably underpaid but nevertheless highly valued members of society bring to our lives. This is in fact the central message of *Dawn of the Dead*. The stuff that we can buy is not enough. We cannot, after all, ever truly buy one other. We need to be with each other regardless of what we can afford. If we are to find satisfaction in our complicated lives, we need company outside of our monetary descriptors. This is why, at the end of the film, the surviving humans leave the relative safety of the shopping mall. They could have secured it again and kept both zombies and dangerous gangs at bay, but these precautions would do nothing to prevent the ennui that existed on the inside once the doors were locked. They would rather take their chances on the outside.

So where does all this lead us?

Zombies are everywhere. There is no better metaphor for the plagues of modern culture than the zombie trope. This is certainly a large part of why zombies refuse to go away. Even today, more than 50 years after Romero's first film, new zombie stories are created with impressive regularity. Something about the metaphor of the zombie speaks to all of us.

This realization, of course, is hardly news to zombie fans. The modern zombie—the shambling, dumb-as-a-box-of-nails and hungry-as-hell cannibalistic ghouls of cinema—provide the perfect blank slate for musing. The zombie story is ripe with symmetrical oppositions. The dead do not live. To be dead and to be alive are literally opposite states, each negating the other. These kinds of dichotomous themes yield an illuminating array of seemingly opposing axioms. For any given zombie scenario, the protagonists of the zombie tale appear compelled to choose among a series of impossibly singular choices:

We must learn to live with the zombies.
We must exterminate the zombies.
The zombies are still human.
The zombies are by definition inhuman.

The almost mathematical logic of these opposing sentiments comprises the backbone of every zombie story worth its salt. Each statement is of course too extreme ever to be truly helpful. Even if we were able to exterminate every zombie, we might never know what caused the zombie outbreak in the first place. If we fail to learn from our mistakes by choosing simply to surrender to the zombies, then we will merely co-exist and never enjoy even the possibility of mutually beneficial existence. If we decide to consider that the zombies are human, then we must assume that the state of zombie-ism is aberrant and we must at least search for a cure. In doing this, we create an automatic self–other dichotomy that is potentially a potent source of health-care disappointment. And yet, if we fail to recognize whatever it is in zombies that seems inhuman, then we run the risk of tolerating their suffering without coming to terms with how they suffer and how to help them to heal. In all cases, we are constrained by the largely all-or-nothing aspects that the zombie story repeatedly puts forth.

In this chapter, I have chosen to argue that zombies are particularly relevant to the travails of health care because these same kinds of questions can be asked of our modern conceptualizations of health and wellness. If we are to posit, with our worried tongues only slightly but nevertheless playfully in our not-yet-eaten cheeks, that the arc of the zombie narrative is akin to the arc of health-care woes, then we must first draw some illuminating parallels. This kind of polemic is exactly why it is entirely appropriate to be discussing zombies in a book that focuses on the relationship to health and humanities. After all, humanities is by definition the search for meaning, whether through irony, metaphor, or comparative analysis. This search allows and even compels us to illuminate important ideas through art that otherwise might very well have stayed outside our field of vision. What happens to zombies and those who live among them is quite similar to what happens to all of us as we suffer through the vagaries of modern health care and well-being. Consider therefore, that we need only to tweak those admittedly extreme notions of zombie films to capture the arenas in which modern health-care delivery potentially falls short. Our rules of flawed health delivery go something like this:

> *We must learn to live with our current system of health and well-being.*
> *We must never accept our current system of health and well-being.*
> *We must require that our current system of health and well-being be entirely humanistic.*
> *We must acknowledge that our current system of health and well-being will never be humanistic at all.*

Just as with the zombie stories, none of these sentiments is particularly helpful. It is unacceptable to live with the lack of humanity in health care. We all recall with hand-wringing nostalgia the professional caregiver who sits at the bedside and understands that simply by truly and mindfully being with someone, care is made immeasurably more human and humane. To reject this memory is to reject the humanity of the patient and the clinician. We also have all increasingly experienced the jaded and numbed professional who instead enacts at best a rather sterile recitation of a scripted interaction with the now impersonalized sick person. If we choose to accept the inhumanity of health care, then we will someday become the inhumanity itself. *The systemic lack of empathy becomes its own zombie, and the pandemic spreads as mindlessly and ruthlessly as any pandemic worthy of a blockbuster film.*

On the other hand, we could choose to exterminate the humanity of health care altogether. Indeed, some would argue that we have begun this already. For example, we can now access our lab test results through patient computer portals, but lacking the knowledge or the emotional wherewithal to interpret these labs without a clinician's guidance, we are left feeling as ill as our labs might indicate, but without the experience of a caring and knowledgeable human interaction to assuage our worries. The plague spreads, and, like the zombies of modern cinema, we become infected with fear without even knowing that we are all, in fact, ill.

These opposing sentiments give rise to a kind of fatalism that, as with all zombie narratives, fails to solve the fundamental crisis at hand. In zombie films, the characters must determine who they will consider human. Is the human a human when she is bitten but has yet to show symptoms? Perhaps she loses her humanity when her fever begins? Or maybe she is gone when she no longer knows who she is or who her loved ones are? In this line of reasoning, the parallels with modern pandemics like dementias and even autism are existentially terrifying. We would never consider these kinds of syndromes to be inhuman, and yet in a zombie film, it is exactly these characteristics that lead us to question the humanity of the afflicted.

But fear not—all is not lost.

Zombie films are horror films. They are designed as cautionary tales. We watch these films and call out to the actors on the screen with predictable frustrations. "Work together," we implore! "Get outside of your comfort zone! Think outside of your imprisoning box." But they never do. *Zombie stories ultimately tell us what not to do.* We can reject the guiding principles of the zombie film just as we can reject the parallels in modern health care. We need only to realize that we are considering these principles in the first place. By realizing what we are becoming, we allow art and all of humanities to mirror what it reflects best— the perils of the path we are on, so that we can choose something better. We *can* do better in health care, and it is through the lessons of art, even the art of the undead, that we will move forward. Otherwise, we will simply shamble about, gnawing without tasting, existing without living, functioning without healing. We owe ourselves more than that. We're better than that. That's what zombie films tell us.

References

Beisecker, A. (1988). Aging and the Desire for Information and Input in Medical Decisions: Patient Consumerism in Medical Encounters. *Gerontologist*, 28: 330–335.

Burki, T.K. (2014). Psychology: Selling Hope: Advertising and Patient Expectation. *Lancet Oncology*, 15(8): 798.

Donne, J. (1633). The Flea. *Poem*. Accessed online at www.poetryfoundation.org/poems/46467/the-flea (accessed 27 November 2019).

Elgin, K.H. and Bergero, C. (2015). Technology and the Bedside Nurse: An Exploration and Review of Implications for Practice. *Nursing Clinics*, 50(2): 227–239.

Friedman, M. (1992). *Capitalism and Freedom*. Chicago: University of Chicago Press.

Krauss, S.E. (2005). Research Paradigms and Meaning Making: A Primer. *Qualitative Report*, 10(4): 758–770.

Romero, G.A. (1968). *Night of the Living Dead*. Film.

Romero, G.A. (1978). *Dawn of the Dead*. Film.

24

FINDING THE SUBJECT IN THE OBJECTIFIED

Problematizing the dependence on metrics for patient care in the United States

Brenda Hall and Paul Kadetz

Introduction

The need to reacquaint the health-care practitioner with the patient as subject may be understood as an outcome of the perfection of the practitioner's (Foucauldian) medical gaze, whose trajectory can be traced to the value of reason and scientific knowledge that flourished from the Enlightenment onward. Such an approach to patient care, in which reason and objectivity are valued over feelings, passions, and subjectivity, may result in the objectification of caring and of the subject of care: the patient. The twentieth-century evidence-based movement, as well as the movements in patient safety and quality care, have resulted in the further demand for a fully quantifiable patient. This ritual of quantification is now believed irrefutably essential to, and inseparable from, biomedicine and contemporary US health care. But how does such quantified health care ultimately impact the understanding and treatment of the patient as a subject? This research, based upon data collected at a large urban academic medical center in the United States, uses the health humanities lens of the patient experience of meaning making in order to identify the assumptions of quantification, as well as to problematize the normative aggregated groupings of patients that are believed to influence the completion of advance directives in the United States. Although addressing one's own mortality may be the most subjective of spaces that can be entered between a health caregiver and a patient, the dominance of objectifying the biomedical patient in the US health-care system has reduced this encounter to an obligation demanded by the facility and a meaningless ritual in which boxes are ticked.

Background

The Patient Self Determination Act of 1990 (PSDA), which went into effect December 1991, sought to provide the legal rights of patients to make decisions concerning their medical care (Wolf et al., 1991). Under this law, patients are able to document their wishes concerning their current and future care, and to designate a surrogate who will make decisions on their behalf, should they become incapacitated or unable to make their own decisions. An advance directive has also been referred to as a living will or health-care power of attorney. American health-care institutions receiving Medicare or Medicaid public insurance funding must demonstrate compliance with this law by developing advance directive policies and procedures, inquiring if patients have an advance directive, documenting or including a copy of the directive in the patient's medical record, and providing advance directive education when requested.

Many hospitals have established policies that require a determination of whether an individual has an advance directive, or would like to execute a directive, be obtained on admission to the hospital. This information is gathered with all other required patient demographic data on intake to the hospital. Under the Affordable Care Act (2010), representatives from the US Department of Health and Human Services, the Office of Management and Budget (OMB), and the Census Bureau developed guidelines and uniform standards for the collection, analysis, and reporting of health data (Parikh and Wright, 2017). These guidelines served as minimum reporting requirements of demographic data from health-care organizations that included information on patient sex, race, and ethnicity. Although the guidelines were intended to minimize or prevent health-care disparities, the potential outcomes of placing individuals in these highly aggregated groupings are questioned in this chapter.

Regardless of the Patient Self Determination Act of 1990, patients and their families have failed to execute advance directives and continue to struggle with a lack of continuity of care and poor communication with health-care practitioners about their treatment wishes. The findings of a "Health Matters" poll, conducted in New Jersey by Rutgers-Eagleton (2016), identifies that although approximately one third of New Jerseyans have thought about end-of-life care, 62% have had a conversation with someone concerning this, and only four out of ten respondents have put their end-of-life care wishes in writing. The reasons for these poor outcomes have been reduced to group stereotypes.

In 2015, the Government Accountability Office (GAO, 2015) was charged with reviewing how the Center for Medicare and Medicaid oversees how covered providers adhere to the regulatory requirements of the Patient Self Determination Act. The study found that the prevalence of advance directives varied according to provider, and according to patient demographics. Furthermore, older individuals were more likely to have advance directives than younger individuals. An estimated "51 percent of individuals 65 years of age and older had advance directives, while among individuals 18 to 34 years old, an estimated 12 percent had advance directives" (Government Accountability Office (GAO), 2015: 23). Specifically, the study identified that advance directives were more likely to be completed among patients with chronic disease, and who were over 65 years old, female, Caucasian, earning $75,000 or more annually, and had completed postgraduate education. Conversely, the completion of advance directives was lowest among males without chronic disease, who were 18–34 years old, had an annual income of $24,999 or less, and had not completed high school. The lowest completion rates were equivalent between African Americans and US Latinos. In general, the literature reviewed has corroborated these findings. A common theme across the studies reviewed were findings of a lack of completed directives among individuals less than 50 years old, and among African Americans, as compared with Hispanics and Caucasians (Anunobi et al., 2015; Huang et al., 2016; Shapiro, 2015).

These aggregated group findings were replicated in other studies. For example, Salmond (2005: 1) found

Table 24.1 Summary of findings

Research question	Statistical test	Statistical finding
Was there a correlation between age and completion of advance directives?	Multi-nominal logistic regression	No significant correlation
Was there a correlation between sex and completion of advance directives?	Chi-square test for Independence	No significant correlation
Was there a correlation between race/ethnicity and completion of advance directives?	Chi-square test for Independence	No significant correlation

> Low completion rates of advance directives among the majority of the population [were] even lower among ethnically diverse individuals despite favourable attitudes toward advance directives, suggest[ing] that there are factors beyond access to information that may influence the decision not to complete an advance directive.

Even though hospital patients were identified to be least likely to have advance directives and nursing home patients were identified as most likely, the assumption for both is that compliance is more of an outcome of the purported traits of the groups to which a patient belongs than to any aspect of the information and communication provided to the patient by the caregiver. In addition to the main categories discussed, retired or disabled status, employment status, educational attainment, religious affiliation, internet access, preferences for physician-centered decision making, and desire for longevity regardless of functional status were independent predictors of advance directive completion (Huang et al., 2016: 150).

Methods

Data was collected during the inpatient admission process and extracted from patient record documentation within a 316-bed acute care academic not-for-profit medical center in Jersey City, New Jersey. This hospital is recognized as having one of the most ethnic and culturally diverse patient populations in the state, which makes it an ideal site for studying the correlations between demographics and the completion of advance directives identified in the literature. The sample (n=70,949) consisted of anonymized individual patient data covering a 4-year period from 2014 to 2017, generated through completed hospital medical records. Inclusion criteria were adult patients, 18 years of age or older. Exclusion criteria included patients admitted to inpatient voluntary and involuntary psychiatric units, and paediatric patients under the age of 18. Sex, race, age, ethnicity, nationality, and county resident status were self-identified by patients. Data was analyzed using the Statistical Package for the Social Sciences (SPSS) version 22. Ethical approval for this research was granted by the Western Institutional Review Boards, with whom the hospital was affiliated.

Results

Overall, this research identified no statistically significant correlations between the factors of age, sex, race, ethnicity, or any combination thereof, and the completion of advance directives (Table 24.1). What minor variations that could be identified directly contradicted the literature. For example, the majority of admissions in this study were in the 75 years of age and older group. The findings revealed that the lowest completion of advance directives was in this age group, followed by the group 55–64 years of age. These findings contradict research maintaining that patients over 75 years old are three-and-a-half times more likely to complete advance directives than those under 30 (e.g., Perleman School of Medicine, 2017; Rao et al., 2014; Shapiro, 2015).

Similarly, although this research found no statistically significant relationship between sex and completion of advance directives, some studies have reported higher completion rates for males (e.g., Anunobi et al., 2015; Yancu et al., 2009) while Rao et al. (2014) reported higher completion rates for females. No explanation was provided for these contradictions in the literature.

Finally, although this study found no statistically significant differences between self-identified race or ethnicity and the completion of advance directives, several studies in the literature imply that non-Caucasian groups are less receptive to end-of-life care planning, palliative care, and hospice use than Caucasians (Bullock, 2011; Giger et al., 2006; Kwak et al., 2005). Similar findings were reported before and after a palliative care consult, in which the rate of completion of advance directives by African American, Asian, and Hispanic individuals was much lower than for Caucasians, both before and after consultation (Zaide et al., 2013).

Discussion

Rationale for differences between the literature and the results of this study

There may be several factors in the study designs and samples selected that can help explain the marked differences between the literature and the results of this study. First, there are differences in sample size. Many of the studies reviewed had significantly smaller samples— from 314 (Yancu et al., 2009) to 2154 (Huang et al., 2016)—compared with the 70,949 records used in this study. Furthermore, the sample in this study was significantly more diverse than in many of the studies reviewed. For example, although this study had markedly equal representation in all age categories over 18 years, the mean age of the sample in the studies reviewed was between 55 and 76 years, with a starting age of 50 years. Similarly, in terms of race and ethnicity, there were either insufficient sample sizes for an adequate comparison, or comparisons were limited to Caucasians and African American patients; or the assumption that the issues African American patients purportedly had with completing advance directives was so strong that only African Americans were studied. Lastly, several studies identified that significant numbers of their samples refused to identify as a particular race/ethnicity. Beyond these important differences that may be leading to different results, in addition to compromised internal validity, marked differences in study designs and data collection can also be identified.

The potential impact of assumptions

But possibly more important than these structural differences between studies is the fact that all of the studies reviewed in some way *assume* a correlation between age, sex, race, and ethnicity, and the completion of advance directives. But this expectation of who might and might not fill out advance directives, by virtue of their demographic category, extends beyond assumptions and bias that may appear in the research and, more importantly, may be influencing practice. For example, if a hospital practitioner anticipates that a young African American male is least likely to complete advance directives, is it more likely that will they target this patient and put more time and energy into communicating the value of advance directives—or is it less likely, in a busy, time-constrained clinical setting, that the practitioner will even broach the subject with this patient beyond the briefest of explanations? Observation during this research tends to suggest that the latter approach is significantly more likely to occur. Thereby, the health-care practices that follow these assumed behaviors of patient groupings may fulfil these assumptions by de-emphasizing the importance of spending time with patients from certain demographic groups and in turn may foster inequitable health-care access to information. The GAO identified a challenge for some providers due to patients' lack of understanding about advance directives (Government Accountability Office (GAO), 2015: 17). Hence, the practice of educating patients about advance directives or any other important health-care knowledge may be thwarted by assumptions influenced by the boxes in which the practitioner is placing the patient, or rather the group identity that the practitioner is imposing on the patient.

The tyranny of metrics

These practices of "imposed identity" facilitate a kind of shorthand that time- and energy-constrained practitioners may believe they must employ in order to accomplish their daily duties within the constraints of profit-driven health care in the United States. However, this objectification of the patient is also very much an inherent outcome of the quantification and scientization of biomedicine and nursing, in which the body and its physiology and pathology is perceived with complexity, while the patient, as a subject, is approached from a simple systems perspective. Even if we employ the seemingly more complex approach of intersectionality—in which we attempt to understand individuals as the outcome of the combined intersections of the social bias and exclusion they experience according to sex, gender, race, ethnicity, sexuality, age, and other categories of identity othering practiced within a given society—we will still at best only approximate the complexity and the uniqueness of the patient as a subject.

   The objectification of the patient is reinforced by what is valued in biomedicine and health care, namely the quantification of evidence-based health care and the centrality of metrics in determining health and well-being. Adams (2016: 8–9) identifies how it is assumed that "numbers will offer unbiased, apolitical truths about health outcomes or health conditions." Even though "numbers are never intrinsically capable of proving anything ... [for] metrical forms of reason often displace other kinds of knowledge, other forms of evidence." Furthermore, the over-reliance on metrics obscures the importance of the two other dimensions of evidence-based medicine—physician experience and patient preferences—arguably the more humanistic elements of evidence.

   This tension in health care between acknowledging the importance of approaching the patient as a subject while relying on the practice of understanding the patient objectively is a division that lies at the heart of Enlightenment modernity and rationality. The philosopher Judith Butler concisely illustrates the issue of representing the complexity of the subject for which "elaborate predicates of color, sexuality, ethnicity, class, and able-bodiedness invariably close with an embarrassed 'etc.' at the end of the list ... these positions strive to encompass a situated subject but invariably fail to be complete" (1990: 143).

   The issue of approaching the subject as a complex subject, rather than as a group of reductive categories, is also illustrated in the parable of the blind men and the elephant. In the well-known story, five blind men are attempting to determine what exactly an elephant is by each examining a part of the elephant. For the man examining the body of the elephant, an elephant is like a wall. The man at the legs of the elephant perceives the elephant as like a tree. And so on. An elephant is like a rope at the tail, like a snake at the trunk, like a fan at the ears and like a spear at the tusk. Yet, in combining these perceived parts of an elephant, an understanding of this animal called an elephant is far from approximated. Hence, in alignment with Aristotle and in contradiction with Descartes, we posit that we *are* greater than the sum of our parts. Similarly, we are unable to see the whole patient in front of us when we do not see beyond the boxes in which we place them.

According to Adams (2016: 9) "the need for numerical data appears as a kind of burden of proof." It is assumed that this burden of proof is the most important aspect of patient care, but as is detailed in this example, much of care may be lost by reducing the patient to numerical values. The point we are trying to make with this research is to emphasize how our categorization and quantification of the patient can prevent us from perceiving and relating to our patients as subjects; and how, in this instance, by not approaching every patient subjectively, we are possibly not affording each the ability to understand the information they need to understand in order to make an informed autonomous decision concerning advance directives, among a multitude of other important health-care decisions.

Hearing the patient and dialoguing

The centrality of interpersonal communication and the demonstration of the value of the patient in this communication is another important distinction to make in this particular case example. In order to treat the patient as a subject, the patient cannot merely serve as a receptacle for the practitioners' information, regardless of how important this information may be to the practitioner. Rather than speaking *at* a patient, patient and practitioner need to engage in a dialogue, where the patient is able to voice their thoughts and concerns and, most importantly, be heard by the practitioner. So, for example, although practitioners may perceive the completion of advance directives as both their responsibility to have the patient complete, as well as the patient's own responsibility, patients may have numerous personal reasons they do not want to complete advance directives at a given juncture. Does this mean the patient should be written off as "non-compliant"? Practitioners may often forget that the patient is not present to be compliant, nor to please the practitioner. Furthermore, as nurses are often the chosen caregiver to communicate with the patient about advance directives, and as nurses are taught that they are fundamentally the patient's advocate, it behooves the nurse to enact their role as advocate by fully engaging with patients in such important decisions as advance directives.

Understanding that being heard is just as important to the therapeutic process as any pharmaceutical is essential to begin to approach the patient as a subject. Hearing the patient also means to engage one's humanity through compassion. *Rachmones* is a Yiddish word that means compassion and "suffering with." Although it may be natural to empathize and suffer with a character in a movie or novel—where social norms allow, and even expect, one to experience feelings—this natural instinct may not be afforded to those who are most in need of our hearing their pain. Central to hearing the patient is the ability to comprehend the patient's meaning.

The need for the health humanities for democratizing meaning making

There is something fundamentally misguided by the deafness that permeates the American health-care system in its disregard for what is a central force of Western societies, namely the denial of one's mortality. The anthropologist Ernest Becker (1973) argued how modern Western lives are obsessed with elaborate rituals of denying our mortality. And yet, somehow, modern American health care expects that the briefest of interludes with a health-care practitioner that results in a signed document will suffice in bridging this inherently complex, existential gulf. More than possibly any other activity, acknowledgement of, and planning for, one's mortality requires time and space for sense making on the part of the patient and the interpretation of this experience with the practitioner. According to Crawford et al. (2015: 4), "Meaning plays a central role in the effort to understand the individual's lifeworld ... their personal and social realities, patterns of action and behaviour." In this example, the understanding for the practitioner to grasp is what end-of-life documents, and, thereby, addressing one's own mortality, mean to this patient at this point in time. Ignoring the meaning attached to such patient decisions is antithetical to the current emphasis in American health care on patient-centered care.

Alternatively, what meaning do the predetermined patient categories of this research communicate to health-care institutions and their practitioners, and how is this then communicated to patients in the actions of their caregivers? Hence, the practitioners' deliberate attempt to understand their patient's "meaning making" can potentially result in a democratizing process for the patient to become an active participant in their own care and care-making decisions. Therefore, hearing, understanding, and attending to the meaning attributed by the patient should ultimately take precedence over the meanings attributed by the practitioner or the institution, or even the government, in order to afford the patient the autonomy to make health-care decisions, particularly concerning end-of-life care.

Conclusion

Almost 30 years after legislation was introduced in the United States to protect a patient's right to determine their medical care, many individuals and families still struggle with end-of-life care planning, a lack of continuity of care, and poor communication with health-care practitioners about their treatment wishes at the end of life. All of these outcomes are often framed by health-care practitioners to be due to the failure of the patient to be compliant and complete an advance directive, particularly as a result of such deterministic factors as sex, age, race and ethnicity, while disregarding the accountability of the caregivers and health-care institutions in this process. It is important to remember that the normative use of these demographic categories was in actuality a minimum requirement from guidelines developed by US governmental organizations of the Department of Health and Human Services, the OMB, and the Census Bureau. Hence, the use of these reified deterministic categories was a directive from the US government that health-care institutions and their practitioners have often followed, albeit uncritically.

Although numerous studies have identified age, sex, race, and/or ethnicity as barriers to completion of advance directives, this research does not support any such correlations and instead suggests that other, often overlooked, variables influence the completion of advance directives. By reducing the reasons that advance directives are not completed to aggregated groupings that serve to create and perpetuate stereotypes, we not only provide a rationale for the unequal treatment of certain groups in health care, but also prohibit any exploration into the actual reasons that are compromising the completion of advance directives and thereby thwart the ability to improve patient care.

This case example illustrates the myriad issues that can arise when a patient is approached by a health-care provider as if the patient possesses predetermined traits as a member of a group. Such objectification prohibits a practitioner's ability to work with a patient as a subject, and may, potentially, dictate the entire practitioner's encounter with the patient, including how much time the practitioner spends with the patient and what the practitioner ultimately communicates to the patient. If we are to achieve equitable health care, we need to seriously rethink the practice of reducing individuals to the purported traits of a group, which ultimately may have the opposite effect.

References

Adams, V. (ed.) (2016). *Metrics: What Counts in Global Health*. Durham: Duke University Press.
Anunobi, E., Detweiler, M.B., Sethi, R., Thomas, R., Lutgens, B. and Detweiler, J.G. (2015). Comparison of Advance Medical Directive Inquiry and Documentation for Hospital Inpatients in Three Medical Services: Implications for Policy Changes. *Journal of Aging and Social Policy*, 27(2): 156–172.
Becker, E. (1973) *The Denial of Death*. New York: Free Press.
Bullock, K. (2011). The Influence of Culture on End-of-Life Decision Making. *Journal of Social Work in End-of-Life and Palliative Care*, 7(1): 83–98.
Butler, J. (1990). *Gender Trouble: Feminism and the Subversion of Identity*. New York: Routledge.
Crawford, P., Brown, B., Baker, C., Tischler, V. and Abrams, B. (2015). *Health Humanities*. New York: Palgrave.
Giger, J.N., Davidhizar, R.E. and Fordham, P. (2006). Multi-Cultural and Multi-Ethnic Considerations and Advanced Directives: Developing Cultural Competency. *Journal of Cultural Diversity*, 13(1): 3–9.
Government Accountability Office (GAO), (2015). *Advance Directives: Information on Federal Oversight, Provider Implementation, and Prevalence*, GAO-15-416: Retrieved 4/5/19 from www.gao.gov/assets/670/669906.
Huang, I.A., Neuhaus, J.M. and Chiong, W. (2016). Racial and Ethnic Differences in Advance Directive Possession: Role of Demographic Factors, Religious Affiliation, and Personal Health Values in a National Survey of Older Adults. *Journal of Palliative Medicine*, 19(2): 149–156.
Kwak, J. and Haley, W.E. (2005). Current Research Findings on End-of-Life Decision Making Among Racially or Ethnically Diverse Groups. *Gerontologist*, 45(5): 634–641.
Parikh, R.B. and Wright, A. (2017). The Affordable Care Act and End-of-Life Care for Patients with Cancer. *Cancer Journal*, 23(3): 190–193.
Perelman School of Medicine at the University of Pennsylvania. (2017, July 5). Two Out of Three U.S. Adults Have Not Completed an Advance Directive. *Science Daily*. Retrieved 5/2/19 from www.sciencedaily.com/releases/2017/07/170705184048.htm.
Rao, J.K., Anderson, L.A., Lin, F-C. and Laux, J.P. (2014). Completion of Advance Directives Among U.S. Consumers. *American Journal of Preventive Medicine*, 46(1): 65–70.
Rutgers-Eagleton/New Jersey Health Care Quality Institute (2016). *Health Matters Poll: End of Life Care in New Jersey – Majority Has Thought About, Discussed Plans But Far Fewer Have Written a Living Will*. Rutgers: State University of New Jersey Eagleton Institute of Politics.
Salmond, S. and David, E. (2005). Attitudes Toward Advance Directives and Advance Directive Completion Rates. *Orthopedic Nursing*, 24(2): 117–127.
Shapiro, S. (2015). Do Advance Directives Direct? *Journal of Health Politics, Policy and Law*, 40(3): 487–530.
Wolf, S.M., Boyle, P., Callahan, D., Fins, J.J., Jennings, B., Nelson, J.L., Barondess, J.A., Brock, D.W., Dresser, R., Emanuel, L., Johnson, S. and Lantos, J. (1991). Sources of Concern About the Patient Self-Determination Act. *New England Journal of Medicine*, 325: 1666–1671.
Yancu, C.N., Farmer, D.F. and Leahman, D. (2009). Barriers to Hospice Use and Palliative Care Services Use By African American Adults. *American Journal of Hospice and Palliative Medicine*, 27(4): 248–253.
Zaide, G.B., Pekmezaris, R., Nouryan, C.N., Mir, T.P., Sison, C.P., Liberman, T., Lesser, M.L., Cooper, L.B. and Wolf-Klein, G.P. (2013). Ethnicity, Race, and Advance Directives in an Inpatient Palliative Care Consultation Service. *American Journal of Hospice and Palliative Medicine*, 11(5): 5–11.

25

ESTABLISHING, PROMOTING, AND GROWING THE HEALTH HUMANITIES IN JAPAN

A review and a vision for the future

Jeffrey Huffman and Mami Inoue

Introduction

The world is healthier than it has ever been before. The population aging phenomenon is often discussed in terms of the problems it brings, but we should not lose sight of the fact that it actually represents a colossal success. Thanks to rapid advancements and consistent efforts in medical science and technology, pharmacology, nursing care and science, epidemiology, and global and local public health efforts, the world has made great progress in improving health as measured by life expectancy, healthy life expectancy, child mortality, and other quantitative indicators.

Japan has been no exception, establishing its universal health insurance system as early as 1961 and consistently ensuring access to a wide array of health services since then. It has continued to do so at a lower cost than most developed countries, and in spite of its rapidly aging society. According to Reich et al. (2011), this has been made possible by a combination of "public health policies, high literacy rates and educational levels, the traditional diet and exercise, economic growth, and a stable political environment" (1051). Japan became the world leader in life expectancy in the 1970s, and more recently it has become the world's first "super-aged" society, meaning that over 20% of the population is 65 or older. Shibuya et al. (2011) state that over the past 50 years, Japan has achieved "good population health at low cost and increased equity between different population groups" (1266). However, they also rightly point out that the financial sustainability of Japan's universal coverage system is by no means guaranteed.

With sustainability of this system and further advances toward healthy longevity in mind, one recent development with great potential to improve Japanese health care is the push toward a "community-based integrated care system." In fact, a law was enacted in 2014 to officially promote the provision of comprehensive community-level support and care for healthy living, with the goal of reducing or delaying hospitalization and instead allowing elderly individuals to continue living in their own home and community for as long as possible (Health and Welfare Bureau for the Elderly, 2016). As Kumakawa et al. (2016) explain it, this system consists of specialized (health-care, nursing care, prevention) and non-specialized (housing, livelihood support) sectors, and the authors propose "social and community prescription" as a way of linking these two sectors. This is indeed very similar, and likely based on, the UK concept of "social prescription"; however, in Japan, the expressive therapies are currently relegated to the non-specialized (livelihood) realm, and they tend to be locally implemented and remain isolated in regional locales. This is a fertile area for the health humanities to contribute in exciting new ways in Japan. The emerging field of health humanities (see Crawford et al., 2015) should seek to document and unify these "non-specialized" activities into a national movement, investigate and accumulate evidence as to their effectiveness, and indeed work to elevate their status to that of a respected specialization. In fact, this may indeed be the missing key that would lead to success of the integrated community-based care system itself.

At the same time, Japan has been attempting to improve its track record in the field of mental health. Kido and Kawakami (2013) point out that Japanese people with mental disorders access mental health services at half the rate of those in other high-income countries, and that stigma toward mental disorders may be higher in Japan. A cross-sectional study conducted by Hamano et al. (2010) indicates that social capital as measured by trust and group membership is associated with improved mental health. Since social connectedness is a prominent area of inquiry in the health humanities, it seems likely that the health humanities will become an important piece of the puzzle in the quest to combat mental disorders in Japan.

Creative solutions will be required to sustain and further these advances in the midst of continued societal aging, while at the same time beginning to address the long-neglected issues of healthy longevity, which includes the maintenance of mental health and well-being throughout the life course. It is our position that the health humanities has great potential to draw on resources, human and otherwise, from outside the traditional health-care professions to maintain and improve individual and societal health moving forward, while at the same time redefining the concept of health itself.

Health humanities is a broadly focused, "big-tent" interdisciplinary field that brings researchers, educators, and students in the arts, humanities, and social sciences together with those in medicine, nursing, dentistry, occupational therapy, public health, and other health-oriented fields to work collaboratively and creatively in the domains of education, research, and practice toward new insights, innovations, and activities that result in the improved health and well-being of individuals, population, and society itself. It embodies an increasingly active field of academic and scientific inquiry, but it should also be seen as an intentional social movement.

In this chapter, we review the current state of the health humanities in Japan and attempt to point out specific areas where it is lacking and where it has potential to contribute to and transform health care in Japan. Finally, we propose concrete steps that need to be taken in order to establish a strong and stable health humanities movement in Japan.

The current state of health humanities in Japan

While admitting there is much overlap, we broadly view health humanities as occurring in the three domains of education (usually of health care professionals, but also for students in the humanities, the arts, etc.), practice (often involving the arts, and including the expressive therapies), and research (investigation of health-related concepts via paradigms and methodologies in the humanities or social sciences) (Huffman and Inoue, 2019).

Education

The US-based medical humanities movement that arguably started with Edmund Pellegrino in the 1970s (Cole et al., 2015) has not made consistent, visible inroads in Japan. Although the concept of liberal arts education and the notion that it benefits medical students is often acknowledged, it is, with the exception of medical ethics, generally given low priority in a tight curriculum. Although some medical schools have indeed made efforts to implement medical humanities, there remains a perception that doctors and dentists would benefit from more training in the area of individual, humanized, patient-centered care. A survey published by Mori and Nishio in 1996 claims that 89% of the medical schools in the study offered "a curriculum in the medical humanities," but a closer investigation reveals that only about 25% of the schools offered more than 30 hours of education in the medical humanities, and that the category of "medical humanities" included "early exposure in the hospital" in addition to bioethics and doctor–patient communication (Mori and Nishio, 1996). One obstacle is a lack of experts who have experience researching and teaching in the medical humanities. This could be remedied in part by a heightened focus on the medical humanities as an emerging field in Japan.

Indeed, in some ways, the field of medicine and nursing in Japan represents fertile ground waiting for a vibrant health humanities movement to take root. The late, great Dr. Shigeaki Hinohara, who spent large parts of his career as director or president of St. Luke's International Hospital and St. Luke's International University in Tokyo (and indeed energetically continued his activities as a physician and public figure right up until his death at age 105), was the most famous and treasured physician in Japan. He was largely responsible for enacting Japan's system of annual medical check-ups, which continues to this day, and he was a strong advocate for patient-centered care, publishing nearly 150 books on topics ranging far beyond the traditional concept of medicine and health (Stafford, 2017). Hinohara was also Japan's most prominent Oslerian, having been so impressed that he decided to translate (together with Hisae Niki) a volume of Osler's essays into Japanese, so that Japanese students "could come to appreciate Osler's perspective on medicine and professional life" (Shedlock, 2002: 352). It seems that Osler's focus on patient-centered and humanistic care attracted and impressed Hinohara. If the medical and health humanities movement indeed burgeons in the coming years, as seems likely, it will in no small part have Dr. Hinohara to thank.

Although nursing education has traditionally focused more on the human side of caring, nursing schools in Japan generally do not offer an extensive liberal arts or humanities program outside of the nursing curriculum. Again, here, bioethics is a notable exception, and it should also be noted that elements of the humanities are often integrated into nursing subjects in ways that may not be immediately apparent from course titles and descriptions. For example, nursing curricula tend to focus on patient-centered (and people-centered) care, end-of-life care, health education and literacy, and non-pharmacological care more than their medical counterparts. The movement toward making nursing education and practice more science oriented and evidence based has proceeded with the intention of elevating the status of nursing as a field and profession, but at the same time it risks going too far and leading to an increased distance between nurses and their patients, accompanied by decreased communication and dehumanization.

Non-nursing related liberal arts courses can be offered to nursing students in two ways. The first, which is common when nursing schools are part of a larger university, is to allow or require nursing students to take courses in other departments. This provides them with a broader education and an expanded view of the world, but it is left up to students themselves to figure out how what they learn in other departments might apply to their future roles in nursing. The second model, which in our view more fully encompasses the integrative and interdisciplinary focus of the health humanities, involves professors from the humanities and social sciences teaching courses specifically designed to enhance the education of nurses. An example of this approach from our own experience at St. Luke's International University would be our non-Japanese simulated patient sessions, in which we draw on principles from applied linguistics and intercultural communication to prepare nursing students for the realities of their future professional role.

There is great potential for further expansion of the health humanities in educational environments in Japan. Experts in health economics, health-care policy, health education and literacy, narratives of disease and suffering, the history of medicine/nursing, etc. should be contributing more and more to the education of nurses, dentists, doctors, physical therapists, and other health-care professionals. And these educational initiatives should be framed as part of a larger shift toward seeing health-care professionals (whether students or practicing) as individual humans first, thoughtful and contributing members of society second, and health experts third.

Practice

Although "health humanities" as a term and as an overarching conceptual framework remains relatively unknown in Japan, the notion that culture and the arts can improve mental health and well-being, as well as foster social connectedness, has been gaining some traction in recent years. So far, it tends to take the form of individual community-based or researcher-led programs and projects that have sprouted up here and there throughout the country.

The closest thing to a clearinghouse for this sort of information is the Welfare and Medical Service Network System (WAM NET), a website run by the Welfare and Medical Service Agency, which provides low-interest loans to private social welfare and medical institutions. In the area of art therapy, for example, WAM NET reports on workshops by an art therapist in Okayama Prefecture that bring together young children and elderly community residents, with the express purpose being the prevention of dementia for the elderly participants and the cultivation of sensitivity and reduction of stress for the children. Nagoya City University has recently launched a Healthcare Art Management project focusing on hospital art. This program focuses on how hospital art can impact the well-being not only of patients and their families, but also of hospital employees themselves. There has also been interest in the area of art by persons with disabilities, following in the footsteps of Dubuffet's *art brut* movement. A large exhibition of art by persons with disabilities was held at the Tokyo Metropolitan Government building in 2006, with over 30,000 attending, and the Tokyo 2020 Olympics/Paralympics committee is also planning to use art and performances inclusive of diverse populations to promote a more unified and connected society leading up to the games.

In the area of music, WAM reports opera-singing workshops in Miyagi Prefecture to promote health among elderly day-care center users, Jamaican ska music being used by a physical therapist in Yamanashi Prefecture to promote stretching and breathing among elderly care center residents, and a professional dancer from a popular music group who developed a dance specifically designed to promote physical movement and prevent dementia among elderly participants at a community center in Saitama Prefecture. These are just a few examples that reveal the beginnings of interest in the health humanities in Japan, even though a coordinated national movement has not yet taken shape. There are currently two organizations offering certification in music therapy in Japan, and a total of over 6000 certified practitioners. Unfortunately, the level of awareness of this certification is still quite low, and job opportunities in this area are few and far between. An important key to promoting music therapy (and other types of expressive therapies) in Japan would be to obtain official recognition and reimbursement under the national social insurance system. It should also be noted here that the grandfather of Japanese health care, Dr. Hinohara (discussed in more detail in the previous section), also promoted music therapy (Stafford, 2017).

Not only are these programs in line with the World Health Organization Framework on integrated people-centered health services and United Nations (UN) Sustainable Development Goal #3 ("Ensure healthy lives and promote well-being for all at all ages"), they are also consistent with Japan's own ten-year national health promotion plan, called Health Japan 21. Among the targets specifically listed in this plan are "maintenance and improvement of functions necessary for engaging in social life" (including mental health, children's health, and elderly health) and "putting in place a social environment to support and protect health" (including strong community ties and health promotion activities). From the examples above, Japan has clearly begun taking steps in the right direction. However, one reason that the "practice" arm of the health humanities remains Balkanized in Japan is that the prevailing opinion seems to be that such activities should be implemented by local municipalities in a regionally autonomous way (Sudo et al., 2018). We feel this is a mistake that will hold back the development and expansion of this field. In Japan, essential government services such as education and health care are generally administered at the national level, and local governments usually closely follow national policies. For this reason, attention to the health humanities at the national level is essential.

Iwagami and Tamiya (2019) note that the "informal sector," including senior clubs, residents' associations, and volunteer groups, has the potential to play an important role in the new community-based integrated care system that is currently being promoted in Japan, and they further state that by helping the elderly maintain their physical and cognitive functions, these activities could help prevent or delay the need for long-term care as well as excessive use of the medical care system. They also point out that Japan maintains massive databases of electronic health records (EHRs) that can be used by researchers to promote evidence-based policy making, in both Japan and other countries that are now also beginning to deal with the challenges presented by their aging populations (by 2050, all regions except Africa are projected to have an average life expectancy over 70, according to the UN's Population Division [2017]). The logical direction, then would be to organize and promote health humanities–related programs such as the expressive therapies and other non–pharmacological approaches under national coordination, have specialists implement them through the local organizations mentioned above, evaluate outcomes, and add all of this data to the existing EHRs for use in coordinated research efforts.

An important prerequisite to the health humanities receiving greater recognition and broader support within the health-care sector is greater emphasis on evaluating the outcomes of such activities, particularly in terms of measurable health indicators. One example of such research is a study by Satoh et al. (2015), which used direct neuropsychological evaluations, functional MRI scans, and interviews with caregivers to investigate the effectiveness of music therapy for Alzheimer's patients. Patients in the experimental group underwent voice training and sang karaoke with professional musicians, and the results indicated improved neural processing. Tabei et al. (2017) investigated the effects of exercise with music versus exercise without music for one hour per week in healthy elderly adults over a one-year period, finding that visuospatial functioning was significantly better in the music group, possibly delaying cognitive decline.

Kamei et al.'s (2010) investigation of an urban intergenerational day program is another example of outcome-focused research in Japan that supports the health humanities. In this longitudinal mixed-methods study, elementary school children interacted with elderly community residents regularly over a six-month period. The participants created traditional Japanese crafts such as quilting, *otedama*, and *netsuke*, played traditional games such as *karuta*, and shared *haiku* poetry. Data collected consisted of ethnographic participant observations as well as widely used questionnaires measuring health-related quality of life, depression, mental status, and fall risk. The study documented a variety of types of interaction between the elderly adults and the children, such as "reminiscing," "handing down regional culture," "teaching each other," and "social interactions expand outside of the program." The quantitative results showed improved mental health among the elderly participants, as well as decreased depression among a subgroup of elderly participants who showed initial depression.

One particularly well considered model of multidisciplinary health care is the ABC conceptual model of cancer care presented by Ueno et al. (2010). Arising out of a partnership between MD Anderson Cancer Center in Texas and St. Luke's International Hospital and Keio University in Tokyo, the authors propose a highly collaborative approach to caring for cancer patients that involves three components. The first component consists of what is traditionally thought of as medical care, delivered by physicians, pharmacists, nurses, and other health-care professionals. The second consists of non-medical support that is personal and direct, such as the emotional support, empowerment, and assistance provided by a psychologist, a spiritual advisor, a social worker, an art/music therapist, or even a family member or friend. The third component is neither direct nor personal, but still essential in its own right. It involves the establishment and maintenance of health-care facilities and infrastructure, research, policy making, and advocating for funding. The model stresses the importance of communication, cooperation, and mutual respect among professionals across the three components in order to complement rather than struggle against each other, with high-quality patient-centered care as the unifying goal. The health humanities represents a broad vision that encompasses both the second and third components of this model.

The challenges that lie ahead for the practice-oriented wing of health humanities in Japan are achieving greater awareness, recognition, funding, and professional expertise. This will require greater unity and a stronger sense of purpose and mission, development of the health humanities as an area of education and research in the university context, and accumulation of various types of evidence regarding its effectiveness.

Research

Under the health humanities umbrella, researchers in fields as varied as anthropology, sociology, literature, history, linguistics, and psychology contribute to a deeper understanding of health, sickness, aging, disability, as well as related cultural and gender-focused issues. Whether their works are read by students and practitioners in the health fields, government policy makers, or the general public, this body of knowledge represents one of the most powerful areas of the health humanities. Regarding Japan specifically, many of the existing contributions in this area have been published by researchers (Japanese or non-Japanese) based outside Japan; however, there are examples of research in this area within Japan as well, some of which parallel existing trends internationally, and others that are relatively unique to Japan.

In the area of medical anthropology, Margaret Lock and John W. Traphagan have made outsized contributions to understanding the intersection of health, medicine, and culture based on ethnographic studies. In addition to writing about the historical and cultural roots and significance of medical practice in Japan in general (1980), Lock also wrote a ground-breaking book about the differing cultural constructions of menopause in Japan and North America, coining the term "local biologies," which drew attention to the intersection of biology and culture (Lock, 1993). Traphagan (2000) has extensively examined aging, cognitive decline, ageism, and social and demographic change in Japan. Danely's (2015) more recent ethnography focuses on aging, death, and grieving in Kyoto. Karen Nakamura's (2013) extensively researched history of psychiatry in Japan, along with her painstaking ethnography of Bethel House, a non-profit organization dedicated to helping people with mental illness live in the community after long-term institutionalization, provides an excellent example of how non-medical and non-pharmacological perspectives can powerfully impact complex public health problems.

In sociology, Kinoshita (2018) has written about how post-retirement Japanese people cope with their transition into a "roleless role," and how they can continue to live meaningful lives marked by contribution to family and society as well as continued personal growth. He also visited Sheffield, United Kingdom to conduct a case study on the University of the Third Age movement, which he proceeded to introduce to his Japanese readership in their own language. Takahashi et al. (2011) similarly focused on how hobbies, enhanced social relationships, and flexible attitudes are the key to meaningful elderly life.

In the realm of literature, Akihito Suzuki's recent chapter on narrative psychiatry in Japan (2017) parallels the renewed attention being given explorations of madness narratives internationally. He argues that the concept of recording the voices of mentally ill individuals was introduced to Japan in the late nineteenth and early twentieth centuries through German academic psychiatry, presenting evidence from both patient case files and contemporary literary works.

Sako and Falcus's (2015) analysis of dementia-related cultural texts spans the areas of literature, feminist studies, film studies, and pop culture studies. Their work delves into three separate cultural texts—a contemporary novel, a film, and a comic book—as cultural representations and explorations of the meaning and reality of dementia in Japan. This work adds to a growing body of scholarship in what the authors themselves term "humanistic gerontology." In their 2019 book, Falcus and Sako discuss the importance of narrative as not only "a therapeutic practice for people with dementia and their carers," but also "central to the public debate over, and understanding of, dementia" (Falcus and Sako, 2019: 3). They also point out that dementia narratives can be a double-edged sword, either reinforcing our discriminatory stereotypes or challenging those same stereotypes and helping us imagine alternative ways of responding to dementia.

Aya Takahashi's history of the development of the nursing profession in Japan (2004) is an excellent example of how important the discipline of history is to both the education of health-care professionals and the continued development of health policy. This book connects its main topic with the Westernization and modernization of Japan as well as the evolving social role of women. Nursing students, like all young people (and perhaps all people), often struggle with the slow pace of social change and become frustrated, but studying history can provide much-needed perspective and even inspiration.

Finally, in the field of linguistics, both Matsumoto (2011) and Hamaguchi (2011) show how sociolinguistics and discourse analysis can shed light on the realities and the lived experience and the human side of aging, challenging our assumptions in the process. The entire volume edited by Matsumoto, *Faces of Aging: The Lived Experiences of the Elderly in Japan* (2011), is a testament to the power of interdisciplinarity in the study of health-related topics. While quantitative, empirical approaches have been and will continue to be essential for the development of safe and effective treatments and medicine, health, and sickness are a core part of who we are as humans, and they are intertwined with every aspect of our lives. This volume shows how contributions from nearly every field imaginable can come together to allow for a richer and "truer" picture of complex health-related issues such as aging and dementia.

The establishment and expansion of health humanities as an academic field and focus of research in Japan would allow for a much greater concentration of effort, creativity, intellect, and financial resources to be focused on a variety of health issues, both urgent and timeless, in ways that both complement and challenge the current focus on medical, surgical, and pharmacological solutions.

A vision for the future of health humanities in Japan

Health humanities has an important role to play in educating health care professionals who can provide people-centered, compassionate care that is grounded in a deep understanding of pain and suffering, a more reflective attitude, and heightened cross-cultural awareness and sensitivity. It can contribute to improved communication skills as well as ethical decision-making ability in clinical settings. It can also improve the health and well-being of health care professionals themselves by reducing stress, providing coping strategies, and to some extent alleviating burn-out. It can even help lay the groundwork for health care professionals to live full and vibrant lives marked by multifaceted, socially conscious, politically active engagement in their communities and societies. To achieve this, medical, nursing, dental, and other health-care-related colleges and universities should increasingly seek to incorporate courses and other educational opportunities that bring the humanities and arts to bear in specifically health- and health-care-focused ways.

Putting the health humanities to work in clinical and community settings can result in improved mental health and well-being of patients, health-care service users, former patients, family carers, and health care professionals themselves. To achieve this, arts programs (visual and performance) should be implemented in hospitals, elderly care homes, and community health centers. The potential of music therapy, art therapy, drama therapy, bibliotherapy, etc. to target specific mental health or other health-related issues and achieve specific outcomes should be explored through various research paradigms, designs, and methodologies. The role of architecture and design in creating health-care and health-oriented facilities that are both efficient and conducive to the well-being of patients, families, and caregivers should also be explored.

The health humanities has the potential to break down some of the walls between the various health professions, uniting them together in a common goal: humanistic, people-centered care. If our health is our most important asset, the responsibility for maintaining it must be carried by a broad coalition of stakeholders rather than leaving it completely up to doctors, dentists, nurses, other health professionals, and patients. We should all be involved in defining, pursuing, and maintaining health. The health humanities can do just this. It can attract the massive potential contributions of students, educators, researchers, and professionals in a wide array of disciplines and occupations to explore how they might be able to play their part toward the goal of healthy people in a healthy society.

The health humanities has great potential to contribute to the sustainability of Japan's successful health insurance system as well as the success of the new community-based integrated care system, particularly in the areas of disease prevention, health education and literacy, mental health and well-being, and non-medical and non-pharmacological interventions. However, in order to accrue these benefits, social investment in the health humanities, in the form of research grants, institutional support, and corporate sponsorship, will be required. The catch-22, however, is that to attract such investment, the benefits of the health humanities will have to be clearly supported by evidence. Thus, an active role by researchers and universities must lead the way.

The way forward

The path toward establishing a vibrant health humanities field and movement in Japan starts with individual researchers. Adachi (2009) has already provided an extensive history and description of the medical humanities in Japanese, and Huffman and Inoue (2019) have published a one-page definition and vision of the health humanities in Japanese. There is a great need for more and more researchers to undertake studies that not only implement health humanities-oriented programs, but also evaluate the outcomes. The next steps will then involve raising awareness and building momentum. Colleges and university departments in both the health fields and the arts and humanities should start developing courses, majors, departments, and research centers focusing on health humanities-related areas. Such institutions are by nature risk averse, so such programs will be small at first, but an "if you build it, they will come" mentality is the only way to build momentum. The next step will be the establishment of a national health humanities organization (presumably with visible focal points and landmarks such as a website, yearly conferences, and a journal) that is both research and action oriented. The steps up to this point will hopefully attract wider interest, and if outcome-focused research yields positive results, the field will begin to attract more funding, leading to further accumulation of evidence. At some point in this process, it is expected that the government will begin to experiment with expanded insurance coverage for evidence-based, non-pharmacological approaches to improving mental health and well-being. At this point, a sturdy research, evidence, policy, implementation, evaluation cycle will have been established. As an attempt to knock over the first domino in this chain reaction, St. Luke's International University will host the 9th International Health Humanities Conference at its campus in Tokyo in October 2020.

Dr. Hinohara once said, "Science alone can't cure or help people. Science lumps us all together, but illness is individual. Each person is unique, and diseases are connected to their hearts" (Kawaguchi, J. in Stafford, 2017: 2). In these words, we feel that his spirit is pushing us toward the establishment and expansion in Japan of this new framework that is equal parts inquiry and action, and equal parts academic field and social movement: the health humanities.

References

Adachi, T. (2009). *Medical Humanities Kyoiku Ni Tsuite—Tojo Haikei to Kyoiku Naiyo* [About medical humanities education: The background of its emergence and its educational content]. *Bioethics Study Network*, 8 (1): 11–22.

Cole, T.R., Carlin, N.S., and Carson, R.A. (2015). *Medical Humanities: An Introduction*. New York: Cambridge University Press.

Crawford, P., Brown, B., Baker, C., Tischler, V. and Abrams, B. (2015). *Health Humanities*. Houndsmills: Palgrave Macmillan.

Danely, J. (2015). *Aging and Loss: Mourning and Maturity in Contemporary Japan*. New Brunswick, NJ: Rutgers University Press.

Falcus, S. and Sako, K. (2019). *Contemporary Narratives of Dementia: Ethics, Aging, Politics*. New York: Routledge.

Hamaguchi, T. (2011). Family Conversation as Narrative: Co-Constructing the Past, Present, and Future. In Y. Matsumoto, ed, *Faces of Aging: The Lived Experiences of the Elderly in Japan*. Stanford, CA: Stanford University Press: 121–137.

Hamano, T., Fujisawa, Y., Ishida, Y., Subramanian, S.V., Kawachi, I. and Shiwaku, K. (2010). Social Capital and Mental Health in Japan: A Multilevel Analysis. *PLoS One*, 5 (10): 1–6.

Health and Welfare Bureau for the Elderly (Ministry of Health, Labour and Welfare) (2016). Long-Term Care Insurance System of Japan. (Accessed August 17, 2019 from www.mhlw.go.jp/english/policy/care-welfare/care-welfare-elderly/dl/ltcisj_e.pdf).

Huffman, J. and Inoue, M. (2019). A Vision for Health Humanities in Japan: A Proposed Definition and Potential Avenues for Application in Nursing Education and Beyond. *Bulletin of St. Luke's International University*, 5: 8–13.

Iwagami, M., & Tamiya, N. (2019). The Long-Term Care Insurance System in Japan: Past, Present, and Future. *JMA Journal*, 2 (1): 67–69.

Kamei, T., Itoi, W., Kajii, F., Kawakami, C., Hasegawa, M. and Sugimoto, T. (2010). Six Month Outcomes of an Innovative Weekly Intergenerational Day Program with Older Adults and School-Aged Children in a Japanese Urban Community. *Japan Journal of Nursing Science*, 8 (1): 95–107.

Kido, Y., Kawakami, N WHO World Mental Health Japan Survey Group. (2013). Sociodemographic Determinants of Attitudinal Barriers in the Use of Mental Health Services in Japan: Findings from the World Mental Health Japan Survey 2002–2006. *Psychiatry and Clinical Neurosciences*, 67: 101–109.

Kinoshita, Y. (2018). *Shinia Manabi no Gunzo: Teinen-go Raifusutairu no Soshutu* [Senior Citizen Learners: Creating a Post-retirement Lifestyle]. Tokyo: Kobundo.

Kumakawa, T., Morikawa, M., Otaga, M., Oguchi, T., Tamaki, Y. and Matsushige, T. (2016). Social and Community Prescription in an Integrated Community-Based Care System. *Japan National Institute of Public Health*, 65 (2): 136–144.

Lock, M. (1980). *East Asian Medicine in Urban Japan*. Berkeley, CA: University of California Press.

Lock, M. (1993). *Encounters with Aging: Mythologies of Menopause in Japan and North America*. Berkeley, CA: University of California Press.

Matsumoto, Y. (2011). Beyond Stereotypes of Old Age: The Discourse of Elderly Japanese Women. In Y. Matsumoto, ed, *Faces of Aging: The Lived Experiences of the Elderly in Japan*. Stanford, CA: Stanford University Press: 194–220.

Mori, C. and Nishio, T. (1996). Survey of Curriculum in the Medical Humanities at Japanese Medical Schools: A Comparative Study Between Initial Survey in 1988 and a Second Survey in 1994. *Igaku Kyoiku* [Medical Education], 27 (3): 155–159.

Nakamura, K. (2013). *A Disability of the Soul: An Ethnography of Schizophrenia and Mental Illness in Contemporary Japan*. Ithaca, NY: Cornell University Press.

Reich, M.R., Ikegami, N., Shibuya, K. and Takemi, K. (2011). 50 Years of Pursuing a Healthy Society in Japan. *Lancet*, 378: 1051–1053.

Sako, K. and Falcus, S. (2015). Dementia, Care and Time in Post-War Japan: *The Twilight Years, Memories of Tomorrow* and *Pecoross' Mother and Her Days*. *Feminist Review*, 111: 88–108.

Satoh, M., Yuba, T., Tabei, K., Okubo, Y., Kida, H., Sakuma, H. and Tomimoto, H. (2015). Music Therapy Using Singing Training Improves Psychomotor Speed in Patients with Alzheimer's Disease: A Neuropyschological and fMRI Study. *Dementia and Geriatric Cognitive Disorders Extra*, 5 (3): 296–308.

Shedlock, J. (2002). Osler's 'A Way of Life' and Other Addresses, with Commentary and Annotations, Sir William Osler. *Journal of the Medical Library Association*, 90 (3): 352–353.

Shibuya, K., Hashimoto, H., Ikegami, N., Tanimoto, T., Miyata, H., Takemi, K. and Reich, M.R. (2011). Future of Japan's System of Good Health at Low Cost with Equity: Beyond Universal Coverage. *Lancet*, 378: 1265–1273.

Stafford, N. (2017). Shigeaki Hinohara: Oslerian Scholar, Prolific Author, and Peace Advocate. *BMJ*, 358: 1–2.

Sudo, K., Kobayashi, J., Noda, S., Fukuda, Y. and Takahashi, K. (2018). Japan's Healthcare Policy for the Elderly Through the Concepts of Self-Help (Ji-jo), Mutual Aid (Go-jo), Social Solidarity Care (Kyo-jo), and Governmental Care (Ko-jo). *BioScience Trends*, 12 (1): 7–11.

Suzuki, A. (2017). Voices of Madness in Japan: Narrative Devices at the Psychiatric Bedside and. in Modern Literature. In: G. Eghigian, eds, *The Routledge History of Madness and Mental Health*. New York: Routledge: 245–260.

Tabei, K., Satoh, M., Ogawa, J., Tokita, T., Nakaguchi, N., Nakao, K., Kida, H. and Tomimoto, H. (2017). Physical Exercise with Music Reduces Gray and White Matter Loss in the Frontal Cortex of Elderly People: The Mihama-Kiho Scan Project. *Frontiers in Aging Neuroscience*, 9 (174): 1–12.

Takahashi, A. (2004). *The Development of the Japanese Nursing Profession: Adopting and Adapting Western Influences*. London: RoutledgeCurzon.

Takahashi, K., Tokoro, M. and Hatano, G. (2011). Successful Aging Through Participation in Social Activities Among Senior Citizens: Becoming Photographers. In Y. Matsumoto, ed, *Faces of Aging: The Lived Experiences of the Elderly in Japan*. Stanford, CA: Stanford University Press: 17–35.

Traphagan, J. W. (2000). *Taming Oblivion: Aging Bodies and the Fear of Senility in Japan*. Albany, NY: State University of New York Press.

Ueno, N. T., Ito, T. D., Grigsby, R. K., Black, M. V. and Apted, J. (2010). ABC Conceptual Model of Effective Multidisciplinary Cancer Care. *Nature Reviews: Clinical Oncology*, 7: 544–547.

United Nations, Department of Economic and Social Affairs, Population Division. (2017). *World Population Prospects: The 2017 Revision*. New York: United Nations.

26

AUSTRALIA AND NEW ZEALAND

A circuitous path to health humanities

Olaf Werder and Kate Holland

Introduction

On the surface, there appears to be no pressing need to dedicate a separate chapter to the trends in health humanities in Australia and New Zealand as, for the most part, the countries follow and mirror developments and debates occurring in their Anglophone cousins, especially those in the United Kingdom and the United States. It is, therefore, quite unsurprising that earlier discussions on the status of health humanities in the United Kingdom (Atkinson et al., 2015; Crawford, 2015), especially the knotty relationship with medical humanities, has featured in the two countries "Down Under" as well.

In fact, the growth of medical humanities programs followed trends in the United Kingdom and United States to expose medical specialists to ideas of philosophy, literature, ethics, and related humanities areas. And, unsurprisingly, medical humanities in Australia and New Zealand operates within comparable medical frameworks that have a long tradition in Anglophone public health. For instance, the University of Auckland in New Zealand offers medical humanities as a program within the Department of Psychological Medicine to provide "an opportunity to study medical issues from the point of view of a humanities discipline ... to enhance the practice of doctors." What makes the situation here unique though are two particular conditions.

First, Australian and New Zealand funding bodies, compared with other Western countries, have subscribed to an outdated science and research framework that skews research priority setting toward the (hard) sciences in terms of benchmarking levels of disciplinary investment. This has roots, as the argument goes, in a traditional underappreciation of the social and economic value the humanities and social sciences can offer the country. Second, unlike the United Kingdom, for instance, Australia has put far less emphasis on organizing programs around issues fundamentally at the core of the humanities at large, such as social inclusion and well-being (Damousi, 2019). In a similar vein, New Zealand universities have reduced their investment in general arts education and support (McWhannell, 2018). Therefore, the growth of health humanities as an area that openly embraces and utilizes the contributions of the arts and humanities to the practice of health (a science) has been a more arduous journey to date.

Ironically, the principles of health humanities, as outlined, among others, by Crawford et al. (2015), still silently prospered to a point as a result of activities from particular organizations and individuals. However, these programs or writings largely run under their own niche heading (e.g., sociology of dying, arts, and Indigenous health) and do not exist in a unified manner under the banner of *health humanities*. The reason they exist at all is a historic openness in the countries to critical cultural (humanistic) ideas derived from a burgeoning cultural studies scene that, following the export of the teachings of the "Birmingham School" of cultural studies, has existed in Australia and New Zealand since the late 1970s (Turner, 1993).

Hence, the critical investigation of social and political dynamics of contemporary culture in all its manifestations has a long-standing tradition among the social sciences, arts, and humanities here. Besides critical approaches to sociocultural phenomena such as class, sexual orientation, gender, and meaning and discourse, it included early on critical reflections on population health and well-being, health and arts, critical health studies, or equitable population health and environment (e.g., the Health Section of the Australian Sociological Association was established in 1967, when it was known as the Medical Sociology Section). True to form, many programs and research projects that can be grouped under the arts/humanities disciplines are isolated, scattered, and often unbeknown to each other and the larger medical field.

After the introduction of the name *health humanities*, usually as a result of visiting international scholars or peer-reviewed publications, a broader engagement with the totality of the connection of the humanities and health commenced, including among those working more with the better-established *medical humanities* concept. By and large, in a parallel pattern to other countries, it led to one of two developments:

(1) The two concepts were blended into the combined title "medical and health humanities" (e.g., it is the name for a pathway for postgraduate master students in bioethics at the University of Sydney, Australia).
(2) The medical humanities were somewhat reconceptualized to incorporate elements of the broader ideas the health humanities are aiming for (see, e.g., the University of Western Australia's Medical Humanities Network, or the "Humanities in Medicine" electives program for third-year medical students at Otago University, New Zealand).

To date, there are still very few programs, groups, or projects that use the health humanities term exclusively, and if so, most exist in an academic environment (e.g., the multidisciplinary Charles Perkins Centre Research Institute at the University of Sydney has a health humanities research cluster; and the Centre for Health Equity—part of the Melbourne School of Population and Global Health—has a health humanities and social sciences research unit). These mostly science-oriented programs profess to work in a multidisciplinary boundary-spanning mode to increase collaborative ideas and practice related to the confluence of health and society. In a similar vein, the Australian National University offers a Master of Culture, Health and Medicine course, which is a joint initiative of its College of Arts and Social Sciences and the College of Health and Medicine. All along, the aforementioned independent activities in different pockets within the social sciences, humanities, and arts disciplines continue their efforts and outputs. In short, as in many other Anglophone countries, the focus on a strict medicalized humanities perspective began to shift but it still has a dominant position here.

Contextual barriers

On average, one would have to argue that the continued existence of programs reflecting the ambitions of health humanities is despite, and not because of, government and academic support. As mentioned, the roadblocks are twofold. On the one side, the HASS (humanities, arts, and social sciences) disciplines at large have traditionally been under-utilized, under-resourced, and marginally regarded by successive governments and the funding bodies. In addition, standard training of future health professionals and promoters continues to follow the biomedical model, as opposed to the bio-psycho-social model of the social sciences and humanities. This narrower education tends to put students out of their comfort zones when exposed to arts and humanities concepts during training modules that broaden a skill set, and may make them hesitant to explore these areas beyond a certain level of understanding (Gaunt, 2016).

Unlike most OECD countries, Australia and New Zealand have largely adopted a vigorously policed definition of science that is restricted to the physical and natural sciences and their applications through technology and engineering, instead of considering the contribution of all research activity to innovation and the national interest regardless of disciplinary cluster (Byron and Howard, 2007). For example, while a 2009 Australian roundtable on the contributions of the humanities and social sciences toward a national science communication strategy delivered a White Paper (Kelly, 2009) that suggested a greater recognition of these disciplines in their expertise to connect science better to society and improve multidisciplinary thinking, the most recent reduction of funding for the humanities by $4.2 million by the Australian Research Council in 2018 revealed a persistent "silo" attitude that not only distinguished between national contributions of STEM (science, technology, engineering, and math) and HASS (humanities and social sciences) disciplines (Damousi, 2019), but also made it more difficult for HASS areas to engage in certain projects due to lack of funding.

Add to that the sizeable number of more than 40,000 medical researchers—all trained under the more traditional biomedical model (Laing, 1971)—who conduct research in medical research institutes, hospitals, and universities across Australia and New Zealand on various perspectives on human health, disease, and best practices of health-care delivery and disease prevention. Subsequently, more often than not any progress in humanistic health concepts is steered by medicine or allied health disciplines. Not surprisingly, Australia's first undergraduate major in Humanities for Health and Medicine at the University of Western Australia in Perth is a creation of its School of Allied Health in collaboration with the Medical School. Its promotional webpage asserts that:

> This field is highly innovative and likely to make a significant impact in shaping the future direction of healthcare for our communities. Increasingly, evidence suggests that inclusion of the humanities and the arts in the sphere of health has the potential to improve individual, health system and population health outcomes.
> *(University of Western Australia, n.d.)*

Here as in other places, humanities and social sciences work is still more in a contributory role toward understanding the meaning of health and disease from the patients', consumers', or lay perspective. That all said though, the trend to involve humanities specialists in work by clinicians, health educators, and medical scientists still has to be regarded as a positive signal for the future.

Pathways for arts and humanities in health

The growing interest among health organizations—both research and practice—in better understanding the lay community's knowledge and opinion of medical procedures and health conditions is palpable. Not many academic or government health district symposia go by in which at least one speaker or panel discusses or asks for a greater inclusion of so-called health consumers or consumer representation. While this inclusiveness has its origin in complying with legal rights of patients within the health-care system, it has expanded the domain of voices deemed to have an important say on health-related projects and processes. For instance, 14 New Zealanders from a mixture of walks of life, ethnicities, age groups, regions, and health status advise the Ministry of Health and working groups delivering eHealth projects within the Digital Health 2020 project in a so-called consumer panel (New Zealand Ministry of Health, 2017).

At the core of these trends is the ongoing struggle with the doctor/health system-to-patient relationship in Australia and New Zealand, more specifically questions of what this relationship entails or should entail, and who it involves (patients, family members, carers, citizens currently not using the health services). With the relationship constantly changing over time and in different contexts as a result of growing diversity among people and ideas, it has moved the human aspect of medicine further to the front here. Although not its sole impetus, it has contributed as an explanation for the growth of medical humanities itself in our countries, as it is precisely this definition of catering to the human aspects of medicine via traditional disciplines like history, philosophy, sociology, and literature as well as the intersection of medicine and the creative arts that allegedly serves to produce more insightful and compassionate doctors (Hooker, 2008).

In October 2018, the Australian Medical Research Advisory Board issued its second set of the Australian Medical Research and Innovation Priorities for the period 2018–2020 (Frazer, 2018). Prominent among the list of strategic priorities were Aboriginal and Torres Strait Islander health, digital health intelligence, comparative effectiveness research, primary care research, consumer-driven research, and public health interventions. It is interesting to note that this document mentioned multidisciplinary collaborative teams, partnerships in research design and practice between researchers, clinicians and consumers, concerted effort in primary care research, and community empowerment for health equity.

Whereas this report did not mention any collaboration with the HASS disciplines (let alone use the term *health humanities*), it does offer a reading that suggests a larger inclusion of diverse contributors and the generation of diverse means of creating a healthier society. Not coincidentally, it corresponds and temporally follows the growth of the medical humanities and health consumer associations in our region.

One aspect of medical and health humanities that appears to be of particular interest here is their focus on "translators" who can make often complex ideas in science and health accessible, using creative arts and culture-specific actions to change perceptions, frame new questions, and direct new discussions that result in more nuanced answers to health issues (Tsampiras and Mkhwanazi, 2019).

The prominent connection that especially the arts have achieved toward health is best illustrated by the creation of the National Arts and Health Framework in Australia. It was endorsed in November 2013 by Ministers of Health and Ministers of the Arts in every Australian state and territory to enhance the profile of arts and health in Australia and to promote greater integration of arts and health practice and approaches (Australian Government, 2013).

A cursive review of the framework document reveals not only a sizeable and growing acknowledgment of the value and benefits of arts for health practice and outcomes, but also budding collaborative partnerships across the health and arts sectors to develop strategies and new approaches. One of the pivotal organizations in the creation of this framework was the Institute for Creative Health, one of the leading not-for-profit arts and health agencies in Australia. Additionally, there is actually a flourishing number of networking and advocacy organizations in the arts and health space, such as Arts and Health Australia,

AccessibleARTS, Arts Health Institute, Australian Indigenous HealthInfoNet, Arts Access Aotearoa, Creative Wellbeing Alliance Aotearoa, to name a few.

Arts and humanities in health: selected activities

Given the relative predominance the arts have achieved among all health humanities fields, it is instructive to commence our overview of some of the various programs and activities that are being undertaken by showcasing a few of the flourishing collaborations between arts and health in Australia and New Zealand. This overview is by no means exhaustive. As Putland (2012a) notes, it is difficult to synthesize work in this area in part because it encompasses such a broad range of practices across multiple disciplines and sectors. We have opted for breadth rather than depth in our overview, with the aim of providing enough information for the reader to follow up specific projects, programs, organizations, websites, and other resources cited.

The arts and humanities are being applied in a variety of health and health-care contexts in Australia and New Zealand. While art therapy is one approach to including arts in health care to improve treatment outcomes, our review is concerned mainly with work within the arts and humanities that focuses on creating communities that are inclusive of and responsive to the needs and values of their members—not just responding to individuals and disease— in a way that aids prevention and promotes health and well-being. In choosing the examples our aim is to illustrate the role of arts and humanities in health intervention efforts in a range of populations and settings.

Programs to support mental health and well-being

One of the more active areas of research and practice is the role of the arts in supporting the mental health and well-being of individuals experiencing ill health or forms of social disadvantage. For example, in the context of our aging population, strategies to improve the quality of life of people with dementia and their carers have become increasingly important. While the majority of dementia care and research continues to be medically oriented, it is notable that arts and health projects and activities are becoming more popular in dementia care and awareness raising.

The Dementia Australia Research Foundation has recently funded projects looking at the potential of group songwriting to improve social connection and mental health and well-being of people with dementia and their carers, the effects of participating in an art gallery program on stress and inflammatory responses of people with dementia, and the role of arts centers in supporting people with dementia in remote Aboriginal communities where prevalence is high and services are lacking (Dementia Australia Research Foundation website).

Partnerships between universities, arts institutions, and health advocacy organizations are evident in a range of contexts in relation to dementia and mental health issues more broadly. In New Zealand, for example, the Auckland Museum in 2014 partnered with Alzheimer's Auckland and the University of Auckland on a program designed to increase the opportunities for socialization, engagement, and creativity for people with dementia and their carers (McGuigan et al., 2015). The six-week program involved a specialist museum volunteer facilitating a variety of activities, including gallery tours, object handling, and discussions of objects and images.

State-based organizations that fall under the Dementia Australia umbrella also offer programs such as Dementia and the Arts, which is based in the Australian Capital Territory and aims to support people with dementia and their carers in both community and hospital settings. Included among its current activities are interactive, discussion-based gallery tours at the National Gallery of Australia and the National Portrait Gallery, reminiscing and objects handling workshops at the Museum of Australia, hands-on arts groups and dance classes (Dementia Australia, n.d., "Dementia and the Arts Program").

Further, members of the Australian Dementia Centre for Research Collaboration have examined the enabling/disabling features of public buildings and spaces for people with dementia. One outcome of this project has been the establishment of the Dementia Enabling Environment Virtual Information Centre, which is described as an "Australian first that translates enabling environments research into practice and focuses on architecture, interior design and gardens" (Dementia Enabling Environments website).

In addition to highlighting increased recognition of the links between built environment, design, and health and well-being, which we touch on later in more general health-care contexts, the above projects and programs highlight the important role the arts and humanities have to play as part of the international movement to create dementia-friendly communities.

The role of the arts in the lives of people experiencing mental health challenges has long been recognized. In Australia, organizations such as the Victorian Mental Health Promotion Foundation (VicHealth) has been something of a leader in arts and health programs, working in partnership with arts organizations since 1987 to promote health and well-being. Its initiatives include the delivery of arts-based programs to celebrate cultural diversity, encourage people to get physically active, and increase social participation and decrease social isolation. Many of VicHealth's programs are targeted at providing opportunities for personal and community development through the arts, particularly for people from disadvantaged communities, in a supportive and collaborative environment (Kelaher et al., 2013).

The benefits of these arts programs (i.e., creative writing, visual arts, music, dance) include the building of self-confidence that can enhance not only individual mental health recovery, but also connection with others, decreased instances of hospitalization, validation as someone who is useful and valuable, a sense of belonging that comes with participating or producing something as part of a group, the opportunity to give and receive social support, learning new skills, and finding a sense of meaning and purpose (Lloyd et al., 2007; Van Lith et al., 2009; Williams et al., 2019).

The creative arts are also being used to assist military personnel experiencing illness or injury. Since 2014 the University of Canberra's Centre for Creative and Cultural Research, in conjunction with the Australian Defence Force (ADF), has been running the Defence ARRTS (Arts for Recovery Resilience Teamwork and Skills) program. Creative arts academics work with the ADF on the delivery of four-week intensive creative arts workshops. Evaluations show "significant psychological and psychosocial benefits" from engaging in the program (University of Canberra website, n.d.).

Similar outcomes have been reported in relation to Ōtautahi Creative Spaces, a New Zealand initiative established in 2015 in response to the high levels of distress and trauma experienced in Christchurch following major earthquakes. The goal of the program was to enhance well-being, social connection, and resilience among community members through the provision of art-making opportunities. Participants reported a range of positive outcomes in areas related to well-being, social connection, strengthened families, cultural connection, community participation, and post-disaster resilience (Savage et al., 2017). Māori artists valued the opportunity it created for them to express their cultural identity and reconnect to important cultural values, aided by the mentorship of knowledgeable Māori tutors: "This reconnection through a strength-based approach was deeply motivating for artists, and encouraged them to learn more about their tribal connections" (Savage et al., 2017: 24). A national network of Creative Spaces has now been established in New Zealand under the leadership of Arts Access Aotearoa (see Arts Access Aotearoa website).

Approaches for Indigenous health and well-being

In Australia and New Zealand it is well recognized that the individualistic focus of Western medicine and the health services and health promotion models it gives rise to are in tension with the holistic perspective on health and social and emotional well-being of Aboriginal and Torres Strait Islander (ATSI) and Māori people. Rather than focusing on deficit, the latter tend to favor a strength-based approach, acknowledge the ongoing impacts of colonization, and emphasize the intimate connections between individual, community, and environmental health. This orientation manifests itself in a variety of ways, from proposals for an alternative epistemology to guide public health practice in line with Indigenous views of health (Warbrick et al., 2016), activism directed at challenging racism within the health sector (Came et al., 2017), and culture-centered, arts-based programs, a selection of which is included in this section.

Since 2005, Indigenous Hip Hop Projects, which is a team of artists with skills in hip-hop, media, entertainment, and performing arts, has worked with Indigenous people in remote, regional, and urban communities across the country to produce health promotion campaigns in areas such as sexual and reproductive health, eye health, ear health, diabetes, alcohol and drugs, smoking, suicide prevention, and dementia, to name a few. Projects of this kind highlight the value of engaging young people in particular in a fun and interactive form of storytelling to enhance their own understanding of health at the same time as creating awareness within their communities and via social media (Indigenous Hip Hop Projects website) An evaluation of one such project found that hip-hop was effectively used to engage young ATSI people about sexual health and to produce and broadcast their performances as part of wider efforts to mobilize community conversation on the issue (Crouch et al., 2011).

The Aboriginal Health and Medical Research Council of New South Wales has also partnered with health services and local health districts in the use of arts-based approaches (creating street art murals) to health promotion around sexual health and alcohol and drug use. Such interactive approaches have proven to be an effective way of engaging young people on topics that could otherwise be a source of shame (Cairnduff et al., 2015). The murals are featured in prominent locations and communicate key messages that reflect the strengths-based language and messages young people had been exposed to in sexually transmitted infection and HIV education.

In Western Australia, another example of arts being incorporated into health programs in Indigenous communities is the Western Desert Kidney Health Project, which focuses on early identification and education around kidney health and reducing diabetes and kidney disease. The action research project combines health and the arts in the form of taking two large vehicles out to communities. One is set up as a clinic where screenings are done and people can receive their results immediately, and the other is set up to run art workshops where the focus is on prevention and teaching people about the causes of diabetes and what they can do about it (Western Desert Kidney Health Project website). Two of the women behind the project write:

> We work with the community to develop their own health promotion materials and the process of that is probably even more important than the materials themselves. The participants absorb the messages and then teach the rest of their community.
>
> *(Stokes and Stokes, in Sayer-Jones, 2011: 35)*

In New Zealand, the art of weaving has been incorporated by maternity staff at Waitakere Hospital Marae as part of a program to reduce the risk of sudden unexpected death in infancy. Expectant mothers are invited to participate in a weaving workshop where they make a flax baby bed (wahakura) while also learning from invited speakers about issues such as safe sleeping, breastfeeding, and smoke-free pregnancies. The program is one aspect of the New Zealand Government's *He Korowai Oranga: Māori Health Strategy* and efforts to encourage Māori participation in the health sector (New Zealand Ministry of Health, n.d.b).

Arts and health programs in ATSI communities have been found to support skills development, foster intercultural and intergenerational dialogue, build social cohesion and inclusiveness, and foster emotional and spiritual healing. Some of the principles to be considered when implementing locally relevant and effective programs in this area include consulting and involving elders, taking a whole-of-community holistic approach, linking to other community services, focusing on creating a positive process more than on the end product, giving careful consideration to program sustainability, and evaluating outcomes, processes, and outputs (Ware, 2014; see also Voyle and Simmons, 1999, on some principles for developing and implementing health programs in Māori communities).

Activities in health-care settings

There is also increasing recognition of the role that art and good design can play in humanizing hospital environments to the benefit of patients and their families, staff, and the wider community. In South Australia, the Flinders Medical Centre (FMC) Arts and Health program, which began in 1996, provides an example of the breadth and diversity of ways in which the arts can be integrated into an acute health-care setting. Over time, programs at FMC have included multiple art forms and collaborations involving artists working intensively with patients and staff, long-term artist residencies, weekly musical performances, an exhibition program, visual artists and musicians working with patients at the bedside, and public and environmental art initiatives (Putland, 2012b).

The Sydney Children's Hospital is another example that shows the importance of the arts as a healing tool, including a range of artwork throughout the hospital with regular exhibitions and the facilitation of art workshops for patients and their families with local artists (Sydney Children's Hospital Art Program website).

A range of arts and health projects have also been undertaken in hospitals in regional Australia. The Orange Health Service in New South Wales, through its Arts and Health Strategy, involved community members in participatory art projects as a way of bridging the gap between the health service and the community and increasing access to health care. Beginning in 2009 with the move of the General Hospital to the Bloomfield Psychiatric Hospital campus, the project involved workshops with a range of participants, including Aboriginal people, mental health consumers, and other community members, to create artworks that adorn the Orange Hospital, making the setting less isolating, and to improve access for Aboriginal communities and people with mental illness (Simpson and Hegyes, 2011). For example, activities included Indigenous weaving and terrazzo workshops where participants worked together with artists and hospital staff to create works that were installed in hospital courtyards. Testimonials from participants reveal the value of learning new skills and being a part of something important and the creation of new opportunities for clinicians to engage with consumers (Simpson and Hegyes, 2011). Other initiatives included a rotating art exhibition at the health service and the employment of an arts curator, a shared position between the Orange Regional Gallery and the Health Service.

Arts OutWest, which was also involved in the above project, is the regional arts development organization of Central West NSW, which in 2014 was also responsible for coordinating a project that involved creating a culturally sensitive health service as part of the Lachlan Health Service's redevelopment of Forbes and Parkes Hospitals in New South Wales. The project involved collaboration with the local Aboriginal community and resulted in the inclusion of the Wiradjuri gugaa (goanna) totem designs on the main entry doors and Wiradjuri signage throughout the hospitals. Stories collected as part of the evaluation reveal the overwhelmingly positive response to the incorporation of Wiradjuri signage and language throughout the hospital (Agency for Clinical Innovation, n.d.). Such has been the success of the program that the Western New South Wales Local Health District Aboriginal Signage and Artwork Strategy was launched at Parkes Hospital in March 2017 and is expected to be rolled out across 36 facilities by the end of 2019 (Arts OutWest, 2017a).

District Health Boards in New Zealand have also sought to increase the visibility of Māori culture in hospital environments through the provision of bilingual signage at the Taranaki Base Hospital, for example, in an effort to make services more inviting and improve Māori health (New Zealand Ministry of Health, n.d.a.).

Hospitals in urban settings are also taking into account the value of arts in their development work. For example, the Blacktown and Mount Druitt Hospitals (BMDH) Expansion Project involved engaging the local community to play an active role in shaping the design of new hospital facilities, with a particular focus on incorporating arts to create welcoming and safe spaces that reflect the values and diversity of the local communities (see the BMDH website for ongoing projects).

Another example of efforts to involve artists in hospital settings is a 2017 Arts OutWest initiative funded by the Lachlan Health Service to provide training to local professional musicians at Parkes Hospital. Six trainees received training on bedside engagement, ethics, suitable repertoires, and working with health professionals, as well as participating in practical sessions within the hospital. Testimonials from musicians reveal how inspiring it was to see the reaction of patients, families, and staff to their music. Arts OutWest is looking for opportunities to expand the project to other hospitals and aged care facilities (Arts OutWest, 2017b).

Community-based programs for empowerment and witnessing

There are numerous examples of the role the arts can play in creating communities that are more inclusive and accepting of difference, three of which will be mentioned here to give a sense of the form these can take. In Wodonga, Victoria, the "dis/assemble dance" multimedia project involved the production of a performance that brought together professional dancers with physically and intellectually disabled dancers. It also provided opportunities for those who did not want to dance to learn new skills, such as working behind the camera and marketing. The artistic director described some of the impacts of the project:

> There have been so many positive changes. For example, physically I've seen things like postural realignment and physical body awareness and confidence. Intellectually, we hear that they've said words they've never said before and they're communicating on a much more positive and clear level. And the emotional changes are significant too.
>
> *(Podesta in Sayer-Jones, 2011: 8)*

"Beyond Roundabouts" is a different kind of community project but one that also involved the use of multimedia to tell stories that break down stereotypes. Situated in Cooma, NSW, it involved a collaboration between a multimedia artist and young parents who had overcome adversity in the form of drug addiction, post-natal depression, abandonment, death, and violence. The project aimed to enable these parents to see their lives in a more positive and less judgmental light by using film and photography to tell their stories in a way that other teenagers could relate to. It culminated in a community exhibition of which the artist who facilitated the project said:

> Once the community viewed the film, and the photographic exhibition, they started to understand this group differently. This goes from the GPs to the school teachers through to just the elderly people walking up and down the street.
>
> *(Nolan, cited in Sayer-Jones, 2011: 26–27)*

The opportunity to exhibit one's artwork in a local community setting is often a critical component of arts and health projects and one that brings benefit not only to the art makers but also to the wider community of which they are a part and in which they interact with health services and professionals.

Another example of the role arts can play in challenging misconceptions and empowering particular groups is the "Art into Health: Puntu Palyarrikuwanpa" [Aboriginal Men Becoming Well] project, which forms part of an Aboriginal men's health project conducted in partnership with Palyalatju Maparnpa Health, a regional community-based cultural health organization in the South East Kimberley, Western Australia. The project involved the publication and exhibition of a collection of paintings by Aboriginal men from the Kutjungka region of Western Australia created between 2002 and 2011. In his commentary on the collection, Mick Adams writes:

> As an Aboriginal man and artist, and as I look at this art and listen to their stories, I am reminded that as health professionals we tend to concentrate on utilising the equipment and techniques that we have learnt in the modern world. We seem to forget the traditional processes of connectedness, of being in tune with our spiritual wellbeing and using alternative ways of healing.
>
> *(in McCoy, 2011: 7)*

With Indigenous males experiencing the worst mortality and morbidity outcomes in Australia, the stories and artworks included in this collection highlight the important role of arts as a medium through which to witness, as Alex Brown writes, "the strengths of Aboriginal men, as a lived reality, as a basis for healing and as a basis for a positive future for our communities" (in McCoy, 2011: 9).

Educational approaches for health professionals

The arts and humanities are also used to inform the education and training of health professionals in a variety of contexts. The University of Melbourne initiated a pilot program at the Ian Potter Museum of Art in 2012 and continues to provide training to students across a variety of health sciences with the aim of getting students "thinking about the importance of a diagnosis that is not just based on physical symptoms, but also on the larger narrative that informs a patient's health story" (Gaunt, 2016). Student feedback has been generally positive, with one observing:

"Every painting is like every patient … they all harbour a story which we need to explore to better appreciate and understand them" (in Gaunt, 2016).

Another example is a partnership between the Broken Hill University Department of Rural Health and West Darling Arts, which aimed to enhance undergraduate health science students' appreciation of non-clinical aspects of healing and of the holistic nature of health care. During their placement students are invited to participate in sessions delivered by local artists, which have included life drawing, photography, Aboriginal art, creative writing, and art observation, in what is described as a "fresh approach to teaching generic skills such as communication, rapport, observation, interpretation and analysis." Post session evaluations of the pilot program have shown positive results (NSW Health and The Arts, n.d.; see also Bolte et al., 2012).

Virtual communities and digital storytelling are also used in innovative ways in the education of health professionals. One example is Wiimali, which is a virtual community developed in 2010 and used in the Bachelor of Nursing program at the University of Newcastle, Australia. The community is designed to engage students about how the philosophy of primary health care is actioned in the real world and to enhance their understanding of concepts such as social justice, person-centered care, and patient safety. It uses digital stories to illustrate social determinants of health and intersectoral collaboration and to incorporate the voices of residents, patients, carers, and health professionals (Levett-Jones et al., 2015). The virtual community learning tool is part of wider curriculum redevelopment that has been enhanced by the input of a variety of disciplinary perspectives (Day et al., 2014). Student feedback has been positive. Wiimali offers an example of the potential of digital storytelling to enrich nursing education and practice.

Mental health is one area in both Australia and New Zealand where consumer involvement in education and training appears to be growing. Following the tradition of health humanities recognizing that a range of people other than clinicians have important knowledge, experience, and skills to bring to health education, policy making, and services, the University of Melbourne's Centre for Psychiatric Nursing offers a unique training program. Recognizing the importance of those with lived experience of and recovery from health challenges (service users or consumers as they are most commonly referred to in Australia and New Zealand), it has a number of "consumer academic" positions, which involve teaching nursing students from a lived experience perspective. Likewise, the Valuing Lived Experience Project is an initiative of the School of Occupational Therapy and Social Work at Western Australia's Curtin University, which is designed to systematically and meaningfully embed mental health lived experience into the social work and occupational therapy curriculum (Dorozenko et al., 2016).

Conclusion

The examples cited in this chapter are merely intended to provide a sense of the range of existing activities and partnerships, some of the aims and outcomes they are reporting, and the ways in which these are being mobilized for community and public health. There is certainly a lot of activity in the arts and health domain involving a range of stakeholders and disciplines tackling a range of health issues in a range of settings. There are also pockets of dedicated art therapy research and practice being undertaken, which are not discussed in this chapter.

In terms of arts and health projects more broadly, it seems that while some involve academics from the creative arts and humanities disciplines, the majority involve traditional health or allied health professionals. This is perhaps a function of the fact that many programs involve partnering with health services and organizations in order to reach those who may benefit from arts activities improving their access to and experience of services, for example. But it also means that much work in this area takes as its starting assumption the benefits of arts to health and well-being while rarely situating the work in a broader humanities context, notwithstanding the fact that critiques of the dominance of a biomedical framework are often implicit.

There is a risk then that arts activities are reduced to a means to an end, namely a tool for promoting public health messages or encouraging people to access particular services rather than playing a more critical role in redefining conceptions of health, illness, and disease in such a way that these alternative conceptions and associated societal responses have more influence on health policy, funding, and service delivery. Similarly, the existence of reports and research programs connected to other humanities fields, such as studies on informal care (Broom et al., 2016), suffering and palliative care (Dragojlovic and Broom, 2017), equity and sociality in health-care settings (Schofield, 2015), critical perspectives on digital health technologies (Lupton, 2014), or cultural competency in health-care delivery (National Advisory Committee on Health and Disability, New Zealand, 1998; National Health and Medical Research Council Australia, 2005) to name a few, are encouraging but tend to also exist in a contributory or counseling role to health research and service.

While it is difficult to know precisely how a more prominent or deciding position can be achieved in light of the clout of medicine and health sciences over health funding, these examples indicate opportunities for further developing the field of health humanities in Australia. These opportunities relate to four key areas:

1. The increasing importance attached to the value of consumer involvement in public health in terms of identifying research priorities and having active input into intervention development, implementation, and the translation of findings has the potential to trickle into regular practice.
2. The level of activity in the "arts and health" area in Australia and New Zealand that is supported by different levels of government is approaching critical mass.
3. The active and diverse field of Indigenous health research that by its nature is community oriented and advocates a holistic approach to health and well-being, including the importance of art and cultural practices, is consistent with the aims of health humanities and can provide a map for other community or sectoral groups.
4. Both countries have a tradition of critical sociocultural scholarship that bodes well for approaches to health and its communication, emphasizing the need to take into account non-medical aspects of health and well-being and the social determinants that shape the realities of individuals and communities, including how they accept, negotiate, or resist public health messages and actions.

In summation, we have to concur with Atkinson et al. (2015) that a more interdisciplinary or inclusive approach is still in a nascent stage. Although we recognize and applaud the influence of a more reflective health humanities logic in the works described above, we are still awaiting a broader interrogation of medicine, health, and illness. For example, it has proven difficult to locate prominent projects outside of arts-connected ones, if we want to look beyond academic research (with or without industry partners). Some of the core fields within the humanities, such as literature, history, religion, and philosophy, play to date still a negligible role in (co-)directing health debates in the countries, aside from being accepted as social determinants.

It is also surprising that the interrogation and exploration of a critical aspect of improving health conditions and debates, namely the field of health communication, has a marginal position when compared with other countries. Unlike here, in the United States and Europe health (care) communication has become more mainstream and spawned academic societies (the US-based Society for Health Communication), not-for-profit organizations (e.g., the UK Healthcare Communication Association), conference themes (e.g., the European conference on health communication series of the European Communication Research and Education Association), and academic programs (there are about 67 degree programs in this field in the United States compared with one in Australia and New Zealand).

Given the centrality of language and communicative sharing in human activity, of which health is a crucial one, it is surprising that among all the disciplines in social sciences, arts, and humanities, communication has not yet played a bigger role beyond health promotion and marketing discussions. To do so has the potential to function as a simple but relevant gateway to advance the role of health humanities in reducing the barriers to more effective health care and outreach.

Resources

- Arts Access Aotearoa: https://artsaccess.org.nz/?src=nav
- Blacktown and Mount Druitt Hospitals Expansion Project: www.bmdhproject.health.nsw.gov.au/
- Dementia Australia Research Foundation: www.dementia.org.au/research/foundation
- Dementia Enabling Environments: www.enablingenvironments.com.au/
- Indigenous Hip Hop Projects: https://www.indigenoushiphop.com
- Sydney Children's Hospital Art Program: http://www.schf.org.au/what-we-do/art-program
- Western District Kidney Project: http://westerndesertkidney.org.au/

References

Agency for Clinical Innovation (n.d.). Mali Marambir Ngurang Lachlan: To Make Better Place Lachlan. Retrieved from www.aci.health.nsw.gov.au/ie/projects/mali-marambir-ngurang-lachlan (Accessed 10/7/2019).

Arts OutWest (2017a). Arts and Health: Wiradjuri Signage Program Expands. Retrieved from http://artsoutwest.org.au/wiradjuri-signage-programs-expands/ (Accessed 12/7/2019).

Arts OutWest (2017b). Training Musicians in Hospitals. Retrieved from http://artsoutwest.org.au/training-musicians-in-hospitals/ (Accessed 12/7/2019).

Atkinson, S., Evans, B., Woods, A. et al. (2015). 'The Medical' and 'Health' in a Critical Medical Humanities. *Journal of Medical Humanities*, 36(1): 71–81.

Australian Government. (2013). *National Arts and Health Framework*. Standing Council on Health and the Meeting of Cultural Ministers. Canberra, ACT: Department of Communications and the Arts.

Bolte, K., Bennett, P. and Moore, M. (2012). ENRICHing the Rural Clinical Experience for Undergraduate Health Science Students: A Short Report on Inter-Professional Education in Broken Hill. *Australian Journal of Rural Health*, 20: 42–43.

Broom, A., Kirby, E., Kenny, K., MacArtney, J. and Good, P. (2016). Moral Ambivalence and Informal Care for the Dying. *The Sociological Review*, 64(4): 987–1004.

Byron, J. and Howard, S. (2007). *Submission to the Productivity Commission Research Study on Public Support for Science and Innovation*. Canberra, ACT: Australian Academy of the Humanities. Retrieved from www.pc.gov.au/inquiries/completed/science/submissions/sub064/sub064.pdf (Accessed 15/7/2019).

Cairnduff, S., Braun, D., and Harrison, K. (2015). HIV Free Generation: AHandMRC Street Art Project. *HIV Australia*, 13(3): 56–58.

Came, H.A., McCreanor, T. and Simpson, T. (2017). Health Activism Against Barriers to Indigenous Health in Aotearoa New Zealand. *Critical Public Health*, 27(4): 515–521.

Crawford, P. (2015). *Health Humanities: We Are Here to Collaborate, Not to Compete*. The Guardian-Australia Edition, March 30. Retrieved from www.theguardian.com/higher-education-network/2015/mar/30/health-humanities-here-to-collaborate-not-compete (Accessed 25/5/2019).

Crawford, P., Brown, B., Baker, C., Tischler, V. and Abrams, B. (2015). *Health Humanities*. Hampshire, UK: Palgrave.

Crouch, A., Robertson, H. and Fagan, P. (2011). Hip Hopping the Gap: Performing Arts Approaches to Sexual Health Disadvantage in Young People in Remote Settings. *Australasian Psychiatry*, 19(Suppl. 1): 34–37.

Damousi, J. (2019). Oh, the Humanities. *Campus Review*, 25(5): 12–13.

Day, J., Levett-Jones, T. and Taylor, A.C. (2014). Using a Virtual Community to Enhance Nursing Student's Understanding of Primary Health Care. *Collegian*, 21(2): 143–150.

Dementia Australia. (n.d.). Dementia and The Arts Program. Retrieved from www.dementia.org.au/support/support-in-your-region/australian-capital-territory/dementia-the-arts-program

Dorozenko, K., Ridley, S., Martin, R. and Mahboub, L. (2016). A Journey of Embedding Mental Health Lived Experience in Social Work Education. *Social Work Education*, 35(8): 905–917.

Dragojlovic, A. and Broom, A. (2017). *Bodies and Suffering: Emotions and Relations of Care*. London: Routledge.

Frazer, I. (2018) *Australian Medical Research and Innovation Priorities 2018–2020*. Canberra, ACT: Australian Medical Research Advisory Board. Retrieved from https://research.unimelb.edu.au/__data/assets/pdf_file/0009/2921499/Australian-Medical-Research-and-Innovation-Priorities-2018-2020.PDF (Accessed 18/6/2019).

Gaunt, H. (2016, Dec 16). Friday Essay: Can Looking at Art Make for Better Doctors? *The Conversation*. Retrieved from https://theconversation.com/friday-essay-can-looking-at-art-make-for-better-doctors-70484 (Accessed 20/6/2019).

Hooker, C. (2008). The Medical Humanities: A Brief Introduction. *Australian Family Physician*, 37(4): 369–370.

Kelaher, M., Dunt, D., Berman, N., Curry, S., Joubert L. and Johnson, V. (2013). Evaluating the Health Impacts of Participation in Australian Community Arts Groups. *Health Promotion International*, 29(3): 392–402.

Kelly, P. (2009). *Inspiring Australia: A National Strategy for Engagement with the Sciences*. Canberra, ACT: Report to the Minister for Innovation, Industry, Science and Research.

Laing, R. (1971). *The Politics of the Family and Other Essays*. London: Routledge.

Levett-Jones, T., Bowen, L. and Morris, A. (2015). Enhancing Nursing Students' Understanding of Threshold Concepts Through the Use of Digital Stories and a Virtual Community Called 'Wiimali'. *Nursing Education and Practice*, 15: 91–96.

Lloyd, C., Wong, S.R. and Petchkovsky, L. (2007). Art and Recovery in Mental Health: A Qualitative Investigation. *British Journal of Occupational Therapy*, 70(5): 207–214.

Lupton, D. (2014). Critical Perspectives on Digital Health Technologies. *Sociology Compass*,8(12): 1344–1359.

McCoy, B.F. (2011). *Arts into Health: Puntu Palyarrikuwanpa [Aboriginal Men Becoming Well]*. The Lowitja Institute, Melbourne. Retrieved from www.lowitja.org.au/page/services/resources/family-and-community-health/mens-health/Art-into-Health (Accessed 5/7/2019).

McGuigan, K.A., Legget, J.A. and Horsburgh, M. (2015). Visiting the Museum Together: Evaluating a Programme at Auckland Museum for People Living with Dementia and Their Carers. *Arts and Health*, 7(3): 261–270.

McWhannell, F. (2018). Oh, the Humanities! On the State of Arts Study at New Zealand Universities. *Spinoff Online Magazine* (1/9/18). Retrieved from https://thespinoff.co.nz/society/01-09-2018/oh-the-humanities-on-the-state-of-arts-study-at-new-zealand-universities/ (Accessed 3/7/2019).

National Advisory Committee on Health and Disability (National Health Committee). (1998). *The Social, Cultural and Economic Determinants of Health in New Zealand: Action to Improve Health*. Wellington, NZ: Ministry of Health Library.

National Health and Medical Research Council. (2005). *Cultural Competency in Health: A Guide for Policy, Partnerships and Participation*. Canberra ACT: Commonwealth of Australia.

New Zealand Ministry of Health. (n.d.a). Bilingual Signage Wins an Award in Taranaki. Retrieved from www.health.govt.nz/our-work/populations/maori-health/maori-health-case-studies/bilingual-signage-wins-award-taranaki (Accessed 15/7/2019).

New Zealand Ministry of Health. (2017). Consumer Panel. Retrieved from www.health.govt.nz/about-ministry/leadership-ministry/expert-groups/consumer-panel (Accessed 15/8/2019).

New Zealand Ministry of Health. (n.d.b). Te Ara Tuarua – Pathway 2: Māori Participation in the Health and Disability Sector. Retrieved from www.health.govt.nz/our-work/populations/maori-health/he-korowai-oranga/pathways-action/te-ara-tuarua-pathway-2-maori-participation-health-and-disability-sector (Accessed 15/7/2019).

NSW Health and The Arts. (n.d.). Arts/Humanities Intervention in Undergraduate Health Education. Retrieved from https://aci.health.nsw.gov.au/ie/health-arts-projects

Putland, C. (2012a). *Arts and Health – A Guide to the Evidence*. Background document prepared for the Institute for Creative Health Australia http://placestories.com/story/26824?_dbg=1 (Accessed 30/6/2019).

Putland, C. (2012b). *Arts in Health at FMC: Towards a Model of Practice*. Report prepared for Arts in Health at FMC. South Australia: Flinders Medical Centre.

Savage, C., Hynds, A.S., Dallas-Katoa, W. and Goldsmith, L. (2017). *Evaluation for Ōtautahi Creative Spaces Trust*. IHI Research. Retrieved from www.ihi.co.nz/what-we-do/otautahi-creative-spaces/ (Accessed 30/6/19).

Sayer-Jones, M. (2011). *Seeded: Great Arts and Health Stories Grown in Regional Australia*. Port Adelaide, South Australia: Regional Arts Australia.

Schofield, T. (2015). *A Sociological Approach to Health Determinants*. Cambridge UK: Cambridge University Press.

Simpson, M. and Hegyes, G. (2011). Orange Health Service Art and Health Project: A partnership between General Health, Mental Health, Drug and Alcohol Service, Orange City Council – Orange Regional Gallery and the community. Retrieved from http://static.placestories.com/pool/story/0007/0019968/lo/doc.pdf (Accessed 28/6/2019).

Tsampiras, C. and Mkhwanazi, N. (2019, Feb 14). New Ways of Thinking on Health, Arts and Humanities are Emerging in Africa. *The Conversation*. Retrieved from https://theconversation.com/new-ways-of-thinking-on-health-arts-and-humanities-are-emerging-in-africa-107305 (Accessed 15/7/2019).

Turner, G. (Ed.) (1993). *Nation, Culture, Text: Australian Cultural and Media Studies*. London: Routledge.

University of Canberra (n.d.). Creative arts and trauma. Retrieved from https://www.canberra.edu.au/research/faculty-research-centres/cccr/research-projects/creative-arts-and-trauma (Accessed 21/7/2019).

University of Western Australia (n.d.). Research at the Intersection of Humanities, Medicine, Health, Education and Science. Retrieved from www.uwa.edu.au/Research/Health-Humanities (Accessed 20/7/2019).

Van Lith, T., Fenner, P. and Schofield, M.J. (2009). Toward an Understanding of How Art Making Can Facilitate Mental Health Recovery. *Australian e-Journal for the Advancement of Mental Health*, 8(2): 183–193.

Voyle, J.A. and Simmons, D. (1999). Community Development Through Partnership: Promoting Health in an Urban Indigenous Community in New Zealand. *Social Science and Medicine*, 49: 1035–1050.

Warbrick, I., Dickson, A., Prince, R. and Heke, I. (2016). The Biopolitics of Māori Biomass: Towards a New Epistemology for Māori Health in Aotearoa/New Zealand. *Critical Public Health*, 26(4): 394–404.

Ware, V.A. (2014). *Supporting Healthy Communities Through Arts Programs*. Resource Sheet no. 28. Produced for the Closing the Gap Clearinghouse. Canberra: Australian Institute of Health and Welfare and Melbourne: Australian Institute of Family Studies.

Williams, E., Dingle, G.A., Calligeros, R. Sharman, L. and Jetten, J. (2019). Enhancing Mental Health Recovery By Joining Arts-Based Groups: A Role for the Social Cure Approach. *Arts and Health*, 2019 May 31:1–13. doi:10.1080/17533015.2019.1624584 [Epub ahead of print]

27

IMAGINATIONS OF HEALTH HUMANITIES IN AFRICAN CONTEXTS

The development of existing critical consciousness and perspectives

Ikem Ifeobu

Introduction: Africa: the continent, its nations, and diverse richness

It is important when considering engagement in Africa to perceive, in accurate detail, the entity known as the African continent. Africa boasts 54 countries covering 30 million square kilometres in five geographical zones: north, south, east, west, and central. It is the second most populous continent after Asia. It is estimated that by 2050 population will be over 2.3 billion; Africa boasts 30% of the world's remaining natural resources (National Geographic, 2013). Equally rich are its cultural and artistic practices, which are arguably obscured in academia (Blier, 1998; Vansina, 2014). Africa has been colonized by the English, French Portuguese, and Spanish in the "Scramble for Africa." Over 240 million of its current 1.2 billion people suffer undernourishment and 40% have not undergone formal Western education. Two thirds of the population are women. The astronomical qualities of this continent justify some speculation about how the rapidly growing international field of health humanities can engage with Africa. Due to the imaginative nature of this conceptualization, the ideas put forward in this chapter are not rigid, but simply provisional, guiding thoughts as to how health humanities might engage in Africa to avoid the imposition of paradigms alien to African culture, as is evident in its history.

Suitability of health humanities: brief review of global engagement and growth

This chapter aims to illustrate the capacity of health humanities to curate, contextualize, extrapolate, display, and celebrate the diverse epistemologies and cultural practices and their values—which remain obscured, underexplored, and still to be more applied in African contexts. The theoretical frameworks of Ronald Barnett (2011) and Paulo Freire (1970, 2018) are used to corroborate the potential of health humanities to collaborate with the human and cultural capitals in the ongoing development and transformation of pedagogic and discursive practices in relation to arts, humanities, health, and well-being across social spaces in Africa. Africa's heritage and deep history of art, humanities, and cultural productions is undoubtedly plenteous, making it a rich context in which to curate unrecognized practices. Yet we need to develop critical perspectives informed by African contexts for contributions to the field to be realized. Health humanities practice indicates the potential to set into action a collaborative, contextual, and culturally needs-based consideration of what can be, from what already exists. This chapter seeks to contribute to what we can call "feasible utopias" that seek to identify the rich resources and social environment conditions of those indigenous to these contexts with the aim to support enhancement therein (Barnett, 2011: 440). This requires the move from imagination to action.

The international scope of health humanities, or what I refer here to as "health humanities international" (HHI), derives from a fast-growing field of research and education that focuses on generating an inclusive, democratizing, and applied approach to applying the arts and humanities in domains related to health care, health, and well-being. Founded by Professor Paul Crawford in 2006, health humanities has consolidated an international appeal, with the institution of annual conferences, undergraduate, and postgraduate courses, research units, partnerships, and funding from high-profile institutions globally. Most impressive, given the field's relative newness, is the forthcoming publication, the *Palgrave Encyclopedia of Health Humanities* (ed. Crawford, P. and Kadetz, P.). The publication of an encyclopedia marks and exemplifies the widespread impact of HHI thus far. However, health humanities has to date only lightly seeded Africa and there is much more to do to advance it in this diverse continent. It is the innovative theoretical framework and practices behind the outputs briefly listed above that spur the imaginations of its operation and subsequent effects in Africa—what I represent here as health humanities in Africa or HHA.

Philosophical imaginations of HHA: a Freirean perspective

Health humanities' efficacy in initiating practical interdisciplinary collaboration across the globe suggests it is timely to consider and to imagine the etiology and ontology of health humanities in the ongoing curation, exposition, and development of the unique human ontologies existing across Africa. The driving question, "how can one use the arts and humanities to improve the human experience?," summarizes the philosophy of HHI and parallels the philanthropic and restorative processes at the core of Freirean ideas of conscientization, liberation, and ultimately humanization. Freire (1970) describes humanization—the conscious and intentional bettering of the human experiences—as the vocation of all peoples, our innate calling. Even without deep comparison of HHI and Freire, their commonality in philosophical perspectives is explicit.

Freire (2018; 1970; 1974) defines conscientization as the process through which an individual becomes aware of the world, their place in it, and their inherent ability to change this position through "human praxis, man's action-reflection on the world" (Freire, 1974: 24). It is the cognitive precursor to humanization because, without it, critical consciousness remains undeveloped and therefore unmanifested as practical development. By it are humans able to address situations of oppression. Therefore, it is of great importance that HHI commits to making sense of the history of African people. HHI needs to engage with Africa's diverse population in a way that assists in reinvigorating their cultures and unique practices, in response to the cultural violence constituted in African history, for "there is no conscientization without historical awareness" (Freire, 1974: 25). HHI boasts a collaborative approach to exploration of new knowledge and practices, and adopting this commitment in approaching Africa would arguably fulfil the Freirean requirement for truly liberatory bodies to act as "beings for another" (Crawford, 2015; Freire, 2018; 1970: 49). I argue that, to be instrumental in African contexts, HHI must engage at grassroots level locally to uncover the indigenous knowledge systems devalued and obscured by the historical events and ongoing globalization. HHI must seek to enliven the cultural reference points that have been lost through the passage of time, to catalyze the growth of African societies through social and human development (Hoppers, 2002).

As the imagined cohesive agent in dialectical and dialogical processes, HHI seeks to construct a metaphorical interactive gallery—a site of curation open to African epistemologies and ontologies as much as any other diverse territory or set of territories—where the interactions between the artistic and humanity-related content and human resources can be harnessed to develop the applicability of the findings in immediate and wider social and academic contexts. HHI as a revolutionary force for social development and change "rejects communiques and embodies communication" by broadening traditional inferential and discursive practices of knowledge formation through implementing dialogical and dialectical methodology (Freire, 2018; 1970: 79); thereby all participants are engaged dually, as student-teacher subjects. This co-intentional education (informed wholly by those in–context) empowers and equips the individuals who exist in-context to become permanent re-creators of intentional realities, as opposed to unconscious, disempowered perpetrators of oppressive realities.

We imagine HHA acting simultaneously as the site and harbinger of progressive restorative practice rooted in exploring the capability of enhancing the human experience through collaborative innovation and shared experience. These shared, place-based, epistemic, and sociocultural explorations position health humanities alongside Africa and her peoples, as they emerge from colonial-postcolonial objectivity to contemporary subjectivity in local, national, and global contexts.

HHA through the lens of Barnett

We can consider the HHA—an ontological imagination—in alignment with some of the tenets on the possibilities of the university as voiced within the musings of Ronald Barnett (2011). This conception seeks to describe the feasible utopias of health humanities in an African context and broadly outlines its purposes, vision, and potential stages of development, illustrating the precepts from the "Coming of the ecological university" that echo with the purpose(s) of health humanities as it expands its horizons.

HHA and the metaphysical university

Drawing again on the fundamental question of how human experience is to be enhanced, we should move to demonstrate how HHA would accommodate the "constellation of ideas" that arise from its operation in Africa (Barnett, 2011: 441). Such ideas would include those concerning holistic and humanizing approaches to learning and inquiry. Delivery of education and research rooted in dialogical relations allows for the emergence of a new paradigm in addressing knowledge formation that inculcates the distinct spiritual, mental, and physical practices inherent in African Beingness. By adopting this approach, HHA would take on the developmental qualities of the metaphysical university, offering a practice that enables those who engage in it to enter a new form of being, thereby transcending the mundane. Unlike the metaphysical university, HHA at this nascent point, should be cognizant of the social class practices in education that mediate stakeholders' perceived and actual notions of accessibility and belongingness in education (Reay et al., 2001); HHA would, by merit of a practically inclusive and contextually focused methodology, deconstruct these barriers and widen potential for engagement of those on the periphery or outside of academia.

HHA and the research university

Like the research university, HHA should be characterized by a focus on knowledge production but aim to do this through culturally congruent, equitable research. One way in which it can achieve this outcome is by moving the inferential processes and resulting knowledge production outside the confines of the academic space (i.e., the university). This would disable the potential of developing a culture of research that exercises control of the physical environment and indigenous peoples (Barnett, 2011; Dei, 2000; Wilson, 2001). I am not suggesting here that any future HHA should isolate its findings and practices from academic institutions in African contexts, but rather by its operations build a platform through which academic institutions can realize their role as collaborative agents in the ongoing conscientization of peoples and local community development. Similarly, HHA should reject the dichotomous categorizations of disciplines in academia by shifting the conventional discursive, and pedagogic practice in academia away from one that relies on STEM (science, technology, engineering, and mathematics) subjects to define health and well-being, to an expanded interdisciplinary approach that includes art and humanities (Academy of Science of South Africa, 2011). This re-characterization of research practice allows for the integration of lay persons, their knowledges, perspectives, and experiences into the exclusive "knowledge economy," previously informed mainly by specialist academic identities (Peters et al., 2009).

HHA and the liquid university

Applications of the liquid university to HHA implicates the vastly distributed and heterogeneous nature of Africa's human and cultural capitals. In realizing the challenge of capturing the diverse knowledge within Africa, imagination of smaller sub-structures within HHA should ensue; its outcome is what we might term "health humanities hubs." These hubs would be "genetically identical" with the preceding imaginations of HHA but liquid in that they would "move of their own volition in response to the world that they encounter" (Barnett, 2011: 447). This imagination is not intended to suggest the continent-wide exploration of Africa but the opposite. By focusing on localized engagements HHA would best serve and accommodate the diversity inherent each single African nation, for example Nigeria, which alone boasts over 250 languages with subdialects and various ethnic tribes and sub-tribes (Blench and Dendo, 2003). In that way, the true richness of the arts and humanities in the African continent to advance health care, health, and well-being, can be made more visible and available through the steady, meaningful illumination of what is possible in each of its many territories.

HHA and the therapeutic university

The final imagination lifted from Barnett (2011) defines the overall ontological disposition of a proposed HHA—the therapeutic university. It reiterates an HHA vision to create spaces for the inclusion of people previously on the periphery or completely detached from creative health and well-being practices. As an advocate for arguably underrepresented peoples and their thoughts, HHA should focus on understanding the sociocultural pathology that mediates associations of well-being in African peoples by "recognizing the authority of the patient" and allowing the same to partake in finding solutions (Garden, 2015). HHA can achieve this through continuing the established HHI practice of including unheard voices in the conversations, thereby relinquishing control of knowledge creation and equit-ably devolving prescriptive control from the academy to include the voices of communities and peoples in its context. Most importantly, HHA as a therapeutic force should denote a staunch commitment to care for those it encounters by ensuring the development of beings capable of navigating a world of endless challenge. This development, based on the African principle of *Ubuntu*, or the commonality of humanness, heals each person's self that will reflect in the environment and society (Le Grange, 2012).

Development in Africa and the university: a brief case study

Africa's quest for development implicates the role of the university, as higher education has a mandate to formulate sustainable development initiatives and practices (UNDP, 2010/ 2011). In turn, an imagination of the role of HHA in consideration of the mandate given to universities follows. The work of Mbah (2019) is foregrounded to inform this potential. Mbah (2019) in his field investigations of a Cameroonian municipality explored the role of universities in local community engagement and development. Through his research he gleaned practices indigenous to the people in a host of domains, for example, agriculture, medicine, and community governance—of all the data collected Mbah (2019) focuses on agriculture. By proxy of the field research, there was an opportunity for formal education to engage with local people, enhancing the local development of sustainable practices. Mbah (2019) demonstrates the capabilities research has to identify and create relationships that encourage development and sustainability in local communities, as well as the potential effects the university may have when focused at local engagement and development. His work depicts a dissonance between the sustainable development goals of the academy and their engagement of local communities, as painted by the voices of local subjects gathered through semi-structured interviews and focus group discussions.

The thematic analysis applied to these interviews and discussions resulted in three key findings. First, local participants realized a need for participation in initiatives driven by the university but expressed a need to have their voices heard and implemented in informing the context and direction of initiatives. Second, engaging local people in dialectical processes within formal spaces allows for sharing of best practices, applicable across various domains (Mbah, 2014); arguably, a bidirectional engagement would be optimum for developing sus-tainable practice in global contexts too. Third, participants recognized an ivory tower quality to the local university justified by its "operating in a cocoon" of its own (Mbah, 2019: 18).

The first point reflects how dialogical processes in research education are conducive to conscientization. Local peoples began to realize how they might interact with the university to achieve sustainable development. The second point is practical evidence of the outcomes of dialectical processes—the sharing of best practices to develop sustainability. The third illustrates a need of the people as relating to universities. Alongside cross-sectional educa-tional engagements with local communities, universities need to develop initiatives that develop an ethos of relatability referred to by participants as "man-know-man" (Mbah, 2019: 18)—a closer, informal relation with individuals (in academic spaces). As a result, clear and identifiable communication pathways between local and academic spaces are created for the sharing of knowledge, questions, and concerns that may frame developmental initiatives. Yet Mbah (2019) rightfully notes that universities do not exist for the sole purpose of serving local concerns.

HHA can act as a cohesive agent between the academy, its peoples, and local communities by seeking to create spaces to foster the development of engaged scholarship (Boyer, 1996), thereby developing a socio-ecologically minded university (Mbah and Fonchingong, 2019). HHA can help ensure that universities work to meet the needs of the ([local) peoples whose future generations it has been mandated to preserve (WCED, 1987).

Conclusion

There is a clear capacity for HHI to be instrumental in cultivating innovative practices in Africa. Africa presents an immeasurable number of contexts in which HHI could operate, contributing to transformative processes already at work on the continent. By working strictly in local contexts across Africa, HHA could develop human identities, unlocking and unveiling art and humanity with those cultures that respond to their needs. Involvement of academic institutions in these processes would certainly bode well for the future of sustainable development in Africa and promote engaged scholarship. In any case, the fruition of HHA anticipates success in improving the human experience through the investigation and discovery of new way of achieving it.

References

Academy of Science of South Africa. (2011). *Consensus Study on the State of the Humanities in South Africa: Status, Prospects and Strategies*. Pretoria: Academy of Science of South Africa.

Barnett, R. (2011). The Coming of the Ecological University. *Oxford Review of Education*, 37 (4): 439–455.

Blench, R. and Dendo, M. (2003). *Position Paper: The Dimensions of Ethnicity, Language and Culture in Nigeria*. Cambridge: DFID.

Blier, S.P. (1998). *Royal Arts of Africa: The Majesty of Form*. London: Laurence King.

Boyer, E.L. (1996). The Scholarship of Engagement. *Bulletin of the American Academy of Arts and Sciences*, 49 (7): 18–33.

Crawford, P. (2015). Health Humanities: We're Here to Collaborate, Not to Compete. *The Guardian Higher Education*. www.theguardian.com/higher-education-network/2015/mar/30/health-humanities-here-to-collaborate-not-compete (Accessed 2/8/19).

Dei, G.J. (2000). African Development: The Relevance and Implications of 'Indigenousness'. In G.J.S. Dei, B.L. Hall and D.G. Rosenberg, eds, *Indigenous Knowledges in Global Contexts: Multiple Readings of Our World*. Toronto: OISE/UT/University of Toronto Press: 70–86.

Freire, P. (1974). Conscientisation. *CrossCurrents*, 24 (1): 23–31.

Freire, P. (2018; 1970). *Pedagogy of the Oppressed*. New York: Bloomsbury Publishing USA.

Garden, R. (2015). Who Speaks for Whom? Health Humanities and the Ethics of Representation. *Medical Humanities*, 41 (2): 77–80.

Hoppers, O.C. (2002). Indigenous Knowledge and the Integration of Knowledge systems. In C.A.O. Hoppers, ed, *Indigenous Knowledge and the Integration of Knowledge Systems. Towards a Philosophy of Articulation* Cape Town: New Africa Books : 2–22.

Le Grange, L. (2012). Ubuntu, Ukama and the Healing of Nature, Self and Society. *Educational Philosophy and Theory*, 44 (2): 56–67.

Mbah, M. (2014). Towards a Model of University-Aided Technologically Driven Community Development. *Community Development Journal*, 50 (3): 463–477.

Mbah, M. (2019). Can Local Knowledge Make the Difference? Rethinking Universities' Community Engagement and Prospect for Sustainable Community Development. *Journal of Environmental Education*, 50 (1): 11–22.

Mbah, M. and Fonchingong, C. (2019). Curating Indigenous Knowledge and Practices for Sustainable Development: Possibilities for a Socio-Ecologically-Minded University. *Sustainability*, 11 (15): 4244.

National Geographic (2013). *Getting to Know Africa: 50 Interesting Facts* ... [online]. *National Geographic.* Available at: https://blog.nationalgeographic.org/2013/10/31/getting-to-know-africa-interesting facts/ (Accessed 5/8/19).

Peters, M.A., Marginson, S. and Murphy, P. (2009). *Creativity and the Global Knowledge Economy.* New York: Peter Lang.

Reay, D., Davies, J., David, M. and Ball, S.J. (2001). Choices of Degree or Degrees of Choice? Class, 'Race' and the Higher Education Choice Process. *Sociology*, 35 (4): 855–874.

Vansina, J. (2014). *Art History in Africa: An Introduction to Method.* London: Routledge.

Wilson, C. (2001). Decolonizing Methodologies: research and indigenous peoples. *Social Policy Journal of New Zealand*, 214–218.

World Commission on Environment and Development (1987). Special Working Session WCED/87/6 Berlin (West) January 29–31. Accessed online (17/08/2019) https://idl-bnc-idrc.dspacedirect.org/bit stream/handle/10625/152/WCED_v17_doc149.pdf?sequence=1

PART 2

Applications

28

INTERVENTION THEATER

Rick Iedema

Introduction

This chapter describes the role of theater in the areas of health-care improvement and patient safety. The chapter draws on *Hear Me*, a 2012 play by Alan Hopgood about an accidental hospital death, to illustrate how sensitive and troubling issues affecting acute care may be rendered discussable. The chapter concludes that theater in combination with targeted discussion about dramatized issues constitutes a powerful resource for addressing complexity in health care.

The dramatization of illness and health-care issues has a long history. The term "operating theatre" originally referred to an amphitheater accommodating spectators of surgical operations. An early theatrical drama is G.B. Shaw's *The Doctor's Dilemma* (1906), which offers a powerful insight into the moral challenges of rationing clinical resources. Another prominent, more recent play is *Wit*, which addresses the care experiences of a female English literature professor dying of ovarian cancer (Edson, 1993).

The shift toward interventionist or "applied" theater that has galvanized social and political advocacy since the 1960s (Boal, 1979) has also become prominent in health promotion and health awareness raising (Hundt et al., 2011). The use of theater in health-care improvement and patient safety is still in its infancy, however, no doubt due to these domains' deference towards conventionally technical conceptions of evidence, knowledge, practice, and change. Given its track record in other health-care domains, the potential of theater to bring about improvements in patient safety should be considerable.

Theater is anchored in narrative, plot, emotion, and real-time communication (MacAuley, 1999). Theater harnesses these resources for audiences to identify with dramatic characters and situations, and to vicariously experience timeless dilemmas to do with faith, justice, and loss (to name only a few). Given the rising complexity of contemporary health care, theater—and more specifically "applied theater"—offers important opportunities for engaging audiences with aspects that defy rationalization and standardization, such as acting amid medical uncertainty, moral-ethical decision making, and managing health-care–caused incidents.

Hear me: engendering discussion about hospital-caused death

Hear Me is a play about the aftermath of a clinical incident that resulted in a young patient's death. *Hear Me* was commissioned from the Melbourne playwright Alan Hopgood in 2011 for the 1st Clinical Incident Disclosure Conference (Sydney, in 2012). The play has since been performed over 100 times to mostly hospital and conference audiences.

Hear Me's overarching tragedy is the death of a young woman who died of a potassium overdose. The problems that led to this tragedy included: the unapproachable behavior of the senior consultant and his illegible writing; the young doctor's reluctance to check their reading of the dose and unwillingness to listen to the nurse; an emergency doctor's lack of attention to the patient's mother, who tried to alert the clinicians to her daughter's deterioration; the senior consultant's inability to acknowledge his role in the tragedy; and, finally, the clinical team's diagnostic error: they failed to establish that the young woman was pregnant and that her disease symptoms (stomach upset, cramps, vomiting) did not warrant their administration of potassium.

The crux of the play is the "incident disclosure" meeting. The meeting is chaired by a high-ranking hospital manager (Mary) who invites the mother (Pam) to discuss how things went wrong for her daughter (Lily). Mary's language includes an invitation to Pam to speak about the incident from her perspective, as well as expressions of sorrow ("I'm so sorry"). The conversation between Mary and Pam unfolds peacefully, until Mary reads the pathologist's report aloud stating that Lily was pregnant. Pam screams in distress, breaks down in tears, and leaves the stage.

The next scene engages Mary, a more junior doctor (James), and the senior consultant (Dr. Henty) in a confronting discussion about people's actions and responsibilities. Dr. Henty refuses to show remorse. He challenges James' analysis that the incident resulted from Dr. Henty being unapproachable and intimidating to trainee doctors. When Pam reappears, Dr. Henty's refusal to apologize and concede responsibility creates a stand-off, and leads to Pam threatening to sue him and the hospital. Instead of acknowledging Pam's distress and her right to an apology, Dr. Henty shrugs and leaves the meeting. Pam then concludes the play:

> I was told I could sue the hospital for a lot of money. But what's money if the system can go on harming people and taking their loved ones away? And that money will only come out of some insurance fund that means nothing to anybody except a group of accountants. So instead, I reached an agreement with the hospital.
>
> *(Hopgood, 2012)*

Pam's last comment addresses Mary and James:

> Okay, here's the deal. I need something good to come from the death of my daughter so that she didn't die in vain. I won't sue if you guarantee to improve communication in hospitals. To get across to clinicians like Dr Henty that they need to listen to patients, junior staff and families. To recognise that families know things that are not in any textbook. That there is diagnosis, drugs and doctors but without patients and families, some of the most valuable resources in medicine are being ignored. So what's it going to be?
>
> *(Hopgood, 2012)*

This redemptive ending shows Pam realizing that suing Dr. Henty and the hospital will make little difference to what happens to future patients and cheapens what happened to Lily. A better outcome is her proposed agreement to change the attitudes and communication of those working at the hospital.

Hear Me's morality therefore centers around two basic principles. The first of these is that health-care service users should be granted the right to inform clinicians about issues important to them, question clinicians about their care decisions, and be respected for raising such issues and questions. The second is that when care goes wrong, service users have a moral right to an apology (Box 28.1), an explanation, and a meaningful program of organizational change aimed at obviating recurrences.

Box 28.1 Linguistics of the apology

In health care, apologizing for clinical incidents is now inscribed into national policy in many countries around the world. But the ways clinicians are instructed to apologize for wrongs are carefully circumscribed. This is to achieve maximum effect on those harmed without incurring excessive legal risk or emotional debt. Such risk and debt can be strategically modulated depending on how we phrase our apology.

In English, apologizing for a wrong can be done in many different ways. A fairly obvious distinction can be made between the formal and the informal apology. The formal version is "I/we apologize for [wrong X]." Its less formal form is "I'm/we're sorry."

A second distinction pertains to the legal status of the apology. In law, the way we express [wrong X] may produce a "full apology" (in which case we attribute responsibility for a specific wrong to ourselves: "I/we apologize for giving you an infection") or a "partial apology" (in which case we limit the attribution of responsibility by leaving the wrong sub-specified: "I/we apologize for what happened").

A third distinction is to do with the apology's level of sincerity. Many tomes have been written on what makes apologies sincere. A common view is that the degree of sincerity is proportionate to the degree of identification with the wrong by the person apologizing. Thus, a marker of low sincerity is not apologizing for the wrong itself, but for how the wronged person feels: "I/we apologize for making you feel you need to complain about our service." An example of an apology that is likely to be heard as more sincere is: "I/we apologize for providing you inadequate service."

A fourth factor is the timing of the apology. Any apology that is issued too late is unlikely to have real effect. Importantly, the choice of timing needs to key in to the level of harm apologized for. If the harm that is apologized for is considerable, an apology that is delivered immediately may not be heard as respecting the severity of that harm.

A final issue is the comprehensiveness of the apology. All things being equal, comprehensiveness depends on two things. First, it depends on whether the apology is given for the whole wrong or only part of it. If the apology fails to address the wrong as the harmed person experiences it, the apology is unlikely to be heard as acceptable. Second, it depends on whether the apology is uttered on its own or is accompanied by a restorative gesture. If the person apologizing is in the position to rectify or mitigate a wrong but restricts themselves to a mere utterance, their apology may also not be taken to be acceptable.

References

Berlinger, N. (2005). *After Harm: Medical Error and the Ethics of Forgivenness*. Baltimore: Johns Hopkins Press.

Lazare, A. (2004). *On Apology*. New York: Oxford University Press.

Tavuchis, N. (1991). *Mea Culpa: A Sociology of Apology and Reconciliation*. Stanford: Stanford University Press.

The way this moral right is met is communicated theatrically, in the sense that specific circumstances conspire against its principles being realized. After Lily's death Pam is invited to a disclosure meeting by the hospital's manager, who listens to her, but Dr. Henty is not inclined to grant her an apology or an acknowledgment of responsibility. Despite this, Pam arrives at the conclusion that it is better to get the hospital (staff) to agree to change than to take them to court. Instead of Pam's anger leading to a decision to sue, the plot has her realizing that a different way of dealing with the hospital's shortcomings may be more effective: establish a change contract. The play finishes with a meeting, nine months later, during which Mary updates Pam about the hospital's achievements, and about Dr. Henty's retraining.

Reprise: *Hear Me* as a resource for making difficult issues discussable

How are we now to understand the impact of a play such as *Hear Me*? First, I should point out that each *Hear Me* performance has included an hour-long audience discussion about the play. These discussions focus on the extent to which the tragedy, problems, and dilemmas presented by the play (could) permeate local care provision. Given the emotional intensity of the play produced mainly through Pam's distress, these audience discussions are often highly charged. Pam's affect invariably infects the audience and radiates through audience members' comments and responses. Her affect raises the energy in the room to such an extent that difficult things become sayable, and challenging issues become addressable.

For example, in one post-performance session that I led, junior doctors were emboldened to speak about "the Dr. Hentys in our hospital." Their comments enabled me to engage management representatives in a discussion about junior doctor support, and commit managers to a process where they would invite junior doctors to regular debriefs. Afterwards, the Chair of this same health service wrote the following on her evaluation of the performance (personal communication):

> Alan Hopgood's powerful, complex and content-rich play "Hear Me" [made me] realise … how simple things such as an inflexion on the voice, a particular body stance or simply a doctor's bad handwriting, can lead to an escalation of events with disastrous consequences. No textbook, learned article or lecture could ever capture what the drama of "Hear Me" has achieved in bringing to us an understanding of truly patient-centred care.

On other occasions I was able to question management's role in allowing the circumstances created by Dr. Henty and his trainees to arise, let alone continue. How is it that managers do not see the kinds of problems portrayed in *Hear Me* coming? Critical questions I was able to raise included: Can managers become more closely involved in scrutinizing care relationships and communication before these descend into disasters such as befell Lily? Or can patients and families become more actively involved in observing and reporting problematic relationships and communication?

In these ways and others, *Hear Me* provided, and still provides, an endless source of discussion opportunities. Its content is, sadly, still highly relevant to how care mishaps are (mis) managed and to the emotional consequences of hospital-caused harm (Bell et al., 2018). These emotional consequences warrant proactive attention and pragmatic responses ensuring that the damage caused by incidents is more appropriately addressed by health-care services than it is currently (Iedema, 2018).

Conclusion

Theater has a critical role to play in raising the emotional temperature of how we respond to clinical incidents and how we deal with people's distress. Indeed, theater introduces a *rigor* to the task of focusing clinicians' and managers' attention on emotional distress caused by incidents:

> The performing arts can have as much rigour as any other experimental set-up, once it is understood that the laboratory, and all the methods that have resulted from it, provide much too narrow a metaphor to be able to capture the richness of the world.
>
> *(Thrift, 2008: 12)*

As Thrift's comment suggests, the theatrical depiction of grief and conflict nets in degrees of (health-care) "richness" and complexity that more established approaches to improvement and safety tend to lack. As has *Hear Me* over the course of its many performances and audience deliberations, theater has the potential to inspire managers and clinicians to reflect on their responsibility for avoiding sub-optimal relationships and interactions, for establishing support mechanisms for novice clinicians, and for engendering receptive attitudes towards patients' and families' knowledge, insights, and preferences.

In short, the rising complexity of health care calls for an *expanded* use of applied theater. Theatrical performance can detail complexities that remain opaque for scientific knowledge and technically oriented methods. The significance of theater for contemporary health care then is precisely its capacity for drawing in professionals and the public to partake in deliberations about difficult and neglected health care dilemmas.

Resources

- Stepping Out Theatre: http://www.steppingouttheatre.co.uk/index.php
- HealthPlay: http://healthplay.com.au/
- Senior Theatre Resource Centre: https://www.seniortheatre.com/

References

Bell, S.K., Etchegaray, J.M., Gaufberg, E., Lowe, E., Ottosen, M.J., Sands, K.E., Lee, B.S., Thomas, E.J., Van Niel, M., Kenney, L. Healing Arm Conference Group. (2018). A Multi-Stakeholder Consensus-Driven Research Agenda for Better Understanding and Supporting the Emotional Impact of Harmful Events on Patients and Families. *US Joint Commission Journal of Quality and Patient Safety*, 44 (July): 424–435.

Boal, A. (1979). *Theatre for the Oppressed*. London: Pluto Press.

Edson, M. (1993). *Wit*. New York: Farrar: Strauss and Giroux.

Hopgood, A. (2012) Hear Me: A play about a clinical incident and its disclosure. [Unpublished resource].

Hundt, G.L., Bryanston. C, Lowe, P., Cross, S., Sandall, J., and Spencer, K. (2011). Inside 'Inside View': Reflections on Stimulating Debate and Engagement Through a Multimedia Live Theatre Production on the Dilemmas and Issues of Pre-Natal Screening Policy and Practice. *Health Expectations*, 14 (1): 1–9.

Iedema, R. (2018). Emotional Harm Following Incidents in Healthcare: What Can Researchers Do? *US Joint Commission Journal of Quality and Patient Safety*, 44: 421–423.

MacAuley, G. (1999). *Space in Performance: Making Meaning in the Theatre*. Ann Arbor: University of Michigan Press.

Shaw, G.B. (1906). The doctor's dilemma. Retrieved from www.gutenberg.org/files/5070/5070-h/5070-h.htm (Accessed 5 December 2019).

Thrift, Nigel. (2008). *Non-Representational Theory*. London: Routledge.

29

GALLERY AND MUSEUM VISITING

Javier Saavedra

Introduction

Museums and galleries (the single term *museum* will be used here throughout) have become essential institutions in our nations. Beside their traditional function of art and culture containers, in recent decades economic and symbolic functions have transformed museums into the motor of economy and symbols that construct the identity of nations and cities: could we imagine Madrid or London without the El Prado Museum or the National Gallery? In the last two decades, a new function has been suggested for these institutions: museums as health and social inclusion resources.

The social function of galleries and museums: arts and culture as health resources

From the perspective of public health, health promotion, psychological well-being, and illness prevention exceed strictly clinical delineations of that field. Moreover, cohesion and social bonds of our communities—what we might call, in other words, social capital—are increasingly understood as determinants of citizens' health. According to Marmot et al. (2010):

> It [social capital] provides a source of resilience, a buffer against risks of poor health, through social support which is critical to physical and mental wellbeing, and through the networks that help people find work, or get through economic and other material difficulties.
>
> *(24)*

By increasing social participation and social bonds in our communities, citizens are empowered to enjoy more control over their health and well-being. In this sense, social prescription is defined as a "mechanism to link patients with non-medical support resources within the community" (Centre Forum Mental Health Commission, 2014: 6). Thus, social prescription works as a resource to improve psychosocial, mental, and socioeconomic states by means of communities' strengthening and enhancing social inclusion (Chatterjee et al., 2018).

Museums may offer valuable contributions to well-being, recovery, and resilience, and in this way can be thought of as a kind of social prescription. To begin with, there is an extensive network of museums and galleries within the European Union, United States, and Canada. This fact makes museums very accessible. Second, while economic and other stigmatizing barriers to the participation do exist, many institutions offer free admission or substantial reductions for vulnerable populations. Finally, museums are spaces increasingly designed for knowledge and learning in which the shared history of communities is condensed and where it is possible to explore objects, information, and stimuli for the learning and reflection (Chatterjee et al., 2018). In this sense, museums are high-density containers of meaning that let us participate in communities of practices. Art, despite the image of the great and unique artist, is rarely practiced in isolation (Saavedra et al., 2017a).

Creative practices as "social prescription"

In the United Kingdom, the crucial role of art as health resource was pointed out by an official political report of the All Party Parliamentary Group on Wellbeing Economics (APPG/WE, 2014). In 2015, The National Alliance for Museums, Health and Wellbeing (MHW) was created, with the objective of sharing information about museums, improving professional practices, and supporting people and institutions that work in this field. Health and museum institutions alike belong to this interdisciplinary consortium.

The MHW identified 603 well-established activities in museums of the United Kingdom, including long- and short-term interventions. Activities addressed to older people, people with dementia, and mental health issues were the most numerous; such activities involved 29.7%, 18.7%, and 17.7% of these groups, respectively (Lackoi et al., 2016). Other interventions addressed to different populations included homeless and unemployed people, or people suffering from illnesses including cancer. In what follows some relevant initiatives are described.

Liverpool House of Memories is a program launched by the National Museums Liverpool, an institution made up of six museums that takes advantage of the museums' experience as collective memory keepers. The program is based on reminiscence work with people who suffer from some level of cognitive deficit. Its activities include telling stories and memories, sharing them with caregivers, family members, and people with dementia, and reconstructing and reviving them thanks to various artistic activities (House of Memories, n.d.). Arts 4 Dementia's Reawakening the Mind project was founded in 2011 in the county of Dorset. It is made up of several artistic, academic, and health institutions. Its primary aim is fostering artistic stimulation for people diagnosed with dementia or cognitive deficit, in order to achieve a life full of meaning and social integration (Gould and Vella-Burrows, 2017).

In terms of cancer-focused initiatives, every year the Foundling Museum and the Great Ormond Street Hospital for Children (GOSH, UK) co-lead the Go Create! program. In this program, invited artists, hospitalized children, and relatives turn into creators, and artistic projects are subsequently exhibited in a hospital gallery. It is worth mentioning that GOSH enjoys a special program addressed to foster artistic activities inside the hospital (Hall et al., 2017).

There are very valuable experiences in the rest of Europe, although these types of interventions are not usually as systematized or institutionally supported as in the United Kingdom. For example, in Seville (Spain) creative workshops addressed to people with severe mental disorders have been held at the Contemporary Art Centre of Andalusia (CAAC) since 2006 through an agreement between the Museum, the Andalusian Health Service, and the

Andalusian Public Foundation for Social Integration of the People diagnosed with Mental Disorders. Every year the CAAC holds three temporary exhibitions by contemporary artists. These temporary exhibitions drive the topics and themes developed within creative workshops conducted by an art mediator each year. Workshops, which are made up of 10–15 participants, consist of two phases. In the first, the art mediator facilitates the discussion about the temporary exhibitions. In the second phase, participants are invited to gather around a large table and use provided materials for painting, drawing, and sculpture. Recently, and in the frame of the Creative Practices as Mutual Recovery project, these workshops have been assessed in terms of impact and outcomes (Saavedra et al., 2017b, 2018).

Why does it work? rationale and evidence

Several studies have found a positive association between the level of participation in cultural activities and a community's health, even controlling for variables like gender or age. Thus, the more cultural activities exist in a community, the more health that community appears to enjoy (Wilkinson et al., 2007). In the last decade, numerous research projects have shown empirical evidence of the positive impact on health of artistic interventions in different populations. However, most of the evidence is qualitative or generated from self-reported data. To establish more robust causal relationships, more experimental designs with control groups are necessary. In addition, it is not easy to discern which creative practices and with which population are the most effective.

One of the most exhaustive, rigorous, and recent efforts to find empirical evidence comes from the project Creative Practice as Mutual Recovery (Crawford et al., 2015). Social prescriptions in museums enjoy the same positive effects that research has shown for creative practices: decreased stress and anxiety, increased psychological well-being, construction of new meanings, improvement of social and communication skills, significant improvement of social inclusion, decrease of obsessive thoughts, and improved cognitive flexibility, among others.

We can turn to guides that help us design and perform artistic projects in museums. For example, Veall et al. (2017), in the frame of the Museums on Prescription project, offer specific recommendations to implement interventions in museums with the aim of promoting health and social inclusion. Without the intention of being exhaustive, what follows are some elementary suggestions for successful implementation of museum and gallery visiting as a health-supporting activity:

- Establish channels of fluid communication between the museum, social, and health institutions involved in the project. Frequently, the aims and communication patterns of these organizations are very different and can lead to misunderstandings. All the time spent building a secure relationship before starting the intervention is well-used time.
- Activities must be designed and directed by a professional specialist in artistic mediation.
- Study the population to which the activity is directed, and select the techniques according to their potential and needs (an activity that is too easy can be boring and a too challenging one can be discouraging).
- Include varied activities in which different senses and psychological processes are involved (for example, interweaving plastic and discursive activities).
- Give opportunities for time-out and breaks. Provide spaces for socialization and meeting: offer drinks, juice or coffee, at break-times.

- When working with traditionally marginalized populations, such as people diagnosed with a mental illness, whenever possible, seek to facilitate integrated, unstigmatized spaces for holding activities.
- Whenever possible, show performed works by participants in public events in order to fight stigma and help participants reconstruct their identity.

References

Centre Forum Mental Health Commission. (2014). The Pursuit of Happiness: A New Ambition for our Mental Health. Retrieved from www.centreforum.org/assets/pubs/the-pursuit-of-happiness.pdf (Accessed 19/2/2019).

Chatterjee, H.L., Camic, P.M., Lockyer, B. and Thomson, L.J.M. (2018). Non-Clinical Community Interventions: A Systematised Review of Social Prescribing Schemes. *Arts and Health*, 10 (2): 97–123.

Crawford, P., Brown, B., Baker, C., Tischler, V. and Abrams, B. (2015). Health Humanities. Basingstoke: Palgrave Macmillan.

Creative Practice as Mutual Recovery (2018). Recuperado de http://cpmr.mentalhealth.org.uk/ (Accessed 19/2/2019).

Gould, V.F. and Vella-Burrows, T. (2017). Reawakening Integrated: Arts and Heritage. Available at: https://arts4dementia.org.uk/wp-content/uploads/2017/10/A4D_REAWAKENING_Integrated-Arts__Heritage_Report_web.pdf (Accessed 31/7/2018).

Hall, S., Layton, S., Biglino B. and Ledgard, A. (2017). Under the Microscope. In J. Saavedra, A. Español, S. Arias-Sánchez and M. Calderón-García, eds, *Creative Practices for Improving Health and Social Inclusion*. Seville: University of Seville: 161–172. Available at: https://idus.us.es/xmlui/handle/11441/65469 (Accessed 19/2/2019).

House of memories (n.d.). Retrieved from www.houseofmemories.co.uk/ (Accessed 31/7/2018).

Lackoi, K., Patsou, M. and Chatterjee, H.J. et al. (2016) *Museums for Health and Wellbeing. A Preliminary Report*, National Alliance for Museums, Health and Wellbeing. Available at: https://museumsandwellbeingalliance.wordpress.com (Accessed 19/2/2019).

Marmot M., Goldblatt, P. and Allen, J. (2010). Fair Society, Healthy Lives: The Marmot Review. Available online at www.instituteofhealthequity.org/(Accessed31/7/2018).

Saavedra, J., Arias, S., Crawford, P. and Pérez, E. (2017b). Impact of Creative Workshops for People with Severe Mental Health Problems: Art as a Means of Recovery. *Arts and Health*, 10 (3): 241–246.

Saavedra, J., Pérez, E., Crawford, P. and Arias, S. (2018). Recovery and Creative Practices in People with Severe Mental Illness: Evaluating Wellbeing and Social Inclusion. *Disability and Rehabilitation*, 40 (8): 905–911.

Saavedra, J., Pérez, E., Español, A., Arias-Sánchez, S., Calderón-García, M., Romero, M.C. and Crawford, P. (2017a). Art Cares for Us: Contributions from Health Humanities. In J. Saavedra, A. Español, S. Arias-Sánchez and M. Calderón-García, eds, *Creative Practices for Improving Health and Social Inclusion*. Seville: University of Seville: 9–18. Available in: https://idus.us.es/xmlui/bitstream/handle/11441/65419/art_cares.pdf?sequence=1 (Accessed 31/7/2018).

Veall, D. et al. (2017) *Museums on Prescription: A Guide to Working with Older People*. Available at: https://culturehealthresearch.wordpress.com/museums-on-prescription. (Accessed July 2018).

Wilkinson, A., Waters, A.J., Bygren, L.O. and Tarlov, A.R. (2007). Are Variations in Rates of Cultural Activities Associated with Population Health in the United States? *BMC Public Health*, 7: 226.

30

POETRY AND MALE EATING DISORDERS

Heike Bartel and Charley Baker

Introduction

"a book must be the axe for the frozen sea inside us."
(Franz Kafka in a letter to Oskar Pollak on January 7, 1904; 1977: 16)

There is great potential for the use of literature in health-care treatment, personal recovery, and health-care education, and for raising greater understanding in the general public of the impact poor health has on people (see Hynes and Hynes-Berry, 1994; Crawford et al., 2015; Mazza, 2017). Literature is used successfully in a variety of therapeutic, educational, and community-building approaches. Hynes and Hynes-Berry (1994), Springer (2006), and Mazza (2017) suggest that bibliotherapy and poetry therapy can offer creative outlets for people struggling or living with ill health, and for carers, friends, and family, enabling them to capture their experiences of the world and aiding in the process of recovery. Literature can also offer medical practitioners and therapists valuable insight into experience of illness and recovery that reaches beyond general perceptions or medical case studies. It enables these readers to link narratives they are reading with their own professional or personal experiences, thus reaching a better self-understanding and understanding of others and strengthening the capacity to support a diverse range of individuals (Crawford and Baker, 2009; Crawford et al., 2015).

The term "literature" is wide ranging. Material can include published or unpublished novels, dramas, or poems as well as other fictional, non-fictional, or autofictional genres such as autobiographies or the narratives of self-help books, to name but a few. Approaches may cover the full range of language arts—reading, writing, speaking, and listening—and can also include cross-cultural and linguistic reflections on texts in translation. The latter may engage for example with attitudes of "foreignization" or "domestication" toward a text and culture (Venuti, 1995: 19; Davies, 2012). Other approaches can include: various forms of bibliotherapy and poetry therapy (for a summary see Harwood and L'Abate, 2010: 59–78); therapeutic writing methods (e.g., Treasure et al., 2010; Pennebaker and Evans, 2014, 150–66); schemes like the "Reading Well" initiative with its "Books on Prescription" available in public libraries and recommended by National Health Service professionals and people living with health problems; or the "prescription" of a poem for specific life situations through *The Poetry Pharmacy* (Sieghart, 2017) or similar published anthologies (e.g., Astley, 2003; Padel, 2004). Texts can be made accessible through a wide range of media: the traditional book format, electronic devices to read online, listening to audio books, attending the communal setting of a book group, and being read to either privately or in more public settings (Davis, 2009), as well as through music and performance. The latter may include the lyrics of songs, hip-hop therapy (Tyson, 2002) or the "poetic dialogue" (Clare, 2010, 127) between author, text, and audience of poetry slams.

While specific therapeutic approaches need expert knowledge and training, and can range from adjunctive and integrative to clinical and informational use (Campbell and Smith, 2003), many ways of engaging with literature in a creative and rewarding way do not require specific expertise beyond "intelligence, intuition, and a good dictionary" and the readiness to be "willing and adventurous" (Astley, 2003: 23). The reader—be it a person affected by illness in any way, a general practitioner, or a member of the wider public—does not have to be a literary theoretician to access texts in a meaningful manner. Particularly the skills of a good medical practitioner or carer who pays attention to the details presented through narrative-based practices bear considerable parallels to that of an attentive reader picking up sensitively on the "what" and "how" of a literary narrative (Astley, 2003; Charon, 2008). The "green shoots" approach as part of the new Maudsley method is one of many examples that employs the approach of detailed text analysis of written experiences in order to understand models of health behaviors and develop coaching methods of training for non-professional carers in collaboration with professionals (Treasure et al., 2010: 88, 198). This method looks in particular for positive features, "green shoots," in the "expressive writings" (Pennebaker and Evans, 2014) produced under guidance by parents and carers of people affected by eating disorders in order to facilitate reflection and change. However, not only texts produced as part of a therapeutic setting, but also published fiction, prose, and poetry can be highly effective additions to the toolkit of health professionals and others. This is highlighted in "Tools of the Trade," an initiative by the School of Medicine at the University of St Andrews, United Kingdom. Here, the "tools" are poems, chosen, read aloud and recorded by medical staff and students. Every graduating doctor is awarded a small anthology with *Poems for New Doctors* to accompany their medical career from the start—literally and metaphorically. The foreword reads:

> Reflecting on poetry, and indeed on all the Arts, can produce a different sort of doctor: one who is richer and deeper as an individual; one who ... has to deliver the products of scientific advance that will transform people's lives, but who also has the ability to relate to and communicate with people ... If you add to the scientific method and evidence-based medicine the stimulation and nurturing of the moral imagination by reflecting on poetry, we will have doctors who will not only have highly tuned clinical skills, but also a more profound understanding of the human condition, and of the psychological and moral subtleties that illness reveals.
>
> *(Fraser et al., 2016: 12)*

The discipline of health humanities can inspire and nurture such approaches that bridge perceived gaps between the arts and humanities and medicine and science, open spaces between the scientific and the creative, and build frameworks for the creative use of literature and other art forms for health and well-being. One example is the "Madness in Literature" network, the result of a Leverhulme-funded project to explore representations of "madness" on

249

post-war UK and US fiction. The series of seminars, online networking, collation of relevant texts, and literary investigation (Baker et al., 2010) offer different ways to explore altered, distressing, or unusual states of mind.

The "Hungry for Words" poetry project on eating disorders

Poems convey to the reader a sensitivity to, and struggle for, language that rarely features in health-care settings where there is an emphasis on fast, effective, matter-of-fact communication. Such poetry is, as Terry Eagleton states in *How to Read a Poem*, "really a kind of spiritual therapy for those … whose words have withered, whose words have become … bland" and "whose experience has become drearily routinised" (2007: 50). It depicts not a harmonized world but, in the words of American poet Emily Dickinson, makes the reader "feel physically as if the top of my head were taken off" (1958: 473).

The research project funded by the Arts and Humanities Research Council (AHRC) "Hungry for Words: an interdisciplinary approach to articulating, communicating and understanding male anorexia nervosa" (PI: Heike Bartel) has collected through a public call for poems on male "disordered eating" 13 poems that fit these descriptions and are openly accessible on the project's website. They are testimony to the power of poetry to articulate and communicate experiences of illness and recovery and perceptions of the world, in this case with regards to diagnosed or undiagnosed "disordered eating." Clinically, this may refer to specifically defined "eating disorders" as per the diagnostic manuals the DSM-V or the ICD-11, or may refer to a wider range of self-defined challenges, struggles, or thoughts about food. In this project, a broad approach included specified eating disorders such as anorexia, bulimia nervosa, and binge-eating disorder, but also other unspecified feeding and eating disorders. In line with the aims of the research project many poems address problematic perceptions of eating disorders as "female only" and focus in particular on men and boys.

The "Hungry for Words" poems center not on the authors, but solely on the poems as artefacts, the insights that can be drawn from reading them closely, and the thoughts they can stimulate about the experiences and perceptions of living with "disordered eating." The project does not follow any specific approaches to poetry therapy, for example structures such as Mazza's RES model (Receptive Expressive Symbolic), where the "receptive/prescriptive" introduction of a poem selected for a particular therapy setting leads to the "expressive/creative" writing of a poem that then culminates in a "symbolic/ceremonial" exploration in discussion or reading (2017: 52). Our 13 intense, open, and often explicit texts have not been collected with concrete therapeutic intentions in mind (compare, e.g., Leedy, 1969) and come with the warning that some readers may find them discomforting or triggering (on potential detrimental effects of creative bibliotherapy on eating disorder patients, see Troscianko, 2018). In their radical openness they are an "axe for the frozen sea inside us," to use the opening quotation from Franz Kafka (1977: 16). They can, as Eagleton attests of modern poetry, rouse the "calloused and anaesthetized" sense of modern life (2007: 50). In their aim to find a language for disturbing and highly individual experiences, which is often hindered by perceptions that eating disorders only affect girls and women, these poems search for unique ways to make sense of the disrupted worlds they convey. In this way they have the potential to bring their readers, particularly health practitioners and carers with limited insight into lived experiences of male eating disorders, new understandings.

The 13 individual poems situate experiences of disordered eating within a wider socio-cultural frame that includes mental health issues, fear, shame, and strained personal or family relationships. Titles like "When Skinny Tastes Good" (Emma Lee), "No One Speaks of It"

(Emma Lee), and "Intolerance" (Derek Parkes) outline the close interconnection between the personal and the public sphere. Others make literary references to sayings, children's stories or nursery rhymes like "Jack Sprat could eat no fat" ("No Sugar" by Selina Burr) and engage with the power of these references to shape (unhealthy) eating habits such as in "The way to a man's heart" (Derek Parkes). Titles like "You Can't Stick to One Smartie" (Juleigh Howard Hobson) and "Keeping Control" (M.T. Taylor) highlight the important issue of control, or lack of it. This is a recurring theme throughout the collection often expressed not only in the content of the poems, but also through the particular form and presentation. "Keeping Control," for example, features deliberate changes from measured "controlled" to free "uncontrolled" rhyme schemes and rhythms. The impact of these poetic elements becomes particularly prominent when this poem is delivered vocally, displaying in its synergy of content, flow, and delivery. Rhythm is also used in several poems to emphasize the desperate pace of running in over-exercising.

Compared with some other health issues, the topic of food and food consumption—that is not limited to clinically diagnosed eating disorders—resonates with most readers. Food is part of daily life, and preoccupations with the body and food consumption, thoughts about our weight, shape, diet, exercise, nutrition, food as celebratory or social, or as isolatory and shameful are part of nearly everybody's life in the Western world. The 13 "Hungry for Words" poems respond in very different ways to such omnipresent concerns and offer a powerful focus on extreme conditions related to food consumption, such as heightened control over food, extreme body images, life-threatening over-exercising, and related personal and health issues. However, there are numerous "entry points" for readers. In "Toxic Poem" by Aéngus Murray, the "I" in this poem—that does not necessarily speak for the author himself but is the "lyrical I" of the poem—expresses an almost scientific knowledge of food and its harmful ingredients that he/she has acquired through continuous bombardment by various sources. This mirrors the widespread (over)information of a highly health-conscious public in the Western world bombarded by scientific and pseudo-scientific food facts circulated in media reports that every reader can to relate to. In "Toxic Poem" these are the "nitrates" in bacon, the "aspartame" in chewing gum, and the high sugar levels caused by the "cellulose in . . . vegetarianism." However, the poem takes the reader beyond these pieces of information to show how they spiral out of control and become "toxic" in the mind and behavior of an individual who is equally food-obsessed and food-fearing. Short phrases at the end of six of the seven stanzas that divide the poem visually and thematically emphasize the threat food presents to this "I" and signal his/her preoccupation with worrying thoughts: "Congealed," "Forever," "In my cells," "Malignant," "Rotten," and the "Toxic" that lends this poem its title. In the last stanza these obsessive, controlling, and fearful thoughts are confronted with the perceived normal eating habits of another person: "Alice tells me when she has a bad day/She cooks a nice healthy meal for herself and feels better." An attentive reader of the poem will understand the vital point the poem makes and that well-meaning "normal" Alice does not comprehend: for this "I" there is no option of a "nice healthy meal" because food presents as a problematic and deeply frightening concept. The last word of the poem is "Nothing." It sums up the inability to communicate fears and the alienation from the "normal" world of "nice" meals. The inability to share any such meals also leads to eating "Nothing," suggesting what clinicians may diagnose as a selective food avoidance disorder. However, the carer or medical practitioner reading this poem will gain much more insight beyond a clinical diagnosis into the world this "I" inhabits: the general feeling of emptiness, isolation, and hopelessness that presents in its urgency both a withdrawal from and a reaching out to the reader.

In comparison, the poem "No Sugar" by Selina Burr uses the sparsity of the words laid out on paper as a formal element to create a skeletal shape that enhances this poem of a sibling about his/her anorexic and over-exercising brother.

No Sugar

My brother won't eat
sugar or fat,
meat or flour.
He runs 18 miles
on a cup of
oatmeal.
His eyes are black
and his fingers
like bone.
I hear his shoes
slapping the pavement
at midnight.
He flies like
a hummingbird
who can't find nectar
For as long
as he can.

The poem employs the image of the hummingbird, which has a long literary history in the poetry of many languages and cultures. Here this image introduces an innovative and original perspective in looking at male anorexia: it brings together grave concerns about the brother's over-exercising and under-eating, the fear of losing him, but also voices love and great tenderness towards him. The tiny bird with the extreme energy expenditure that beats its wings at ferocious frequency evokes the thrill of almost weightless flight and the beauty of flashing brightness. It is situated in a world apart where intervention does not seem possible: "He flies like/a hummingbird." The backdrop of the brother's "black" eyes, "fingers/like bone," the fact that he "won't eat" and "can't find nectar" and his relentless running "at midnight," without regard for any boundaries or limitations, darken the hummingbird image metaphorically and literally with the danger of overexertion and starvation with fatal consequences. The last stanza "For as long/as he can" mimics the movement of the bird, the seeming temporary stillness of hovering in mid-air suspended between being there and vanishing. The poem is a delicately balanced structure holding still at the moment before tipping point between fulfilment and starvation, high energy and burning out, hope and grief, life and death. For the carer or family member of someone affected by anorexia and over-exercising it may open a pathway to engage with the mixture of diverging emotions they may experience.

Outlook

The 13 poems of the project share with many other poems a "hunger" for words, the striving to articulate, communicate, and make sense of the troubled and troubling world—here of male disordered eating. The "Hungry for Words" open-access website features performative video readings of these poems to encourage current and future health professionals, carers, and members of the public to engage further with the insights they offer and to stimulate informal yet managed online discussion. Areas of further potential exploration are to utilize these powerful poems through performative and/or shared reading, as evidenced through the "Get Into Reading" schemes where reading aloud in groups has been shown to offer therapeutic and well-being benefits (Davis, 2009; Davis et al., 2016). This could then offer a way for medical and health educators, as well as eating disorders charities such as the project's partner First Steps Eating Disorders, to "teach" about disordered eating in males (and others) through the medium of poetry—read aloud or distributed for more quiet contemplation proceeding discussion. Further, therapists could use such an approach, either as a springboard for creative writing or using poetry to find the words that cannot otherwise be spoken (Roe and Garland, 2011).

Resource

• www.nottingham.ac.uk/research/groups/hungry-for-words/index.aspx (Accessed 16/10/ 2018).

References

Astley, N. ed., (2003). *Staying Alive. Real Poems for Unreal Times*. New York: Miramax.

Baker, C., Crawford, P., Brown, B.J., Lipsedge, M. and Carter, R. (2010). *Madness in Post-1945 British and American Fiction*. Basingstoke: Palgrave.

Campbell, L.F. and Smith, T.P. (2003). Integrating Self-Help Books in Therapy. *Journal of Clinical Psychology: In Session*, 59: 177–186.

Charon, R. (2008). *Narrative Medicine: Honoring the Stories of Illness*. Oxford: Oxford University Press.

Clare, T. (2010). Slam: A Poetic Dialogue. In T. Chivers, ed, *Stress Fractures: Essays on Poetry*. London: Penned in the Margins: 127–131.

Crawford, P. and Baker, C. (2009). Literature and Madness: A Survey of Fiction for Students and Professionals. *Journal of Medical Humanities*, 30: 237–251.

Crawford, P., Brown, B., Baker, C., Tischler, V. and Abrams, B. (2015). Health Humanities. Basingstoke: Palgrave Macmillan.

Davies, E. (2012). Translation and Intercultural Communication: Bridges and Barriers. In C. Bratt Paulston, S. Kiesling and E. Rangel, eds, *The Handbook of Intercultural Discourse and Communication*. Malden, MA/Oxford: Wiley-Blackwell: 367–388.

Davis, J. (2009). Enjoying and Enduring: Groups Reading Aloud For Wellbeing. *Lancet*, 373 (9665): 714–715.

Davis, P., Magee, F., Koleva, K., Tangeras, T., Hill, E., Baker, H. and Crane, L. (2016). *What Literature Can Do*. Liverpool: University of Liverpool. Online: www.liverpool.ac.uk/media/livacuk/institu teofpsychology/researchgroups/CRILSWhatLiteratureCanDo.pdf (Accessed 10/09/18).

Dickinson, E. (1958). *Letters 1870–1874*, ed. by T.H. Johnson. Cambridge, MA: Harvard University Press.

Eagleton, T. (2007). *How to Read a Poem*. Oxford: Blackwells.

Fraser, L., Gillies, J., Hendry, K., Morrison, L. and Newell, A. eds. (2016). *Tools of the Trade. Poems for New Doctors*. Edinburgh: Scottish Poetry Library.

Harwood, T.M. and L'Abate, L. eds (2010). *Self-Help in Mental Health a Critical Review*. New York/Heidelberg/London: Springer.

Hynes, A.M. and Hynes-Berry, M. (1994). *Biblio/Poetry Therapy. The Interactive Process: A Handbook*. St Cloud: North Star.

Kafka, F. (1977). *Letters to Friends, Family and Editors*, transl. from German by Richard and Clara Winston. New York: Schocken.

Leedy, J. (1969). *The Use of Poetry in the Treatment of Emotional Disorders*. Philadelphia: Lippincott.

Mazza, N. (2017). *Poetry Therapy: Theory and Practice*. New York/London: Routledge.

Padel, R. ed., (2004). *52 Ways of Looking at a Poem. A Poem for Every Week of the Year*. London: Vintage.

Pennebaker. J. and Evans, J. (2014). *Expressive Writing. Words that Heal.* Enumclaw, WA: Idyll Arbor.

Roe, C. and Garland, A. (2011). The Use of Poetry in the Construction of Meaning in Cognitive Behavioral Psychotherapy and Mental Health Studies. *Mental Health Review Journal*, 16 (3): 93–101.

Sieghart, W. ed., (2017). *The Poetry Pharmacy. Tried and True Prescriptions for the Heart, Mind and Soul.* London: Particular Books.

Springer, W. (2006). Poetry Therapy: A Way to Heal from Trauma Survivors and Clients in Recovery from Addiction. *Journal of Poetry Therapy*, 19 (2): 65–71.

Treasure, J., Schmidt, U. and Macdonald, P. (2010). *The Clinician's Guide to Collaborative Caring in Eating Disorders: The New Maudsley Method.* London/New York: Palgrave.

Troscianko, E.T. (2018). Literary Reading and Eating Disorders: Survey Evidence of Therapeutic Help and Harm. *Journal of Eating Disorders*, 6 (8) doi: https://doi.org/10.1186/s40337-018-0191-5.

Tyson, E. (2002). Hip Hop Therapy: An Exploratory Study of a Rap Music Intervention with at-Risk and Delinquent Youth. *Journal of Poetry Therapy*, 15 (3): 131–144.

Venuti, L. (1995). *The Translator's Invisibility: A History of Translation.* London/New York: Routledge.

31

PHOTOGRAPHY

Susan Hogan

Introduction

Since its conception in the nineteenth century, photography had been used to interrogate the human condition: from mistaken attempts at physiognomy (the judgment of character from facial characteristics), to Muybridge's illuminating high-speed photographic sequences in the late nineteenth century, which elucidated animal and human movement in an unprecedented way. Human rights organizations also seized on photography to campaign for social reform, illustrating unhealthy and unsanitary conditions in both urban and rural locations. The UL National Society for the Prevention of Cruelty to Children (NSPCC), for example, had a formal role to bring prosecutions for neglect and cruelty under the provisions of the Prevention of Cruelty to, and Protection of, Children Act (1889), and produced shocking photographs of malnourished infants in its work in the latter part of the nineteenth century against "baby farms."

The twentieth century saw the rise of the popularity of the family album. This compilation of photographic prints represented the self-identity, and even the ideals, of families across the United Kingdom, forming a social talking point within families: something to show visiting friends and relatives to stimulate reverie and exchange. The album was often regarded as a very precious object; it imbued the essence of the humans involved having developed talismanic qualities. In many families just one person (often dad) would take the photos and children might not be allowed to touch the camera, let alone express themselves taking pictures. Producing photos meant posting the role of film, or dropping it into a local chemist, to be developed and then waiting for the return of the prints (many of which were thrown away, as blurry, or otherwise disappointing). From the twenty-first century onward, mobile phone technology incorporating digital cameras made photography both ubiquitous and democratic. It also changed the way we take photos, allowing us to make instantaneous decisions about which photos to keep and which to dispose of.

The physical photo album was displaced as a primary mode of exchange by social media platforms. Facebook launched in 2004, and now has over 2 billion monthly active users. Profile and cover pictures have become an import aspect of self-presentation. It permits sharing of images on one's timeline with "friends" (with optional accompanying explanatory commentary), allowing friends to respond in a variety of ways, with remarks, images, "likes," or other automatic responses. Getting fairly instant responses to photographs from friends is potentially gratifying, while a lack of response can prove unsettling. Settings can be altered, but most users allow themselves to be "tagged" in others' photos, and these images of themselves in social settings are shared to their own timeline and friends (with potentially embarrassing consequences). Photo sharing is a central aspect of Facebook and images can also be shared in "albums."

Another predominant platform, Twitter, enables users to post messages up to 140 characters, and upload pictures and short videos. Twitter operates on the basis of non-reciprocal "following." Posts are known as "tweets." There are many social networking sites operational now. Flickr hosts images, and allows users to follow one another and comment on the images of others, creating "communities of practice" (Wenger, 1998). Private messages can also be sent. Unlike Facebook, Flickr has relaxed censorship allowing a wider range of imagery to be reproduced. Images are classified as one of three categories: "safe," "moderate," and "restricted" in order to separate family-friendly and pornographic or otherwise disturbing content.

WhatsApp (2009), Instagram (2010) and Snapchat (2012) are simpler ways of communicating images to others, incorporating the opportunity to send an image and comment instantaneously and are favored by young people as quicker to use than Facebook (although Instagram, an online mobile photo and video-sharing social media platform, also offers the capacity to follow others, comment and like their content, so shares some similar features with Facebook; it has a younger user group). This spontaneity does have the disadvantage that some people may post images they then later regret having shared. Sexting is the exchange of erotic or explicitly pornographic imagery primarily between couples in intimate relationships and is a practice that has been encouraged by magazines such as Cosmopolitan to improve and spice up relationships; however, these supposedly private images are often shared. One survey suggested that over 20% of such imagery is routinely shared, as some enjoy sharing "private" sex photos (Kinsay Institute, 2016). Revenge porn (intimate images of an ex-lovers posted as an act of psychological violence and retribution) is another unfortunate feature of these sites.

Mobile phone technology comes replete with a palate of editing tools to remove imperfections, or even make us look thinner. Louis Theroux's "Talking to Anorexia" (2017) noted the pervasiveness of perceived feelings of "powerlessness and lack of self-worth" among those young women he spoke to. Grogan and Wainwright (1996) argued that girls as young as eight recognize and internalize dominant cultural pressures to be thin. We are bombarded with highly idealized and sexual digitally manipulated images of women, leading to astonishing levels of body dissatisfaction among women and girls and to epidemics of self-mutilation, or self-starvation. The proliferation of the "selfie" as a dominant mode of self-presentation for young people has contributed to body dissatisfaction and cyber-bullying.

Within the health humanities, art therapy (incorporating the use of photography), therapeutic photography, and photography as part of visual research methods used to explore health topics are all noteworthy developments.

Photographic research methods

The International Visual Sociology Association (IVSA) was formed in 1981, originally concerned with photography and documentary filmmaking within a sociological context, but now more broadly interested in the contribution of visual research methods to the "study of society, culture, and social relationships" (IVSA website). A photograph is persuasive because "it appears to permit the rapid and faithful recording of visual phenomena" (Ball and Smith, 1992: 4). In *Working Across Disciplines Using Visual Methods in Participatory Frameworks* (2017),[1] I elaborate ten reasons to use visual images in research, which I summarize here, though I am referring to visual images in general, including collage, as well as photography.

Pictures can be used to represent and explore the ineffable

That which is hard to put into words, including mood tones and feeling states, can often be expressed eloquently by images. Symbols, analogies, and metaphors can be sophisticated, and metaphors used in conjunction with one another create complex reverberations within a pictorial frame. Feelings that are indefinable can find expression in a moment of ontological revelation in the act of making. The image and process of production is potentially illuminating. Subsequent interactions with it may become of significance. The images created in photo-documentation have been argued to encapsulate "the textures and tactilities, smells, atmospheres and sounds of ruined spaces, together with the signs and objects they accommodate, [which] can be emphatically conjured up by the visual material" (Edensor, 2005: 16).

Images can convey an all-at-oneness (Eisner, 1995)

Images can produce a holistic depiction of ideas or feelings. They can also encapsulate eloquently. As images are not linear sequences as are utterances, different levels of meaning can be conveyed simultaneously and contradictory sentiments expressed instantaneously. Equally, images can be used to convey complicated concepts and complex data. The developing field of informatics uses diagrams and images to summarize chunks of information, which would be hard to digest if simply heard, but which are immediately evident when seen. Complicated concepts can be condensed in simple visual formulations, or extended ones such as animations or cartoons.

Images can make us attentive to things in new ways

When visual anthropologists or sociologists photograph mundane practices, we are able to see these in a new light. The image can draw attention to previously unnoticed details, but can also enable us to look at objects afresh (Pink, 2011; 2015). The images can help us to refresh our sensibilities and to highlight culturally distinctive, but often taken for granted, cultural practices. In her photo-elicitation practice, Ruth Beilin has used images to *reveal* landscape conservation issues. In my discussion of this work (Hogan, 2012: 58), I note that the images are absolutely revelatory to the viewer who is not used to seeing the land in such a way, and the images and text combine to open out a new consciousness to the reader.

Images can be memorable

From billboards to news footage, it is often iconic images that stay with us. In *The Birth Project*[2] particular images stayed in participants' minds and triggered particular memories and emotions relating to their experience of childbirth.

Images can develop empathetic understanding and generalizability

While issues of mass migration or civil war in some far corner of the globe might feel abstract and remote, images can be used to make these issues feel much more immediate. Often this is done by the depiction of individual people to highlight the issues of many, so the story of one family's migration journey stands for many such journeys, for example. Charities such as Oxfam or Amnesty International often use this approach. Through the photograph of the individual, the humanitarian issue is given weight and meaning.

Images can be used to look at changes over time

Photo-elicitation techniques have been used to look at how neighborhoods change over time, but also as an ethnographic tool to look at specific cultural phenomena. Clayden et al. (2015) for example, used time-lapse photography to examine the ways that people use space and build informal memorials in natural burial sites. As a sequence, complex changes, which would be laborious to describe, are easily illuminated. We can *see* how people are changing the space.

Images may be more comprehensible than most other forms of academic discourse

People who might not read a broadsheet newspaper or academic article can still engage with images; also as a "stimulant" to research interviewing, asking a respondent to talk about a photo can provide useful results, replacing abstract or interrogatory questioning (Prosser, 2006).

Images provoke action for social justice

Images are often used to provoke social change. More recent photographs of police brutality in the United States and in Greece have been used prominently in campaigns for reform and retribution, and are useful to researchers in lending weight to justifications for research activity.

Image making can foster the exploration of embodied knowledge

Images can be affecting almost as though through a process of "emotional contagion" (Hogan and Coulter, 2014: 95). Nor should the kinesthetic aspects of art or image making be overlooked: Bourdieu, for example, speaks of embodied knowledge as "habitus." Others refer to "muscular knowledge" (see Martens et al., 2014, for a discussion of embodied research practices). The kinesthetic qualities of both producing and viewing artwork are of potential importance. One characteristic of an installation exhibition format, for example, is that it uses the total space and invites the viewer to move within it. This physical moving into the discursive space is slightly different qualitatively to simply looking at something on a wall or plinth; it is a more bodily engagement with the artwork and offers a more immersive experience. It is potentially more challenging in its theatrical invitation to the viewer to engage with the subject matter in an embodied way. How the narrative flow unveils itself depends on the participant's movement through the space; one perspective may necessarily cut off another, and new configurations are generated by being at different vantage points in the space. The format evokes uncertainty, anxiety perhaps, and the entire work cannot be viewed from any particular vantage point. In certain conceptual frameworks, such as one that seeks to emphasize heterogeneity, this might be a very appropriate format to prevent the foreclosure of meaning.

Image making can be vitalizing

Artworks can be made in a manner that can jolt our mundane sensibilities, using materials in ways that can refresh our outlooks and capture our enthusiasm. There is the opportunity to be immersed (in the flow) using intuition, serendipity, spontaneously enjoying the tactile embodied nature of the experience—what many call "creativity" (though often without defining what they mean). In this indeterminate space individuals or groups of people can become highly attuned to what is emerging—it is an emergent space. If working collectively, there are also potentially productive opportunities to explore interpersonal dynamics (for instance, within teams) or to reflect upon the nature of personal authorship. These are spaces of being and becoming, of ontological uncertainty, spaces in which ways of knowing are explored.

Arts and health: therapeutic photography and photography within art therapy

Health humanities is an umbrella term increasingly being used to include medical humanities and the arts in health (Clift and Stickley, 2017). The arts in health incorporate a range of practices from community-based participatory arts (using techniques such as photo diaries) to confidential therapeutic group work. Therapeutic photography, which is part of art therapy practice (Hogan, 2001), is used in several models of art therapy today, particularly the use of photographic collage (Hogan, 2016).

Phototherapy has its antecedents in the work of Jo Spence and is interested in social critique. Spence explicitly suggested that photography should be used as "one of the healing arts" and went on to develop re-enactment phototherapy with Rosy Martin. Spence described her practice as a form of cultural "sniping" (Stanley, 1995). Re-enactment phototherapy is interested in challenging dominant stereotypes and creating new, more empowering narratives that are told in a pictorial sequence and are frequently publically exhibited as part of the process—indeed, the work is displayed as a proclamation (Martin, 2003, 2019). This work straddles the line between social science research, political activism, and art. The work of Jo Spence was notable from a health humanities perspective for its interrogation of her experience of being a cancer patient. She said, "I used the camera as a third eye, almost as a separate part of me which was ever watchful: analytical and critical, yet remaining attached to the emotional and frightening experience I was undergoing" (Spence, 1995: 130).

This method is a cultural critique and therapeutic practice as one. Sherlock describes Spence's legacy thus: "Taking aim at certain personal and political myths – the family snapshot, the domestic goddess, the cancer victim – her work asks unflinching questions about the power structures of visibility, of who can be seen under whose terms and in what light" (Sherlock, 2012: 1).

Brief case example

Representing Self-Representing Ageing used creative arts to negotiate and challenge images of aging and explore their contribution to participatory approaches to research in social gerontology. The initiative brought together researchers from gerontology and art therapy with a cultural development agency that uses the transformative power of the arts to make a difference to people and places. Photo-diaries, re-enactment phototherapy, arts elicitation and photography were all used by different groups of women interrogating their experience of aging.

Notes

1 An example of an arts-based research project is www.derby.ac.uk/media/derbyacuk/assets/research/research-groups/documents/65835-The-Birth-Project.pdf.
2 This is an abridged list which originally appeared in further detail in Pink et al.'s edited volume *Theoretical Scholarship and Applied Practice* (2017) in a chapter entitled Working Across Disciplines Using Visual Methods in Participatory Frameworks. This in turn, was based on a list produced by Weber (2008: 44–47). As I felt Weber's categorisations lacked sufficient distinction, I used her list as a starting point and acknowledge her work as the initial inspiration.

Resource

* *Representing Self, Representing Ageing.* Go to: http://www.newdynamics.group.shef.ac. uk/assets/files/194.pdf

References

Ball, M.S., and Smith, G.W.H. (1992). *Analyzing Visual Data*. London: Sage.
Clayden, A., Green, T., Hockey, J., and Powell, M. (2015). *Natural Burial: Landscape, Practice and Experience*. London: Routledge.
Clift, S. and Stickley, T., eds, (2017). *Arts, Health and Wellbeing*. Cambridge: Cambridge Scholars Publishing.
Edensor, T. (2005). *Industrial Ruins: Space, Aesthetics and Modernity*. Oxford: Berg.
Grogan, S., Wainwright, N. (1996). Growing Up in the Culture of Slenderness: Girls' Experiences of Body Dissatisfaction. *Women's Studies International Forum*, 19(6): 665–673.
Hogan, S. (2001). *Healing Arts: The History of Art Therapy*. London: JKP.
Hogan, S. (2012) Ways in which Photographic and Other Images are used in Research: An Introductory Overview. *International Journal of Art Therapy: Formerly Inscape*, 17(2): 54–62.
Hogan, S. & Counter, A. (2014). *The Introductory Guide to Art Therapy*. Abingdon, Oxon: Routledge.
Hogan, S. (2016). *Art Therapy Theories. A Critical Introduction*. Oxon: Routledge.
Kinsay Intitue: Garcia, J. R., Gesselman, A. N., Siliman, S. A., Perry, B. L., Coe, K., Fisher, H. E. (2016). Sexting among singles in the USA: prevalence of sending, receiving, and sharing sexual messages and images. *Sexual Health* 13: 428–435.
Martens, L., Halkier, B. and Pink, S. (2014) Researching Habits: Advances in Linguistic and Embodied Research Practice, *International Journal of Social Research Methodology*. 17(1): 1–9.
Martin, R. (2003). Challenging Invisibility: Outrageous Agers. In: S. Hogan, ed., *Gender Issues in Art Therapy*. London: Routledge: 194–227.
Martin, R. (2019). Look at Me! Representing Self: Representing Ageing: Older Women Represent Their Own Narratives of Ageing, Using Re-enactment Phototherapeutic Techniques. In: S. Hogan, ed., *Arts Therapies and Gender Issues: International Perspectives on Research*. Abingdon, Oxon: Routledge: 188–209.
Pink, S. ed., (2011). *Advances in Visual Methodology*. London: Sage.
Pink, S., Mackley, K. L. & Moroşanu, R. (2015). Hanging out at home: Laundry as a thread and texture of everyday life. *International Journal of Cultural Studies*, 18(2): 209–224.

Pink, S., Fors, V. and O'Dell, T. eds., (2017). *Theoretical Scholarship and Applied Practice*. London: Berghahn.

Prosser, J. (2006). Researching with visual images: Some guidance notes and a glossary for beginners. Working Paper. Real Life Methods, Manchester. ESRC National Centre for Research Methods. http://hummedia.manchester.ac.uk/schools/soss/morgancentre/research/wps/3-2006-07-rlm-prosser.pdf (Accessed 30/11/19).

Sherlock, A. 2012. Jo Spence. *Freize* (online Magazine, Issue 149). https://frieze (addressed 30/11/19).

Stanley, J. (1995). ed. Jo Spence. *Cultural Sniping: The Arts of Trangression*. London: Routledge.

Theroux, L. 2017. *Talking to Anorexia. BBC Documentary. First shown October*, 29: 2017.

Warren, L., Gott, M., Hogan, S. and Richards, N. (2012). *Representing Self-Representing Ageing: Look at Me! Images of Women and Ageing*. Project Report. New Dynamics of Ageing, Sheffield.

Weber, S. 2008. 'Using Visual Images in Research' In: J.G. Knowles and A.L. Cole (eds.) *Handbook of the Arts in Qualitative Research: Perspectives, Methodologies, Examples and Issues*. London: Sage: pp. 41–54.

Wenger, E. (1998). *Communities of Practice: Learning, Meaning & Identity*. Cambridge: Cambridge University Press.

32

FASHION AND TEXTILES

Rebecka Fleetwood-Smith

Introduction

The purpose of this chapter is twofold: to outline the significance of clothing and textiles to the individual, and to explore the capacity of clothing and textiles as tools for engagement and creativity within dementia care settings. Dementia is an umbrella term used to describe a number of diseases that affect the brain, the most common of these is Alzheimer's disease. There is currently no cure for dementia, yet creative approaches have been found to improve the lives of those living with the condition.

Clothing, the body, and identity

Fashion and clothing, although not synonyms, are often terms that are used interchangeably. To quote Joanne Entwistle, "Fashion is about bodies: it is produced, promoted, and worn by bodies. It is the body that fashion speaks to" (Entwistle, 2015: 1). Drawing upon the argument that the body is at the center of how we may consider and discuss fashion, Entwistle (2015) suggests that fashion can be explored both at the macro-level (i.e., global corporations designing, manufacturing, promoting, and selling fashion) and at the micro-level, whereby we focus on the individual's experience of their clothing. For the purpose of this chapter I focus on fashion at the micro-level of the individual.

Western culture is a culture of clothed bodies: we all engage with clothing and wear it on a daily basis. Wearing clothing involves the intimate proximity of body and material, influencing a person's movement, and the way they sit and stand. As Bovone (2012) notes, clothing not only functions in connection to our needs (e.g., to keep us warm) but is also appreciated as something that enriches our lives. Thus, we can form relationships with our clothing. Attempts to unravel and explore such relationships can be found in examples ranging across: Emily Spivack's book *Worn Stories* (2014), containing a collection of over 60 items of clothing, each with their accompanying narrative; the artist Marcia Farquhar and her "Acts of Clothing" (2013), in which she modeled countless items of clothing on stage, emotively narrating tales about each to the audience; and the 2018 "Fashion Unraveled" exhibition at the Fashion Institute Technology Museum, New York, where the emotional value of clothing was explored through exhibiting worn, imperfect, and flawed garments (Fashion Unraveled, 2018).

The notion that what we wear is significant is not a new phenomenon. In 1890, psychologist William James posited that clothing was more important than a man's other possessions. James believed clothing to be a fabric extension of the flesh and, as such, inextricably connected to a person's identity and their sense of self. This physical and intangible proximity of clothing to a person's identity was explored by Sophie Woodward in her book *Why Women Wear What They Wear* (2007), in which she interrogated women's everyday dress. She found that, through clothing, women were able to engage with and carefully construct their identity. She also highlighted the complex assemblage of selecting an outfit, whereby women considered whether the clothing was *really* "them," and whether the outfit was suitable for the occasion, and also considered how others may perceive them. The suitability of an outfit, or item of clothing, can affect the way a person feels, as wearing inappropriate clothing can make a person feel uncomfortable and out of place, while wearing the "right" clothing can make a person feel at ease and empowered (Entwistle, 2015). The notion of what constitutes the "right" item of clothing is not only informed by the style and design of the clothing, but also the meanings associated with the garment.

Clothing and associated meanings

The capacity for an item of clothing or outfit to, for instance, enable a person to feel empowered, has been studied by social psychologists, who have investigated the ways in which meanings associated with item(s) of clothing can affect the wearer. Studies have found that the color of an item of clothing can affect both the behavior of the wearer and the way in which the wearer is perceived (Elliot and Niesta, 2008; Pazda et al., 2014). Similarly, Elliot et al.'s (2013) research demonstrated that through wearing red items of clothing, participants were able to access and take on the symbolic associations of attractiveness and sexual receptiveness surrounding that color. The notion that an item of clothing can be imbued with meanings, and that these meanings can be accessed by and affect the wearer, is strengthened by the findings of Adam and Galinsky (2012), who coined the term "enclothed cognition." Enclothed cognition is defined as the systematic effect on the wearer's psychological processes through physically wearing a garment imbued with meaning. Moreover, in their study, Fleetwood-Smith et al. (2019) found that participants wearing clothes that they described themselves as being emotionally attached to reported feelings of enhanced well-being due to being able to take on and access the personal meanings that they associated with their specific items of clothing. Therefore, the capacity for an item of clothing to make a person feel comfortable resides not only within the material or physical sensation of wearing it, but also within the meanings associated with that garment.

The significance of clothing in health and social care settings

The effect that clothing has on the wearer can be particularly significant when considering the care of those in health and social care settings. There has been increased recognition reflecting this from both the social sciences and design literature (Buse and Twigg, 2015, 2018; Chan et al., 2018; Iltanen-Tähkävuori et al., 2012). For example, the interdisciplinary project Garment+ (Chan et al., 2018) sought to explore the potential of clothing in the care of people with musculoskeletal conditions, for example, conditions such as rheumatoid arthritis. Such conditions can cause difficulties in dressing due to restricted joint mobility, pain, and fatigue. The project, a collaboration between designer Alexa Chan, academics from King's College London, and adults from a rheumatology outpatient clinic in London, tested the role of fashion to promote positive well-being in patients. Employing a collaborative design process, clothing prototypes were developed and tested with patients to address their concerns with clothing fastenings, comfortable fabrics, and the accessibility of garments (how easy they were to put on). Findings reported that patient participants felt a sense of empowerment for having their views heard and considered throughout the design process. They also began adapting their existing clothing based on designs developed within the project.

Not only can the design of clothing in health and social care settings be considered important, but research has also demonstrated that the type of clothing people wear in such settings can be significant. In their study, Topo and Iltanen-Tähkävuori (2010) found that clothing provided in hospitals created limited possibilities for being active and symbolized the low status of patients within the hospital setting. Notably, in April 2018, the National Health Service (NHS) launched its 70-day #EndPJParalysis campaign. The initiative, founded by Professor Brian Dolan, a visiting Professor of Nursing at Oxford Institute for Nursing, Midwifery and Allied Health Research, aimed at achieving 1 million days of patients being up, dressed, and moving. During the campaign it was reported that 710,468 patients were up and mobile, with 703,161 of those patients dressed. Stories collected from patients during the campaign highlighted feelings of dignity and autonomy when being dressed in their own clothes (End PJ Paralysis, 2018). These examples demonstrate some of the ways in which clothing can be considered important within the psychosocial care of people in health and social care settings.

Clothing as creative practice

Clothing, and the way it is used by the individual, can be considered a form of creative practice (Bellass et al., 2018). For example, Buse and Twigg (2018) found that people with dementia used handbags to create privacy in the care home environment. They also found that people with dementia used their coats or jackets to signify that they wanted to leave the care home and go outside. This form of creativity, referred to as "little-c" creativity, is the engagement with creative practice in ways that are meaningful to everyday life (Kaufman and Beghetto, 2009). Drawing upon this notion, the findings of Buse and Twigg (2018), and current creative approaches in dementia care, in which sensory and material objects are used to promote calm, alleviate distress and anxiety, and enable well-being (Treadaway and Kenning, 2016), I present an approach that uses clothing and textile handling sessions as a method for creative engagement in the dementia care setting.

Clothing and textile handling sessions

Clothing and textile handling sessions derive from object handling sessions carried out with people with dementia (Camic et al., 2017; Griffiths et al., 2019; Johnson et al., 2017), but use solely items of clothing, textiles, and accessories. The sessions have been devised to explore items at a multisensory level (e.g., via touch), to encourage people to discuss potential meanings associated with the clothing, sharing their likes and dislikes, and to create or share stories. Due to the sensory properties of the items, the sessions allow for flexible participation, as they do not necessitate talking. This can be particularly empowering for those who may struggle with verbal communication, an issue common in those living with dementia.

Facilitation of clothing and textile handling sessions

Before carrying out a clothing and textile handling session, the facilitator would collate items thematically. Theming the sessions was found to be particularly useful in providing focus and structure. For example, a 'wedding'-themed session resulted in sourcing fabrics such as silk, lace, embellished, and ornate textiles. The sessions were carried out with small groups of between four and six residents and care home staff. During the sessions the facilitator would invite those taking part to interact with the items and to share any thoughts and feelings that they might wish to. Each person in the session would have the opportunity to handle, discuss, and even try on the item (where appropriate) if they wished. There were instances where some people chose to discuss, and share stories associated with the items, while some people engaged with the items through handling and exploring different tactile qualities, for example the clasp of a handbag. Throughout the session the facilitator asked open-ended questions such as: "How do you feel about the item? What does the object feel/look/smell like?" Once all the items had been handled and discussed, participants were invited to select their favorite item and, if they chose to, they could then share why that item was their favorite.

Overcoming barriers to facilitating clothing and textile handling sessions

Successful facilitation of the clothing and textiles sessions involved a facilitator who was able to adapt creatively and sensitively to the needs of residents living with dementia. A flexible approach was necessary when considering where the sessions took place, although a public space in the care home could allow for residents to access the session on a drop-in basis. The sessions were more successful when carried out in a separate room or quiet area of the care home. The support of care home staff in assisting residents to attend the sessions was therefore integral, while including staff in the sessions was a powerful way in which to encourage residents to join and participate in the sessions. Close involvement with care home staff also assisted in tailoring the sessions to the preferences of those residents attending.

Sourcing items for the sessions

Accessing items of clothing and textiles to use in the sessions can be challenging, as time and resources are required. Low-cost methods can be used, however—for example, local charity shops and thrift stores can be an effective way to find items. Moreover, residents and members of care home staff can be asked to bring in and share personal items, such as wedding photos and other items such as accessories. Images or photographs can be used effectively to provide alternative opportunities for engagement.

Developing the sessions

The clothing and textile handling sessions inspired a series of making workshops, whereby care home residents designed and constructed wearable fabric corsages. Residents were invited to wear their finished corsages; these then provoked opportunities for engagement and communication with other residents who offered compliments and critiqued each other's designs. The sessions could therefore be developed to sit alongside making workshops.

The clothing and textile handling sessions could be developed to work with different groups of people, and to be held within different settings. Moreover, the sessions could be used to facilitate engagement and conversations around different topics, as demonstrated in the work of the Marie Curie–funded "Design to Care" project (2018), in which sensory objects were found to be powerful tools with which to explore and envision end-of-life-care.

Conclusion

This chapter has sought to explore the ways in which clothing can be considered important to the individual. The type of clothing worn, the design of the clothing, and meanings associated with the clothing can all impact upon on the wearer. Therefore, the scope for clothing to be considered within the care of those in health and social care settings is vast, as is the potential for clothing to be used as a tool for creative and multisensory practice and engagement.

References

Adam, H. and Galinsky, A. (2012). Enclothed Cognition. *Journal of Experimental Social Psychology*, 48(4): 918–925.

Bellass, S., Balmer, A., May, V., Keady, J., Buse, C., Capstick, A., Burke, L., Bartlett, R. and Hogson, J. (2018). Broadening the Debate on Creativity and Dementia: A Critical Approach. *Dementia*. 18(7–8): 2799–2820.

Bovone, l. (2012). Fashion, Identity and Social Actors. In A. González and L. Bovone, eds, *Identities through fashion: a multidisciplinary approach*. London: Bloomsbury: 67–93.

Buse, C. and Twigg, J. (2015). Materializing Memories: Exploring the Stories of People with Dementia Through Dress. *Ageing and Society*, 36(6): 1115–1135.

Buse, C. and Twigg, J. (2018). Dressing Disrupted: Negotiating Care Through the Materiality of Dress in the Context of Dementia. *Sociology of Health and Illness*, 40(2): 340–352.

Camic, P., Hulbert, S. and Kimmel, J. (2017). Museum Object Handling: A Health-Promoting Community-Based Activity for Dementia Care. *Journal of Health Psychology*. 24(6): 787–798.

Chan, A., Lempp, H., Peabody, G., Simpson, C., Souza de, S., Galloway, J., Milasevic, M., Prout, L., Ellam, I., Esterine, T. and Gillingwater, E. (2018). Garment+ Challenging the Boundaries of Fashion for Those with Long-Term Physical Disabilities. *Journal of Dress History*, 2(1): 26–43.

Design for Care. (2018). Retrieved from www.mariecurie.org.uk/professionals/working-in-partnership/design-to-care (Accessed 19/2/2019).

Elliot, A. J., Greitemeyer, T. and Pazda, A. D. (2013). Women's Use of Red Clothing as a Sexual Signal in Intersexual Interaction. *Journal of Experimental Social Psychology*, 49(3): 599–602.

Elliot A.J. and Niesta D. (2008). Romantic Red: Red Enhances Men's Attraction to Women. *Journal of Personality and Social Psychology*, 95: 1150–1164.

End PJ Paralysis. (September, 2018). Retrieved from www.endpjparalysis.com/ (Accessed 19/2/2019).

Entwistle, J. (2015). *The Fashioned Body*. 2nd ed. Cambridge: Polity Press.

Farquhar, M. (2013). *Acts of Clothing*. (Performance). Palazzo Zenobio, Venice 55.

Fashion Unraveled. (September, 2018). Retrieved from http://exhibitions.fitnyc.edu/fashion-unraveled/ (Accessed19/2/2019).

Fleetwood-Smith, R., Hefferon, K. and Mair, C. (2019). "It's Like . . . It's Me . . .": Exploring the Lived Experience of Attachment Clothing. *International Journal of Fashion Studies*, 6(1): 41–62.

Griffiths, S., Dening, T., Beer, C. and Tischler, V. (2019). Mementos from Boots multisensory boxes – Qualitative evaluation of an intervention for people with dementia: Innovative practice. *Dementia*, 18(2): 793–801.

Iltanen-Tähkävuori, S., Wikberg, M., and Topo, P. (2012). Design and dementia: A case of garments designed to prevent undressing. *Dementia*, 11(1): 49–59.

Johnson, J., Culverwell, A., Hulbert, S., Robertson, M., and Camic, P. M. (2017). Museum activities in dementia care: Using visual analog scales to measure subjective wellbeing. *Dementia*, 16(5): 591–610.

Kaufman, J. C. and Beghetto, R. A. (2009). Beyond big and little: The four C model of creativity. *Review of General Psychology*, 13(1): 1–12.

Pazda, A. D., Elliot, A. J. and Greitemeyer, T. (2014). Perceived sexual receptivity and fashionableness: separate paths linking red and black to perceived attractiveness. *Color Research & Application*, 39(2): 208–212.

Topo, P. and Iltanen-Tähkävuori, S. (2010). Scripting Patienthood with Patient Clothing, *Social Science & Medicine*, 70(11): 1682–1689.

Treadaway, C. and Kenning, G. (2016). Sensor e-textiles: person centered co-design for people with late stage dementia, *Working with Older People*, 20(2): 76–85.

Woodward, S. (2007). *Why women wear what they wear*, Oxford: Berg Publishers.

33

CLASSICS

Peter Meineck

Introduction

Greek and Roman materials, particularly philosophical and medical texts, are continuing to be applied to modern medical practice by providing historical and cultural contexts to contemporary bioethical issues. These include topics such as the Hippocratic influence on Western medicine, concepts of plagues, gender and sexuality, medical terminology, ideas about anatomy, experimentation, mental illness, and the role of spirituality and belief systems in ancient medical practice. The academic study of such topics has become part of the wider scholarly field of medical or health humanities. Furthermore, under the aegis of narrative medicine, which seeks to combine the study, appreciation and empathetic effects of literary narratives with clinical medical practice, texts such as Homer's *Iliad* and *Odyssey*, ancient Greek plays, Virgil's *Aeneid*, and Ovid's *Metamorphoses* have provided fertile ground for the kind of joint close readings and collective reflections central to the effectiveness of many of these programs.[1]

The notion that certain classical works contain inherent themes, motifs, narrative structures, and performative devices intended to provoke some sort of healing response can be traced back to Aristotle. In *Poetics* he makes a series of rather enigmatic statements about the role of drama in provoking affective states that could, in turn, produce a state of *catharsis* in the spectator. The meaning of *catharsis*, which Aristotle does not elaborate on, has been debated, but by examining the term's usage in fifth-century Greek drama and in other texts of Aristotle, it seems safe to say that he means some sort of psychological purgation or healing through emotional response. Aristotle famously names *eleos* and *phobos* as two emotions, among others he does not name, as often most prone to induce *catharsis*. Most translators render *phobos* as fear, which is quite straightforward, but *eleos* tends to get translated as "pity," which is possibly misleading: perhaps the term "empathy" is more apt. This would certainly make sense with the little we do know of the ways in which drama was received in the classical period. Although we possess no contemporary critical responses or accounts of the performances themselves we do hear from Isocrates, Plato, and Aristotle that tragedy in particular was *pyschagogia*: it possessed the power to "move the soul."[2]

We can see powerful moments of performative *catharsis* in action within the Homeric texts, which predate Athenian drama by at least 100–200 years and probably existed far longer within a vibrant oral tradition. At the end of the first book of *The Iliad*, Zeus and Hera are both depicted quarrelling over the secret visit of Achilles' mother Thetis to

Olympus to plead with Zeus to help her son. Hera knows that Thetis is dangerous, and in the argument that follows, Zeus threatens his divine wife with physical violence. The anger of Zeus and Hera's fearful reaction casts a pall of despair over Olympus, which threatens the delicate celestial balance of power. The cure is to call on Hephaestus, the disfigured god of the forge and only son of Hera, to perform a rendition of his own story of how he was thrown off Olympus by Zeus. In the telling of this story, which was later enshrined as "The Return of Hephaestus" and performed at festivals to Dionysos throughout Greece, Hephaestus performs a little comedy, mocking his own disability (caused by Zeus) and changing the mood of the gods from gloom to pure glee. Hephaestus' comic turn produced the healing effects of laughter, refreshing a communal bond and restoring harmony to the world of the gods.

The second example comes from Book 8 of *The Odyssey* and is indicative of how classical texts have been used in programs aimed at the veteran community in the United States (and, to a much lesser extent, the United Kingdom). Here Odysseus is in disguise at the court of King Alcinous after 19 years away from home. The king's bard, Demodocus, begins to sing of the Trojan War, and the disguised guest tried to hide his tears as the warrior hears about the men he served with and their campaign. At the moment when the bard sings of the triumph of the Greeks, Odysseus lets out a cry of grief and cannot control his tears. The image Homer presents at this moment is of a Trojan woman mourning over her dead husband being forced away by the end of a Greek spear into a life of slavery. At this moment Odysseus reveals himself and because of his cathartic reaction to the song of the bard he is induced to tell his own story, which produces, in turn, a sense of empathy among the Phaeacian listeners and a desire to bring him safely home.

There are other links that have been found which indicate the close connection between the theater, performance, and healing in ancient Athenian society—for example, the establishment of the sanctuary of Asclepius, the god of healing, next to the Theatre of Dionysos on the southeastern slope of the Acropolis. The content of many of these plays often depicts the after effects of some kind of trauma, return from conflict or social upheaval. This may be indicative of the fact that throughout much of the fifth century BCE, Athens was at war and under the active threat of destruction. Veteran's Administration Psychiatrist Jonathan Shay, who applied Homer's works to mainly Vietnam War veterans in a clinical setting beginning in the 1990s, has correctly described Athenian drama as "theatre by combat veterans, performed by combat veterans for an audience of combat veterans" (Shay, 2002: 152–153). Shay proposes that the works of Homer and Greek drama may have been offering a kind of cultural therapy to a society that was itself traumatized by conflict and war. Perhaps this is why one of the most prolific applications of classics in a health humanities context has been by combat veterans of today.

Three programs have garnered a good deal of attention in the United States since 2007. These are: Homer for Veterans, led by Roberta Stuart, a classics professor at Dartmouth College in New Hampshire and based in New England; Theater of War, a national program that uses celebrity actors to read scenes from Greek drama to provoke discussion, led by Bryan Doerries; and the Warrior Chorus, a veteran participatory theater arts and public engagement program led by Aquila Theatre (see the chapter "Post-Conflict Resolution and the Health Humanities: The Warrior Chorus Program" in this volume).

Roberta Stewart's program began as a class at Dartmouth in 2008 when she noted how a veteran in that class was deeply affected by the content. Through this and further interactions with other veterans, and a first reading group organized at the Veteran's Affairs hospital in White River Junction in Vermont, her small local grass roots program has developed into a New England-wide project with the subtitle "Homer Can Help You." The basis of this program is using Homer to develop empathy and provide a place for a supportive environment where veterans can feel free to discuss their issues related to a classical text. Stewart has proposed that teaching empathy through Homer has enabled many veterans to create their own self-narrative that can help them overcome trauma by creating small community groups focused on reintegration of the veteran to civilian and home life.

Stewart's program has been expanding to other colleges and into their surrounding communities and using classics scholars to forge new local groups. She has also helped develop workshops with clinicians who work directly with veterans, including Army suicide prevention managers, and other such health workers where clinicians, academics, veterans, and military personnel work together to explore best practices for these kinds of programs.[3]

Bryan Doerries' Theater of War has perhaps garnered the most attention due to the program's use of celebrity actors such as Adam Driver, David Strathairn, Frances McDormand, Jake Gyllenhaal, Reg E. Cathey, and Ty Jones. Originally a vehicle for Doerries' translation of Sophocles' *Philoctetes*, the program partnered with the US Department of Defense to present its work on military bases throughout the United States and abroad. In it four actors perform a table reading of select scenes from the play, narrated by Doerries, and afterwards Doerries introduces a group of experts, usually military officers who take part in a "town hall"-type meeting where audience members can ask questions of Doerries and the panelists. Theater of War describes itself as offering theater-based projects that address public health issues, rather than as being direct therapy based, but it has been criticized as being too reductive, scripted, promoting an overly simplistic idea of PTSD, and too willing to conform to Pentagon-directed guidelines. That said, the program has shown how ancient drama can be an excellent and popular resource in health humanities programs.

Aquila Theatre pioneered work with combat veterans and the medical practitioners who care for them as part of their US-based national public programs, which have been running since 2007. These programs (Page and Stage, Ancient Greeks/Modern Lives, You|Stories, and the Warrior Chorus) have used ancient works to create community and dialogue between combat veterans and the wider American public. In addition, they developed training to that end with workshops, book groups, film clubs, public lectures, staged dramatic readings, filmmaking, and full theater productions mounted throughout the United States in venues as diverse as local public libraries, museums, and arts centers to the Metropolitan Museum of Art, the Obama White House, and the United States Congress at the US Capitol. In contrast to Theater of War, which used celebrities to generate interest and audiences, Aquila's programs, funded by the National Endowment for the Humanities, have placed veterans at the center of their programming, having them perform, moderate, advise, devise, and lead programming. Like Roberta Stewart's work, Aquila's programming is grassroots based, although with a national reach, and the program often partners with local public libraries, arts centers, theaters, museums, and galleries, particularly in underserved urban and rural communities.[4]

An offshoot of this public programming has been the development of special initiatives aimed at medical professionals who work with veterans. These have included programs with the psychiatry faculty at the Yale School of Medicine, the student therapists and New York University medical school, and participatory workshops with a number of Veterans Administration hospital staff at several VA hospitals throughout the United States. In addition to the public engagement parts of this programming, the work has also led to an academic conference and publication (*Combat Trauma and the Ancient Greeks*; Meineck and Konstan,

2014) that collected several articles on whether or not the issues of combat trauma could be identified in ancient texts.

One of the many positive results of this kind of programming was the development of a large and diverse community of veterans, who had mainly served in Vietnam, the Cold War, Iraq, and Afghanistan (although veterans from World War II and Korea also attended). Several of the program events were also held at a number of Veteran's Administration hospitals, where it soon became clear that the medical staff treating the veteran population would also benefit from this kind of programming. Following on from these events, the You|Stories and Warrior Chorus programs mounted events at a number of medical schools, including Yale and New York University, aimed at psychiatrists, psychologists, and therapists who specialized in the care of the veteran population. This volume included pieces by leaders in the field of trauma studies in antiquity such as Larry Trittle, an ancient historian and Vietnam War veteran, and Nancy Sherman, who has written on the issue of moral injury and trauma and how literature and drama has been used to address this. As a result of the applied nature of Aquila's work in this area, two chapters, one by philosopher and Vietnam Veteran Paul Woodruff, and another by Texas classicist Tom Palaima, examined the use of classical material by veterans in performative and public settings.

Notes

1 For example the Program in Narrative Medicine at Columbia University. www.narrativemedicine. org/about-narrative-medicine/ (accessed October 20, 2018).
2 Plato *Minos* 231a; Isocrates *Evagoras* 2.10 and 2.49; Aristotle *Poetics* 1450b. 16–21.
3 https://classicalstudies.org/amphora/ancient-narratives-and-modern-war-stories-reading-homer-combat-veterans-0 (last accessed November 11, 2018).
4 www.warriorchorus.org/ (last accessed November 11, 2018).

References

Meineck, P. and Konstan, D. (2014). *Combat Trauma and the Ancient Greeks*. Basingstoke: Palgrave.
Shay, J. 2002. *Odysseus in America: Combat Trauma and the Trials of Homecoming*. New York: Scribner.

34

HISTORY

Anna Greenwood

Introduction

When American neurosurgeon Harvey Cushing (1869–1939) allegedly stated that "a physician is obligated to consider more than a diseased organ, more even than the whole man—he must view the man in his world," he was indirectly asserting the importance of history in caring and health care (Dubos, 1965: 345). It is no linguistic coincidence that doctors, therapists, and carers take detailed patient *histories* as a routine part of their assessments for care, and it is without doubt that both the practice of health care and attitudes to what it means, and how it feels, to be well or unwell rest on thousands of years of precedent and experience. (In this contribution I speak about Western medicine, although I acknowledge that other important medical systems exist simultaneous to, or instead of, it in many non-Western contexts.) How humans navigate poor health, or caring for others who are ill, curiously simultaneously touches both deeply personal physiological and psychological histories (genetic and experiential) but also intricately draws upon the broader shifting landscape of contemporaneous values, fashions, and language. Furthermore, how we react, or how we might be treated, when unwell depends upon the historically rooted political and economic structures of the world in which we find ourselves reaching out for care.

Although an age-old connection, this recognition of the role of history in human health and society has only begun to be regularly articulated within the last decade. Its precedents lie within a historiographic movement that has debated since the 1980s why history is taught, written, and researched. This heralded the acknowledgement that history provides not only pleasure and insight into past events and experiences, but also has a definite social and political role to play in allowing people to critically understand the present. In John Tosh's words, to be a good citizen living as an integral part of a representative democracy, people should be "deliberative, for which a certain level of relevant knowledge and critical acumen is required" (Tosh, 1984: 140).

Growing out of these debates over the utility of history have been a number of initiatives, but perhaps none so successful and high profile as the History and Policy network founded in 2002, which seeks to explicitly stream policy recommendations and opinion pieces written by historians directly to the desks of journalists and government officials. With the UK National Health Service (NHS) at 70 years old, health has become one of the lead features on the website, although it should be noted that the specific cause of channelling historical research as a relevant means to improving health-care policies has been tirelessly championed within academic journals for over a decade by Virginia Berridge and Sally Sheard (Berridge, 2008, 2018; Sheard, 2008, 2018; see also Madsen, 2018).

These initiatives are to be loudly applauded, but the importance of history for human health is even broader than the guidance it might offer future policy design. History can also be a powerful source of inspiration and creativity, with the ability to nurture and console, and in some cases even heal. Analyzing previous experiences of illness and disease can impact positively upon both patients and carers, shaping the form, or attitude, of care given or received. Furthermore, this impact should not be limited to bodily health. Connecting with history can be a formidable way of helping people over trauma through reconciling memories, rationalizing pain, or contextualizing modern-day experiences against those of relatives, or preceding generations. Above all history shows us that we are not alone. Voices unearthed from the archive, material displays in cabinets and experiences shared in "witness" seminars all help to attach patients and carers to the past. As Helen Chatterjee, for example, has shown in her ground-breaking research on the role of museums in psychosocial health, this connectivity can help to rationalize experiences and be a powerful source of empowerment and cure.

History, health, and well-being

The evidence showing the importance of history in improving health and well-being is abundant and varied. When historian Emily Michelson found herself a patient in the Victoria Hospital, Kirkcaldy, she noticed that her historical training meant she "accepted nothing, and questioned everything," giving her "comfort with ambiguity" in a scientific environment which was typically accustomed to looking for clear-cut answers (Michelson, 2017). This lesson of embracing uncertainty taught to her through her historical research, Michelson felt, could usefully be absorbed by carers as well as patients in a variety of healthcare settings. Very recently Glen McGee has also asserted the importance of understanding history to improve clinical encounters, and cautioned that those practicing medicine are in danger of becoming "utterly unable to cope with a changing world because they lack roots in the history of their profession" (McGee, 2018:533).

History gives more than just a broader perspective and an ability to question and contextualize, however. Examples can be seen where engagement with history has become a "crucial part in legitimating new research protocols" (Kushner, 2008: 553). Researchers looking at Tourette syndrome and Kawasaki's disease, for example, have highlighted how an examination of past research hypotheses has influenced modern scientific research on these conditions (Kushner, 2008). Without reference to history, many practical health improvements in society would not have been implemented. Water and food safety, sanitation, vaccination, car safety, malaria prevention, and the installation of anti-suicide barriers, to name just a few disparate examples, all relied on testimony gleaned through historical experiences before their widespread employment.

Most prominently, evidence from historians has been sought in major legal cases or public enquiries, which in turn have informed attitudes to both somatic and mental health. Leading this trend were two historians of occupational health, Author McIvor and Ronnie Johnston, who in 2001 published their interviews of 31 people who had worked with asbestos between 1940 and 1990 to create a vivid picture of the way this exposure impacted the health of individuals and families. Evidence from this historical survey was then mobilized as part of the national campaign to ban asbestos in Scotland, which lobbied government to bear some responsibility for the high asbestos death toll "because of the sheer inadequacy of workplace regulation" (Johnston and McIvor, 2001).

Similarly, American historian Allan Brandt made ground-breaking contributions as an expert witness in a landmark 2006 court case involving tobacco companies, in which he explained how they had manipulated the scientific debate over the risks of smoking in the 1950s (Brandt, 2004, 2009). More recently, the mobilization of historians in the British High Courts has helped to bring justice to several Kenyan individuals, the brutality perpetrated against whom had been hitherto swept under the carpet by British colonial regime (Anderson, 2005; Elkins, 2005, 2014). Closer to home, historians have helped in inquiries to bring psychological peace to those who have previously had none, such as the contextual evidence provided by historians for the inquiry into the serial abuse conducted by TV presenter Jimmy Savile, released February 2015 (Lampard and Marsden, 2015).

These formal avenues for activism reveal just one route whereby history can demonstrate its power to improve health and well-being. Another important use of the discipline can be seen via the numerous websites listed at the end of this section, signposting multiple initiatives using history as the disciplinary glue to connect communities. Oral history has been particularly important in this regard providing archives of health experience as resources for compassion and support. Oral history, furthermore, does not only act a supportive reference point for modern sufferers; it can also be active therapy. One particular scheme inviting the production of audio life histories, undertaken at the Sheffield Macmillan Unit for Palliative Care, conducted an analysis of the benefits for terminally ill individuals participating in their project and found them to be numerous. The process of remembering stimulated by inviting patients to make their own histories through audio recordings not only reinforced people's "sense of identity, at a time when circumstances may have changed their identities out of recognition," but was valuable in terms of enhancing "their own sense of dignity" (Winslow et al., 2009: 128). Benefits were also reported as accruing to the practitioners and carers who worked on this project, in that it gave staff a better understanding of "the impact of life-threatening disease on patients' identities and lifestyles" (Winslow et al., 2009: 130). In short, history projects such as this one can be powerful training tools for those administering care as well as cathartic for the sufferers and their families.

One immensely successful case study illustrating the role of history in health can be seen in the "Diabetes Stories" project lead by David Matthews of Oxford University, funded by the Wellcome Trust. This project recorded over 100 oral histories of diabetes, collected mostly from patients, but also from patient family members and health-care professionals using interview techniques that encouraged participants to indulge in "a freedom to recall the mundane and the routine." The project was ground-breaking because of its large chronological coverage, moving from the period when insulin treatment began in 1923, through to the modern day. As such, the resource provides a valuable window into changing attitudes and practices over a transformative period in diabetes care. Furthermore, since diabetes is largely managed by patients within their own homes, these experiences make a vital contribution to the historical record, by giving a rare insight into health management within the domestic sphere.

The benefits of this sort of project were immediately celebrated by visitors to the project's website. One American with diabetes declared that "[t]he interviews gave me a sense of myself in time, an appreciation for modern technologies, and they make me feel more grounded, less alone." Another diabetic man in the United Kingdom confessed that he had always worried "whether it is truly possible to lead a long and normal life," but felt comforted that "[u]pon reading and listening to some of the accounts ... I realised this was more than possible" (Jonah Berele, Chicago, United States and Lee Hawley, Bromley, United Kingdom; see http://www.diabetes-stories.com/research-transcript.asp (accessed November 30, 2019). These, and many other testimonies like them, prove the usefulness of approaches beyond science to deal with sickness, injury, and anxiety. They illustrate the multifarious ways that history can deepen sympathies, extend imaginations, and create therapeutic communities beyond the customary restrictions of geography and time.

Resources

- An archive of historical accounts of mental illness compiled by Gail A. Hornstein, Mount Holyoke College, United States: http://phsj.org/wp-content/uploads/2007/10/Narratives-of-Mental-Illness-Gail-Hornstein1.pdf (accessed November 30, 2019).
- The "Making Cancer History Voices Oral History Collection" of the University of Texas M.D. Anderson Cancer Center, United States: http://cdm16333.contentdm.oclc.org/cdm/ (accessed November 30, 2019).
- Personal histories from Sheffield Macmillan Unit for Palliative Care, UK: www.sheffield.ac.uk/snm/research/oralhistory/main (accessed November 30, 2019).
- The National Alliance for Museums, Health and Wellbeing, UK founded by Professor Helen Chatterjee: https://museumsandwellbeingalliance.wordpress.com (accessed November 30, 2019).
- Using historical objects for people with dementia, a project led by Liverpool Museums, UK: https://houseofmemories.co.uk/things-to-do/my-house-of-memories-app/ (accessed November 30, 2019).
- History and Policy Network: www.historyandpolicy.org (accessed November 30, 2019).
- Ronnie Johnston and Arthur McIvor, "Oral Histories of the Asbestos Tragedy in Scotland", International Ban Asbestos Secretariat, 8 June 2001 http://ibasecretariat.org/eas_rj_am_scotland.php (accessed November 30, 2019).

References

Anderson, D. (2005). *Histories of the Hanged: the Dirty War in Kenya and the End of Empire*. New York and London: W.W. Norton.

Berridge, V. (2008). History Matters? History's Role in Health Policy Making. *Medical History*, 52: 211–226.

Berridge, V. (2018). Why Policy Needs History (and Historians). *Health, Economics, Policy, and Law*, 13: 369–381.

Brandt, A.M. (2004). From Analysis to Advocacy: Crossing Boundaries as a Historian of Health Policy. In F. Huisman and J.H. Warner, eds, *Locating Medical History*. Baltimore: Johns Hopkins University Press: 460–484.

Brandt, A.M. (2009). *The Cigarette Century: The Rise, Fall and Deadly Persistence of the Product that Defined America*. New York: Basic Books.

Dubos, R. (1965). *Man Adapting*. New Haven: Yale University Press.

Elkins, C. (2005). *Imperial Reckoning: the Untold Story of Britain's Gulag in Kenya*. New York: Henry Holt and Co.

Elkins, C. (2014). *Britain's Gulag: The Brutal End of Empire in Kenya*. London: Bodley Head.

Johnston, R. and McIvor, A. (2001). Oral Histories of the Asbestos Tragedy in Scotland. International Ban Asbestos Secretariat, 8 June 2001. http://ibasecretariat.org/eas_rj_am_scotland.php (Accessed 30/11/2019).

Kushner, H. (2008). History as a Medical Tool. *Lancet*, 371(9612): 551–553.

Lampard, K. and Marsden, E. (2015). *Themes and Lessons Learnt from NHS Investigations into Matters Relating to Jimmy Savile, Independent Report for the Secretary of State for Health*. London: Department of Health and Social Care. https://assets.publishing.service.gov.uk/government/uploads/system/uploads/attachment_data/file/407209/KL_lessons_learned_report_FINAL.pdf (Accessed 19/2/2019).

Madsen, W. (2018). History in Health: Health Promotion's Underexplored Tool for Change. *Public Health*, 154: 118–122.

McGee, G. (2018). The Importance of Medical History in Medical Education. *BMJ*, 324: 533.

Michelson, E. (2017). Historians Make the Best Healthcare Workers. *Times Higher Education*, January 22, 2017. https://www.timeshighereducation.com/blog/historians-make-best-healthcare-workers (Accessed 30/11/2019).

Sheard, S. (2008). History in Health and Health Services: Exploring the Possibilities. *Journal Epidemiology Community Health*, 62: 740–744.

Sheard, S. (2018). History Matters: The Critical Contribution of Historical Analysis to Contemporary Health Policy and Healthcare. *Healthcare Analysis*, 26(2): 140–154.

Tosh, J. (1984). *The Pursuit of History: Aims Methods and New Directions in the Study of Modern History.* London: Longman.

Winslow, M., Hitchlock, K. and Noble, W. (2009). Recording Lives: The Benefits of an Oral History Service. *European Journal of Palliative Care*, 16(3): 128–130.

35

LIFE-WRITING

Frances Cadd

Introduction

The fundamental purpose of life-writing, or writing in any form, is communication in order to facilitate understanding of a certain subject. Both the practice of writing and the reading of writing are tools for sense-making; the process through which an individual interprets and gives meaning to his or her experiences (Varner Gunn, 1982; Gring-Pemble, 1998). Through life-writing, then, one can find meanings in experiences and circumstances, and come to a better understanding of themselves and their place in the world they inhabit (Roper, 2001; Walton, 2014). Other chapters in this volume have discussed the therapeutic purposes and cathartic effects that sense-making through writing or storytelling, in various forms, can have on individual producers and consumers of writing. This chapter is concerned with how life-writing can provide an understanding of how both the physical and social environments that individuals engage with impact and influence health and well-being. It analyzes how life-writing provides access to three types of information that are particularly useful for understanding present and future health and health care practices and attitudes:

1. "Everyday" or "ordinary" practices and processes.
2. Mentalities and attitudes.
3. Subjective perspectives and connections.

Each section will begin by providing an overview of how life-writing materials have been used by researchers to obtain information, followed by suggestions for how these methods can be applied to inform our understanding of health and well-being-related subjects and practices. The sections conclude with illustrative examples drawn from my research into the British nurse and political campaigner Avis Hutt (1917–2010), using her oral testimonies about her experiences as both nurse and patient to indicate how the ideas and methods described might be put into practice in the health humanities. While this chapter presents a distinctively historical perspective, the ideas, methods, and techniques applied to access information from the life-writing of individuals are transferable and can be used in contemporary research in a multitude of fields of scholarly and practical health-care research.

"Everyday" or "ordinary" practices and processes

Life-writing materials are particularly valuable for recovering information, details, or accounts that would have otherwise been lost due to having been disregarded for being "mundane," "ordinary," or "everyday" (Grele, 1992, Cauvin, 2016; Thomson, 2016). From the 1960s, scholars began to turn away from examining the lives and achievements of well-known, established, and usually "extraordinary" individuals and instead towards recovering the voices and reconstructing the everyday, routine lived experience of "ordinary" men and women (Thompson, 1963; Zemon Davis, 1984; Steedman, 1987, 2009, 2013; Renders et al., 2017). Diaries and letters are particularly useful for recovering the "everyday" and "ordinary"; their immediacy and proximity to historical events ensures that details, which may be forgotten in later accounts, are more likely to be recorded. Their ephemerality, brevity, but also practicality has meant that they were more widely practiced forms of life-writing by ordinary men and women (Dobson and Ziemann, 2009). Meanwhile, the distance from the historical moment oral testimony and autobiography provides makes them useful for illuminating daily experiences and activities, since data that can be recalled many years later usually indicates routine or "norms," being remembered as a result of its frequency, repetition, or reoccurrence. Accounts recorded a significant length of time after the event also allow the individual to compare and contrast their previous and present experiences, drawing attention to change—or perhaps lack of change—over time (Abrams, 2010). Capturing the "ordinary" and the "everyday" is of particular benefit to the health humanities as it can reveal micro-processes and ephemeral factors and situations that impact on health and well-being. It also records the way that ordinary individuals managed ill-health, or maintained good health, on a day-to-day basis, reminding us that health is not a constant state and can fluctuate, not only day by day but also minute by minute.

An extract from an interview with Hutt, conducted in 1998 by nursing historian Stephanie Kirby, demonstrates how everyday perspectives found in life-writing can provide valuable information which can inform health-care practices. When asked what care and treatment she received if she became ill or injured during her nursing training in the late 1930s, she responded:

> Well I can remember now the septic fingers I went home with … I would go home and my mother would put bread poultice, she was a country girl remember, and I would go on duty and do dressings with it.
>
> *(Kirby, 1998)*

This apparently simple memory provides much information about the day-to-day health of nurses and treatments of minor ailments in the 1930s. First, Hutt's description of her septic fingers illustrates how her everyday working environment and routine could impact her health. The casual way that she refers to these septic fingers indicates that Hutt accepted that these sorts of injuries and ailments were part and parcel of her nursing work: they were not extraordinary or especially significant. Second, the passage reveals how, rather than taking her to hospital, her mother would use an old folk remedy, a bread poultice, to draw out the infection. She notes the irony of this by explaining how she would "go on duty and do dressings with it," providing more "modern" medical care despite using traditional methods herself. Later in the interview, Hutt remarks that these kinds of practices were common, since not many people went to hospitals for treatments "because of the financial thing" (Kirby, 1998). This draws attention to how privatized health care in the 1930s, before the UK National Health Service (NHS), meant that ordinary men and women would often treat themselves at home with traditional remedies rather than seeking expensive medical treatment from their local doctor or hospital.

Mentalities and attitudes

Anthropologist Clifford Geertz argued that "signs," such as language, gestures, clothes, buildings, and objects, hold specific meanings for the members of a society that use them. An analysis of these languages, actions, and objects can therefore uncover "cultural scripts," or shared mentalities, attitudes, and practices held by a community and accepted as the norm (Geertz, 1973; see also Thomas, 1963; Lüdtke, 1995). British cultural historian Matt Houlbrook has demonstrated how individuals drew on these cultural scripts to shape the stories they told about themselves in order to aid communication with others. These stories are therefore specific to the time and place in which they took shape and act as "mirrors in which we might see reflected the worlds through which [that individual] moved" (Houlbrook, 2016 :17; see also Israel, 1999; Lepore, 2001). The stories individuals tell about their lives, and the language and techniques they use to do so, can illuminate shared mentalities or attitudes a society or group hold towards a certain subject.

Understanding how groups think and the beliefs they hold is clearly vital for communication between health-care practitioners and policy makers and the communities among which they seek to enact positive change or spark development; life-writing is one tool for accessing such insights. For example, when reviewing practices and policies it would be useful to understand the mentalities and behaviors of those treating and caring for patients in order to consider how changes to their working environment or practices can affect their work. Avis Hutt, discussing the ethos of the nursing profession in the 1930s, explained that:

> If you were ill you had to report, and of course … we got very ill, [so if] we went on duty, we caused, you remember Florence [Nightingale]'s famous expression 'the hospitals who do the patient no harm' … My first ward was a ward of … tuberculosis young men beautiful young men, shiny eyes, high male flush, coughing; they'd all be dead in two weeks … whole ward of them … So that when I think of the risks we took, it didn't seem a hardship because we were doing a job which was important, and the patients were so in need.
>
> *(Kirby, 1998)*

Although Hutt is describing her own experience, she uses the collective "we" and the hypothetical "if you were" to demonstrate that these behaviors and attitudes were shared among nurses in the 1930s. Hutt remembers the rules and regulations that guided her approach to her own health, noting how if she was ill she "*had to*" report it to matron, not for her own safety and well-being but in order to prevent her from causing the patient harm either due to her impaired abilities while ill or from passing on infections and diseases. Moreover, she was willing to risk her own health by working on the tuberculosis ward, believing that caring for those dying patients took priority. She reveals the profession's "patient first" and "patient-centred" approach to care, advocated by Florence Nightingale in *Notes on Nursing* (1860), whereby the nurse should act solely in the best interests of the patient, not themselves, ensuring the patient received the best care. This highlights the belief in nursing as a vocation—requiring absolute dedication to the cause of relieving suffering, even to the extent of self-detriment and self-sacrifice. Understanding the values that underpin and influence the work of nurses is useful when implementing structural changes to health-care systems and practices, as it will highlight possible ways those changes will impact the work nurses carry out.

Subjective perspectives and new connections

The subjectivity of individual life-writing can provide a specific and unique frame through which to view and understand a time and place (Koven, 2014). Fields of study that examine marginalized groups, such as gender, race, or disability studies, have been particularly influential in demonstrating how diverse past experiences intersect to form an individual subjectivity, which impacts and shapes their understanding of present and future events and experiences (see Kafer, 2013; Crenshaw, 1989, White, 2001). Life-writing can therefore illuminate the complexities of human experience and how a time and place can be experienced, interpreted, and understood differently by each individual. This can alert readers to new connections between different events, forces, and factors, and it can also challenge generalizations made about a specific subject, providing alternative perspectives (Stanley, 1987; Palmer, 2014).

Life-writing therefore can facilitate a holistic approach to care as by considering the individual not just as a body that requires treating, but as a human interacting and being influenced by the world around them, awareness can be raised about different social and cultural factors that can impact health and well-being. In gender historian Joan Scott's words, individuals and their life-narratives "remind us of the strangeness that refuses to be systematized by the order we want to impose on things. In their particularity they resist the simplicity of universal assumptions based on sameness" (Scott, 2011: 207; see also Zemon Davis, 2011). The individuality of each patient is crucial for health-care practitioners to consider; what works for one person may not work for all due to physiological and circumstantial differences, but also because each person will experience and manage an illness or condition subjectively, interpreting the present from past experiences in a way that makes sense to them.

Interestingly, Hutt provides an example of this in practice as she explains in her interview how her own subjective experience of moving from a comfortable middle-class upbringing in suburban Surrey to working as a nurse in the slums of Stepney allowed her to connect various social, economic, and political factors that impacted the health of patients in London's East End in the 1930s. Her move to the East End was "a bit of a culture shock," since while growing up in Surrey she was never "deprived in the way that I saw when I became a nurse in Stepney, that social deprivation, material deprivation, and also spiritual deprivation" (Morgan, 2002). She identified the connection between such deprivation and the patients she saw and whose case histories she took on the wards, speaking of "a revolving door," Hutt explained how when treating patients with marasmus, or malnutrition, "we would give them good basic nursing care, ensure that they took their meals ... get them better, send them home, they'd be back again" (Holder, 1998; Kirby, 1998). The medical system was operating independently of public health and social welfare whereas, in Hutt's view, they needed to work together. This experience encouraged her to join campaigns for a universal, comprehensive health-care system free at the point of use in the 1930s, which would later evolve into ideas for the National Health Service in Britain, as she believed this type of health-care system would respond better to the needs of the patients whose lives she had witnessed in the East End. In terms of health care and welfare today, Hutt's subjective experience is useful for reminding us how various social factors can impact on health and that inequality in health standards and provisions exist.

In summary, this chapter has presented three key ways in which the study of individual lives and subjectivities through their life-writing can be used to help inform understandings of health, well-being, and health-care practices in the past, present, and future. These uses of life-writing and individual lives provide insight into how an individual is both impacted by and impacts on the milieu they inhabit, illuminating causes and effects over time and space and presenting opportunities for changes and developments to improve the experience of health and the prevision of health care today and tomorrow.

References

Abrams, L. (2010). *Oral History Theory*. London: Routledge.

Cauvin, T. (2016) *Public History: A Textbook of Practice*. New York: Routledge.

Crenshaw, K. (1989) Demarginalizing the Intersection of Race and Sex: A Black Feminist Critique of Antidiscrimination Doctrine, Feminist Theory and Antiracist Politcs. *University of Chicago Legal Forum*, 139–167.

Dobson, M. and Ziemann, B. eds, (2009). *Reading Primary Sources: The Interpretation of Texts from Nineteenth- and Twentieth-Century History*. London: Routledge.

Geertz, C. (1973) *The Interpretation of Cultures*. New York: Basic Books.

Grele, R. (1992) Useful Discoveries: Oral History, Public History, and the Dialectic of Narrative. *The Public Historian*, 13(2): 61–84.

Gring-Pemble, L.M. (1998). Writing Themselves into Consciousness: Creating a Rhetorical Bridge Between the Public and Private Spheres. *Quarterly Journal of Speech*, 84(1): 41–61.

Holder, S. (1998) Avis Hutt interviewed by Stanley Holder, *Royal College of Nursing Archive*, T123/B (1998).

Houlbrook, M. (2016). *Prince of Tricksters: The Incredible True Story of Netley Lucas, Gentleman Crook*. Chicago: University of Chicago Press.

Israel, K. (1999) *Names and Stories: Emilia Dilke and Victorian Culture*. Oxford: Oxford University Press.

Kafer, A. (2013). *Feminist, Queer, Crip*. Bloomington, Indiana: Indiana University Press.

Kirby, S. (1998) Avis Hutt interviewed by Stephanie Kirby. Royal College of Nursing Archive, T123/A. London: RCN.

Koven, S. (2014). *The Match Girl and the Heiress*. Princeton: Princeton University Press.

Lepore, J. (2001). Historians Who Love Too Much: Reflections on Microhistory and Biography. *The Journal of American History*, 88(1): 129.

Lüdtke, A. (1995) *The History of Everyday Life: Reconstructing Historical Experiences and Ways of Life*. Princeton, NJ: Princeton University Press.

Morgan, K. (2002) Avis Hutt interviewed by Kevin Morgan, *British Library*, C1049/70. T1-T2 (29 November 2002).

Palmer, J. (2014). Past Remarkable: Using Life Stories to Trace Alternative Futures. *Futures*, 64: 29–37.

Renders, H., de Haan, B. and Harmsma, J. (2017). The Biographical Turn: Biography as Critical Method in the Humanities and in Society. In: H. Renders, B. de Haan and J. Harmsma, eds, *The Biographical Turn: Lives in History*. London: Routledge Taylor & Francis: 3–12.

Roper, M. (2001). Splitting in Unsent Letters: Writing as a Social Practice and a Psychological Activity. *Social History*, 26(3): 318–339.

Scott, J.W. (2011). Storytelling. *History and Theory*, 50(2): 203–209.

Stanley, L. (1987). Biography as Microscope or Kaleidoscope? The Case of "power" in Hannah Cullwick's Relationship with Arthur Munby. *Women's Studies International Forum*, 10(1): 19–31.

Steedman, C. (1987). *Landscape for a Good Woman: A Story of Two Lives*. New Brunswick, NJ: Rutgers University Press.

Steedman, C. (2009). On Not Writing Biography. *New Formations*, 67: 15–24.

Thomson, A. (2016). Life Stories and Historical Analysis. In: S. Gunn and L. Faire, eds, *Research Methods for History*. 2nd edition. Edinburgh: Edinburgh University Press: 104–121.

Steedman, C. (2013) *An everyday life of the English Working Class: work, self and sociability in the Early Nineteenth Century*. Cambridge: Cambridge University Press.

Varner Gunn, J. (1982) *Autobiography: Toward a Poetics of Experience*. Philadelphia, PA: University of Pennsylvania Press.

Thomas, K. (1963) History and Anthropology. *Past & Present*, 24(1): 3–24.

Thompson, E.P. (1963) *The Making of the English Working Class*. New York: Pantheon Books.

Walton, H. (2014) *Writing Methods in Theological Reflection*. London: SCM Press.

White, D.G. (2001) Nationalism and Feminism in the Black Atlantic. In: Grimshaw, P., Holmes, K., and Lake, M. (eds.) *Women's Rights and Human Rights: International Perspectives*. London: Palgrave.

Zemon Davis, N. (1984) *The Return of Martin Guerre*. Massachusetts: Harvard University Press.

Zemon Davis (2011). Decentering History: Local Stories and Cultural Crossings in a Global World. *History and Theory*, 50(2): 188–202.

36

READING

Philip Davis and Josie Billington

Introduction

This chapter focuses on a specific model of shared reading, developed and delivered by The Reader, a UK national charity dedicated to extending literary reading to hard-to-reach communities. The Reader began life as a small outreach unit of the School of English at the University of Liverpool, taking serious literature out of the tutorial room, into the wider world, for people who typically were not literature students and often, although literate, were not habitual readers at all (Davis, 2011; Macmillan, 2010). Shared reading groups are distinct from the conventional book clubs, which have enjoyed a revival in recent decades (Hartley, 2002).[1] The material is not read in advance, nor confined to contemporary works or a restricted (middle-class) demographic. The literature is not chosen for its targeted relevance as in self-help bibliotherapy (Hicks, 2006) or reading interventions that seek to treat particular cases, conditions, or moods (Bate et al., 2016; Berthoud and Elderkin, 2013). Rather, poems, short stories, and novels from the whole range of the literary heritage down the ages are read aloud, together, live, and the reading is regularly interrupted for group members to share thoughts and responses (Billington, 2016; Davis, 2013).

Shared reading thereby resurrects or continues two time-honoured Western traditions. First is the practice of reading aloud, a culture successively overtaken by print, televisual, and digital cultures (Ong, 2012; Wolf, 2008). Second is a faith in literature's intrinsic capacity to affect mental and emotional states and make them available to further thought. The earliest authenticated library, founded by Pharaoh Rameses II in ancient Thebes, bore the inscription over its portals, "the house of healing for the soul" (Lutz, 1978). The Reader re-activates these traditions in particular from two periods of renewal in English poetry. Renaissance poetics, in its revival of ancient and classical culture in the Elizabethan age, offered a lyric model for the contemplation and consolation of human sorrow through aesthetic achievement. George Puttenham, in *The Art of English Poesy* (1589), drew a direct analogy between the poet and the physician, claiming that the poem, as a repository of intense private pain, offers, cathartically, "one short sorrowing" as "the remedy of a long and grievous sorrow" (Davis and Billington, 2016a:. 397). For The Reader these qualities are further developed in a second period of poetic revolution marked by the "Preface to *Lyrical Ballads*" (1802) with its democratic ambitions for the uses of poetry in the common world—above all in Wordsworth's "sorrow that is not sorrow to hear of" (Wordsworth et al., 1979). But there is a third period that also forms an essential part of The Reader's ethos, with particular relation to far-reaching social issues beyond the world of literature, arising out of the Industrial Revolution and the crisis of meaning involved in secularization (MacIntyre, 1981). The Reader's shared reading model consciously builds on the twin literary ambitions of Victorian realism in its broad humanizing endeavor: to represent ordinary life, through the development of prose fiction as well as poetry, and to reach *into* the real life of the reader, transformatively (Rose, 2010).

Shared reading and mental health: research findings

Currently, there are 500 Reader groups across the United Kingdom and in Europe, in health and social care contexts, and community and secure settings, including drug and rehabilitation centers, prisons, hospitals, drop-in centers in local medical practices, dementia care homes, facilities for looked-after children, schools, and libraries. It works through three stages comprising initial involvement with the text, then sustained engagement with it both textually and personally, until some individual change or realization freely arises out of the immersion: in brief "Getting In, Staying In, and Breaking Through." Published studies from the Centre for Research into Reading, Literature and Society (CRILS, University of Liverpool, UK) have shown its value in relation to mental health in community and health-care settings (Hodge et al., 2007), specifically depression (Dowrick et al., 2012), dementia (Billington et al., 2013a) and chronic pain (Billington et al., 2016a, 2014).

The benefits of Reader groups include: literature's offering of a language for the triggered feelings and a stimulus to mental agility in a way that few activities demand with equivalent directness and immediacy (Billington, 2012); slowed deep thinking in intrinsic relation to personal emotion, where the text is not a two-dimensional manual but a voiced living presence (Billington et al., 2013b); and the memory or recovery of lost aspects of being, where the reading matter helps bridge the gap between a current unwell self and a past healthy self, and enables integration of fragmented parts of the self into a functioning whole (Gray et al., 2016). The group setting and the literature offered within it by a Reader Leader provide a compassionate alternative (and partial antidote) to the experience of being judged, exposed, or disregarded within the world, enabling the compression of lived experience in moments of sudden reflection and verbal realization (Longden et al., 2015).

Related research in the field of reading and neuroscience has suggested that the inner neural processing of language when a mind reads a complex line of poetry has the potential to re-excite and modify existing brain pathways and shift reading acts from left-hemisphere automaticity to areas in the right hemisphere that some neuroscientists have interpreted as being implicated in recognition and autobiographical involvement (e.g., Ciaramelli et al., 2008), influencing emotion networks and memory function away from habitual or depressed defaults (Davis et al., 2012; Jacobs, 2015; O'Sullivan et al., 2015; Peters et al., 2017). Current research suggests how literary reading addresses, through very specific felt instances, meaning-of-life issues or the sense of lost purpose, stimulating high-level mentalization, and shows that it does so with a freedom of immediate individual response not offered in the prescribed stages of a step-by-step top-down therapeutic agenda (Billington et al., 2016a, 2016b).

A brief case history

Laura, a woman in her early twenties, is attending a weekly community reading group. She is suffering significant neurological impairment resulting from an accident with an electric fence during a gap-year in South Africa. The group have been reading Robert Frost's "The Road Not Taken," in which the speaker recalls walking through a wood and coming to a fork in the pathway. The choice of one path and not the other, he concludes in retrospect, is what, ever since, "has made all the difference" (Lathem, 1988: 105).

Here, for the first time, Laura speaks about the difference her accident made to her life.

> A lot of my health problems started when I went to South Africa ... But if I hadn't gone I would still probably be like: wanting to go here, want to go there. At the same time, would I have the same mentality as now? Perhaps something worse could have happened. Or I could have been worse if it had been easier.

Then, suddenly:

> But if anyone was thinking of going and doing exploring, I'd say, don't do it, don't do this, don't do that. I'd be awful if if ... I'd be awful if I ever had ... if I ever had ... if I ever had ... if I ever had ... if I ever had ... children. Because I'd be like, you're not doing *that*.

Laura's neurological impairment means that she has occasional difficulty with fluent speech. But it is here statistically that her stutter lasts longest in all the recorded sessions, when her intermittent speech difficulty comes under most emotional strain. She stutters five or more times "if I ever had" before poignantly managing to complete the sentence with "children." To Laura, in her condition, despite her youth, the possibility within that "if" must seem unlikely. And "if" is itself a key word of the poem: in the closing line of the penultimate stanza, the speaker doubts "if" he will be coming back. That feeling of "if" has to do with the negotiation of painful areas of feeling, through unanswered questions and unresolved matter. That is how literature offers a holding-ground for experiences otherwise hard to contain or investigate (Davis, 2013). Laura's condition only makes more evident what other participants experience: a creative inarticulacy, triggered by literary reading, wholly distinguished from the norms of automatic opinion and habitual cliché, or the set languages of diagnosis and therapy (Billington, 2016).

In a later session, in relation to Robert Herrick's seventeenth-century lyric "To Anthea, Who May Command Him Anything," Laura (with no formal experience of studying literature since school) saw how important sonically was the poem's repeatedly minute use of the comma: "Bid me to live, and I will live," "Bid me to weep, and I will weep" (Ricks, 1999: 144) in making the lover's pledge freely weighed rather than automatically given. When the CRILS team showed her selected clips of this session and asked about her suddenly fixing on that little thing the comma, she said she had learnt a lot about the working of the brain in acts of communication since her accident. At the neurological support center, they had told her about how much percentage in every act of communication is due to body language and tone, more than the words themselves.

> But here you've only got the words on the pages. Which is why you need to be careful if you write a letter or a text. You don't have all the hand gestures; there is a lot more when in person. You only can give clues, like that comma, as to how it should be heard said. When something is well written, your head understands all the extra stuff which it looks for in communication, it *reads* from it. But when you're reading something badly written, or too literal, your brain is unable to fill in the blanks.

The challenge of literature, especially in areas of still vital emotional concern taken from the strong language of an earlier age, offers an alternative discourse to (often predictable or stereotypical) modern forms of expression, enabling a move away from safe, habitual, or default positions. Close attention to the difficulty and linguistic depth of the literary text works as a profitable obstacle to simple facility, literal explanation, or automatic opinion— accessing areas of experience for which readers have no ready language yet which they need to get out and work at.

Implementation and impact

The Reader has a national and international mission to develop a reading revolution for the sake of mental health in the deepest sense. There are related organizations and partnerships in Denmark, Belgium, Sweden, Norway, Germany, Australia, and New Zealand. Research and evaluation attract funding but the major barrier to further widespread growth is the economic cost of training and funding reader group leaders. With the support of Big Lottery funding, The Reader has therefore developed a national network of trained volunteers—to work as "Reader Leaders" within health, business, or community-led projects to address the needs of those at risk of loneliness or poor mental health across the age range, from children to older people living with dementia.[2]

Assessment of the benefit of shared reading includes potential savings from decreased use of national health facilities; increased sense of purpose and meaning in life measured by the Ryff scale of psychological well-being (Longden et al., 2015); and individual evidence from research interviews stimulated by filmed excerpts of participants' reading group sessions (Davis et al., 2016b). "With books and poems, it makes you look at things honestly," says one member of a reading group held within a drug and alcohol rehabilitation center, "It's harder to lie around them. In other therapy groups you're often just talking about actions and behaviours. But this is about feelings" (9). "It is therapy by stealth," another member adds (51).

Notes

1 Arts and Humanities Research Council study, Cultural Value (AH/P014356/1), in which Shared Reading groups were filmed and sound-recorded (see Longden et al., 2015). The study was conducted according the University of Liverpool research ethics protocols, including informed consent by participants. Pseudonyms are used.
2 For information on The Reader's Read to Lead training courses and a suite of online training films, developed by CRILS and funded by Arts and Humanities Research Council (AHRC), see: www.thereader.org.uk.

References

Bate, J., Byrne, P., Ratcliffe, S. and Schuman, A. (2016). *Stressed/Unstressed: Classic Poems to Ease the Mind*. London: William Collins.
Berthoud E. and Elderkin, S. (2013). *The Novel Cure: An A–Z of Literary Remedies*. Edinburgh: Cannongate.
Billington, J. (2012). Prison Reading Groups in Practice and Theory. *Critical Survey*, 23(3): 67–85.
Billington, J. (2016). *Is Literature Healthy?* Literary Agenda Series. Oxford: Oxford University Press.
Billington, J., Carroll, J., Davis, P., Healey, C. and Kinderman, P. (2013a). A Literature-Based Intervention for Older People Living with Dementia. *Perspectives in Public Health*, 133(3): 165–173.

Billington, J., Davis, P. and Farrington, G. (2013b). Reading as Participatory Art: An Alternative Mental Health Therapy. *Journal of Arts and Community*, 5(1): 25–40.

Billington, J., Farrington, G., Lampropoulou, S., McDonnell, K., Jones, A., Ledson, J., Humphreys, A.-L., Lingwood, J. and Duirs, N. (2016a). A Comparative Study of Cognitive Behavioural Therapy and Shared Reading for Chronic Pain. *Journal of Medical Humanities*, 43(3): 155–165.

Billington, J., Humphreys, A.-L., Jones, A. and McDonnell, K. (2014). A Literature-Based Intervention for People with Chronic Pain. *Arts and Health: An International Journal for Research, Policy and Practice*, 8(1): 13–31.

Billington, J., Longden, E. and Robinson, J. (2016b). A Literature-Based Intervention for Women Prisoners: Preliminary Findings. *International Journal of Prisoner Health*, 12(4): 230–243.

Ciaramelli, E., Grady, C. L. and Moscovitch, M. (2008). Top-down and bottom-up attention to memory. *Neuropsychologia*, 46(7): 1828–1851.

Davis, J. (2011). The Reading Revolution. In: M. Haddon, M. Rosen, Z. Smith, C. Callil, J. Winterson, T. Parks, B. Morrison, M. Wolf, M. Barzillai, N. Carr and Davis, J. eds, *Stop What You're Doing and Read This!* London: Vintage: 115–136.

Davis, P. (2013). *Reading and the Reader.* Literary Agenda Series. Oxford: Oxford University Press.

Davis, P. and Billington, J. (2016a). The Very Grief a Cure of the Disease. *Changing English Special Issue: Uses of Poetry*, 23(4): 396–408.

Davis, P., Keidel, J., Gonzalez-Diaz, V., Martin, C. and Thierry, G. (2012). How Shakespeare Tempests the Brain: Neuroimaging Insights. *Cortex*, 48(5): 21–64.

Davis, P., Magee, F., Hill, E., Baker, H. and Crane, L. (2016b). *What Literature Can Do.* University of Liverpool: Centre for Research into Reading, Literature and Society. www.liverpool.ac.uk/media/livacuk/iphs/researchgroups/CRILSWhatLiteratureCanDo.pdf (Accessed 19/2/2019).

Dowrick, C., Billington, J., Robinson, J., Hamer, A. and Williams, C. (2012). Get into Reading as an intervention for common mental health problems. *Medical Humanities*, 38(1): 15–20.

Gray, E., Kiemle, G., Billington, J. and Davis, P. (2016). An Interpretative Phenomenological Analysis of Experience of a Reader Group. *Arts and Health*, 8(3): 248–261.

Hartley, J. (2002). *The Reading Groups Book.* Oxford: Oxford University Press.

Hicks, D. (2006). *An Audit of Bibliotherapy/Books on Prescription Activity in England.* London: Arts Council England and the Museums Libraries and Archives Council.

Hodge, S., Robinson, J. and Davis, P. (2007). Reading Between the Lines: Experiences of a Community Reading Project. *Medical Humanities*, 33(2): 100–104.

Jacobs, A.M. (2015). Neurocognitive Poetics: methods and models for investigating the neuronal and cognitive-affective bases of literary reception. *Frontiers in Human Neuroscience*, 9: 186.

Lathem, E.C. ed., (1988). *The Poetry of Robert Frost.* New York: Henry Holt.

Longden, E., Davis, P., Billington, J. and Corcoran, R. (2015). Shared Reading: Assessing the Intrinsic Value of a Literature-Based Intervention. *Medical Humanities*, 41(2): 113–120.

Lutz, C. E. (1978). The Oldest Library Motto: ψγχησ Iatpeion. *The Library Quarterly: Information, Community, Policy*, 48(1): 36–39.

MacIntyre, A. (1981). *After Virtue.* London: Duckworth.

Macmillan, A. ed., (2010). *A Little, Aloud.* London: Chatto and Windus.

O'Sullivan, N., Davis, P., Billington, J., Gonzalez- Diaz, V. and Corcoran, R. (2015). The Neural Basis of Literary Awareness, and its Benefits to Cognition. *Cortex*, 48(5): 21–64.

Ong, W. J. (2012). *Orality and Literacy: The Technology of the Word.* 3rd ed. London: Routledge.

Peters, A., McEwen, B. S. and Friston, K. (2017). Uncertainty and Stress: Why It Causes Diseases and How It Is Mastered by the Bain. *Progress in Neurobiology*, 156: 164–188.

Ricks, C. ed., (1999). *The Oxford Book of English Verse.* Oxford: Oxford University Press.

Rose, J. (2010). *The Intellectual Life of the British Working Classes.* 2nd ed. New Haven: Yale University Press.

Wolf, M. (2008). *Proust and the Squid: The History and Science of the Reading Brain.* Cambridge: Icon Books.

Wordsworth, J., Abrams, M. H. and Gill, S. eds, (1979). William Wordsworth, *The Prelude: 1799, 1805, 1850.* New York: W. W. Norton and Company, [1805] V. p. 627; XII: 245–247.

37

DANCING

Sara Houston

Introduction

Dancing stands across cultures and histories as being a medium for living well, or living badly, within artistic, social, and cultural environments. As a collection of complex movement systems, the way dancing converses with health and ill health is immensely varied (Kaeppler, 2000). Even using the terms "dance" and "health" may do disservice to some rituals and social practices, which connote "dancing" and "health" to an outsider's eye, but fail to match local understanding of those practices (Williams, 2004).

Historical accounts of dance are numerous, from cave paintings to diary entries, from written stories to paintings, from religious texts to film, from carvings to murals. Among these, there are a few accounts that explicitly or implicitly document dance's association with health or ill health. Take, for example, medieval documentation of tarantism (dancing after being bitten by a poisonous spider; Hanna, 2006), and of choreomania, or St. Vitus's Dance (the medieval phenomenon of large groups of people dancing for days, even months at a time in the countryside). Often linked to artwork of *La Danse Macabre*, where dancers followed the skeletal, black-robed Death, some historians point to a connection between dancing, the plague, societal disorder, and poverty (Nohl, 1961; Camporesi, 1989).

In the contemporary world, anthropologists have identified some traditional healing rituals. These include dances to appease evil spirits, to exorcize demons, and to promote human and animal fertility (Hanna, 2006). Each ritual will use and characterize the moving body differently——sometimes as a container to possess or to trap the evil spirit, sometimes to purge the body of negativity, to embody a supernatural deity, or to induce a trance, for example.

Alternative contemporary conceptions of health, which center on the psychological integration of the person, have allowed for alternative dance approaches. For instance, dance movement psychotherapy is a creative movement form of psychotherapy. It is grounded in clinical assessment and works through the creative relation between the therapist and patient. The belief here is that non-verbal, bodily creativity may allow the patient to become more aware of the integration of their body and mind, which may help develop the person's health and well-being (Beardall, 2017).

When dancing is characterized as art, entertainment, or a leisure pursuit it can also play an important, often informal, part in promoting health or assisting with health-related issues. Unavoidably, because of its physicality, dancing is often assessed as a physical activity. There are benefits to doing this in that dancing has proved to be a reliable source for fitness, aerobic capacity, and strength, particularly for those who do not participate much in other sports, such as teenage girls (Quin et al., 2007; Connolly et al., 2011; Burkhardt and Brennan, 2012) and older adults (Keogh et al., 2009; Connolly and Reading, 2010). In fact, Keogh and colleagues add to the list of benefits for older people citing positive changes in balance, flexibility, and lower body muscle endurance too.[1] Evidence suggests that physical activity helps prevent some of the major chronic diseases, such as heart disease and diabetes, and as an enjoyable activity, dance is an attractive pursuit to incorporate into everyday life (Warburton et al., 2006; WHO, 2007).

Dancing is both a complex physical and cognitive activity. Verghese and colleagues (2003) saw in their study on dementia that dancing was the only physical activity examined that showed a significant reduction in risk. It stood alongside other cognitive activities (such as board games, reading, and playing a musical instrument) as a good way to reduce risk of dementia. Additionally, a study on pain reduction in children after surgery showed that 92% of patients who engaged with improvised somatic dance showed a reduction in pain, with 80% reducing that pain by half (Dowler, 2016).

Well-being is often used to describe personal growth and satisfaction, as well as feeling capable (Crossick and Kaszynska, 2016). Outcomes from dancing that may point to well-being growth could be increased confidence, better self-esteem, and developing social relations for example, and there is evidence of these outcomes for recreational dancers. In a study of 475 non-professional dancers, the emotional impact of their hobby was strong and also led to better coping strategies and augmented self-esteem (Quiroga et al., 2010). Other reports note that dance in particular helps older people combat loneliness, promoting social integration, and creativity (McLean et al., 2011; Mowlah et al., 2014). The evidence includes specific studies, which detail how dance reduces stress (Wilbur et al., 2015), and develops self-belief, confidence and trust, as in the case of dance for young people with psychosis (Optimity Advisors, 2016).

Since the medium of expression is the body, there is no need for specialist equipment, such as paint and canvas or a musical instrument. Normally, however, the activity requires open space to move in safely. An exception to this requirement would be if working with people at their hospital bedside.

Despite the ease of "just bringing yourself" to a dance session, there are assumptions about dance that mean the art form often struggles to make a big impact in arts and health initiatives. First is the assumption that dance is only for people who are fit, flexible and co-ordinated. Second is the assumption that dance is for girls and not boys. Third is that dance is only for young people. These assumptions have been damaging to the growth and interest in dance for the wider population. Many people think dance "is not for them." Some who may be interested are prevented from trying or continuing by carers, teachers, or peers.

The above assumptions can be counteracted. The community dance movement has developed a set of values: diversity, inclusion, and the idea that everyone can be an artist. The first assumption of physical dexterity and fitness is counteracted by dance offered to people with, for example, diabetes, breathlessness, cancer, or fibromyalgia. In these instances and others dance can be tailored to accommodate needs. Specialist dance sessions will take into account fatigue or balance issues, for example, by setting some of the dancing from a seated position.

Tailored dance sessions are made to make people feel capable too. The art of dance is stressed: it is not about how high one can lift one's leg, but about the imaginative, creative, and interpretive nature of the movement done, and valuing even the smallest movement someone might be able to make.

The second assumption has proved difficult to crack. Female dancers still outnumber male and other-gendered dancers. Some dance artists advertise their classes as "exercise" rather than "dance" to be more appealing to men; others start with street dance, as seen in popular music videos where young men are seen. Others have male-only sessions. The third assumption about age is still pervasive, but steadily is being eroded, with a growing number of older dancer groups. An increasing body of research suggests that dancing may be one of the most useful activities for interested older people because of its ability to be gentle or challenging, to decrease the risk of falls (Connolly and Reading, 2010) and to be sociable and tactile (Houston and McGill, 2015).

Methods of engagement in health and well-being projects vary according to the population with which the dance artist works. Dance and health initiatives take place in dance studios, community halls, doctors' waiting rooms, hospitals, and the outdoors. For those living with Parkinson's disease, many specialist classes start seated to integrate those with balance issues or wheelchair users. They will also move across the floor, dance with partners, and create work themselves. There is a Dance for Parkinson's program at the English National Ballet, United Kingdom. The repertory of the company is used to establish themes as a stimulus to dance. Alongside the weekly session, there are subsidized visits to the theater to see the company perform. The program became a case study in "cultural commissioning." The local National Health Service (NHS) health commissioning service funded the program for a year because it recognized the gap in post-diagnosis support for people with Parkinson's disease and their carers that the dance program could give (Houston and McGill, 2013, 2015).

The participants in English National Ballet's Dance for Parkinson's program to date have not performed to others in a showcase, but there are some dance projects that also incorporate performance into the process. Theatre Freiburg, Germany, created a project for women affected by cancer. Using ideas from the women themselves, a performance was created to show at the state-run theater. The two facilitators wove the women's stories and movement ideas into a show that confronted the discomfort people feel talking about the disease. With women from the age of 17 to 80, it was an intergenerational project linked by an experience of cancer either as a family member or in themselves. Again, the emphasis was on artistic creation in a supportive environment.

Dance and health projects do not just focus on people with specific diseases (and there is a question to be asked about why the label "dance and health" should be applied just because the project is for those with a particular condition). Dance has aided people in stressful situations, such as those seeking asylum in another country. Dance Well, Bassano del Grappa. Italy, was set up to provide artistic engagement for citizens with and without Parkinson's disease. After the city began to take in a number of women and men seeking asylum, Dance Well welcomed them to the group. The dance initiative offered a safe, creative environment where skills and ideas were shared among a diverse yet vulnerable group of people. The mode of engagement in this example takes into account the physical and cultural diversity of individual participants by using improvisation and contributions in people's own movement and cultural idiom.

Resources

- www.communitydance.org.uk People Dancing's website has to be the first port of call internationally for those working in dance, health, and well-being. The strategic organization for community dance in the United Kingdom, it has a wealth of information on projects, training, professional development, and further reading.

- The Dance for Parkinson's Partnership UK is housed on the People Dancing site, where details of UK-wide dance initiatives for people living with Parkinson's are documented. www.communitydance.org.uk/creative-programmes/dance-for-parkinsons
- www.communitydance.org.uk/developing-practice/animated-magazine For further reading, look up *Animated*, the People Dancing's industry magazine that has articles in the area of dance and health.
- https://admp.org.uk The Association of Dance Movement Psychotherapists.
- www.ydance.org The national dance organization for children and young people in Scotland.

Note

1 The literature on professional and pre-professional dancers' health is much more extensive, but deals with a population that has significantly different issues than the recreational dancer. The literature tends to focus on studies investigating the impact of intensive dancing, for example effects of overtraining on the body, injuries and injury prevention, and psychological effects. The pursuit of dancing as a professional occupation has brought with it unhealthy working practices, such as bullying, dancing through injury, as well as mental illness, such as anorexia nervosa and bulimia (Buckroyd, 2000; Jola and Calmeiro, 2017).

References

Beardall, N. (2017). Dance/Movement and Embodied Knowing with Adolescents. In V. Karkou, S. Oliver and S. Lycouris, eds, *The Oxford Handbook of Dance and Wellbeing*. New York: Oxford University Press: 459–478.

Buckroyd, J. (2000). *The Student Dancer: The Emotional Aspects of the Teaching and Learning of Dance*. London: Dance Books.

Burkhardt, J. and Brennan, C. (2012). The Effects of Recreational Dance Interventions on the Health and Wellbeing of Children and Young People: A Systematic Review. *Arts and Health*, 4 (2): 148–161.

Camporesi, P. (1989). Bread of Dreams, *History Today*, 39, April., www.historytoday.com/piero-camporesi/bread-dreams (Accessed 19/2/2019).

Connolly, M.K., Quin, E. and Redding, E. (2011). Dance 4 Your Life: Exploring the Health and Well-Being Implications of a Contemporary Dance Intervention for Female Adolescents. *Research in Dance Education*, 12 (1): 53–66.

Connolly, M.K. and Reading, E. (2010). *Dancing Towards Wellbeing in the Third Age: Literature Review of the Impact of Dance on Health and Wellbeing Among Older People*. London: Trinity Laban Conservatoire of Music and Dance.

Crossick, G. and Kaszynska, P. (2016). *Understanding the Value of Arts and Culture: The AHRC Cultural Value Project*. Swindon: Arts and Humanities Research Council.

Dowler, L. (2016). Can Improvised Somatic Dance Reduce Acute Pain for Young People in Hospital? *Nursing Children and Young People*, 28 (9): 20–25.

Hanna, J.L. (2006). *Dancing for Health: Conquering and Preventing Stress*. New York: AMS Press.

Houston, S. and McGill, A. (2013). A Mixed-Methods Study into Ballet for People Living with Parkinson's. *Arts and Health*, 5 (2): 103–119.

Houston, S. and McGill, A. (2015). *English National Ballet Dance for Parkinson's: An Investigative Study 2, A report on a Three Year Mixed-Methods Research Study*. London: English National Ballet. Research Report 2. http://roehamptondance.com/parkinsons/articles (Accessed 19/2/2019).

Jola, C. and Calmeiro, L. (2017). The Dancing Queen: The 'Feel-Good Effect' in Dance. In V. Karkou, S. Oliver and S. Lycouris, eds, *The Oxford Handbook of Dance and Wellbeing*. New York: Oxford University Press: 13–40.

Kaeppler, A. (2000). Dance Ethnology and the Anthropology of Dance. *Dance Research Journal*, 32 (1): 116–121.

Keogh, J.W.L., Kilding, A., Pidgeon, P., Ashley, L. and Gillis, D. (2009).Physical Benefits of Dancing for Healthy Older Adults: A Review. *Journal of Aging and Physical Activity*, 17: 479–500.

McLean, J., Woodhouse, A., Goldie, I., Chylarova, E. and Williamson, T. (2011). *An Evidence Review of the Impact of Participatory Arts on Older People*. Edinburgh: Mental Health Foundation.

Mowlah, A., Niblett, V., Blackburn, J. and Harris, M. (2014). *The Value of Arts and Culture to People and Society: An Evidence Review*. Manchester: Arts Council England.

Nohl, J. (1961). *The Black Death: A Chronicle of the Plague*. London: Unwin.

Optimity Advisors (2016). *The Alchemy Project Evaluation Report*. London: Optimity Advisors. www.gsttcharity.org.uk/sites/default/files/Final%20Report%20-%20The%20Alchemy%20Project%20Evaluation%2021%2002%202016.pdf (Accessed 19/2/2019).

Quin, E., Redding, E. and Frazer, L. (2007). *The Effects of an Eight-Week Creative Dance Programme on the Physiological and Psychological Status of 11–14 Year Old Adolescents: An Experimental Study*. London: Hampshire Dance and Laban.

Quiroga, C., Kreutz, G., Clift, S., and Bongard, S. (2010). Shall we dance? An exploration of the perceived benefits of dancing on well-being. *Arts & Health*, 2(2): 149–163.

Verghese, J., Lipton, R.B., Katz, M.J., Hall, C.B., Derby, C.A., Kuslansky, G., Ambrose, A.F., Sliwinski, M. and Buschke, H. (2003). Leisure Activities and the Risk of Dementia in the Elderly. *New England Journal of Medicine*, 348: 2508–2516.

Warburton, D., Nicol, C.W. and Bredin, S.S.D. (2006). Health Benefits of Physical Activity: The Evidence. *Canadian Medical Association Journal*, 174 (6): 801–809.

WHO (World Health Organization). (2007). *Steps to Health: A European Framework to Promote Physical Activity for Health*. Denmark: WHO Regional Office for Europe.

Wilbur, S.M., Meyer, M.B., Baker, M.R., Smiarowski, K., Suarez, C.A., Ames, D. and Rubin, R.T. (2015). Dance for Veterans: A Complementary Health Program for Veterans with Serious Mental Illness. *Arts and Health*, 7 (2): 96–108.

Williams, D. (2004). *Anthropology and the Dance: Ten Lectures*. 2nd edition. Chicago: University of Illinois Press.

38

MASKS

Peter Meineck

Introduction

Masks have long been associated with healing in many cultures where they have acted as objects of cult practice and performance, and are associated with shamanistic rites, spiritual purgation, emotional projection, and the enactment of staged narratives. Recently in the United States, masks, a longstanding and effective tool in drama therapy, have been placed into service in health humanities programs working with combat veterans suffering from the symptoms of post-traumatic stress disorder (PTSD) and dealing with the challenges of homecoming. Broadly, such programs have used masks in two distinct ways: as self-constructed objects that act as a kind of physical fetish for the treatment of traumatic memories, or as character masks in performance works where they can become intense focalizers of strong emotional states and a means of enacting powerful narratives.

The use of masks in performance by combat veterans was put into practice during Aquila Theatre's Ancient Greeks/Modern Lives project, which was a national public engagement program, started in 2010, that visited 100 sites in the United States and was based around ancient Greek texts. This program, which I helped develop, sought to bring veterans and the public together to explore certain themes found in the ancient works that still resonated today. These included the return of the warrior, the ethics of war, women in combat, and the concept of the hero. One main element of the program was the live staged reading of four short scenes from Homer and ancient drama by actors and veterans, each introduced by a scholar who then moderated a public discussion. One such scene was the messenger speech from Euripides' *Herakles*, where a witness to the madness of Herakles tells how the hero went "berserk" and killed his entire family. This harrowing scene, although extreme in its content, provoked much discussion about homecoming, family, mental illness, and violence, and many found it striking that one of the most famous of all Greek mythological heroes would be presented in this way and with so many points of contemporary connection for the veteran community. As a result, at the culmination of the program a decision was made to present the work in its entirety as a stage production, using reconstructions of ancient Greek classical theater masks based on new research. This supported the premise than the Greek masks were entirely capable of seeming to change their affective aspect and were used as a highly effective means for the projection of emotions.

In many ways these reconstructions resembled Japanese Noh masks, in that they were full-face masks, about the same size as a normal human head, with naturalistic features, a small mouth aperture with slightly larger eyes and foreheads, and rendered with a larger bottom lip. They were attached to the head with a soft skullcap with realistic hair attached and were lightweight. These reconstructions were made from silicone rubber that had been molded over specially commissioned sculpted forms (by David Knezz), whereas the originals (all now lost) were probably made of linen. When used in coordination with choreographed gestures and movements, this type of mask had the ability to seem to change its emotional state, at least through most commonly recognized facially displayed "basic emotions" (such as fear, anger, joy, grief, contempt, and surprise). When worn by the combat veterans who participated in the production, these masks in workshops and rehearsal became remarkable tools for emotional exploration by the wearer and projection by the observer. However, this could sometimes be overwhelming, especially when dealing with the traumatic memories of many combat veterans. This is a case where humanities programs that deal with people suffering from post-traumatic stress need support from specialist therapists and mental health experts.

One important health-related factor of this kind of mask work came about in the act of taking off the mask at the end of a workshop or rehearsal session. What at first seemed like the ordinary task of taking off a costume at the end of a work session became something that took on much more significance, as the emotional weight of the character just played was "removed" and stored until its next use. This quickly became something of a ritual act, which held great significance for the veteran/actor who had worked in that mask. There was also often a moment of reflection where the wearer would gaze on the mask before placing it in its storage container. We see this scene in many of the representations of masks found in antiquity, where the actor is depicted holding the mask and staring at its face as the mask seems to look back at the actor. This act was repeated at the start of each day when the mask was removed from its box; it also became evident that no one else should wear or even handle that particular mask. What was quite uncanny is that after around a week, the mask, treated this way, started to look like the veteran/actor who was wearing it. We also see this on certain ancient Greek vase paintings where the face of the actors closely resembles the mask he is holding.

This strange feature of mask work may have much to do with the fact that the mask places the viewer's visual emphasis on the performer's gestures and body movements, even enhancing the kinesthetic empathy of the spectator, increasing and personalizing their affective responses. The mask then becomes a distinctive part of the whole-body schema of the performer and when disembodied is still somehow reflective of their particular mannerisms and movements. From the perspective of the audience the mask can make for compelling visual theater, although there is some evidence to suggest that masks were cognitively processed somewhat differently in antiquity. This may have been due to the connections between the neural networks of the brain for facial processing and language comprehension and production, in that literate people see faces less emotionally and more contextually than illiterate or semi-literate people (the bulk of the ancient audience) (Meineck, 2017). If anything, then, masks were even more affecting in the Greek theater than they are to audiences now.

Yet masks are still powerful tools in performance today, from both the audience's and the performers' perspectives. Herakles, when he awakens from his mania, is devastated, covers his head in shame, and just sits, unable to move. He says that no one must look at him for fear that they will suffer his *miasma*, or pollution. Yet at the end, his friend, Theseus, unveils him, looks his straight in the eye and proclaims that his comradeship is far more powerful than what has afflicted Herakles. At this moment in Aquila's production the mask of Herakles was lifted to reveal Brian Delate, a Vietnam War combat veteran and actor. This was an intense moment of emotionality that resonated powerfully for Delate and many of the veterans who witnessed it in performance, and in the ancient moment of *catharsis*, was made new again.

Another way masks have been used productively in arts and humanities health settings is as objects of projection and reflection on the psychology of the person who has made them. One such application forms part of the Art Therapy program at the National Intrepid Center of Excellence, at the Walter Reed National Military Medical Center, in Bethesda, Maryland. Here, veterans enroll in a four-week intensive outpatient program, which includes a variety of art therapy programs alongside medical and psychiatric care. One of these components is a mask-making group therapy session, where veterans are asked to paint any aspect of their experience or identity on the surface of a blank mask. The results are often striking, for example representations of veterans' physical injuries have included a mask showing part of the brain exposed, a head being squeezed by a large vice, or a grimacing face secreting blood being gripped at the sides by clenched fingers. Other masks represent psychological injuries, such as a face wrapped in barbed wire with a lock on the mouth indicating the inability to articulate trauma, or a broken face stitched back together embodying the pain of multiple deployments and the difficulties of homecoming. There are also masks rendered to display cultural indictors, such as movie characters like the Joker or Hannibal Lecter; others are painted with American flag imagery, positive and negative, or represent extreme versions of unit crests. Another theme identified by researchers was of the conflicted or divided self, with masks painted with two faces, an obvious split, or question marks (Walker et al., 2017).

The progress of one patient who took part in the mask therapy program at Bethesda was documented in the journal *The Arts in Psychotherapy* (Walker et al., 2016). This senior military officer had been diagnosed with traumatic brain injury (TBI), the symptoms of which can include depression, mood swings, anxiety, aggressive behavior, substance abuse, and PTSD, along with sleep disorders, hypervigilance, and difficulties adjusting to home life. The particular patient had been in good mental and physical health before deployment to a war zone seven years prior. On that tour he had been rendered unconscious by a mortar round, and on that same deployment he reported feelings of survivor guilt over the loss of close comrades and witnessing death first hand. On eventually being diagnosed with TBI and PTSD some years later he enrolled in the mask therapy program as part of a wider system of treatment. On seeing the masks made by other veterans he recalled that he had often seen a bloody face. Eventually, encouraged by the therapist, he began to render this face on a mask, a haunting image with large bulging eyes, a deep crimson complexion, and a look of horror made manifest by the mouth. He was encouraged to create a box for the mask and a place to put it as a means of attaching his traumatic memory to real object and then removing it, physically, and perhaps psychologically. At first the patient demurred, not quite ready to live without the image, although it haunted him. He felt that the mask could be an expression of himself and that externalizing this image as a mask had been beneficial. He reported seeing the image far less and that it was now less terrifying. He told how this and the other therapies offered to him were helping him sleep and better manage his symptoms.

For the patient at Walter Reed who had painted the crimson mask, the way in which his mask operated for him as an enactive embodiment of his trauma and even survivor's guilt is similar to the mask of Herakles worn by Brian Delate in Aquila's *Herakles*. Both took on a deep emotional and therapeutic significance for the maker/wearer, but they also communicated something vital and meaningful in a non-verbal manner to whosoever viewed the mask. Masks have proven to be valuable tools in the engagement, community building, and treatment of veterans, and a means by which inhibitions are lessened, emotions are channeled, alternate characters are developed, and stressful narratives told, shared, and understood. We may never fully understand the uncanny attributes of the mask, nor its abilities to seem to change expression, channel extreme affective states, and capture something essential about the maker and/or wearer. Perhaps this is why masks are found in every human culture and still persist today, and why novelist and playwright Oscar Wilde once wrote "give [a man] a mask, and he will show you the truth" (Wilde, 2015: 36).

References

Meineck, P. (2017). *Theatrocracy: Greek Drama. Cognition and the Imperative for Theatre*. London: Routledge.

Walker, M.S., Kaimal, G., Gonzaga, A.M., Myers-Coffman, K.A. and DeGraba, T.J. (2017). Active-Duty Military Service Members' Visual Representations of PTSD and TBI in Masks. *International Journal of Qualitative Studies on Health and Wellbeing*, 12(1): 126731.

Walker, M.S., Kaimal, G., Koffman, R. and DeGraba, T.J. (2016). Art Therapy for PTSD and TBI: A Senior Active Duty Military Service Member's Therapeutic Journey. *The Arts in Psychotherapy*, 49: 10–18.

Wilde, O. (2015). *The Critic as Artist (Upon the importance of doing nothing and discussing everything)*. New York: Mondial.

39

PUPPETRY

Marina Tsaplina and Cariad Astles

Introduction

Puppetry is a radical theatre art form that has a unique capacity to work across borders; to connect the unusual and the mainstream; to enable discussion about metaphysics, neuroscience, emotions, anatomy and mechanics; narrative ... and almost any field you can imagine. It is a particular fusion of the material and immaterial; of physical presence haunted by ghosts of past and future; of vivid existence in an immediate world and of multiple, communal voices singing collective songs of shared culture and memory.

(Astles, 2012: 70)

Over the last ten years, puppetry has become increasingly recognized as a powerful medium to interrogate and understand medical practices, histories, experiences of illness, disability, and the medical gaze. This is largely due to its unique capacity to foreground, challenge, and deconstruct understandings of the body and the power relations that are imprinted upon bodies.

Puppetry is an embodied praxis for the theoretical frameworks of disability studies (Goering, 2015; Linton, 2010), critical disability studies (Berghs, 2007; Connell, 2011; Reaume, 2014), phenomenology (Carel, 2016; Merleau-Ponty, 2015; Toombs, 1992, 2001), science and technology studies (Latour, 2004; Despret, 2004), and affect theory (Blackman, 2013). Embodiment can be understood as "the moment to moment process by which human beings allow awareness to enhance the flow of thoughts, feelings, sensations, and energies through our bodily selves" (Aposhyan, 2004: glossary). Puppetry explores embodiment (the body as it is lived) in all of its dimensions: personal, social, cultural, political, historic, and poetic. It also provides pathways to investigate the application of power of one being over another, serving patient intervention, health-care provider training, and public health.

Creating the illusion of life

We propose that a puppet can be experienced as a material site of imagination and invocation. The puppetry artist animates a constructed, material body with her breath, body, and voice by imagining the world of the puppet and invoking an imagined world through the object. The puppeteer then evokes the imaginative perception of the participant/witness to join in this world with the puppet. When this meeting is successful, the puppet-object (*it*) transforms, in the witness's perception, into a subject (*you*) that is able to hold and expand the relationship to it. This can be perceived as an "enchanted" phenomenological space of complicity and connection, leading to responses of profound beauty, sorrow, and joy in puppet theater while playing in the space between "life" and "non-life."

Where the medical gaze (Good, 1994; Mol, 2002) claims to form objective seeing through biology, in puppetry there is a careful negotiation of the act of perception and the role of the imagination within it. The puppet embodies *poetic materiality*. Imagination is essential to animate a physical constructed puppet-body, and to find meaning in that act. Focusing on puppetry's *intrinsic construction* of the "illusion of life" allows for training the practice of *perception*, where *body* and *being* emerge as a *process* (Tsaplina et al., 2018). This brings into question fundamental notions of what it means to be a body in the world and the role of one's own affected, articulate body (Despret, 2004; Latour, 2004). It enables the deconstruction of the notions of "otherness" as related to disability and disease, as well as the relationship between science, nature, and ethics, and the structural foundations of health (Metzl and Hansen, 2014). Puppetry's success in achieving these aims depends on the space (Kumagai and Thirusha, 2015) in which it is performed and the way it is taught, because "puppets, as bodies that are materially constructed, can both reinforce and rupture [cultural] constructions [of the disabled body]" (Purcell-Gates and Fisher, 2017: 363).

The practice of puppetry can ontologically be associated with questions of control and manipulation. The authors, both practicing puppeteers, take the position that although it may appear otherwise, the puppeteer does not *control* the puppet: the "illusion of life" of the object is guided by its physical materiality, and the task of the animator is to *find* the life and breath of the form (to animate, from Latin *animatus*, past participle of *animare*: "give breath to"). In this way, it mirrors a therapeutic encounter between the person-in-care and the caregiver that is guided by shared presence and not by domination or force (Bleakley, 2017; Shapiro, 2018). Indeed, ritual puppetry has traditionally been thought of as a channel for the shared encounter between gods, ancestors, and marginalized voices. This provides further creative exploration into the nature of agency, interdependence, and imagination in the experiences of illness, definitions of health and healing, and practices of health care.

Transitional objects

Scholars of ritual puppetry (Darkowska-Nidzgorski, 1976; Geertz and Lomatuway'ma, 1987; Houdart, 2004; Jurkowski, 1988; Pimpaneau, 1977) note that humans in all cultures throughout the world have made effigies of themselves that accompany them through major rites of passage. We know of puppets to assist women in childbirth; puppets to support the process of fertility; puppets that are or were buried with the dead to assist them into the otherworld; puppets to represent marriage, violent death, childhood, and old age. In its intersections with health, the body, and illness, puppetry trespasses into sensitive or unknown areas of the psyche and of consciousness. Performance examples of this include *Hooray for Hollywood* by Raven Kaliana, which explores child sexual abuse, and Kate James-Moores' *Ophelia's Revenge*, a piece about mental health.

Puppetry's liminal status, between the states of life and non-life, enables it to be perceived as a transitional object, capable of accompanying others in the successful passage through the rite into the next stage of life, whether this is an operation, illness, transition into other identities following change, or death itself. The puppet is recognized as an intermediary, which gives it a particular place within health contexts.

Global overview

Below are some examples of areas where puppetry has been used in relation to health and health-care contexts; these fields are not intended to be finite or exclusive, but to provide case studies and models of practice.

Health education

Puppetry has been used all over the world with remarkable results to educate communities about specific areas of health, notably in sex education, healthy eating programs, drug use, safe water education, vaccinations, breastfeeding education, and others. These programs have often been funded by overseeing organizations seeking to achieve concrete results in the modification of behavior in relation to key health objectives. On the African continent the use of puppetry in health education is widespread. The Kenya Institute of Puppet Theatre is a good example of this. Eighteen puppet troupes were set up to tour Kenya with health education messages; initially, these focused on the prevention of HIV/AIDS. The company continues to work extensively, engaging in dialogue about the benefits and barriers to health education initiatives. Similar projects have been run in Southern Africa, Madagascar, and Vietnam, among others.

Training in health care

The puppet, as alternative body, offers the scope for caregivers to engage with systems of care, ranging from handling of bodies to enabling and exploring empathy. Matt Jennings of the University of Ulster runs a program with life-sized mannequins that trains health-care providers in skills of empathy, manual handling, and care for the body, through training in puppetry skills that require profound care for another, attention to the breath, weight, and movement of another body, and so on. The puppetry company Dotted Line Theatre has trained surgeons in puppetry as a means to improve their dexterity. A project was set up between Exeter University and Torbay Hospital where therapists working on the stroke ward were trained in puppetry skills in order to be able to communicate better with patients through the use of "mood puppets." All of these projects are examples of how handling and communicating with a puppet and giving care to another body can assist with the development of care practices.

Accompaniment

In this scenario, puppets are used as companions to the child, elderly person, or patient through a process of transition, for example: to accompany children going into surgery; in work with people with dementia, where a puppet can offer powerful companionship, testimony, and witness to their existence without pressure; and as a figure that explores loss and complications in chronic illness in The Invisible Elephant Project by Marina Tsaplina (www.thebetes.org). CadLab in Birmingham, United Kingdom, run by Persephone Sextou, has specialized in bedside stories for children in hospital (www.newman.ac.uk/article-categor ies/community-applied-drama-lab-cadlab). Similarly, at the RDE hospital in Exeter, Cariad Astles and the University drama department are working with the children's ward to create puppet doctors and nurses that accompany children through transitions, and with people with dementia at West Bank Healthy Living Centre, where puppets are used as partners in daily activities.

Entertainment or distraction

This use of puppetry, primarily for children or young people in health-care situations, may provide distraction from pain, fear, and distress while maintaining the potential to discuss or represent fears, concerns, or identities.

Therapy

In formal contexts, the puppet is used as a means to express things that cannot be easily discussed, particularly in play therapy or in therapy for sufferers of political, domestic, or sexual abuse. The puppet here is used not only as a means to talk, but also as a process of empowerment. A fascinating example of this work is Muñecoterapia in Chile, which specializes in puppets to explore trauma experienced by families of the disappeared in Chile. People who lost members of their families in the political violence of the 1970s and 1980s are enabled to create puppets of the "disappeared" in order to mark their lives and absence in a process of recovery from grief (www.munecoterapia.cl). Puppets have also been used extensively in play therapy and for people suffering post-traumatic stress, functioning as uninhibited mediators of emotion, memory, and trauma to enable them to create a safe space for examination of traumatic issues, characters, and situations.

To interrogate and understand scientific and medical research

The puppet acts as a model for new discoveries and models. The company Theatre Rites in London, United Kingdom, was involved in a neuroscience project that examined the brain through a series of experiments carried out with neuroscientists and manifested through performance interventions. Also in the United Kingdom, the Wellcome Trust funded a series of creative encounters called Objects of Emotion where puppets were used to demonstrate perception, the performance of emotion, and thinking itself. Puppets, as imagined but articulate beings, are able to represent the human condition poignantly and powerfully.

Future directions: embodiment, presence, attention, imagination

In 2017 The Broken Puppet symposium was the first gathering of its kind to bring together puppetry artists working in contexts of health care to discuss their approaches, contexts, and projects. A collaboration between Mary Immaculate College Limerick, the University of Cork, and UNIMA (the international puppetry organization) Research Commission, the symposium led to widespread interest, with subsequent symposia focusing on puppetry and disability and questions of training and institutional support.

In 2018–2019 a new program for medical/health training at Duke University, Reimagine Medicine, includes Embodiment and Puppetry as one of its central pedagogies. Students encounter body-based practices from diverse theatrical pedagogies that are interwoven into puppetry exercises. Students grow a sensibility of the *relationality* of illness, body, and person while eliciting and disrupting assumptions of how a "normal" body moves. Three key principles of puppetry practice were distilled from this work as training objectives specifically relevant for health-care providers: *presence, attention, imagination.*

The poetic materiality of the puppet is inseparable from its physical materiality, just as the testimony of the patient's body is not simply a neutral account of biometrics but an entangled account of embodiment—embodiment as "bodily doubt" (Carel, 2013), as the inseparability of the technical and metaphysical (Nancy, 1999), as holding imprints of racialized, gendered, and structural violence, and as an articulate body that has learned to be affected (Latour, 2004). A practice of embodied health care that will move beyond the abstraction of the medical gaze requires the integration of one's breath, body, thought, feeling, and imagination, the tangible with the intangible. The puppet can offer a safe space for negotiation of emotion, identity, and experience. The *practice* of puppetry offers a direct engagement with training a specificity of imaginative reach needed for both health-care providers and patients.

We would like to highlight the idea that holistic views of healing and healing practices that involve material performative practices offer much to medical research and practice. In some cultures, the concept of healing through ritual objects, including puppets, forms part of a worldview that we have not addressed here directly. Research into the reclaiming of puppetry as a profoundly holistic practice that affects body, emotion, and spirit is at an early stage; how this vision of puppetry can speak to contemporary questions of the body, illness, and disability holds huge potential. It is hoped that from these initiatives more documentation, analysis, and understanding will be generated, which will in turn lead to formal recognition of puppetry as a discrete and unique form to use alongside other approaches in health-care training, prevention, discussion, and healing.

References

Aposhyan, S.M. (2004). *Body-Mind Psychotherapy: Principles, Techniques, and Practical Applications*. New York: W.W. Norton.

Astles, C. (2012). Between Worlds. *Moin-Moin: Revista de Estudos sobre Teatro de Formas Animadas*, 12(16): 54–77.

Blackman, L. (2013). Immaterial Bodies. Affect, Embodiment, Mediation. London: Sage. 2012.

Berghs, M., (2007). Disability as Embodied Memory? Questions of Identity for the Amputees of Sierra Leone. *Wagadu*. Available at: http://sites.cortland.edu/wagadu/wp-content/uploads/sites/3/2014/02/berghs.pdf (accessed 18/1/2019).

Bleakley, A. (2017). Force and Presence in the World of Medicine. *Healthcare*, 5(3): 58.

Carel, H. (2013). Bodily Doubt. *Journal of Consciousness Studies*, 20(7–8): 178–197.

Carel, H. (2016). *Phenomenology of Illness*. Oxford: Oxford University Press.

Connell, R. (2011). Southern Bodies and Disability: Re-thinking Concepts. *Third World Quarterly*, 32(8): 1369–1381.

Darkowska-Nidzgorski, O. (1976). *Théâtre Populaire de Marionnettes en Afrique Noire*. Paris: Paris VIII-Vincennes.

Despret, V. (2004). The Body We Care for: Figures of Anthropo-zoo-genesis. *Body & Society*,10 (2–3): 111–134.

Geertz, A.W. and Lomatuway'ma, M. (1987). *Children of Cottonwood: Piety and Ceremonialism in Hopi Indian Puppetry*. Lincoln: University of Nebraska Press.

Goering, S. (2015). Rethinking Disability: The Social Model of Disability and Chronic Disease. *Current Reviews in Musculoskeletal Medicine*, 8(2): 134–138. Available at: www.ncbi.nlm.nih.gov/pmc/articles/PMC4596173/ (accessed 29/1/2019).

Good, B.J. (1994). How Medicine Constructs Its Objects. In: B.J. Good, ed, *Medicine, Rationality and Experience: An Anthropological Experience*. Cambridge: Cambridge University Press: 65–87.

Houdart, D. ed., (2004). *Les Rituels de la Marionnette*. Lyon: Musée Gadagne.

Jurkowski, H. (1988). *Aspects of Puppet Theatre*. London: Puppet Centre Trust.

Kumagai, A.K. and Naidu, T. (2015). Reflection, Dialogue, and the Possibilities of Space. *Academic Medicine*, 90(3): 283–288.

Latour, B. (2004). How to Talk About the Body? The Normative Dimension of Science Studies. *Body & Society*, 10(2–3): 205–229.

Linton, S. (2010). *Claiming Disability: Knowledge and Identity*. New York, NY: New York University Press.

Merleau-Ponty, M. (2015). *Phenomenology of Perception*. London: Forgotten Books.

Metzl, J.M. and Hansen, H. (2014). Structural Competency: Theorizing a New Medical Engagement with Stigma and Inequality. *Social Science and Medicine*, 103: 126–133.

Mol, A., and Duke University Press. (2002). *The body multiple: ontology in medical practice*. Durham, NC: Duke University Press.

Nancy, J.-L. (1999). L'Intrus. Available at: www.maxvanmanen.com/files/2014/10/Nancy-LIntrus.pdf (Accessed 19/2/2019).

Pimpaneau, J. (1977). *Des Poupées à l'Ombre. Le Théâtre d'Ombres et de Poupées en Chine*. Paris: Université Paris VII, Centre de Publication Asie Orientale.

Purcell-Gates, L. and Fisher, E. (2017). Puppetry as Reinforcement or Rupture of Cultural Perceptions of the Disabled Body. *Research in Drama Education: The Journal of Applied Theatre and Performance*, 22 (3): 363–372.

Reaume, G. (2014). Understanding Critical Disability Studies. *Canadian Medical Association Journal*, 186 (16): 1248–1249.

Shapiro, J. (2018). "Violence" in Medicine: Necessary and Unnecessary, Intentional and Unintentional. *Philosophy, Ethics, and Humanities in Medicine*, 13(1). Available at: https://peh-med.biomedcentral. com/track/pdf/10.1186/s13010-018-0059-y (Accessed 6/5/2019).

Toombs, S.K. (1992). *The Meaning of Illness: A Phenomenological Account of the Different Perspectives of Physician and Patient*. Dordrecht: Kluwer Academic Publishers.

Toombs, S.K. (2001). Reflections on Bodily Change: The Lived Experience of Disability. In: S.K. Toombs, ed, *Philosophy and Medicine: Handbook of Phenomenology and Medicine*. Berlin: Springer: 247–261.

Tsaplina, M., Odendahl-James, J., and Bend, T. (2018). Attending to the 'Illusion of Life': Reimagining Medicine Through the Art of Puppetry Practice. *Puppetry International*, 44(Puppetry Social Action/ Social Justice special issue): 16–19.

40

DRAWING

Curie Scott

Introduction

Drawing is defined here as "mark-making for meaning." Mark-making is a well-recognized convention for drawing (Petherbridge, 2012) and "meaning-making" aligns well with exploring issues in health and well-being through the arts and humanities. Mark-making encompasses drawing as a noun (the physical drawn artefact) and verb (the process of drawing) (Jonson, 2002; Rohr, 2012). Drawing is deftly woven into the fabric of society but its value has shifted over the years. Drawing as mark-making pre-dates written language by thousands of years (Massironi, 1973). The oldest accepted drawings are in the Ardèche valley caves in Southern France, although this has been recently contested by archaeologists who have discovered ochre abstract marks in caves in Cape Town, South Africa (Henshilwood et al., 2018). We do not know what the cave drawings communicate (Schirato and Webb, 2004) but graphic communication can be dated to 25,000 years earlier than we believe writing originated (Ravilious, 2010; von Petzinger, 2016).

In Western history, non-artists drew in everyday life for both aesthetic pleasure and utility, with drawing being a legitimate "tool of accurate and universal communication" indispensable in the scientific revolution (Bermingham, 2000: 73). Although children readily probe various intellectual capacities of drawing, unfortunately "drawing has [now] lost its connection to everyday life" (Bermingham, 2000: 246). Children make meaning of their world visually (Cox, 1992; Malchiodi, 1998; Bornholt and Ingram, 2001; Jolley, 2010; Theron et al., 2011). However, this self-directed drawing starts dwindling at approximately 8–12 years when children aspire to produce "realistic" reproductions (Cox, 1992; Jolley, 2010). At the same time, the corresponding emphasis in the school curriculum on text-based literacy and numeracy means that increasing intellectual capacity is tacitly associated with word-based outputs (Mirzoeff, 1999; Jewitt, 2008).

The practice of drawing occurs more with children than adults. This may be because it is "natural" for children to draw (Yuen, 2004; Jolley, 2010); communication via drawing may be better developed than language skills (Malchiodi, 1998; Hopperstad, 2008; Jolley, 2010) and children tend to communicate about things they have made (Hope, 2008). However, it may also stem from our cultural preference for locating drawing with "art," which is a disservice to the bigger picture of drawing (Farthing, 2011). With supremacy afforded to written and verbal text, unless one is deemed artistic, or uses drawing professionally, or draws as part of art therapy, drawing becomes marginalized in adulthood.

Deanna Petherbridge, an acclaimed drawing practitioner, academician, artist, writer, and curator, advocates drawing as an accessible practice for everyone useful for intellectual activity:

> [Drawing is a] universally ubiquitous means for generating and critiquing ideas and forms and for investigating the world. It is entirely democratic: belonging to everyone, blurring distinction between art and everyday usage.
>
> *(Petherbridge, 2010: 432)*

From various frameworks of drawing (Farthing, 2005; Adams et al., 2006; Simmons, 2011; Riley, 2012) Adams et al.'s work (2006) is probably the most practical translation for health care.

The value of drawing for health care, health, and well-being

Drawing is beneficial for exploring the lived experience of children (Cox, 1992; Hopperstad, 2008; Jolley, 2010), artists (Cain, 2008; Rogers, 2008; Cain, 2010; Macdonald, 2010) and those engaging with expressive therapies (Malchiodi, 2005). This section summarizes examples of objective and subjective drawing in health care. Objective drawings are informational drawings with a skew towards being "more rational and logical" whereas subjective drawings are "expressive and intuitive" (Sale and Betti, 2008: 10). Objective drawings can be documentary, schematic, or represent the item being copied. Drawing may be routinely embedded in everyday health-care practice but not even considered "drawing" (Wright and Shah, 2011).

Objective drawing

All diagrams are drawings and these are common in print and web material for education and explanation. Examples include biochemical or structural pathways and line drawings to simplify complex anatomical structures (such as in Ellis and Mahadevan, 2013; Neal, 2016). For surface anatomy drawings, the skin of the person is pressed on, or palpated, by another in order to map out anatomical structures. Once landmarks are identified, marks are made directly on the skin. For example, surface anatomy helps students learn anatomical structures (Douglas et al., 2013) and drawings are used as markers for surgery. Drawings can provide a visual record of surgical procedures (Rose and Sammut, 2013). More familiar are graphical portrayals of heart rate and blood pressure that are drawn on patient observation charts. Note taking can include abstract marks to denote respiratory sounds on auscultation. Pain maps or charts record the patient's pain level, location, and radiation.

Health educators or professionals may draw to explain concepts to students (Ridley and Rogers, 2010) or for patient/client education (Houts et al., 2006; Lyon and Turland, 2016). In one example, students worked together to transform teaching materials and word-based information into a drawing, which helped consolidate knowledge by concretization and visualization (Chan, 2013).

Observational drawing in health care is claimed to facilitate a deeper attentive seeing (Lyons, 2009; Ridley and Rogers, 2010; Fougner and Kordahl, 2012; Allen, 2016). This is what most adults think of as "drawing": something is copied and there is a desire to create a convincing likeness to the original (Eisner, 2002). For example, Allen (2016), an artist, works with medical students to draw cadavers; Fougner and Kordahl's (2012) integrated 12 hours of nude life drawing into a physiotherapy curriculum; and life drawing was one of several drawing processes in a module for third-year craft students and medical students (Lyon et al., 2013, 2016). Another artist, Lucy Lyons (2009), created detailed drawings of skeletons of people who had fibrodysplasia ossificans progressiva. Observational life drawing facilitates critical looking, a multisensory process provoking questions on the meaning of the body (Lyons, 2009; Fougner and Kordahl, 2012; Lyon et al., 2016).

There was significant correlation with the drawn size of the heart, anxiety measures, and clinical markers of illness severity when Reynolds et al. (2007) analyzed the size and areas of damage on drawings patients made of what their heart looked like before heart failure and at the time of the study. Elsewhere, women mapped their pain on printed body outlines and the findings demonstrated that pain distribution was more widespread than assumed by clinicians (Türp et al., 1998).

Subjective drawings

Subjective drawings are more expressive and not as concerned about producing accurate facsimile images (Eisner, 2002; Sale and Betti, 2008). They can capture a "sense" of the situation and are open-ended, intuitive, provisional, expansive, evocative, and experimental (Kaupelis, 1992; Aimone, 2009). The "draw-and-write" and "draw-and-tell" methods are common methods where people draw and then write or talk about their drawing and are used to research the lived experience (Locsin et al., 2003; Guillemin, 2004a, 2004b; Rollins, 2005; Driessnack, 2006). Guillemin (2004a, 2004b) interviewed women and then asked them to create a drawing on how they visualized their condition. They then described the content of their drawings and offered reasons for the colors, spatial organization, and composition. Strong color linkages were noted and natural metaphors of trees, seasons, and clouds denoted transition periods.

The draw-and-write/tell method requires the individual to know what they want to depict before drawing it. Drawing can be also used for visual thinking, exploration, and making new knowledge. This builds on sketcherly or designerly thinking. Darwin and Da Vinci worked through the drawing to visually think, investigate, and problem-solve (Zimmer, 2009; Rohr, 2012). Leonardo created "*pensieri*" sketches (in Italian, "thoughts"), which contained "untidy indeterminacies" (Fish and Scrivener, 1990: 117) "demonstrating a dialogue with himself, and also communicating to others" (Gray and Malins, 2004: 93). I designed a Drawing Program (DP) using this form of intuitive drawing, and one of these activities is expanded upon next.

A short case presentation on drawing in health care

In the DP, health professional students and people over 60 came together for three hours weekly for one month to think about their future aging. Drawings were generative with revelations of embedded and unscrutinized beliefs on aging and resultant shifts of self-agency towards future aging (Scott, 2018).

Participants were introduced to drawing materials and facilitated through different experimental mark-marking techniques. Drawing materials included pencils (of different graphite densities), biros, felt tips, torn magazines, paint, watercolor pencils, and art-bars (blocks of colored pigments). Each week there was a drawing activity linked to a prompt about aging (five in total) which became progressively more personalized. People created an individual drawing, shared the meaning of their drawing with one another, and asked questions. The core interest focused on *what happened* during the drawing process. People displayed their drawings at home and provided reflections on the drawing and on aging.

The second drawing activity was a "Landscape of Life" (Figure 40.1) which has since been used with groups of health professionals, educators, and students, and within one-to-one coaching. It is easy to adapt and transfer into different settings and the equipment is cheap and portable. Graphite pencils and felt tips are used on A2 paper to create a line that works in relationship to the horizontal and vertical.

Timelines with annotations have been successfully used in research to gain rich narratives (Sheridan et al., 2011; Adriansen, 2012). The Landscape of Life drawing is relatively uncomplicated and familiar due to its graphical format to reflect upon personal experiences. In addition to visually time lining past events, there is the added dimension of projecting into the future. Participants were asked to reflect on their life experiences to the present time and then continue the line to predict life experiences till the age of 99. The drawing expresses the emotional hills and valleys of life with a simple line. The explanation here is from the DP, where participants were thinking about their future aging.

This 20-minute drawing has two parts. The paper has a pre-drawn horizontal pencil line and is folded in half vertically. Each person is given one folded sheet, presented as a backward-opening book. Each person jotted any feelings, reactions, and responses to drawing on sticky notes that functioned as discussion aide-mémoires.

Part A takes five minutes and can be discussed or not (time pending). People plot significant points in their life, connect these with a line, and draw annotations (Figure 40.1). The higher the point, the more positive the experience, and vice versa. Some helpful prompts are to plot marks first in pencil and then connect them; work backwards in time; start with

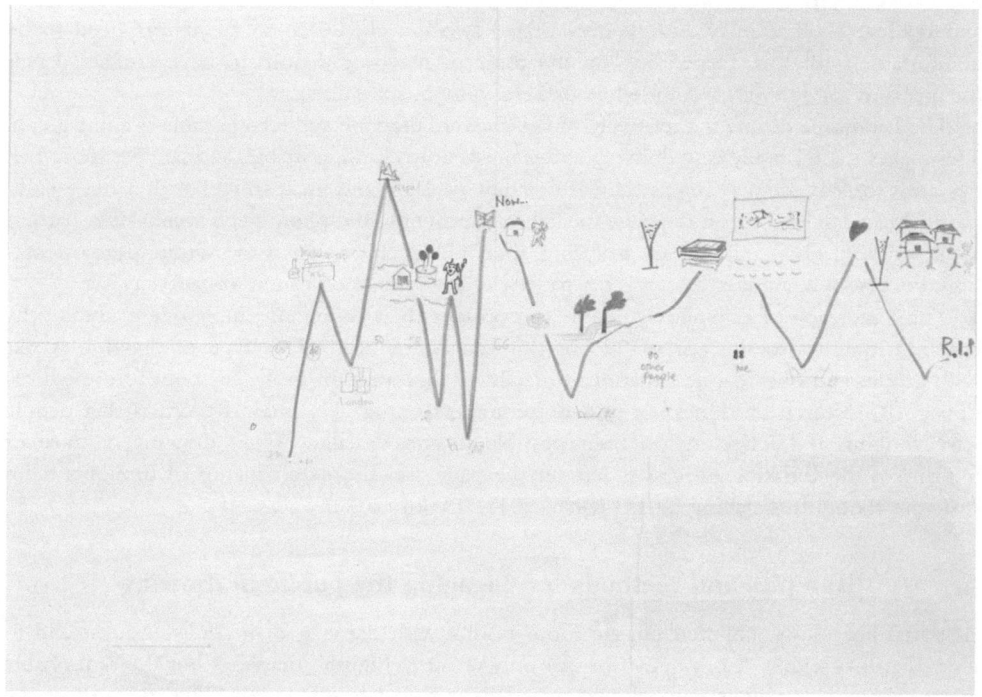

Figure 40.1 Landscape of Life exemplar ("Pat", research participant in Scott, 2018)

significant points in life (e.g., first job, career move, birth of a child, relocation, etc.) or use a framework of age bands such as working in decades.

For part B, the folded sheet is opened. From the midpoint (their current age) they now project forward into the future till the age of 99. Participants were primed that part (B) would be discussed and were asked to consider the possible "highs and lows" of their future life with the proviso that, of course, they were just forecasting as nobody knows the future. They were encouraged to be as honest and open as possible. They might be considering things that they may not have thought about before.

For the discussion, each person had five to ten minutes to tell the group about their Landscape of Life and what they thought might occur in the future. They were also asked whether there was something they wanted to capture in the drawing that they were unable to. Although others offered interpretations, the meaning of the drawing resided with the creator. These line drawings, like the other drawing activities in the research, were taken home by the participants and put up in order to reflect on them. Over time, the meaning of some of the drawings altered.

Barriers and promoting factors

When adults are asked to draw they are anxious, self-conscious, and apologetic about their drawing skills (McCarthy and Sherlock, 2001; Guillemin, 2004b). Therefore, the biggest barrier is potential anxiety about drawing. It is important to be encouraging, to watch for people looking "lost" or "stuck" and to be explicit that drawing skills will not be judged. I used the phrase "There is no good drawing or bad drawing, there is just drawing." Drawing can evoke a variety of unexpected memories, analogic associations, and emotions (Prosser and Loxley, 2008; Ridley and Rogers, 2010; Lyon et al., 2013) so facilitators need to be comfortable with this. Depending on the topic, it maybe judicious to have contact details for specialist services (e.g., counsellors or bereavement specialists).

The Landscape of Life is a relatively straightforward drawing and recognizable as a line graph. This makes it a relatively easy drawing and it needs only cheap, portable, and familiar tools. Felt tips are excellent for drawing as they are readily available and inexpensive, with a huge color range. They can be seen on the page (pencils often cannot) and photograph well. Other barriers are practical: if photographing or analyzing, then add labels or arrows to indicate page orientation. For research, another barrier is the paucity of analytical tools to interrogate drawing.

The Landscape of Life allows people to consider their future. In the above example, the timeline stretches to the age of 99 but this can be reduced. This type of drawing works with groups and one-to-one situations to facilitate thinking, for example about future education goals, research deadlines, or post-retirement planning. The main benefit is that people start thinking and reflecting on their possible futures visually. When drawing, a trace or imprint of the thinking process is left on the page and the externalizing of thoughts helps structure thoughts (Farthing, 2011; Kirsh, 2011; Taylor, 2012).

Examples and methods for engaging the public in drawing

As stated previously, children engage more readily with drawing than adults. Adults tend to insist that they either "can't draw" or can only create "childish" drawings but this is probably due to drawing development being curtailed in mid-to-late childhood. The majority of the drawings detailed above were research practices in institutions such as universities and hospitals.

Working alongside galleries and exhibitions by inviting people to draw is another option. Rachael Allen (2014) ran evening drawing workshops during the Body Worlds Vital exhibition of Dr Gunther Von Hagen's plastinated human bodies. I ran drawing workshops for health professional students and staff during the Georgie Meadows (2016) exhibition of stitched drawings.

The Year of Drawing project (2018) had participatory elements such as drop-in drawing workshops and courses that culminated in public exhibitions to challenge the stigma surrounding mental health issues. To develop objective drawing skills, there are numerous day and evening drawing courses. On a lighter level, various local groups, such as Drink and Draw, gather socially to draw in public spaces.

When engaging the public, it is useful to have a large space with open drawing prompts and ample materials. Facilitators can lead relaxed drawing techniques such as drawing with the non-dominant hand or both hands, using extended fingers by strapping crayons on long sticks, or using mirrors to draw. Of course, observational drawings can be set to draw specimens and objects. It is beneficial to have an array of drawing materials and an emerging exhibition of participants' drawings. Finally, drawings are excellent prompts to start discussions which will need facilitators.

Conclusion

In summary, drawing is very versatile. There is increasing interest in using drawing within health humanities. It is readily engaged with by children and has proven value with adults. The commonest method is the draw-and-write or draw-and-tell process. As adults may be out of practice with drawing and anxious, it is worthwhile spending time playing and exploring the bounds of drawing.

Acknowledgements

This chapter on the value for drawing is derived from my as first person doctoral thesis, entitled "Eliciting perceptions of ageing through participatory drawing: A phenomenographic approach."

Resources

- There is a freely accessible resource detailing the myriad ways that drawing can be incorporated into Health and Social Science Education (Ridley and Rogers, 2010).
- Although not directly targeted for health care, the Power Drawing publications (Adams et al., 2005 is one example) include useful drawing case studies.
- The Campaign for Drawing (2014) exists to make drawing accessible for all. People are invited to tender projects using public spaces to draw for their Big Draw annual event.
- There are a few specialist drawing research groups with good representation from those allied to health and well-being. TRACEY (2018) incorporates diverse perspectives on drawing and visualization and their website hosts an open-access journal, Project Space and the Drawing Research Network. Another is Thinking through Drawing (2018), which hosts annual symposia and workshops.

References

Adams, E., Baynes, K. and the Guild of St George. (2005). Power Drawing: Lines of Enquiry, Worthing: Campaign for Drawing. www.bigdrawshop.co.uk/collections/power-drawing-books (Accessed 19/2/2019).

Adams, E., Baynes, K. and the Guild of St George. (2006). *Professional Practices*. Lancing: Campaign for Drawing.

Adriansen, H.K. (2012). Timeline Interviews: A Tool for Conducting Life History Research. *Qualitative Studies*, 3(1): 40–55.

Aimone, S. (2009). *Expressive Drawing: A Practical Guide to Freeing the Artist Within*. New York: Lark Crafts.

Allen, R. (2014). *BODY WORLDS Drawing Evenings. BODY WORLDS Vital*. Newcastle: Centre For Life, Newcastle. 26 June to 30 October.

Allen, R. (2016). The Body Beyond the Anatomy Lab: (Re)Addressing Arts Methodologies for the Critical Medical Humanities. In A. Whitehead and A. Woods, eds., *Edinburgh Companion to the Critical Medical Humanities*. Edinburgh: Edinburgh University Press: 186–208.

Bermingham, A. (2000). *Learning to Draw: Studies in the Cultural History of a Polite and Useful Art*. New Haven: Yale University Press.

Bornholt, L. J. and Ingram, A. (2001). Personal and Social Identity in Children's Self-concepts about Drawing. *Educational Psychology*, 21(2): 151–166.

Cain, P., 2008. *Drawing as coming to know: how is it that I know I make sense of what I do?* Ph.D. University of Glasgow. Available at: http://ethos.bl.uk/Home.do [Accessed:7 February 2013].

Cain, P. (2010). *Drawing: The Enactive Revolution of the Practitioner*. Bristol: Intellect.

Campaign for Drawing. (2014). [online] Available at: https://thebigdraw.org/the-campaign-for-drawing (Accessed 18/9/2018).

Chan, Z.C.Y. (2013). Drawing in Nursing PBL. *Nurse Education Today*, 33(8): 818–822.

Cox, M.V. (1992). *Children's Drawings*. St Ives: Penguin Books.

Douglas, G., Nicol, F. and Robertson, C. (2013). *Macleod's Clinical Examination*. 13th edition. London: Churchill Livingstone Elsevier.

Driessnack, M. (2006). Draw-and-Tell Conversations with Children About Fear. *Qualitative Health Research*, 16(10): 1414–1435.

Eisner, E.W. (2002). *The Arts and the Creation of Mind*. New Haven: Yale University Press.

Ellis, H. and Mahadevan, V. (2013). *Clinical Anatomy: Applied Anatomy for Students and Junior Doctors*. 13th edition. Chichester: Wiley Blackwell.

Farthing, S. (2005). *Plan de Dessin: A Drawing of the Bigger Picture of Drawing*. London: The Drawing Gallery. [pdf]. Available at: http://stephenfarthing.com/pdf/map.pdf (Accessed 6/3/2016).

Farthing, S. (2011). The Bigger Picture of Drawing. In A. Kantrowitz, A. Brew and M. Fava, eds., *Thinking Through Drawing: Practice Into Knowledge*. New York: Columbia University: 21–26. [pdf]. Available at: http://ttd2011.pressible.org/files/2012/05/Thinking-through-Drawing_Practice-into-Knowledge.pdf (Accessed 3/7/2013).

Fish, J. and Scrivener, S. (1990). Amplifying the Mind's Eye: Sketching and Visual Cognition. *Leonardo*, 23(1): 117–126.

Fougner, M., and Kordahl, H.L. (2012). Nude Drawing: A Relevant Tool in Health Professions Education? Developing Skills in Observation Method for Reflective Physiotherapy Practice. *Arts and Health: An International Journal for Research, Policy and Practice*, 4(1): 16–25.

Gray, C. and Malins, J. (2004). *Visualising Research: A Guide to the Research Process in Art and Design*. Aldershot: Ashgate.

Guillemin, M. (2004a). Embodying Heart Disease Through Drawings. *Health: An Interdisciplinary Journal for the Social Study of Health, Illness and Medicine*, 8(2): 223–239.

Guillemin, M. (2004b). Understanding Illness: Using Drawings as a Research Method. *Qualitative Health Research*, 14(2): 272–289.

Henshilwood, C.S., d'Errico, F., van Niekerk, K.l., Dayet, L., Queffelec, A. and Pollarolo, L. (2018). An Abstract Drawing from the 73,000-Year-Old Levels at Blombos Cave, South Africa. *Nature*, 562 (7725): 115–118.

Hope, G. (2008). *Thinking and Learning Through Drawing: In Primary Classrooms*. London: Sage Publications.

Hopperstad, M.H. (2008). How Children Make Meaning Through Drawing and Play. *Visual Communication*, 7(1): 77–96.

Houts, P.S., Doak, C.C., Doak, L.G. and Loscalzo, M.J. (2006). The Role of Pictures in Improving Health Communication: A Review of Research on Attention, Comprehension, Recall, and Adherence. *Patient Education and Counselling*, 61(2): 173–190.

Jewitt, C. (2008). *The Visual in Learning and Creativity: A* Review *of the Literature – A Report for Creative Partnerships.* [pdf]. Available at: http://judyrobertson.typepad.com/files/the-visual-in-learning-and-creativity-168.pdf (Accessed 22/ 10/2013).

Jolley, R.P. (2010). *Children and Pictures: Drawing and Understanding.* Singapore: Wiley-Blackwell.

Jonson, B. (2002). Sketching Now. *International Journal of Art and Design Education,* 21(3): 246–253.

Kaupelis, R. (1992). *Experimental Drawing Techniques.* 30th edition. New York: Watson-Guptill Publications.

Kirsh, D. (2011). Using Sketching: To Think, To Recognize, To Learn. In A. Kantrowitz, A. Brew and M. Fava, eds., *Thinking Through Drawing: Practice into Knowledge.* New York: Columbia University: 123–125 [pdf]. Available at: http://ttd2011.pressible.org/files/2012/05/Thinking-through-Drawing_Practice-into-Knowledge.pdf (Accessed 3/7/2013).

Locsin, R.C., Barnard, A., Matua, A.G. and Bongomin, B. (2003). Surviving Ebola: Understanding Experience Through Artistic Expression. *International Nursing Review,* 50(3): 156–166.

Lyon, P., Letschka, P., Ainsworth, T. and Haq, I. (2013). An Exploratory Study of the Potential Learning Benefits for Medical Students in Collaborative Drawing: Creativity, Reflection and "Critical Looking". *BMC Medical Education,* 13(1): 86–96.

Lyon, P., Letschka, P., Ainsworth, T. and Haq, I. (2016). Drawing Pedagogies in Higher Education: The Learning Impact of a Collaborative Cross-disciplinary Drawing Course. *International Journal of Art and Design Education.* 37(2): 221–232.

Lyon, P. and Turland, M. (2016). Manual Drawing in Clinical Communication: Understanding the Role of Clinical Mark-Making. *Visual Methodologies,* 5(1): 39–44.

Lyons, L. (2009). *Delineating Disease: A System for Investigating Fibrodysplasia Ossificans Progressiva.* Ph.D. Sheffield Hallam University. Available at: www.academia.edu/1432515/Delineating_disease_a_system_for_investigating_Fibrodysplasia_Ossificans_Progressivan (Accessed 14/2/2013).

Macdonald, J. (2010). *Drawing Around the Body: The Manual and Visual Practice of Drawing and the Embodiment of Knowledge.* Ph.D. Leeds Metropolitan University. Accessed from www.julietmacdonald.co.uk/phd_files/I_Overview.pdf (Accessed 14/2/2013).

Malchiodi, C.A. (1998). *Understanding Children's Drawings.* New York: Guildford Press.

Malchiodi, C.A., 2005.Art therapy. In: C.A. Malchiodi, ed. *Expressive Therapies.* New York: The Guilford Press; pp. 16–45.

Massironi, M. 1973. The psychology of graphic images: seeing, drawing, communicating. Translated from Italian by N. Bruno. 2013. New York: Psychology Press.

McCarthy, P. and Sherlock, G. (2001). Drawing: An Image-Making Approach. *International Journal of Art and Design Education,* 20(3): 343–351.

Meadows, G. (2016). *Stitched Drawings on Tour from the Wellcome Collection* [exhibition]. The Beaney House of Art and Knowledge, Canterbury, 24–27 November.

Mirzoeff, N. (1999). *An Introduction to Visual Culture.* London: Routledge.

Neal, M.J. (2016). *Medical Pharmacology at a Glance.* 8th edition. Chichester: Wiley-Blackwell.

Petherbridge, D. (2010). *The Primacy of Drawing.* London: Yale University Press.

Petherbridge, D. (2012). Nailing the Liminal: The Difficulties of Defining Drawing. In S. Garner, ed., *Writing on Drawing: Essays on Drawing Practice and Research.* Bristol: Intellect Books: 27–41.

Prosser, J. and Loxley, A. (2008). Introducing Visual Methods [pdf]. Available at: http://eprints.ncrm.ac.uk/420/1/MethodsReviewPaperNCRM-010.pdf (Accessed 25/3/2013).

Ravilious, K. (2010). Discovered: The Prehistoric Code. *New Scientist,* 205(2748): 30–34.

Reynolds, L., Broadbent, E., Ellis, C. J., Gamble, G. and Petrie, K. J. (2007). Patients' Drawings Illustrate Psychological and Functional Status in Heart Failure. *Journal of Psychosomatic Research,* 63(5): 525–532.

Ridley, P. and Rogers, A. (2010). *Drawing to Learn: Clinical Education, Health and Social Care.* Brighton: Centre for Learning and Teaching, University of Brighton. Available at: http://about.brighton.ac.uk/visuallearning/drawing (Accessed 4/12/2017).

Riley, H. (2012). Drawing: Towards an Intelligence of Seeing. In S. Garner, ed., *Writing on Drawing: Essays on Drawing Practice and Research.* Bristol: Intellect Books: 152–167.

Rogers, A. (2008). *Drawing Encounters: A Practice-Led Investigation into Collaborative Drawing as a Means of Revealing Tacit Elements of One-to-One Social Encounter.* Ph.D University of the Arts. Available at: http://ualresearchonline.arts.ac.uk/4926 (Accessed 30/ 11/2012).

Rohr, D. (2012). Imagining Truth: The Role of Drawing Within the Creation of Knowledge. *TRACEY: Drawing and Visualisation Research* [pdf]. Available at: www.lboro.ac.uk/departments/sota/tracey/journal/edu/rohr.html (Accessed 30/ 11/2012).

Rollins, J. A. (2005). Tell Me About It: Drawing as a Communication Tool for Children with Cancer. *Journal of Pediatric Oncology Nursing*, 22(4): 203–221.

Rose, C. and Sammut, D. (2013). *Drawing in Craft and Surgery: A Conversation* [video]. Available on https://vimeo.com/77975872 (Accessed 15/7/2014).

Sale, T. and Betti, C. (2008). *Drawing: A Contemporary Approach*. 6th edition. Belmont: Thompson Wadsworth.

Schirato, T. and Webb, J. (2004). *Understanding the Visual*. London: Sage Publications Limited.

Scott, C. (2018). *Elucidating Perceptions of Ageing Through Participatory Drawing: A Phenomenographic Approach*. Ph.D. University of Brighton.

Sheridan, J., Chamberlain, K. and Dupuis, A. (2011). Timelining: Visualizing experience. *Qualitative Research*, 1(5): 552–569.

Simmons, S. (2011). Philosophical Dimensions of Drawing Instruction. In A. Kantrowitz, A. Brew and M. Fava, eds., *Thinking Through Drawing: Practice into Knowledge*. New York: Columbia University: 39–44. [pdf] Available at: http://ttd2011.pressible.org/files/2012/05/Thinking-through-Drawing_Practice-into-Knowledge.pdf (Accessed 3/7/2013).

Taylor, A. (2012). Foreword. In S. Garner, ed., *Writing on Drawing: Essays on Drawing Practice and Research*. Bristol: Intellect Books: 9–11.

Theron, L., Mitchell, C., Smith, A. and Stuart, J. eds., (2011). *Picturing Research: Drawing as Visual Methodology*. Rotterdam: SensePublishers.

Thinking through Drawing. (2018). [online] Available at www.thinkingthroughdrawing.org/(Accessed 18/9/2018).

TRACEY. (2018) [online] Available at www.lboro.ac.uk/microsites/sota/tracey/index.html (Accessed 18/9/2018).

Türp, J.C., Kowalski, C.J., O'Leary, N. and Stohler, C.S. (1998). Pain Maps from Facial Pain Patients Indicate a Broad Pain Geography. *Journal of Dental Research*, 77(6): 1465–1472.

von Petzinger, G. (2016). *The First Signs: Unlocking the Mysteries of the World's Oldest Symbols*. London: Atria books.

Wright, J. and Shah, N. (2011). Evolving Dialogues Between Surgeon and Drawing Practitioner. In A. Kantrowitz, A. Brew and M. Fava, eds., *Thinking Through Drawing: Practice into Knowledge*. New York: Columbia University: 109–113 [pdf]. Available at: http://ttd2011.pressible.org/files/2012/05/Thinking-through-Draw-ing_Practice-into-Knowledge.pdf (Accessed 3/7/2013).

Year of drawing. (2018). www.makeyourmarknhs.co.uk/A Year of Drawing: Public Drawing Events (Accessed 19/2/2019).

Yuen, F.C. (2004). "It Was Fun . . . I Liked Drawing My Thoughts": Using Drawings as a Part of the Focus Group Process with Children. *Journal of Leisure Research*, 36(4): 461–482.

Zimmer, C. (2009). Drawing from Darwin. *Nature*, 458(7239): 705 [online] Available at: www.nature.com/articles/458705a (Accessed 15/9/2017).

41

PAPERMAKING

Drew Luan Matott and Gretchen M. Miller

Introduction

People across a range of cultures and traditions have long used their hands to express themselves and tell their stories. Cave paintings, stone carvings, clay tablets, papyrus scrolls, parchment codices, and paper broadsides are just some of the media used throughout history to record human experience. Art production by hand offers a profound personal connection between the process and the maker, and fosters important opportunities for rich expression connected to the self, others, and our communities.

Kaimal et al. (2016) cite numerous examples of how handmade craft production such as woodworking, pottery, sewing, fiber arts, and the like have a strong link to improving and enriching emotional health and informing societal and cultural experiences. Likewise, Kapitan (2011) speaks to the personal, sensory-based temperament that carefully creating a product by hand can positively have on our entire being, spirit, and personal consciousness. Lambert (2006) also supports the physical and repetitive use of our hands as a neurobiological means to decrease and manage depression, anxiety, and stress. These studies show the strong connection between the arts, handcrafted processes, and its validating impact on well-being.

The ancient tradition of hand papermaking is an excellent example of the value of handmade expression and creation on well-being. With specific attention to our involvement in the Peace Paper Project (2018), we outline how papermaking can be applied as means for transformation, reclamation, and restoration related to communicating experiences and emotions, especially as these involve encounters with mental wellness, trauma, and loss.

Origins of papermaking

While papermaking arrived comparatively late in the scheme of human expression, it nevertheless has a long history. Paper was invented in China in the second century BCE, by combining hemp fish netting and mulberry bark. The materials were pounded with mallets into a pulp, suspended in water, and formed into a sheet. The papermaking process was a much-protected secret and remained so until the eighth century, when the Samarkand paper mill was taken during the Battle of Talas (Hunter, 1974). From that time onward, paper became an important resource for the developing Arab-Muslim world and flourished as an open market industry (Bloom, 2001).

In the eleventh century, Christian armies seized a factory in Spain where paper was being produced and, with it, gained their first glimpse at how paper was manufactured. At this time paper was not in common use for books in Europe, where manuscripts were often written on treated animal skins called vellum or parchment (Hunter, 1974). The invention of the printing press in the fifteenth century brought paper to the forefront since there was not enough animal skin to keep up with book production. Almost overnight papermaking replaced the more laborious practice of making parchment (Diringer, 1982).

With the continued industrialization of Europe and America, there was an increased demand for paper now used in books, newspapers, and packaging materials. As a result, rag supplies grew scarce and producers looked to other sources of plant material for papermaking. In the northern states of America, where industrialists owned immense tracts of forested lands, the method for making paper out of trees was developed and a new era of papermaking was born. Almost immediately the nearly 2000-year-old industry of making paper from old rags disappeared (Hunter, 1974).

Today, papermaking is additionally recognizable as a vehicle for art therapy. Hand-papermaking is in the midst of a renaissance, brought on by a growing interest in the haptic qualities of the process: cutting rags, beating pulp, and pulling sheets (Hiebert, 2000). Not only has papermaking established itself as an interdisciplinary art throughout the United States, it has also piqued the interest of the international art therapy community, becoming an agent for deep personal expression and exerting a meaningful impact on the lives of people around the world (Peace Paper Project, 2018).

The therapeutic process of papermaking: benefits and challenges

The first steps of creating paper invites the maker into a safe environment to explore experiences, emotions, and sense of self through the process of cutting rags into small postage-stamp-size pieces. This tearing, ripping, and pulling apart is a powerful creative act to honor, acknowledge, bring closure to, or explore experiences associated with these materials. Rag can come in the form of clothing, such as a military uniform, a hospital gown, a special T-shirt, or another emotionally significant garment. Cotton-based textile items such as a family tablecloth, meaningful fabric, or paper-based material like photographs and letters can also be powerful to use in this process. There is something extraordinary that occurs when one begins breaking down the fiber. Participants may begin to share stories, memories, and important details connected to the material being altered. Common with other handmade art practices, reclaiming these fibers in this way helps translate the participant's memories, struggles, and feelings into a process of survival and restored life (Kapitan, 2011). This process of releasing and reforming is a fundamental step to help transform the papermaking experience as a means for personal expression, engagement, and renewal, and as a representation of recovery and healing.

The final step to "breaking rag" is to mix the pieces with water in a Hollander beater (if using fabric or cloth rag) or a household blender (if using paper rag). Here the fiber material is beaten into a slurry pulp and ready to form into paper sheets with papermaking tools such as a mould and deckle. When the deckle is removed from the mould, the sheet is transferred onto an interface such as felting and then pressed to make the wet paper flat and strong. Techniques such as pulp printing, creative writing, bookmaking, collaging, and more can be used with the formed paper once sheets are dry.

The therapeutic process of papermaking includes purposeful, concrete, and repetitive steps to safely engage the maker in stages that ultimately resolve in meaning-making and reconstruction of experiences and emotions through the pulled paper sheet and created artworks (Paper Peace Project, 2018). Some benefits of using papermaking to enhance well-being include:

- Strengthening resilience through a tangible manifestation of change and the value of breaking something down in order to create something new.
- Empowerment and inner awareness through a process of transformative change of letting go and reconstruction of self, emotions, experiences, and memories.
- Sensory-based integration that activates a mind–body connection for safely expressing and processing thoughts/feelings in a mindful, here-and-now orientation.

However, challenges to creating a successful and meaningful papermaking experience also exist in both health care and community-based settings located outside the ideal art studio environment. These can include appropriately adapting and simplifying tools, applications, and the milieu to meet the needs of population, their surroundings, or the location being used for papermaking. Access to equipment, a power source, water management, and special safety precautions including sharps handling, keeping the floor dry from wet and slippery surfaces, as well as supervising the use of the Hollander beater or blender are also important considerations to carefully think through and plan in advance (Miller et al., 2015).

In a hospital or similar health setting, bedside papermaking requires mobile materials that are easy to clean, discard, or disinfect while effectively making paper in a small space. In a carpeted indoor space, being mindful of how to handle water (or obtain water if a sink is not readily available) and the wet nature of papermaking can necessitate additional preparation. The use of scissors to break down rag may involve close monitoring, or materials may have to be torn by hand using paper. Having access to, the means to obtain, or space for a Hollander beater may present a real challenge to pulping fabric, and adapting the papermaking experience for use with paper in a household blender may be more realistic and practical. For some populations and settings, the process may need to be divided into smaller amounts of time, taking place over a few groups or sessions. As with most arts-based and therapeutic activities, advance organization and troubleshooting are well worth the effort to create a productive and empowering papermaking experience for everyone involved.

Peace Paper Project

Peace Paper Project, co-founded in 2011 by Drew Matott, Margaret Mahan, and Gretchen Miller, serves as "an international community-arts initiative that utilizes traditional papermaking as a form of trauma therapy, social engagement, and community activism" (Paper Peace Project, 2018). Peace Paper Project's directors, toolmakers, and collaborators include a diverse body of artists, professors, university students, municipal officials, social activists, and engineers. Each institution or individual contributes to the practice of engaging communities in the expressive and empowering process of hand-papermaking. This interdisciplinary group champions the vast potential of adapting papermaking to suit the individual needs and interests of communities, integrating elements of portability, social engagement, community empowerment, education, and healing into their paper-related projects.

In addition, Peace Paper Project is a direct collaboration with credentialed art therapists and has spread the therapeutic benefits of papermaking throughout the United States and abroad. Populations served include military service members, refugees, service providers, individuals in mental health recovery, at-risk youth, and survivors of trauma. Peace Paper Project's collaboration with the art therapy community has inspired art therapists to incorporate papermaking into their work with veterans, individuals with eating disorders (Richard, 2013), at-risk youth, and adults living with epilepsy, to name a few examples (Miller et al., 2015). Peace Paper Project serves as an extensive resource for art therapists interested in developing papermaking programs, recommending appropriate equipment and materials, and providing education about the technical process and therapeutic application of papermaking. Peace Paper Project also travels internationally and domestically to work alongside and onsite with art therapists in group and workshop settings.

Two case studies

Papermaking for substance abuse recovery

One example of Peace Paper Project's collaboration with art therapists has included conducting workshops at veteran hospitals throughout the United States. The Edward Hines Jr. Veterans Administration Hospital in Chicago, Illinois, is one program model where the credentialed art therapist on staff, Erin Mooney-Simkus, LCPC, ATR-BC, engages both inpatient and outpatient veteran communities in the therapeutic process of papermaking.

The primary focus at this site includes working with adult patients in substance abuse recovery. Promoting emotional expression and creating opportunities for self-awareness and discovery is one of the workshop objectives. At first, participants are often hesitant to get involved or "do art," often with their focus scattered, uncertain what to do. For some participants, this initial apprehension may come from thoughts that they "are not artistic" or the expectation that they "need to be good at art" to participate. Communicating that this experience is a safe and non-judgmental space for emotional expression, and not focused on skill, but on the process, can support participants to feel more comfortable and encourage engagement. By the end of the group, many participants are often deeply engaged in the papermaking process.

The participants begin with cutting personal or unserviceable donated military uniforms while learning about the history of papermaking, sharing memories and telling stories inspired by the cloth, their service, or life experiences. The group then loads the cut uniforms into a Hollander beater, watching the rag and their recollections connected to the fabric gradually change before their eyes into a blended pulp, releasing the old and reforming it into a new form. Next, group members take turns immersing moulds and deckles into the slurry pulp to pull and form multiple sheets of handmade paper. After the paper has enough time to dry, the group continues to work with the art therapist, further transforming their paper into new art. Papers from these workshops have created mandalas, papier-mâché masks, journals, and collages reflecting on past experiences, present situations, and future goals.

For the last half an hour of the workshop, group members gather around a table and have an opportunity to discuss their experience: how the process helped illustrate their feelings, relieve their stress, and boost their self-confidence. The papermaking sessions also provide a time for the individuals to get their mind off of being hospitalized, use their hands creatively, enjoy learning something new, and feel in control. A common response from patients is that for the first time they were able to forget about their addiction and feel validated as a whole person.

Papermaking for eating disorder recovery

Another example inspired by the Peace Paper Project was Transfiguration, a papermaking workshop that invited a group of men and women in treatment and recovery for disordered eating. Credentialed art therapists Genevieve Camp, MA, ATR-BC, LMHC, and Amy

Bucciarelli, MS, LMHC, ATR-BC, in collaboration with artist Amy Richard, the University of Florida and Shands Eating Disorder Recovery Center, initiated the workshop. The offering included participants of varying ages (from adolescents to older adults) to create handmade paper from personal clothing significant to their experiences of living with an eating disorder. Articles of clothing such as "skinny" jeans, or wardrobe items symbolizing old ways of unhealthy and destructive behaviors, distorted views of self, and past memories, were used. The process of breaking down these materials served as an opportunity for participants to let go of and transform difficult emotions and experiences specifically associated with the fibers (Camp, 2013; Miller et al., 2015).

Participants in the Transfiguration project embedded words into their newly formed paper sheets, expressing positive messages related to healthy body image, such as energy, peace, health, strength, and love. Once the sheets were dry and ready to make art with, we invited the group to draw their own images inspired by these words onto pieces of the handmade paper. The paper was then sewn together to create clothing for a size 16 mannequin. Group members also wrote personalized letters to their bodies and used these reflections to create paper beads and form a necklace for the mannequin.

Camp (2013) described this about the papermaking process and its therapeutic significance to recovery and healing for this population:

> This cycle of taking articles of clothing strongly associated with the eating disorder and literally breaking them down to their very fibers, reintegrating the fibers to make paper, and then sewing the paper to make a new garment, serves as a metaphor for the profound transfiguration that happens during the healing process. Part of recovery is recognizing that true beauty exists in our imperfection and brokenness. By accepting and honoring the broken fibers of our being we rediscover our sacred wholeness.

In summary, papermaking has an intriguing history, spanning two millennia of cultural development. This chapter has described recent innovations of adapting the processes to be used as a form of art therapy and social engagement with a variety of populations. The benefits of this handmade creative process are many, including the opportunity to transform emotions, experiences, and sense of self towards a path of recovery and healing.

References

Bloom, J. (2001). *Paper Before Print: The History and Impact of Paper in the Islamic world*. New Haven, CT: Yale University Press.

Camp, G. (2013). *Transfiguration: Making Peace with Our Bodies*. Retrieved from www.peacepaperproject. org/transfiguration.html (Accessed 19/2/2019).

Diringer, D. (1982). *The Book Before Printing: Ancient, Medieval, Oriental*. New York, NY: Dover Publications.

Hiebert, H. (2000). *The Papermaker's Companion: The Ultimate Guide to Making and Using Handmade Paper*. North Adams, MA: Storey Publications.

Hunter, D. (1974). *Papermaking: The History and Technique of an Ancient Craft*. New York, NY: Dover Publications.

Kaimal, G., M.L. Gonzaga, A. and Schwachter, V. (2016). Crafting, Health and Wellbeing: Findings from the Survey of Public Participation in the Arts and Considerations for Art Therapists. *Arts and Health*, 9(1): 81–90.

Kapitan, L. (2011). Close to the Heart: Art Therapy's Link to Craft and Art Production. *Art Therapy*, 28(3): 94–95.

Lambert, K.G. (2006). Rising Rates of Depression in Today's Society: Consideration of the Roles of Effort-Based Rewards and Enhanced Resilience in Day-to-Day Functioning. *Neuroscience and Biobehavioral Reviews*, 30: 497–510.

Miller, G., Mims, R., McMackin, M., Bucciarelli, A., Camp, G. and Havlena, J. (2015). *Art, Transformation, and Trauma: Papermaking as Art Therapy*. Panel presentation at the Annual Conference of the American Art Therapy Association, July 2015. Minneapolis, MN.

Paper Paper Project. (2018). Retrieved from www.peacepaperproject.org/arttherapy.html (Accessed 19/2/2019).

Richard, A. (2013). Recipe for Healing: Key Ingredients of an Arts in Medicine Papermaking Workshop. *Hand Papermaking*, 28(1): 26–27.

42

MAKING MUSIC

Rosie Perkins, Daisy Fancourt and Aaron Williamon

Introduction

Music is a fundamental human pursuit. It features in spiritual rituals, media such as television and film, interactions between parents and infants, shops and railway stations, festival stages and concert halls, and in a whole plethora of ways that contribute to what it is to experience life as a human. Indeed, music has also long been linked with health. As early as the Palaeolithic period, there is evidence that music contributed to health and healing rituals (Fancourt, 2017). Over time music has become widely acknowledged as contributing to mental, physical, and social health (MacDonald et al., 2012). Simultaneously, music has become more accessible, with technology changing how we can make and receive music and opening up a myriad of ways in which we can engage with music in everyday life. In this chapter, we explore the evidence for how and why making music supports health, before presenting two case presentations of music being applied to support mental health: first with mental health service users, and second with women experiencing symptoms of postnatal depression (PND). We conclude with practical examples and tips for engaging with music for health. In what follows we focus not on music therapy—that is, music used in specifically therapeutic contexts—but, rather, on music use in everyday life, communities, and interventions for specific patient groups and clinical settings.

Music and health

The health impacts of music are thought to be manifold, supported by a large and international body of research. Based on recent reviews of the evidence base, we can summarize a wide range of benefits for both psychological and physical health.

Music and psychological health

- Music and singing—both listened to and made—can reduce or prevent depression and enhance well-being across the adult life span. In particular, regular music engagement among older adults can prevent depression and social isolation, and music can also support well-being in specific groups such as young adults, pregnant women, and prisoners (Daykin et al., 2018).

- Among adults with chronic health conditions, group singing may enhance health-related quality of life and have beneficial effects on anxiety, depression, and mood, although further research is required (Reagon et al., 2016). Music interventions can have beneficial effects on quality of life, pain, fatigue, and anxiety for people with cancer (Bradt et al., 2016).
- Group music making can support social inclusion and cohesion among young people, as well as supporting emotional expression. It can also help to build resilience and healing in children who have experienced challenge or trauma (Hallam, 2015).

Music and physical health

- Recorded and live music can reduce post-operative pain—as well as distress and anxiety—in children undergoing surgery (van der Heijden et al., 2015).
- In adults, music has been shown to reduce post-operative pain as well as analgesia use, and enhance patient satisfaction, with no outcome differences according to choice or timing of music (Hole et al., 2015).
- Rhythm-centered music, such as drumming, can improve pain tolerance, balance, pulmonary function, blood pressure, and immunological profiles (Yap et al., 2017).
- Music can have a positive impact on psychoneuroimmunological responses, perhaps linked in particular with music's ability to reduce stress (Fancourt et al., 2014; Finn and Fancourt, 2018).

It is clear that music can have multiple health benefits, among many different groups of people. But why does this happen? According to MacDonald et al. (2012: 4–6), there are several properties of music that support health: it is ubiquitous, emotional, engaging, distracting, physical, social, and communicative, and can affect behavior and identities. A number of studies have focused specifically on drumming, finding that it offers a grounding experience, a form of relaxation, a means of emotional expression and release of trauma, and a safe space for risk-taking (Burnard and Dragovic, 2014; Newman et al., 2015; Perkins et al., 2016; Winkelman, 2003). Further research has suggested that music may elicit an emotional response that can support the particular needs of groups such as new mothers (Perkins et al., 2018a), while others have demonstrated that music can strengthen interpersonal social bonds (Kreutz, 2014), as well as change physiological states (Fancourt et al., 2016a, 2016b).

While the mechanisms of health change associated with music are still under investigation, music has the potential to take a central place in holistic health care. Two examples of music-making being applied successfully to enhance mental health follow, detailing a summary of the context, music, and people involved, the health outcomes of engagement, and the reasons why the music appeared to be effective.

Applying music 1: group drumming and mental health

Context, music, and people

In 2014 a series of group drumming workshops were held in London, United Kingdom, for mental health service users and their informal/formal carers. The workshops were held in a community setting and ran for 90 minutes once a week for either six or ten weeks. Djembe drums were provided for participants, and there was no fee for attendance. The sessions included learning the basics of how to use the drum, "call-and-response" exercises where participants copied the leader, learning rhythmic patterns to create a larger drumming piece, and small sections of free improvisatory drumming. The workshops were led by a professional workshop leader and supported by specially trained students from the Royal College of Music (RCM).

Outcomes

Researchers monitored participants' psychological and social well-being throughout each program, using questionnaires, saliva samples to measure stress response and immune function, and interviews. The findings showed that, compared with control non-musical activities, group drumming led to significant improvements in measures of anxiety (by 20%), depression (by 38%), social resilience (by 23%), and well-being (by 16%), maintained at a three-month follow up. Analyses of immune function showed that drumming was also associated with a shift away from an inflammatory immune profile, a finding that is comparable with results from studies involving antidepressant medication and psychotherapies (Fancourt et al., 2016a, 2016b). Participants reported that the drumming facilitated positive emotions, increased their sense of agency and accomplishment, provided a means of engagement, enhanced self-awareness, and fostered social connections (Ascenso et al., 2018).

Mechanisms and promoters

Three properties of the intervention were identified as important factors in supporting recovery: the drumming itself, which provided a unique form of non-verbal communication, a connection with life through its rhythmic properties, and a grounding experience that both generated and released energy; the group environment in which the drumming took place, which was set up to allow for a space of connection and of belonging, acceptance, safety, care, and new social interactions; and the learning processes, which framed music learning as an inclusive activity where there can be no mistakes and where there is musical freedom supported by an embodied (rather than cognitive) learning process. The skills and compassion of the expert musical facilitator were also essential (Perkins et al., 2016).

Applying music 2: group singing and postnatal depression

Context, music, and people

In 2016 a series of ten-week group singing programs and group creative play programs were held for mothers experiencing symptoms of PND in London, United Kingdom. The workshops were held free of charge in community Children's Centres, and ran for 60 minutes, once a week. Mothers attended with their babies. Singing workshops involved mothers listening to songs sung by the leader, learning and singing songs with their babies, and creating new songs together reflecting aspects of motherhood. Creative play workshops involved mothers engaging in sensory play with their babies, doing arts and crafts, and playing simple games together. The workshops were led by a professional workshop leader and supported by specially trained students from the RCM.

Outcomes

When they joined the project, women were randomly allocated either to the singing group, the creative play group, or care as normal (with an option to join a singing program after ten weeks). Their symptoms of PND were monitored by questionnaire at the start of the program, after six weeks, and at the end of the ten weeks. The findings showed that women with moderate-to-severe symptoms of PND who took part in the singing classes had a significantly faster improvement in symptoms than mothers having their usual care. By the sixth week, they had a 35% decrease in their symptoms. There was not a significant difference in recovery speed between mothers taking part in singing versus creative play, or between mothers taking part in creative play versus care as normal (Fancourt and Perkins, 2018a).

Mechanisms and promoters

Five features of the singing group appeared to promote the women's recovery:

- The perceived authenticity of the musical engagement, which drew on the women's multicultural backgrounds to provide a meaningful and social creative experience.
- The ability of singing to help calm and sooth babies.
- The "me time" that the singing provided for mothers.
- The feelings of achievement and identity that being part of a singing group elicited, especially when motherhood was experienced as challenging.
- The ways in which singing can support the perceived mother–infant bond (Perkins et al., 2018a).

Singing was also found to have specific psychophysiological effects, including lowering stress hormones in the mothers and reducing anxiety (Fancourt and Perkins, 2018b).

Further research with the workshop facilitators and assistants highlighted the need for the creative leaders to plan for both structure and flexibility, as well as to provide women with autonomy and opportunities for bonding. A strong team of facilitators and a progressive ten-week structure were seen as key features enabling the successful intervention, and support structures are required to care for those leading interventions that can have strong emotional impacts (Perkins et al., 2018b).

How to engage in music-making

Music is something that can be made individually or with others, at home, in the community, and in clinical, work, or educational settings. There are many different types of music, including pop, rock, hip-hop, jazz, classical, contemporary, and many more. This section outlines some of the ways in which music-making can be accessed.

Musical experience is not needed in order to join in with music-making. Local libraries often advertise a range of different activities suitable for beginners as well as more experienced musicians. It is also possible to search online for music instrumental lessons or local amateur groups such as bands or choirs, many of which do not have auditions. Two useful starting points in the United Kingdom are:

- "Find a music group" at Making Music: https://www.makingmusic.org.uk/resources/find-a-group-list
- "Practical help" at Music for All: https://musicforall.org.uk/practical-help/

Music can also be made at home. For example, if you have young children you can use baby-safe everyday items around the house to make sounds and music, or sing to them. You do not need to worry about what you sing or how you think you sound—your child will enjoy made up songs, nursery rhymes, lullabies, or songs that you like. There are also phone apps designed to make and share music, such as Figure, GarageBand, or Magic Piano.

For music-making with specific groups of people, the following organizations provide activities and support across the United Kingdom, and there are similar programs in many parts of the world:

- Live Music Now delivers interactive music programs for people that rarely experience live music: www.livemusicnow.org.uk.
- Musical Futures aims to make music making accessible to all young people: www.musicalfutures.org.
- Youth Music creates music-making opportunities for disadvantaged children: www.youthmusic.org.uk
- Music Man Project provides music for children and adults with learning disabilities: http://themusicmanproject.com.

Resources

- The 2019 World Health Organization Scoping Review of evidence on the role of the arts in improving health and well-being at http://www.euro.who.int/en/publications/abstracts/what-is-the-evidence-on-the-role-of-the-arts-in-improving-health-and-well-being-a-scoping-review-2019

Further reading

For an overview of the role of music in health and well-being, including from community, therapeutic, educational, and everyday contexts see: MacDonald, R., Kreutz, G., and Mitchell, L. (Eds.). (2012). *Music, Health, and Wellbeing*. Oxford: Oxford University Press.

For an overview of the use of music and wider arts in health, including how to develop and evaluate music interventions in health care, see: Fancourt, D. (2017) *Arts in Health: Designing and Researching Interventions*. Oxford: Oxford University Press.

For current research into music, health and well-being, visit the Centre for Performance Science's website: http://performancescience.ac.uk/musichealth/

To read more about how the arts in general, including music, can support health and well-being, access the 2017 All-Party Parliamentary Group on Arts, Health and Wellbeing Inquiry Report at: www.artshealthandwellbeing.org.uk/appg-inquiry/Publications/Creative_Health_Inquiry_Report_2017_-_Second_Edition.pdf

References

Ascenso, S., Perkins, R., Atkins, L., Fancourt, D. and Williamon, A. (2018). Promoting Wellbeing Through Group Drumming with Mental Health Service Users and Their Carers. *International Journal of Qualitative Studies on Health and Wellbeing*, 13(1): 1484219. https://doi.org/10.1080/17482631.2018.1484219.

Bradt, J., Dileo, C., Magill, L. and Teague, A. (2016). Music Interventions for Improving Psychological and Physical Outcomes in Cancer Patients. *Cochrane Database of Systematic Reviews* (8): 1–156. Art. No.: CD006911.

Burnard, P. and Dragovic, T. (2014). Collaborative Creativity in Instrumental Group Music Learning as a Site for Enhancing Pupil Wellbeing. *Cambridge Journal of Education*, 45(3): 371–392. https://doi.org/10.1080/0305764X.2014.934204.

Daykin, N., Mansfield, L., Meads, C., Julier, G., Tomlinson, A., Payne, A. and Victor, C. (2018) What Works for Wellbeing? A Systematic Review of Wellbeing Outcomes for Music and Singing in Adults. *Perspectives in Public Health*, 138(1): 39–46. https://doi.org/10.1177/1757913917740391

Fancourt, D. (2017). *Arts and Health: Designing and Researching Interventions*. Oxford: Oxford University Press.

Fancourt, D. and Perkins, R. (2018a). Effect of Singing Interventions on Symptoms of Postnatal Depression: Three-Arm Randomised Controlled Trial. *British Journal of Psychiatry*, 212(2): 119–121. https://doi.org/10.1192/bjp.2017.29

Fancourt, D. and Perkins, R. (2018b). The Effects of Mother–Infant Singing on Emotional Closeness, Affect, Anxiety, and Stress Hormones. *Music and Science*, 1: 1–10, 205920431774574. https://doi.org/10.1177/2059204317745746.

Fancourt, D., Ockelford, A. and Belai, A. (2014). The Psychoneuroimmunological Effects of Music: A Systematic Review and a New Model. *Brain, Behavior, and Immunity*, 36: 15–26. https://doi.org/10.1016/j.bbi.2013.10.014

Fancourt, D., Perkins, R., Ascenso, S., Atkins, L., Kilfeather, S., Carvalho, L.A. and Williamon, A. (2016a). Group Drumming Modulates Cytokine Activity in Mental Health Service Users: A Preliminary Study. *Psychotherapy and Psychosomatics*, 85(1): 53–55. https://doi.org/10.1159/000431257

Fancourt, D., Perkins, R., Ascenso, S., Carvalho, L. A., Steptoe, A. and Williamon, A. (2016b). Effects of Group Drumming Interventions on Anxiety, Depression, Social Resilience and Inflammatory Immune Response among Mental Health Service Users. *PLOS ONE*, 11(3): e0151136. https://doi.org/10.1371/journal.pone.0151136

Finn, S. and Fancourt, D. (2018). The Biological Impact of Listening to Music in Clinical and Nonclinical Settings: A Systematic Review. *Progress in Brain Research*, 237: 173–200. https://doi.org/10.1016/bs.pbr.2018.03.007

Hallam, S. (2015). *The Power of Music: A Research Synthesis of the Impact of Actively Making Music on the Intellectual, Social and Personal Development of Children and Young People*. London: UCL Institute of Education.

Hole, J., Hirsch, M., Ball, E. and Meads, C. (2015). Music as an Aid for Postoperative Recovery in Adults: A Systematic Review and Meta-Analysis. *Lancet*, 386(10004): 1659–1671. https://doi.org/10.1016/S0140-6736(15)60169-6.

Kreutz, G. (2014). Does Singing Facilitate Social Bonding? *Music and Medicine*, 6(2): 51–60.

MacDonald, R., Kreutz, G. and Mitchell, L. (Eds.). (2012). *Music, Health, and Wellbeing*. Oxford: Oxford University Press.

Newman, G. F., Maggott, C. and Alexander, D.G. (2015). Group Drumming as a Burnout Prevention Initiative Among Staff Members at a Child and Adolescent Mental Healthcare Facility. *South African Journal of Psychology*, 45(4): 439–451. https://doi.org/10.1177/0081246315581346

Perkins, R., Ascenso, S., Atkins, L., Fancourt, D. and Williamon, A. (2016). Making Music for Mental Health: How Group Drumming Mediates Recovery. *Psychology of Wellbeing*, 6(1): 1–17. https://doi.org/10.1186/s13612-016-0048-0

Perkins, R., Yorke, S. and Fancourt, D. (2018a). How Group Singing Facilitates Recovery from the Symptoms of Postnatal Depression: A Comparative Qualitative Study. *BMC Psychology*, 6(41): 1–12. https://doi.org/10.1186/s40359-018-0253-0

Perkins, R., Yorke, S. and Fancourt, D. (2018b). Learning to Facilitate Arts-in-Health Programmes: A Case Study of Musicians Facilitating Creative Interventions for Mothers with Symptoms of Postnatal Depression. *International Journal of Music Education*, 36: 644–658. https://doi.org/10.1177/0255761418771092

Reagon, C., Gale, N., Enright, S., Mann, M. and van Deursen, R. (2016). A Mixed-Method Systematic Review to Investigate the Effect of Group Singing on Health Related Quality of Life. *Complementary Therapies in Medicine*, 27: 1–11. https://doi.org/10.1016/j.ctim.2016.03.017

van der Heijden, M.J.E., Oliai Araghi, S., van Dijk, M., Jeekel, J. and Hunink, M.G.M. (2015). The Effects of Perioperative Music Interventions in Pediatric Surgery: A Systematic Review and Meta-Analysis of Randomized Controlled Trials. *PLOS ONE*, 10(8): e0133608. https://doi.org/10.1371/journal.pone.0133608

Winkelman, M. (2003). Complementary Therapy for Addiction: "Drumming out drugs." *American Journal of Public Health*, 93(4): 647–651. https://doi.org/10.2105/ajph.93.4.647

Yap, A.F., Kwan, Y.H. and Ang, S.B. (2017). A Systematic Review on the Effects of Active Participation in Rhythm-Centred Music Making on Different Aspects of Health. *European Journal of Integrative Medicine*, 9: 44–49. https://doi.org/10.1016/j.eujim.2016.11.011

43

SHARED MUSIC LISTENING

Claire Garabedian

Introduction

Modern Western societies are facing a curious dilemma: average life expectancy is increasing, but so too is the prevalence of age-related conditions such as dementia (Birch and Draper, 2008; Chatterjee, 2008; Hennings et al., 2010; Small et al., 2007). "Dementia" is an umbrella term used to describe a cluster of terminal degenerative disorders of the brain usually affecting older people (Chatterjee, 2008; De Vries, 2003; Small et al., 2007).

Discovering new ways of effectively connecting with people living with advancing dementia (who may also be physically frail) has become a primary aim of dementia researchers and practitioners. Creative arts have repeatedly been shown to be especially effective for reaching people living with dementia (Brotons, 2000), although there has been little progress in determining and evidencing the mechanisms for these effects.

Music interventions are generally organized either towards "curing" (therapy) or toward "healing" (therapeutic) the recipient(s). Although often used interchangeably, the ethos behind these two terms is actually quite different: "curing" is synonymous with "fixing" or "repairing" the "patient," while "healing" focuses on providing comfort and improving well-being of recipients by meeting them as they are in the moment (Boudreau et al., 2007; Hutchinson et al., 2009). Although both objectives are equally valid, "healing" can benefit all people regardless of their health status (Fachner, 2007).

Sharing the activity of listening to "receptive" music listening

This chapter speaks directly to the shared activity of receptively listening to music. Receptively listening to music signifies being present and open to the music and the person with whom you are listening to music with. This receptive standpoint enables the music to create an internalized "haven" wherein external concerns, disabilities, and inequalities dissipate; basic human needs of comfort, identity, attachment, inclusion, occupation, and love (Kitwood, 1997) are met; and connecting or perhaps reconnecting with others who are sharing the experience can be realized (Garabedian, 2019; Garabedian and Kelly, 2018).

Case studies

People who come together through musical activity are people who, potentially, can be transformed.

(DeNora, 2013: 139)

My PhD thesis (Garabedian, 2015) focused on the impact that receptive listening to personalized music had on dyads consisting of (1) a care home resident with dementia thought to be within the last six months of life, and (2) a family or care staff member closely connected to the care home resident. During six weekly sessions, I played familiar favorite music, either live or pre-recorded (three sessions each), on the solo cello in each resident participant's private bedroom. To summarize for the purposes of this brief chapter, there was a marked increase in engagement and connection within each participating dyad over the course of these music sessions. Several specific examples drawn from these findings are provided below.

Maggie (resident) and Jean (daughter)

There was little doubt regarding the initial disconnect Jean felt toward her mother Maggie, when she described her mother as: "anti-social ... never relaxed in company ... very strict and cold ... severe," adding, "I've got a lot of issues with Mum, which I've come to terms with."

Throughout their initial three recorded music interventions, Jean's body language reflected her disconnection: sitting on the furthest edge of her chair with her arms and legs tightly crossed facing away from Maggie. Meanwhile, Maggie engaged with the recorded music, frequently naming the played tunes to Jean, who generally made no reply.

Conversely, the tone of their interactions made a dramatic improvement from the start of their live-music interventions (sessions 4–6), primarily as they received my live cello playing as an extra-special occasion. Maggie spontaneously clapped her hands as most tunes ended, exclaiming, "This is like a dream!" Jean also became very animated and began interacting with Maggie. Over the course of these three live-music interventions, their ostensibly disaffected connection metamorphosed into one of a closely unified unit. They greatly enjoyed their shared experience of my playing the cello live for them, expressing their delight through lengthy exchanges about the music, shared reminisces, shared physical affection, and copiously showering me with compliments and appreciation.

Below is a representative sample of with virtually constant interactions occurring between them during their three live-music interventions.

Maggie: It was lovely [Maggie looked over at me smiling broadly, and Jean reached out her hand and fondly patted Maggie's head]

During their second live-music intervention:

Maggie: Well this is lovely! [Laughing and looking at Jean who looks back at her, smiling broadly]
Jean to Maggie: [reaching out and again putting her hand on Maggie's arm] It's worth getting out of bed for isn't it?
Maggie: Oh, I would, I would say so! [Maggie and Jean are looking at each other]
Maggie to Jean: It's wonderful isn't it! [Maggie smiled broadly and Jean laughed]

> Maggie to Jean: This is a dream Jean!
> Jean: [smiled and reached over to pat Maggie's arm] Well, it's real.

At their final live-music intervention, Maggie and Jean's interactions began even before the music started:

> Maggie to Jean: [gesturing around the room] I can't believe this is all happening!
> Jean: I know [Jean reaching over and stroking Maggie's hair]. [Jean looking at Maggie who is looking towards her] And you, you absolutely adored Claire's music ... [Jean patting Maggie's hand]
> Maggie: I can't believe this is happening!
> Jean: Well, this is special.
> Claire: Thank you.
> Jean to Maggie: [smiling and gently rubbing Maggie's arm] This is special, isn't it?
> Maggie to Jean: [grinning broadly] Oh! Special! Very, very special!

I left their final two live-music interventions feeling that I had been given an opportunity to contribute to, and to witness, a truly magical transformation in the connection (whether fleeting or long-lasting) between a previously estranged mother and daughter.

Aileen (resident) and Tommy (nephew)

Aileen and Tommy exhibited an affable, if somewhat detached, rapport from the beginning of their interventions—as expressed through their occasional exchanges and brief comments when tunes ended. During their first session, I noted that Tommy's demeanor suggested he was somewhat disengaged: sitting with folded arms, looking down or around the room, and sporadically looking towards Aileen. Verbally articulate, Aileen was attentive and clearly indicated her responses to each tune played. Tommy grew increasingly relaxed and engaged throughout each successive intervention, and by their second (recorded music) intervention, he and Aileen were already settling into a pleasant camaraderie:

> Aileen to Tommy: I'm enjoying it more than the last time! What changed?
> Tommy to Aileen: We're getting jigs and things now; getting faster stuff.

The use of the word, "we," suggests a sense of a shared experience. When I played a familiar hymn during their third (recorded music) intervention, Aileen gave a nod of recognition before singing along, while Tommy looked over at Aileen and at me before humming along—when this hymn ended, Tommy said to Aileen: "You probably learned this at [Sunday] school about 90 years ago."

By their fourth (live-music) intervention, Tommy and Aileen were regularly sharing brief exchanges and reminiscences after nearly every tune. When I played, "My Bonnie Lies Over the Ocean" they sang along together in full voice.

Near the start of their fifth (live-music) intervention, Aileen named the tune, "Scotland the Brave" as I began playing, and Tommy smiled, saying, "Spot that tune!" Later in this same intervention, after I played the hymn, "All Things Bright and Beautiful":

> Aileen to Tommy: Do you know that one Tommy—"All Things Bright and Beautiful"?
> Tommy to Aileen: Oh yes, yes, yes, yes, "All Things Bright and Beautiful." Yes.

Still later in this same intervention when I played, "My Bonnie Lies Over the Ocean," Tommy said to Aileen: "You like this one." Aileen nodded, smiled and replied, "Yes!" and from the first refrain through two entire verses they both sang and waved their arms and hands along with the music.

Although Aileen was especially tired during their final (live-music) intervention, she and Tommy sang together for part of "All Things Bright and Beautiful." This intervention ended with them singing together and looking towards one another while I played "Auld Lang Syne."

When I asked Tommy if he had noticed any changes in their interactions, he replied: "at times I think we almost played a game of 'Spot that tune' (an old UK television show)!" and "We had other things to talk about." Aileen's keyworker (staff member who provided care for Aileen) later validated what I had witnessed:

> Well what I did see was it has given . . . families an opportunity to come together a little bit more . . . [Tommy] has been quite a bit more involved since meeting with you; in a few different aspects of her [Aileen's] care . . . Because it's a nice wee relationship she's [Aileen] got with [Tommy] as well and that's something that they can share.

This dyad's experience suggests that the repeated format of a familiar pleasurable shared event can create a comfortable and safe environment in which interactions can increase.

Discussion

The above examples provide only a glimpse of the increased connection experienced by those sharing the act of receptively listening to music. This finding is supported by Nolan et al. (2003: 289):

> Collaborating was associated with supportive interactions between carer and care recipient in which both demonstrated that they still cared for and valued the other . . . couples successful in this were subsequently able to 'evolve' and create shared meanings which in the best situations, brought them closer together and allowed a new perspective on life to emerge.

Fortunately, there is considerable guidance for how to determine and find favorite, familiar music via the Playlist for Life website (www.playlistforlife.org.uk), and there are a number of helpful resources available through the website of Linda A. Gerdner (https://gerdnerlinda.wix site.com/musicalmemories)—a pioneer in developing individualized music for people with dementia.

Important considerations

While many of the participants in this study enjoyed and engaged with pre-recorded versions of the music, live music generally evoked more bonding and connection between listeners. The quality of the music being played is also a critical consideration: in order to capture and hold the attention of a person with advancing dementia, the quality of the music played must be of the highest level. Also, having appropriate training in non-verbal communication and in dementia is key. Music is powerful: it can reach people on many levels, and while music can engender wonderful thoughts, feelings, and memories, the opposite responses may also be engendered. Therefore, one must be constantly vigilant for any indication that the music being played is disliked or causing upset to other listeners, along with instantly responding by changing or ceasing the music.

It is never acceptable to leave someone listening to music on their own if they are unable to change or stop the music at any time. Playing music is about encouraging connection and reconnection. It is important to not rely solely on familiar music and reminiscence; although a sense of comfort and identity can be fostered by listening to familiar music, all too often people with dementia are wrongly denied the experience of growing and expanding through exposure to new things—including unfamiliar music. While there is not scope in this brief chapter to discuss its importance, knowing about the power that matching the mood and rhythm of the music to expressed the emotional state of the listener has been shown to have considerable impact on the successful capturing and holding of attention—including those who are living with dementia (Black and Penrose-Thompson, 2012; Fachner, 2007; Khalfa et al., 2008).

Conclusion

Researchers have found that the frequency of visits made to care home residents with dementia is largely predicated on the perceived success of their previous visit (Martin-Cook et al., 2001; Piechniczek-Buczek et al., 2007). Sharing the simple activity of receptive music listening could help to enhance these visits, which can feel disappointing and frustrating to visitors when there is seemingly no connection or response during their visit. This finding also echoes Goffman's (1959) observation that when repeated visits take place between people within the same location, a social relationship is likely to arise even when one has not previously existed—or, as in the case of this current study, the relationship has deteriorated due to diminished communication and other changes resulting from the progression of dementia.

It should be noted that each person with dementia is an individual, bringing their individual personalities, histories, and thus responses to each piece of music listened to—responses that will likely change from day to day and indeed hour to hour. Thus, time, resilience, compassion, kindness, and open curiosity are required in order to benefit through the experience of shared receptive listening to music.

Resources

- Claire Garabedian: "I'D RATHER HAVE MUSIC!": the effects of live and recorded music for people with dementia living in care homes, and their carers http://hdl.handle.net/1893/21757
- Playlist for Life website: www.playlistforlife.org.uk/
- Linda A. Gerdner, PhD, RN, FAAN https://gerdnerlinda.wixsite.com/musicalmemories

References

Birch, D. and Draper, J. (2008). A Critical Literature Review Exploring the Challenges of Delivering Effective Palliative Care to Older People with Dementia. *Journal of Clinical Nursing*, 17(9): 1144–1163.

Black, B.P. and Penrose-Thompson, P. (2012). Music as a Therapeutic Resource in End-of-Life Care. *Journal of Hospice and Palliative Nursing*, 14(2): 118–125.

Boudreau, J. D., Cassell, E. and Fuks, A. (2007). A Healing Curriculum. *Medical Education*, 41(12): 1193–1201.

Brotons, M. (2000). An Overview of the Music Therapy Literature Relating to Elderly People. In D. Aldridge, ed, *Music Therapy in Dementia Care*. London and Philadelphia: Jessica Kingsley: 33–62.

Chatterjee, J. (2008). End-of life Care for Patients with Dementia. *Nursing Older People*, 20(2): 29–34.

De Vries, K. (2003). Palliative Care for People with Dementia. In A. Innes, C. Archibald and C. Murphy, eds, *Dementia Care*. London: Arnold: 114–135.

DeNora, T. (2013). *Music Asylums: Wellbeing Through Music in Everyday Life*. England: Ashgate Publishing, Ltd.

Fachner, J. (2007). Wanderer Between Worlds: Anthropological Perspectives on Healing Rituals and Music. *Music Therapy Today*, 8(2): 166–195.

Garabedian, C.E. (2015). I'D RATHER HAVE MUSIC!: The Effects of Live and Recorded Music for People with Dementia Living in Care Homes, and Their Carers. https://dspace.stir.ac.uk/bitstream/1893/21757/3/POSTVIVA%20THESIS%2013%20FINAL%20May%202015.pdf (Accessed 19/2/2019).

Garabedian, C. E. (2019). Dementia: When Music is the Only Way In: An Emergency Intervention: Innovative Practice. *Dementia*, 1471301219835078.

Garabedian, C. E. and Kelly, F. (2018). Haven: Sharing Receptive Music Listening to Foster Connections and Wellbeing for People with Dementia Who are Nearing the End of Life, and Those Who Care for Them. *Dementia*, 1471301218804728.

Goffman, E. (1959). *The Presentation of Self in Everyday Life*. Harmondsworth: Penguin Books.

Hennings, J., Froggatt, K. and Keady, J. (2010). Approaching the End of Life and Dying With Dementia in Care Homes: The Accounts of Family Carers. *Reviews in Clinical Gerontology*, 20(2): 114–127.

Hutchinson, T. A., Hutchinson, N. and Arnaert, A. (2009). Whole Person Care: Encompassing the Two Faces of Medicine. *Canadian Medical Association Journal*, 180(8): 845–846.

Khalfa, S., Roy, M., Rainville, P., Dalla Bella, S. and Peretz, I. (2008). Role of Tempo Entrainment in Psychophysiological Differentiation of Happy and Sad Music? *International Journal of Psychophysiology*, 68(1): 17–26.

Kitwood, T.M. (1997). *Dementia Reconsidered: The Person Comes First*. Buckingham: Open University Press.

Martin-Cook, K., Hynan, L., Chafetz, P. K. and Weiner, M. F. (2001). Impact of Family Visits on Agitation in Residents with Dementia. *American Journal of Alzheimer's Disease and Other Dementias*, 16(3): 163–166.

Nolan, M., Lundh, U., Keady, J. and Grant, G. (2003). New Directions for Partnerships: Relationship-Centred Care. In M. Nolan, U. Lundh, G. Grant and J. Keady, eds, *Partnerships in Family Care*. Philadelphia: McGraw-Hill International: 257–291.

Piechniczek-Buczek, J., Riordan, M. E. and Volicer, L. (2007). Family Member Perception of Quality of Their Visits With Relatives With Dementia: A Pilot Study. *Journal of the American Medical Directors Association*, 8(3): 166–172.

Small, N., Froggatt, K. and Downs, M. (2007). *Living and Dying with Dementia: Dialogues About Palliative Care*. Oxford and New York: Oxford University Press.

44

CLAY MODELING

Elaine Argyle

Introduction

The human relationship with clay has been integral to traditional cultures and religions for centuries. The process of clay work effectively unites the elements of earth, water, air, and fire, enabling the creator to feel a direct affinity with their natural environment (Sherwood, 2004). While the use of clay vessels for practical purposes dates back to pre-historic times, clay, pottery, and ceramics have also gained worldwide recognition as an effective therapeutic medium that can be used to promote health and well-being in many different settings and with diverse user groups (Henley, 2002; Sherwood, 2004). Working with clay has been used to reduce the somatic symptoms of people with disabilities and to improve their spatial thinking and self-esteem (Henley, 2002), while for children, clay can be used as a means of self-expression (Oaklander, 1978). Furthermore, within mental health practice, clay therapy is widely used to apparently great effect (Waldman, 1999).

So what is it about working with clay that is "therapeutic"? The three-dimensional nature of clay modeling lends itself well to the use of symbolism and the expression of both the individual and collective unconscious (Jung, 1959) and is particularly apparent in the use of clay models. These expressive and symbolic features are enhanced by the tactile and regressive qualities of clay work. In contrast to many other forms of creative practice, most people will have gained childhood experiences of working with clay or with similar materials. Added to this is the uniquely kinesthetic nature of this work involving direct manual contact and manipulation. Combined, these qualities help to link participants to their formative experiences and promote their ability to engage with their emotions, which can be subsequently explored through the use of verbal therapy. As such, while clay modeling has traditionally been associated with Freudian approaches and the anal stage of childhood development (Aruffo et al., 2000), more socially orientated perspectives are becoming increasingly popular (Sherwood, 2004).

Examples of these social perspectives on the process and outcome of clay work include the fact that it is potentially more accessible and less intimidating than other forms of creative practice. Clay work does not necessarily require high levels of skill from participants and the raw material is relatively cheap and easily obtained. Furthermore, with regard to the emotional impact of clay work, this can be enhanced when carried out in a group setting and with the shared experiences that this facilitates (Argyle and Winship, 2015). It can also reinforce the supportive capacities of these groups that have themselves been found to have a significant impact on the well-being of individual members (Argyle and Winship, 2018). The sense of achievement, increasing confidence, and skill acquisition that can result from this practice can also be beneficial. This recognition has been reflected in the growth of arts for health programs that aim to promote community integration and development through such things as the public display of completed work, with an emphasis on this work rather than on the process of creating it (Argyle and Bolton, 2004, 2005).

Clay transformations

In spite of the potentially broad impact of creative practice with clay—not only on individual well-being, but also on the groups and communities in which this work is located—most research in this area has tended to adopt an individualized approach and a primary concern with mental health issues (Argyle and Winship, 2015, 2018). This is reflected and reinforced by the long-standing link between the therapeutic use of clay and psychotherapeutic techniques and Freudian theory. These omissions have been recognized in the more recent concept of "mutual recovery," which extends the concept of recovery beyond individual clients to include those who work with them and the groups and communities in which they are located: thus integrating strategies and understandings that have previously been separated (Crawford et al., 2013). Accompanying this development has been recognition of the value of engagement in creative practice in promoting this recovery and its role in transcending divides and enhancing the incidence of reciprocal exchange and the co-production of creative capital (Argyle and Winship, 2018). Consequently, as part of the Creative Practice as Mutual Recovery program, it has been the purpose of an innovative project called Clay Transformations to explore these issues and the way in which involvement in clay workshops can promote well-being among diverse groups of participants (Argyle, 2015).

The project included three blocks of eight-week clay workshops that were run by a local community arts provider. Forty-two voluntary participants took part, attending one block each and including mental health service users, artists, and practitioners. Sessions were facilitated by two separate artists, with one taking the first four weeks and the other taking the last four weeks of each block. All 24 workshops were attended by the project researcher, whose role was to evaluate the sessions and their impact upon participant's well-being (Argyle, 2015). Mixed methods were used in this evaluation, including two questionnaires measuring social inclusion and mental well-being. Both measures were administered to participants during the first, middle, and last session of each block of workshops. In order to find out *how* as well as *whether* well-being was impacted by attendance at the clay sessions, qualitative methods were also used. These methods included ongoing reflective logs, one-on-one interviews with participants during week one and week eight of each block, and a focus group in the final session of each block.

Statistical analysis of questionnaires showed that participants' social and psychological well-being improved significantly as a result of attending the sessions (Argyle and Winship, 2018). Qualitative data indicated that particular benefits of attendance included being in a group, involvement in both the process and outcome of art creation, the potentially sustained and lasting impact of workshop attendance, and the unique features of working with clay. For example, one participant felt that clay work was more forgiving and "tactile" than other forms of creative practice:

> What I really like about the clay is that it's really tactile. If you don't like what you've done you can just start again. It's not permanent. It's fun as well. It's a bit like being back at school. (Practitioner)

These tactile benefits were enhanced by the shared experience of being in a group and the reduced social isolation and "mutual recovery" arising from this:

> Throughout the sessions we have developed help and support from and for each other, not only with regard to the work but also in other aspects of our lives and some particular bonds have developed. (Mental health service user)

The project also had a wider impact beyond the individual and the group, with many participants going on to further pursue their clay work:

> I've loved working with clay and this will inspire my future creative process. (Artist)

After the workshops finished, three public exhibitions of clay work were held. Uncollected work was then sold at a charity fundraising event held at the host research institution.

Routes to engagement

The exhibiting and sale of work produced in traditional art therapy sessions has long been a subject of debate, with some believing that this encourages a misplaced assessment of the aims of the activity. However, it can also have a beneficial impact on individual participants as well as on wider group and community settings (Argyle and Bolton, 2005). Participants in the case presented here expressed a great sense of pride and achievement to see their work on display, much of which was accompanied by their individual narrative on the per-ceived meaning of this work and their experience of creating it.

This pride was compounded by the positive and significant public engagement in these exhibits. Obviously, there can be ethical issues involved in the sale of such work: placing a monetary value on this work could not only marginalize its therapeutic value, but also be per-ceived as judgmental and divisive. However, these issues were minimized by the fact that par-ticipants were consulted on this process and a flat fee was charged for all the sold work, with the proceeds going to charity. All of the sold clay work was "fired," which involves heating it to a very high temperature in order to ensure its long-term preservation. In order to perform this firing a specialist oven or kiln is required. For this project, a kiln belonging to one of the facilitating artists was used, but gaining access to a kiln can sometimes be challenging given cost and space considerations. This potential barrier can be overcome by accessing communal firing facilities, by photographing the work before it is destroyed, or by attempting to preserve unfired items through the use of such things as papier-mâché moulds.

The inclusion of a diverse group of participants in creative practice workshops can help to access "hard to reach" or marginalized users by facilitating a broad-based level of engage-ment, and has been found to minimize the hierarchal divisions often apparent in more trad-itional therapeutic sessions (Argyle and Winship, 2015). However, when working with diverse groups, the similarly diverse needs and aspirations of individual members should be recognized and addressed. Thus, with regard to Clay Transformations, there was a huge variation in the skill levels and aspirations of those taking part, with mental health service users tending to want to acquire basic skills in creative practice.

In contrast, artists and practitioners in the group who already had these basic skills were more concerned with experiencing an art intervention in a non-pressurized environment and from a participant's perspective. These potential conflicts were addressed by the employment of two different artists who adopted flexible and contrasting approaches to their sessions, with the first focusing on clay modeling and mask making, while the second was a more traditional "potter."

In order for an experience to be genuinely therapeutic, its impact should transcend the session and be broad and sustained (Argyle and Bolton, 2004, 2005). With regard to the participants in the Clay Transformations project, this was achieved through such things as enhanced creative confidence, personal and professional networking and development, and an increased awareness of relevant opportunities. In order to further facilitate these sustained impacts, participants can be given attendance certificates and signposted to further relevant activities. Project dissemination and social media can also be used to establish this impact and to promote public engagement. Shown below are links to examples of these activities used in the Clay Transformations project, including a video of sessions that continues to be shown at relevant conferences and other meetings, as well as a project Facebook page.

Challenges and conclusions

The achievement of this sustained impact and engagement is inevitably compromised by the short-term funding of creative practice interventions and the lack of statutorily provided alternatives. This highlights the persisting marginality of these interventions to health and social care provision in spite of their evident effectiveness in promoting recovery (Crawford et al., 2013) and the role of the community as well as the group context in helping or hindering this recovery. This in turn suggests the need for more sustained and widespread funding for this cost-effective, versatile, and accessible means of health promotion. However, the efficacy of these interventions must be proven if appropriate funding is to be obtained and maintained, and further research is needed. For example, questions remain on the relative benefits of different forms of creative practice and the optimal way in which these benefits can be delivered and sustained, as well as on the therapeutic impact of being in a group on one hand and in engaging in creative practice on the other.

Resources

- International magazine for ceramic art: www.ceramicreview.com
- Earth and Fire International Ceramic Fair: www.earthandfire.co.uk
- Clay Transformations Video: www.youtube.com/watch?v=Lmx3jqXfC9o
- Clay Transformations Facebook: www.facebook.com/claytransformations/

References

Argyle, E. (2015). A Potter's Day. *Ceramic Review*, 272: 79.

Argyle, E. and Bolton, G. (2004). The Use of Art Within a Groupwork Setting. *Groupwork*, 14(1): 46–62.

Argyle, E. and Bolton, G. (2005). Art in the Community for Potentially Vulnerable Mental Health Groups. *Health Education*, 105(5): 340–354.

Argyle, E. and Winship, G. (2015). Creative Practice in a Group Setting. *Mental Health and Social Inclusion*, 19(3): 141–147.

Argyle, E. and Winship, G. (2018). Creative Practice with Clay: A Mutual Route to Recovery? *Journal of Applied Arts and Health*, 9(3): 385–397.

Aruffo, R, Ibarra, S and Strupp, K. (2000). Encopresis and Anal Masturbation. *Journal of the American Psychoanalytic Association*, 48(4): 1327–1354.

Crawford, P; Lewis, L. Brown, B and Manning, N. (2013). Creative Practice as Mutual recovery in mental health. *Mental Health Review Journal*, 18(2): 55–64.

Henley, D. (2002). *Clay Works in Art Therapy*. London and USA: Jessic Kingsley.

Jung, C. (1959). *The Archetypes and the Collective Unconscious*. 2nd edition. London: Routledge.

Oaklander, V. (1978). *Windows to Our Children*. USA: Gestalt Journal Press.

Sherwood, P. (2004). *The Healing Art of Clay Therapy*. Melbourne: ACER Press.

Waldman, J. (1999). Breaking the Mould. *International Journal of Art Therapy*, 4(1): 10–19.

45

ARCHITECTURE

Santiago Quesada-García and Pablo Valero-Flores

Introduction

Many external physical stimuli affect human beings and accumulate, little by little, within our bodies and minds. Sensory factors (e.g., noises, smells, colors, and so on) and extrasensory factors (e.g., air quality, chemical agents, and electromagnetic fields) condition human comfort levels and, consequently, quality of life. These factors can promote human physical and mental well-being, but they may also precipitate the loss of physical, psychological, and cognitive capacities, or the onset of possible diseases. Well-being is closely linked to the perception of how a person relates to and interacts with their environment. This perception is influenced by individual preferences, beliefs, and culture, as well as by spatial characteristics. Given the proof that particular spatial configurations can impact certain aspects of human conduct (Aries et al., 2010; Lawson, 2010), the extent to which a person experiences a sense of agency and coherence within a space significantly influences the nature of those feelings. Architecture is the art form responsible for imposing a sense of coherence and meaning upon places and, at the same time, it builds increasingly healthy spaces that can prevent diseases. For that reason, architecture has an important role in the health field.

Architecture, health, and human well-being

Since the mid-nineteenth century, architecture has assumed a key role in improving human health. The first such architectural response emerged during the Industrial Revolution and its consequent urban agglomerations, which triggered the social demands of the hygienist movements.

One highlight in the evolving healthiness of buildings involved programmatic claims by the European architectural avant-garde of the beginning of the twentieth century. A paradigmatic example is the introduction of the bath into homes. Founded on the basic premise that all buildings must satisfy minimum hygienic standards, architects proposed the need for an architectural aesthetic to be a faithful expression of a structure's intended use (Benévolo, 1974). This represented an important step in the quest to design increasingly healthy spaces that would successfully prevent the onset of diseases. At first, architecture focused on achieving standard benchmarks related only to issues of health, accessibility, and safety, omitting consideration of the emotional component: how would the inhabitants feel when they experienced and lived in the space?

Following the Second World War, amid European reconstruction, the human being was situated at the center of any design plan. The ninth CIAM (*Congrès Internationaux d'Architecture Moderne*, or International Congresses of Modern Architecture) was held in 1953 on the theme "The Human Habitat." The conference considered habitat "as the area best suited to meet the inborn and future needs of man" (Gideon, 1982). Therefore, architecture had to come to terms with the social and emotional expectations of people, attending to factors such as identity and feeling of belonging. As a result, architects started to integrate relevant emotional factors into the designing of buildings and cities. To meet these growing social needs, in the last quarter century new disciplines such as salutogenesis and neuro-architecture have emerged. Salutogenesis, developed by doctor and sociologist Aaron Antonovsky, was articulated in his book *Health, Stress and Coping* (Antonovsky, 1979). He focused his study on the origin of health and health assets, and it was regarded as a supplement to the pathogenic focus aimed at tackling the origins and risk factors of a disease. In 2003, on the basis of recent discoveries related to the plasticity of the brain, American neurobiologist Fred Gage presented a key concept at a conference held by the American Institute of Architecture—that is, that changes in the environment modify the human brain, thereby modifying people's behavior. Gage's presentation sparked the inception of a cutting-edge interdisciplinary relationship between neuroscience and architecture.

A practical understanding of neuroscientific principles guides and facilitates efforts to design the constructed environment, improve spatial awareness, strengthen cognitive abilities, and enable positive emotions and motivation. This approach bore fruit in a new field named neuro-architecture (Dance, 2017; Eberhard, 2008; Mallgrave, 2010; Robinson and Pallasmaa, 2015). It aims to understand how habitats impact the physical and mental health of human beings, as well as their moods and behavior. Researchers of neuro-architecture have been concerned with the possible link between a spatial configuration and some aspects of human conduct and understanding the mode by which an architectural environment can influence certain brain mechanisms including stress, emotion, memory, and learning (Edelstein, 2008).

Meaningfulness: the main value of architecture

These innovative disciplines satisfy society's new demands, which are oriented less toward health and medical healing—now regarded as essential rights—and more toward the overall maintenance of emotional equilibrium, self-identity, and maximal levels of personal autonomy and independence.

Architecture can do that, first, by designing and constructing safe, accessible, healthy, flexible, and comfortable environments, empowering persons to control them through modifying their spaces, changing distributions, removing and installing partitions, adapting the furniture, and creating places to introduce natural plants (Calkins, 1988). In general, this is done by generating an environment that enables individuals to govern their day-to-day physical reality effectively and by designing spaces that enable them to maintain their homoeostasis (i.e., the regulation of body temperature, blood glucose levels, hydration, and so forth). Second, architecture can render a space significant and in that way the inhabitants can identify narrative meaning within their physical surroundings. To achieve this, it is necessary to engender accurate, appropriate, and identifiable itineraries, orientations, and urban patterns, among other factors. (Marshall, 2014). Last and very important, architecture functions as a source of meaning, given its ability to establish attachments between an individual and communal values (e.g., society, friends, and family) and links to more abstract ideals and pursuits that arts such as painting, drawing, and sculpture, among others, provide. Through the meaning with which architecture infuses spaces and structures, it manages to attach people to values that transcend them (Quesada-García and Valero-Flores, 2017a).

More definitively, the value that architecture can potentially contribute to health consists, on the one hand, of its ability to construct increasingly healthy buildings, spaces, and environments that prevent the onset of diseases. On the other hand, such value more importantly attaches to architecture's potential to personalize and endow spaces with meaning, in accordance with specific needs, for people, healthy or ill (Dominiczak, 2013). It does so in a way that allows people to strengthen their cognitive faculties and enable their positive emotions and motivation, with the ultimate objective of simultaneously maintaining a physical and emotional equilibrium (Degremont, 1998).

Designing for the absence of memory: architecture for Alzheimer's patients

As is in the field of psychology, memory is perhaps best understood through the study of its opposite: from oblivion, from forgetfulness. The value of the architectural contribution to human health and well-being is better understood by analyzing the extent to which certain types of architecture influence specific groups, each suffering from a particular disease or physical or cognitive impairment.

Since 2016, the Healthy Architecture and City research group at the University of Seville, Spain, has been pursuing a line of research called "Designing for the Absence of Memory," the objective of which is to determine precisely how the physical environment influences the spatial awareness, memories, sensations, and experiences of people afflicted with Alzheimer's disease. Based on the conventional wisdom regarding their specific needs and demands, we tried to establish precise patterns and implementation practices in the design of spaces and environments. To this end, we created a methodology to ascertain, interpret, and analyze some components of the spatial memory that characterizes an inhabitant suffering from Alzheimer's disease, with the ultimate aim of quantifying, measuring, and using data to evaluate which elements of the environment are most capable of evoking emotions and memories (Quesada-García and Valero-Flores, 2017b).

To date, some of the results obtained in the above tests demonstrate that via the use of natural light and the control of spatial temperatures, 77% of people suffering from Alzheimer's-related dementia experienced improved conditions of comfort and well-being. The location of a building and its relationship with the surrounding environment was regarded by 68% of the sample population as the element with the most influence on the extent to which they could remember the space they inhabited. Another aspect worth noting is that 61% of individuals participating in the trials associated the functionality of a room with the existence of personal and recognizable elements linked to some activity of daily life.

This research emphasizes the importance of designing environments that evoke emotions and stimulate feelings, because in a way those buildings arouse a certain level of identification and sense of belonging. These are very positive emotions because they amplify feelings of autonomy that strengthen self-esteem.

Despite the great value that architecture can manifestly contribute to the daily lives of citizens, whether healthy or ill, one of the main barriers that it faces for its application in the field of health is that its conception and priorities as a discipline or as an art generally do not meet the interests, needs, and desires of the users. It is our contention that this fact produces results that fail to meet expectations and a lack of functionality.

On the other hand, architecture is an art based on techniques that traditionally involve a state of constructive inertia; to wit, changes in certain practices or processes take time to be implemented and subsequently verified. This quality renders the introduction of healthy materials and practices into the construction process at a slower pace than many would prefer. Moreover, construction processes are closely linked to economic and production factors within which contexts, priorities, and interests do not always coincide. To these circumstances is added the lack of a regulatory framework for healthy architecture, an aspect that would contribute to organizing and encouraging the use of healthy techniques in the field of construction.

However, as a promotional measure for integrating architecture into the field of health, it must be noted that construction has been recognized by the Commission on Social Determinants of Health established by the World Health Organization (2008) as one of the four determining factors of a given population's health, along with genetic factors, individual behavior, and the quality of medical care. This consideration should encourage and promote the design of spaces and environments as fundamental components of any actions to implement improved health, along with disease prevention, recovery, and rehabilitation.

Another important component of the situation concerns the development and implementation of emergent and innovative technologies. Through concepts such as Digital Home, Ambient Assisted Living (AAL), and Ambient Intelligence (AmI), architecture is well positioned to design safer, more accessible, and increasingly personalized spaces, rendering them healthier and of higher quality, while providing symbolic meaning to facilitate greater personal, physical, and intellectual equilibrium.

Promoting healthy architecture

Architecture is a discipline in which numerous agents must intervene to initiate implementation: clients, public administrators, technical experts, suppliers, builders, and end users. Therefore, it is difficult to suggest practical examples that the users can put into practice themselves. However, a series of simple architectural practices can be prescribed that, endorsed by trials and research, can be undertaken by the inhabitants of a home, such as the following:

- Natural lighting can be enhanced by increasing its presence indoors, since natural light has a positive impact on physical and emotional well-being and encourages concentration and performance (Heschong et al., 2002).
- The proper use of artificial light can be effective by choosing appropriate light fittings, with recommendations for when to switch them on and off, and on standby times. Deficient or poorly studied and situated artificial light does not help the brain to exert itself.
- The human brain is very sensitive to temperature; therefore, this factor has repercussions at cognitive, emotional, and physical levels. The temperature range that stimulates attention ranges from 20°C to 23°C, with relative humidity around 50% (Lewinski, 2015). A good-practice would be to implement suitable zoning that allows for the regulation of air conditioning levels via the introduction of thermostats per areas of use (bathrooms, kitchens, bedrooms, etc.).

- On an emotional level, color powerfully influences people and neural processes, stimulating, producing, and even intensifying certain emotions. The careful study of the color treatment of walls, as well as their textures and materials, is another domestic practice to bear in mind.
- Inhabitants should try to allow the presence or a view of green areas into the house because they evoke greater calm, tranquillity, and attention levels and also reduce stress (Li and Sullivan, 2016). Space in a home can be organized and oriented towards windows or terraces that introduce open spaces into the house, inviting the presence of green areas or incorporating plants into interior domestic spaces.
- The architecture must also have enough flexibility to allow inhabitants to meet their needs by having high autonomy, customizing ambience, creating new spaces, and modifying boundaries of their close spaces.

In conclusion, spaces must not only function, resonate emotionally, and be beautiful, but must also be healthy, comfortable, safe, and accessible. Well-being is the ultimate objective of healthy architecture.

Resources

Among the international bodies and institutions that promote and incentivize the participation of architecture in the field of health are the following:

- Academy of Neuroscience For Architecture (http://anfarch.org/).
- International Academy for Design and Health (www.designandhealth.org).
- Healthy Architecture and City (www.grupo.us.es/hac)

References

Antonovsky, A. (1979). *Health, Stress, and Coping*. Michigan: University of Michigan Press.

Aries, M.B., Veitch, J.A. and Newsham, R. (2010). Windows, View, and Office Characteristics Predict Physical and Psychological Discomfort. *Journal of Environmental Psychology*, 30: 533–541.

Benévolo, L. (1974). *Historia de la Arquitectura Moderna*. Barcelona, Spain: Gustavo Gili.

Calkins, M. (1988). *Design for Dementia: Planning Environments for the Elderly and the Confused*. Owing Mills, MD: National Health Publishing.

Commission on Social Determinants of Health (2008). *Closing the Gap in a Generation: Health Equity Through Action on the Social Determinants of Health: Final Report of the Commission on Social Determinants of Health*. Geneva, Switzerland: World Health Organization.

Dance, A. (2017). The Brain Within Buildings. *Proceedings of the National Academy of Sciences: Science and Culture*, 114(5): 785–787.

Degremont, N. (1998). *Soins Palliatifs et Architecture: de l'Hôpital vers l'Homme*. European Journal of Palliative Care, 5(4): 127–129.

Dominiczak, M. (2013). Illness and Culture: Maggie's Centres. *Clinical Chemistry*, 59: 333–334.

Eberhard, J. (2008). *Brain Landscape: The Coexistence of Neuroscience and Architecture*. Oxford: Oxford University Press.

Edelstein, E.A. (2008). Building Health. *Journal of Health Environments Research*, 1(2): 54–59.

Gideon, S. (1982). The International Congresses for Modern Architecture (CIAM) and the Formation of Contemporary Architecture. In A. Gideon and V. Clay-Gideon, eds, *Space, Time and Architecture. The Growth of a New Tradition*. 5th edition. Cambridge, NH: Harvard University Press: 696–702.

Heschong, L., Wright, R. L. and Okura, S. (2002). Daylighting Impacts on Human Performance in School. *Journal of the Illuminating Engineering Society*, 31: 101–114.

Lawson, B. (2010). Healing Architecture. *Arts and Health*, 2(2): 95–108.

Lewinski, P. (2015). Effects of Classrooms' Architecture on Academic Performance in View of Telic Versus Paratelic Motivation: A Review. *Frontiers in Psychology*, 6: 746.

Li, D. and Sullivan, W.C. (2016). Impact of Views to School Landscapes on Recovery from Stress and Mental Fatigue. *Landscape and Urban Planning*, 148: 149–158.

Mallgrave, H.F. (2010). *The Architect's Brain: Neuroscience, Creativity, and Architecture*. Malden: Wiley-Blackwell.

Marshall, M. (2014). *Designing Mental Health Units for Older People*. Stirling: Dementia Services Development Centre, University of Stirling.

Quesada-García, S. and Valero-Flores, P. (2017a). *Architecture as a Creative Practice for Improving Living Conditions and Social Welfare for Alzheimer's Patients*. Paper presented at the 5th International Health Humanities Conference, Seville, 15–17 September.

Quesada-García, S. and Valero-Flores, P. (2017b). Proyectar espacios para habitantes con alzhéimer. Una visión desde la arquitectura. *Arte, Individuo y Sociedad*, 29: 89–108.

Robinson, S. and Pallasmaa, J. eds, (2015). *Mind in Architecture: Neuroscience, Embodiment, and the Future of Design*. Cambridge: MIT Press.

46

DIGITAL STORYTELLING

Carla Rice

Introduction

Much of health discourse is premised on the belief that there exists a normative or prototypical human, and that it is the work of health-care providers and systems to return people who embody difference to a mythical normal or ideal human state. This state is mythical since, as disability, fat, and aging studies scholars have shown, norms are determined through the stories that statisticians tell about numbers and calculations that divide populations into normal and outlier or deviant groups—through the bell curving of a given population's traits and capacities (Davis, 1995).

The notion of a norm or standard also ignores the fact that many people who are born with or acquire differences early in life have never inhabited bodies deemed as ordinary, and so a species' typical body is itself often an alien state (Clare, 2017). Feminist scholars working on questions of sex and other difference have layered this analysis by tracing how the human has been conflated with the male form in Western scientific and medical research. Embodiment philosopher Margrit Shildrick (1997) notes that from the inception of early modern anatomy, Western science has taken the male as the stand-in for the human; many women's health researchers have since shown how such conflation continues in conventional biomedical research.

Most recently, post-humanist feminist Rosi Braidotti (2013) argues that the imagined human at the center of humanist thought "is very much a male of the species: it is a he. Moreover, he is white, European, handsome and able-bodied ... an ideal of bodily perfection" (13), who is "heterosexually inscribed in a reproductive unit and a full citizen of a recognised polity" (65), as well as "a rational animal endowed with language" (141). This framing ensures that some of us are more human than others, and that many are excluded from the category. Those considered Other to such a limited conceptualization of humanity are positioned to fail, never fully enacting the bodily selves held up in both humanist and biomedical images and scripts as archetypal (Rice et al., 2018a).

Rather than accept that those of us with differences must live marginal lives, how do we disrupt the normative standard at the center of scientific and humanistic scholarship, and expand our thinking about what a body can do and become? The artistic work cultivated by the Re•Vision Centre for Art and Social Justice at the University of Guelph, Canada, is dedicated to investigating this question by creating new and multiple representations of difference and studying what happens when these are loosened into the world. At the heart of our method is "the 'coming together' of storytelling and social change"—creating and sharing of new representations via audio and video that shift taken-for-granted understand-ings to advance social justice (Rice and Mündel, 2018: 215).

Re•Vision workshops enable participants (artists/non-artists, researchers/communities, health-care providers/recipients, students/teachers) to create digital/multimedia stories: short videos that pair narratives with visual, oral, aural, and other sensory modes including photos, artwork, video, ambient sound, music, movement, and more. Developed in the 1990s as a digital adaption of the radio and theater genres of autobiographical monologue (Benmayor, 2008; Lambert, 2013), digital storytelling has since evolved into an arts-based research and pedagogical tool for critical and creative theorizing, and for autoethnographic storytelling. While a growing number of researchers use digital storytelling as a method for centering marginalized perspectives (Gubrium et al., 2014), Re•Vision's turn to the video arts is borne out of the understanding that when we change how difference is storied, we also change how difference is experienced and responded to—in health care and society.

Since Re•Vision's inception in 2011, our research has oriented to speaking back to the ways that disabled people have been viewed as "not quite human" in a world that marginal-izes individuals with outlier bodyminds, such as those who use wheelchairs or sign language to act and interact (Rice et al., 2015, 2017, 2018a); to the ways that Indigenous peoples have been cast as wards of the state and as "less than" human in settler-colonial systems that equate Indigeneity with the primitive/immature/naïve; to how bodies classified as "obese" have been framed as unfit and unproductive through the equating of fat with disease and excess (Rinaldi et al., 2016); and to how in the genealogy of sexual science LGBTQI people have been cast as deviant and degenerate for a perceived failure to contribute to the reproduction of the species and of the polity/nation (Rinaldi et al., 2017). What ties all these groups together are that they are regarded as failing to qualify as "fully human," as lacking vitality, productivity, and the capacity to contribute to culture and society.

Since scholars in feminist, disability, and other interdisciplinary areas of study have taught us to trouble the normative human that marginalizes bodies of difference, and that haunts medical research as much as it does humanistic inquiry, I contend that these critical fields have much to offer health humanities researchers seeking to avoid reproducing the norma-tive and wanting to put new visions of the human into the world. Using Re•Vision's meth-odology as a case study, I briefly describe one way that story-based researchers might incorporate critical theory into different dimensions of digital storywork, by taking an orien-tation that foregrounds community making and invites failure as integral to learning and transformational change.

Making community

Re•Vision's work is situated in the methodological tradition of critical arts-based research—which emphasizes political, participatory, and process-oriented approaches (Conquergood, 2002; Finley et al., 2014)—and its main pulse is to bring together stakeholders from advan-taged and disadvantaged groups to collaboratively re-story difference. In our neoliberal, hyper-individualizing world, we desperately need to scaffold spaces and methods that make dialogue across pressing social issues possible, but to do this in ways that do not erase power or collapse difference. This work is necessary because the twin problematics of relating across difference and addressing power differentials are at the core of challenging the impulses that fuel oppression, and that lead to war and conflict.

We have held hundreds of digital/multimedia storytelling workshops where participants ranging from senior policy makers to people with lived experiences of homelessness (as an example) come together for one to five days to learn digital storytelling methods and explore issues of power and difference relating to race, class, indigeneity, age, disability, body size, gender, and beyond.

To mitigate tendencies to reproduce dominant narratives, we begin every workshop with: an in-depth framing of the issues that bring storytellers together (designing new curricula for all projects) and provide examples of how artists and activists have intervened in conventional scripts; a story circle where participants share initial ideas around an experience or moment they wish to develop and consider how they might use their stories to unsettle the dominant account; and writing exercises and tutorials on audio, video, and editing methods to allow participants to experiment with creative ways of telling stories; and technical, writing, and conceptual support to help them from script development to finished video.

For me, this methodology is distinctive not only in how it brings majority and minoritized storytellers together and into creative and accountable spaces, but also in how it brings into being new communities of practice. When diversely positioned people share personal stories, this invites vulnerability among those who are typically perceived/expected to perform as disembodied experts (doctors, educators, policy makers, and professors), thus briefly disrupting the notion of the autonomous, rational self that is the basis of Western law/institutions/professions, and foregrounding the vulnerable self as integral to human experience and relationship (Fineman, 2008). Further, centering difference, both in terms of the workshop foci and the bodies occupying leadership positions (as researchers and facilitators) temporarily repositions members of justice seeking groups as experts who possess valued knowledge that is needed to re-story difference and remake systems. This coming together incites a "becoming together" where individuals' stories begin to bleed and breathe together and, through the connections made in the workshop space, to make/remake community.

While many discussions of storytelling for social change focus on individuals telling their stories in DIY style, what we find so powerful about group process is how it re-centers the necessity of listening, of taking responsibility for the stories we share and hear, and, in so doing, of remaking our relationalities with each other. Through being shared beyond the workshop space, the stories play an important part in remaking policy and practice (Rice and Mündel, 2018).

Welcoming failure

Like many critical arts-based research approaches, Re•Vision draws from social justice principles to purposely set up our workshops to be spaces of radical relationality, accessibility and accountability, and to be intimate, nourishing, and safe(r) spaces to tell stories. With each project, researchers work together to modify Re•Vision procedures (theoretical framings, curricula, workshop activities) to suit the context; in this sense I understand storytelling methods as processual—as continually under construction—and recognize with ethnographer Sarah Pink (2015: 11), how "methods themselves have biographies, they evolve through different projects." Pushing against overly prescriptive methods, I further take from narratologist Arthur Frank (2010: 1) the insight that "stories are too lively and too wild to be tied up."

When we approach storytelling methodology as open-ended, we re-orient to anticipating, preparing for (to the extent possible), and welcoming the disruption that occurs in each project's unfolding. Here new knowledge, in addition to emerging from the stories created, surfaces provisionally from the insights acquired, and the meanings and mistakes made, throughout the process of giving life to them.

Despite researchers' effects to anticipate the needs of participants, whether those needs are for accessibility or for ideological openness to varied perspectives on politically charged issues (such as ensuring access to gender-neutral washrooms, comfortable chairs for diverse bodies, and room for wheelchair users, as well as providing nuanced, culturally safe curricular materials/processes), we inevitably confront the unknown and unexpected that comes with working across differences and, with this confrontation, failure. One powerful example of the rub of difference was in a workshop with Indigenous participants, who collectively pushed against the individualizing emphasis of the digital storytelling genre through joining together to improvise "a collective (re)telling and (re)turning of the colonial gaze" (Rice and Mündel, 2018: 227).

Another example was found in a workshop with disabled storytellers, whose seemingly incommensurate accommodation needs (such as fluorescent lights that needed to be dimmed to prevent migraines in some participants and to be turned up for others to access sign language interpretation) made us realize that we were approaching access in the way that inclusion, under neoliberalism, is typically taken up: as a zero sum game where one person's "loss" is another's "gain."

While in both cases the researchers and facilitators re-negotiated the terms of the workshop, these rubs made me wonder whether we could revision research processes premised on non-competitive, non-zero-sum (and anti-colonial) logics, and if so, how these might be enacted (Rice and Mündel, 2019). These and other experiences have impacted my research practice by orienting me to welcome the unexpected; to work improvisationally to make processes and spaces work for those in the room; to practice reflexivity in response to failure; and to recognize how, at its best, storytelling as method is shape-shifting, continuously moving and changing along with subjectivities and social worlds (Rice et al., 2018b).

Following the workshops, Re•Vision researchers commit to sharing the stories created beyond academic circles, notably with audiences of policy makers, practitioners, and others, following the belief that art and story can teach in non-didactic ways (Rice et al., 2018a, 2018b). I have witnessed how social change happens through the relational reconfigurations that occur within workshop spaces and, with these, the intersectional and intersectoral alliances that storytellers forge for intervening in systemic inequities. Change making continues after the workshops, through where and how the stories travel and how researchers and community members engaged in various projects use them to influence policy and practice.

Through re-storying experiences and alliances across differences, Re•Vision creates new communities and captures the conditions under which these are made possible. Together, researchers and storytellers rethink what counts as knowledge, who can be a knower, whose stories matter, and how we can re-imagine the human in more expansive and affirming ways.

References

Benmayor, R. (2008). Digital Storytelling as a Signature Pedagogy for the New Humanities. *Arts and Humanities in Higher Education*, 7(2): 188–204.

Braidotti, R. (2013). *The Posthuman*. Cambridge, UK: Polity Press.

Clare, E. (2017). *Brilliant Imperfection: Grappling with Cure*. Durham, NC: Duke University Press.

Conquergood, D. (2002). Performance Studies: Interventions and Radical Research. *TDR/The Drama Review*, 46(2): 145–156.

Davis, L. J. (1995). *Enforcing Normalcy: Disability, Deafness, and the Body*. London: Verso Press.

Fineman, M. (2008). The Vulnerable Subject and the Responsive State. *Yale Journal of Law and Feminism*, 20(1): 1–22.

Finley, S., Vonk, C. and Finley, M.L. (2014). Critical Arts-Based Research as Public Pedagogy. *Cultural Studies ↔ Critical Methodologies*, 14(6): 619–625.

Frank, A. (2010). *Letting Stories Breathe: A Socio-Narratology*. Chicago, IL: University of Chicago Press.

Gubrium, A., Krause, E. and Jernigan, K. (2014). New Ways of Seeing and Being Seen as Young Mothers Through Digital Storytelling. *Sexuality Research and Social Policy*, 11: 337–347.

Lambert, J. (2013). *Digital Storytelling: Capturing Lives, Creating Community*. 4th edition. New York: Routledge.

Pink, S. (2015). *Doing Sensory Ethnography*. 2nd edn. Thousand Oaks, CA: Sage.

Rice, C., Chandler, E., Harrison, E., Ferrari, M. and Liddiard, K. (2015). Project Re•Vision: Disability at the Edges of Representation. *Disability and Society*, 30(4): 513–527.

Rice, C., Chandler, E., Rinaldi, J., Liddiard, K., Changfoot, N., Mykitiuk, R. and Mündel, I. (2017). Imagining disability futurities. *Hypatia: A Journal of Feminist Philosophy*, *32*(2), 213–229.

Rice, C., Chandler, E., Liddiard, K., Rinaldi, J. and Harrison, E. (2018a). The Pedagogical Possibilities for Unruly Bodies. *Gender and Education*, 30(5): 663–682.

Rice, C., LaMarre, A., Changfoot, N. and Douglas, P. (2018b). Making Spaces: Multimedia Storytelling as Reflexive, Creative Praxis. *Qualitative Research in Psychology*. https://doi.org/10.1080/14780887.2018.1442694.

Rice, C. and Mündel, I. (2018). Storymaking as Methodology. *Canadian Review of Sociology*, 55(2): 211–231.

Rice, C. and Mündel, I. (2019). Multimedia Storytelling Methodology: Notes on Access and Inclusion in Neoliberal Times. *Canadian Journal of Disability Studies*, 8(2): 118–146.

Rinaldi, J., Rice, C., LaMarre, A., McPhail, D. and Harrison, E. (2017). Fatness and Failing Citizenship. *Somatechnics*, 7(2): 218–233.

Rinaldi, J., Rice, C., LaMarre, A., Pendleton Jiménez, K., Harrison, E., Friedman, M. and Tidgwell, T. (2016). Through 'Thick and Thin'. *Psychology of Sexualities Review (PoSR)*, 7(2): 63–77.

Shildrick, M. (1997). *Leaky Bodies and Boundaries: Feminism, Postmodernism and (Bio) Ethics*. London: Routledge.

47

HEAVY METAL MUSIC

Charley Baker and Alex Bishop

Introduction

This chapter builds upon previous work by one of the authors (Baker and Brown, 2016) and our dual longstanding affinity with heavy metal music, both musically and subculturally. Specifically, we aim to reflect on some of the potential mental health *benefits* of metal in its broadest form. Recent work (Hughes et al., 2018) has once again drawn attention to the tentatively supported relationships between belonging to a heavy metal subculture and an increased risk of self-harm and/or suicidality. What is not clear, and is under-explored, is whether this is a possible unidirectional or bidirectional relationship: it is likely neither in any simple sense (Olson, 2015) and is beyond the scope of this chapter to fully critique the studies that suggest increased sensitivity towards mental ill health or expressions of potential distress within metal subcultures.

The evidence base for this association remains relatively small, yet Hughes et al.'s article attracted a significant amount of media attention (e.g., Knapton, 2018), much like that which occurred following Young et al.'s (2006) study, which also purported to find a relationship between metal affiliation and mental health difficulties (see also Curtis and Carvel, 2006). More rarely acknowledged are the potential mental health *benefits* of such a belonging, however (see, for example, Hill, 2011; Baker and Brown, 2016; Ro, 2016). Additionally, the metal community at large has increasingly sought to draw attention to modes of support available for younger (and older) fans who may be struggling, encouraging them to reach out, seek support (You Rock Foundation, 2018), and look after one another (as indeed happens in the pit at any gig where the ethos is usually a variation of "fall down, get picked back up").

This chapter reviews recent discussions around the relationship between suicidality and heavy metal affiliation and reflects on the experiences inherent in metal affiliation, including the music itself and gig attendance. While the precise roots of the term "heavy metal" are unknown, it can be traced to bands of the late 1960s, who began mixing blues and rock music, creating a thick, heavy, guitar-and-drums-centered sound (Weinstein, 2000). The evolution of this sound over the decades has led to the rise of various subgenres, each with characteristic elements, but all based around the use of highly amplified guitar sound distortion. To this end, the term "heavy metal" (or "metal") has become a catch-all for music across this range of subgenres. In this chapter we use "metal" in its broadest sense, covering the range of subgenres including "metalcore," "emo," and "goth."

Metal and mental health: research and directions within health humanities

In spring 2018 the debate around metal-related subcultural suicidality and self-harm was reignited with the publication of a systematic review examining this association (Hughes et al., 2018). Hughes et al. present some important findings, summarizing the oft-held argument that there may be a small-to-modest increase in the risk of self-harm or suicidality among people who identify with any of the metal-related subcultures. Less clear, however, is whether it is possible to evidence precisely "what it is about alternative subculture affiliation (or alternative music preference) that could contribute to the risk of self-harm" (18). This review includes 12 studies (ten quantitative, two qualitative) over a timeframe of 25 years. The individual studies have mixed findings, often with modest or small sample sizes or limited generalizability.

Previously, metal affiliation (in particular "goth" or "emo" sub-subcultural identification), has attracted media headlines in a way that actively fuels unhelpful stereotypes of the suicidal goth or emo teen, at risk from indulging in such depressing, angry, or aggressive music, never mind attending live music venues with their violent approaches to "dancing." One such example is the UK-based newspaper *Daily Mail*, whose headline "Why no child is safe from the sinister cult of emo" (Rawstorne, 2008) is an exemplar of this kind of "moral panic" (see Olson, 2015; Baker and Brown, 2016). Such a drawn-out and hyperbolic association played out in the media is far from likely to encourage young people to speak to their parents or a trusted adult, fueling further stigma in an already "different" group of people.

The reasons behind self-harm and suicidality in the metal community (as in any group of people) are unique, highly individual, and driven by a multitude of factors; narrative accounts of people's own lived experience of self-harm highlight these diverse reasons as well as the survival function that self-harm (as *distinct* from suicidality) can have (Pembroke, 2003; Baker et al., 2013). There seems to be a drive, lasting over two decades, toward establishing whether people who may already be struggling are drawn towards music that undeniably has dark imagery, focusing on more difficult emotional states, or whether the metal scene *itself* normalizes or validates self-harm as a coping strategy (Hughes et al., 2018). In recent research, the strength and survival aspects that people find within supportive metal communities has been researched in more systematic detail (Rowe and Guerin, 2018).

Health humanities (Crawford et al., 2010, 2015) as a discipline might interpret this *potential* interaction as a source of opportunity, therapeutically and pedagogically. That is, metal may offer a creative vision—for practitioners, scholars, academics, people who are struggling, and their carers or friends—of a particular mental health experience. While examples of the portrayal of different mental states and struggles are in abundance across the spectrum of different metal subgenres, we focus only on one here, namely that of Australian metalcore band The Amity Affliction.

The Amity Affliction

The Amity Affliction's Joel Birch has been open across social media and in interviews about his own struggles with depression, anxiety, and addiction. Ahren Stringer, Birch, and various members of the band have produced a range of albums praised for their engagement with both mental health, starkly screamed, *and* recovery, including *Chasing Ghosts* (2012), *Let The Ocean Take Me* (2014) and most recently *Misery* (2018). Such powerful and stark portrayal of depression, addictions, and suicidality might offer both a catharsis and an identification (Baker and Brown, 2016), but at a potential cost. Taylor (2014) quotes Birch describing how he "wrote an open letter to fans coinciding with the release of The Amity Affliction's song 'Don't Lean On Me,' which deals with the difficulties of being confronted with his fans' pain" (Taylor, 2014). Birch, in this interview, notes the healing power of music:

> Music is such a healing, therapeutic release for me ... I know a lot of people are out there saying this and that saved my life, but for real, without music I don't know what I would be doing, music saved my goddamn life.
>
> *(Taylor, 2014)*

In this song, the lyrics draw on both the need to support each other and the challenges that can occur in responding to fan's distress as metal icon. The bridge in "Don't Lean on Me" (The Amity Affliction, 2014) speaks to listeners to *hold on*.

From Birch's interview, it is clear that the sense of (potentially mutual) identification available for listeners at a point of struggle, distress, or desperation may *promote* reaching out and provide encouragement that things can and do feel differently with time. In a more recent interview, when asked what the music industry could do to better support people's mental health, Birch replies:

> The answer is a long and sustained campaign to educate people who aren't depressed about what people who are depressed are going through. People need to be given the tools to empathise with people ... We're at the beginning, it's positive and we just need to make sure it keeps going and just becomes a part of life in the music industry. It's a discussion that needs to be had.
>
> *(Joel Birch in interview with Leviers, 2018)*

Communities of metal musicians and fans, both in and out of the gig arena, then, may hold important keys to the way in which such benefits might be harnessed more broadly.

Community

Any identified "causal" mechanisms between metal affiliation and increased risks of mental health difficulties and/or self-harm are likely to be as complex and multifaceted as are suicidality, self-harm, and psychological distress themselves. Feelings of stigma and marginalization from others may contribute of a sense of "minority stress" (Hughes et al., 2018), where fans of heavy music seek comfort and community among those who share a common passion in a "protective" community (see Rowe and Guerin, 2018). Indeed, one product of affiliation with alternative subculture can be an active and deliberate reaction against perceived norms. Often the very distinct appearance (clothing, tattooing, and body modification) chosen by fans of heavy music acts to celebrate and affirm their membership of a community that is routinely misunderstood and demonized. Strong or even violent reactions from outside the community can lead people to seek sense and affirmation solely from within, as might be identified in ethnographic, anthropological, and sociological disciplines. Externally abusive responses to subcultural association are perhaps most brutally affirmed in the death of Sophie Lancaster, who was horrifically murdered and her boyfriend seriously injured for looking "different." (See the Sophie Lancaster Foundation, 2018 for the work that her family has done in promoting subcultural abuse as a hate crime.) When people feel alienated by erroneously promulgated assumptions from outside their scene, they are left with little choice but to look inwards for support; such support abounds in the music itself, the lyrics, the wider culture, and the gig itself.

Social media has increased connectivity to others within a subculture, and with this comes increased access to those with similar experiences and outlooks. While this has undoubtedly provided a platform to spread the kind of awareness that Birch refers to, there may also exist the potential for exposure to themes and experiences that some fans may not be adequately prepared or supported to encounter. Given the increasing rates of mental health difficulties and self-harm (e.g., Morgan et al., 2017; Griffin et al., 2018) among young people, and associated increased media and social media mental health awareness campaigns (for example, Time to Talk, 2018), it may be that those who are *already* feeling in a state of distress and struggle find solace and support in communities where such distress is heard, understood, and validated. This is most actively played out in the process of attending a gig, a setting that might look dark and dangerous from the outside but which offers a uniquely welcoming, supportive, and closeknit community.

Personal reflections: on the emotionality and physicality of metal gigs

Metal's gig experience can be thought of as a dichotomy between shared experience and personal involvement. A crowd witnessing the same set list on stage will be absorbing the content in any number of ways. As a communal experience, there is a degree of anonymity that comes with being part of a crowd, all convened for a common cause. It provides an opportunity to detach from the stresses of real life to come together and participate in a mutual recognition of the performers on stage. Even down to the clichéd yet true uniform appearance of metal fans—black band T-shirts, denim and leather, tattoos, piercings, dyed hair—there is a tacit understanding that everyone is there for the same reason. It is an arena free of the judgment that many have to deal with away from that environment. Within this safe space, each individual is free to experience—and interact with—the music in the way they choose. This may be metaphorically true in any music concert attendance, and where metal gigs differ is through the physicality of the mosh pit, a different experience to that seen with other concerts and dancing.

Those that opt to go to the front and get involved in the more physical aspects of concerts—mosh pits—do so in the knowledge they enter an allotted space, and that they are among others who will observe an unwritten code of etiquette and mutual respect. Looking out for those around you ("fall down, get picked back up") has long been considered a prerequisite of moshing. Often misunderstood by those taken aback at the physicality and seeming violence of the mosh pit, there is a security that comes from knowing others have your security in mind.

That is not to say that gigs are always safe environments. Instances of "crowd killing" at hardcore shows—unprovoked attacks towards those on the periphery of the pit, who have chosen to not actively engage in moshing—show something of a more selfish participation in the gig-going experience. While there can be swift summary justice against these perpetrators (again under the ethos of pit etiquette), it is evidence of an unpredictability that excites some while giving credence to the concerns and criticisms of others. Hardcore dancing (violent and unpredictable movements, largely isolated from what others around are doing) can be seen as an almost *antisocial* way to react to music. At that time, that person's experience is centered on what they are doing and is largely unconcerned with fellow gig goers. Even though this can be seen as the antithesis of what many see as the primary appeal of gigs, it is still the case that at a given show, in a given space, this behavior may be seen as either "unacceptable" or "acceptable."

The community aspects though are key here; metal is in many ways a self-policing culture where the rituals of the pit (the "wall of death" or "circle pit"), the gig, and the music offer a simultaneously shared and radically individualized experience. The stratospheric rise of bands such as Architects, Slipknot, Trivium, and Bring Me The Horizon, who now play sell-out stadium tours, offer a wide-scale connectivity with over 10,000 people in attendance. What is different then is that the larger scale might impact on the more traditionally sized venues of 500-person capacity upwards, where a smaller crowd offers a more personal or intimate connection within the crowd and with the band.

While not specific to metal, one recent study has demonstrated how subjective well-being scores were found to be "significantly higher for those who engaged with music via dancing or attending musical events, compared to those who did not engage with music in those forms" (Weinberg and Joseph, 2017: 264). As Ambrose wrote in 2001: "There is more fraternity and harmony in the pit than outsiders can possibly imagine" (Ambrose, 2001: 5). From a gendered point of view, the gig space offers an increasingly safe(r) space for female attendees, in the era of #MeToo where the extent to which (predominantly) women experience sexual assaults has been laid bare like never before. Despite the hyper-masculinized environment of the metal mosh pit, musicians have spoken out when witnessing gropes in the crowd. Sam Carter of UK-based band Architects (O'Connor, 2017) received significant positive attention for calling this behavior out. Girls Against, a group of teens dedicated to fighting assault at gigs, were noted as NME People of the Year in 2016 (Cooper, 2016). Steps are being taken not only to protect the fraternity, but also to promote safety and respect for all.

Conclusion

When we return to the words of The Amity Affliction in their 2012 album *Chasing Ghosts*, the beauty of survival in struggle is played out through the song "Open Letter," with lines that could be read as a finding of hope, beauty, and meaning and an offering to creatively show the pain inherent behind some of the best of metal songs.

This writing-through of depression, suicidality, and addiction continues in their most musically diverse album to date *Misery* (2018), which shows Birch singing a range of clean vocals, the pain stark and frank but—for us—perhaps less claustrophobic than in earlier work.

Those into metal are far from a homogenous group and divisions related to genre can be fiercely fought in the YouTube sections of bands pages and across social media. However, our reflections here—that being both different *and* accepted in a way not otherwise seen elsewhere is common to metal, where mental health is written into the very fabric of the songs themselves—offers an understanding of the mental health benefits of metal that extend beyond the lyrical, the musical, and the identificatory. The metal scene more broadly is actively engaging with the mental health of the fans and the crowds, seen in the You Rock Foundation, where crisis helpline numbers are available on the same page as videos from metal icons (Corey Taylor of Slipknot and Randy Blythe of Lamb of God among them) sharing their own stories of mental health struggle, surviving, and thriving. UK-based suicide prevention charity Samaritans offer a Festivals Branch who attend festivals up and down the country, offering the potential for a person to reach out at a critical juncture.

There is a further opportunity to begin to consider the experiences of older and aging metal fans. We know that music has a profound impact on the well-being of people with dementia, for example, and focusing in the future on prior musical preference and the impact of later music-based approaches to care would be instructive. Further ethnographically informed research with fans themselves around the mechanisms of survival drawn from the lyrics and (increasingly) engagement with the bands at gigs or on social media is essential to destigmatize further self-harm, suicidality, and mental health in populations where their difficulties have become acute, urgent, and widespread.

References

Ambrose, J. (2001). *The Violent World of Moshpit Culture*. London: Omnibus Press.

The Amity Affliction (2012). *Chasing Ghosts* (Roadrunner Records).

The Amity Affliction (2014). *Let The Ocean Take Me* (Roadrunner Records).

The Amity Affliction (2018). *Misery* (Roadrunner Records).

Baker, C. and Brown, B. (2016). Suicide, Self-Harm and Survival Strategies in Contemporary Heavy Metal Music: A Cultural and Literary Analysis. *Journal of Medical Humanities*, 37: 1–37.

Baker, C., Shaw, C. and Biley, F. (2013). *Our Encounters with Self Harm*. Ross-on-Wye: PCCS Books.

Cooper, L. (2016). NME People of The Year 2016: Girls Against For Fighting Sexual Assault One Gig at a Time. *NME*, 7th December 2016. Available at: www.nme.com/blogs/nme-blogs/people-year-2016-girls-against-1898817#F3HcThzEjv166CUh.99 (Accessed 22/09/18).

Crawford, P., Brown, B., Baker, C., Tischler, V. and Abrams, B. (2015). *Health Humanities*. Basingstoke: Palgrave.

Crawford, P., Brown, B., Tishler, V. and Baker, C. (2010). Health Humanities: the future of medical humanites? *Mental Health Review Journal*, 15(3): 4–10.

Curtis, P. and Carvel, R. (2006). Teen Goths More Prone to Suicide, Study Shows. *The Guardian*, 14th April 2006. Available at: www.theguardian.com/society/2006/apr/14/socialcare.uknews (Accessed 22/09/18).

Griffin, E., McMahon, E., McNicholas, F., Corcoran, P., Perry, I.J. and Arensman, E. (2018). Increasing Rates of Self-Harm Among Children, Adolescents and Young Adults: A 10-Year National Registry Study 2007–2016. *Social Psychiatry and Psychiatric Epidemiology*, 53(7): 663–671.

Hill, R. (2011). "Emo saved my life": Challenging the Mainstream Discourse of Mental Illness around My Chemical Romance. In C.A. McKinnon, N. Scott and K. Sollee, eds, *Can I Play with Madness? Metal, Dissonance, Madness and Alienation*. Oxford: Oxford University Press: 143–153.

Hughes, M.A., Knowles, S.F., Dhingra, K., Nicholson, H.L. and Taylor, P. (2018). This Corrosion: A Systematic Review of the Association between Alternative Subcultures and the Risk of Self-Harm and Suicide. *British Journal of Clinical Psychology*, 57(4): 491–513.

Knapton, S. (2018). Young Heavy Metal Fans Five Times More Likely to Self Harm or Attempt Suicide. *The Telegraph UK*, 4th April 2018. Available at: www.telegraph.co.uk/science/2018/04/04/young-heavy-metal-fans-five-times-likely-self-harm-attempt-suicide/ (Accessed 22/09/2018).

Leviers, D. (2018). The Amity Affliction: If This Doesn't Work, We're F*cked. *Loudersound*. Available at: www.loudersound.com/features/the-amity-affliction-if-this-doesnt-work-were-fcked (Accessed 22/09/18).

Morgan, C., Webb, R.T., Carr, M.J., Kontopantelis, E., Green, J., Chew-Graham, C.A., Kapur, N. and Ashcroft, D.M. (2017). Incidence, Clinical Management, and Mortality Risk Following Self Harm Among Children and Adolescents: Cohort Study in Primary Care. *BMJ*: 359.

O'Connor, R. (2017). Architects Singer Sam Carter Calls Out Man 'Who Grabbed Fan's Breast While She Was Crowdsurfing. *The Independent UK*, 19 August 2017. Available at: www.independent.co.uk/arts-entertainment/music/news/architects-gig-sam-carter-crowdsurfer-video-lowlands-festival-sexual-assault-grope-latest-a7901606.html (Accessed 22/09/18).

Olson, R. (2015). Suicide, Rock Music and Moral Panics. *Centre for Suicide Prevention: Editorial*. Available at: www.suicideinfo.ca/resource/musicandsuicide/ (Accessed 14/01/19).

Pembroke, L. (2003). *Self Harm: Perspectives from Personal Experience*. London: Chipmunka Publishing.

Rawstorne, T. (2008). Why No Child Is Safe from the Sinister Cult of Emo. *Daily Mail*, 18 May 2008. Available at: www.dailymail.co.uk/femail/article-566481/Why-child-safe-sinister-cult-emo.html (Accessed 14/01/2019).

Ro, C. (2016). The Positive Psychology of Metal Music: Shredding Assumptions About Heavy Metal Music and Its Fans. *Smart Set*, 13 June 2016. Available at: https://thesmartset.com/the-positive-psych ology-of-metal-music/ (Accessed 22/09/18).

Rowe, P. and Guerin, B. (2018). Contextualizing the Mental Health of Metal Youth: A Community for Social Protection, Identity, and Musical Empowerment. *Journal of Community Psychology*, 46(4): 429–441.

Sophie Lancaster Foundation (2018). Available at: https://sophielancasterfoundation.com/ (Accessed 22/09/18).

Taylor, R. (2014). Music Exploring Mental Illness Strikes Chord with Fans: The Amity Affliction Praised for Tackling Issue. *ABC News*, 9 October 2014. Available at: http://mobile.abc.net.au/news/2014-10-09/amity-affliction-mental-illness-strikes-chord-with-fans/5799884?section=news (Accessed 22/09/18).

Time to Talk (2018). Available at: www.time-to-change.org.uk/about-us/about-our-campaign/time-to-talk (Accessed 22/09/2018).

Weinberg, M.K. and Joseph, D. (2017). If You're Happy and You Know It: Music Engagement and Subjective Wellbeing. *Psychology of Music*, 45(2): 257–267.

Weinstein, D. (2000). *Heavy Metal: The Music and its Culture*. New York: DaCapo.

You Rock Foundation (2018). www.yourockfoundation.org/ (Accessed 22/09/18).

Young, R., Sweeting, H. and Young, P. (2006). Prevalence of Deliberate Self Harm and Attempted Suicide within Contemporary Goth Youth Subculture: Longitudinal Cohort Study. *British Medical Journal*, 332: 1058–1061.

48

GRAPHIC MEDICINE

MK Czerwiec and Brian Callender

Introduction

The term *graphic medicine* was coined in 2008 by Ian Williams, a physician working, at the time, in North Wales. As he tells the story in *The Graphic Medicine Manifesto* (2015), Williams was contemplating a thesis idea for a Master's degree in the medical humanities, and his topic was an inquiry into whether or not comics could have a serious role in the discourse of health and illness. This exploration was inspired by a graphic memoir, *Mom's Cancer* by Brian Fies (2006), that he discovered at the Tate Modern bookstore in London.

In *Mom's Cancer*, Fies shows us a family member's perspective on cancer treatment, how health-care providers present patients with grossly conflicting messages, and what happens to patients and their families when they step out of clinical settings and go home. Reading *Mom's Cancer*, with its insightful graphic depictions of experiences in the health-care system, Williams wondered about the possible impact this book could have if used in teaching medical and nursing students. He also wondered if there could be a benefit in sharing this kind of book with patients and families going through similar experiences. The possibilities for using this text in teaching and learning about health care seemed loaded with potential. Noting the comic potential of this genre in the medium of comics, he proposed the term *graphic medicine*: "Could the graphic be the medicine?"

Williams was not alone. Scholars, cartoonists, practitioners, teachers, librarians, and others had already been contemplating the possibilities of using comics in health care. At Penn State College of Medicine, Michael Green had been teaching comic-making to fourth-year medical students; and at nearby Pennsylvania State University Susan Squier had begun using them as text in her literature scholarship (see her chapter in this volume). After Williams established the Graphic Medicine website (www.graphicmedicine.org) to catalog comics that covered health and illness, he was contacted by these and other like-minded people, who decided to host the first conference on Graphic Medicine in London, United Kingdom, in 2010. In less than ten years, the field has exploded online, in clinics, and in classrooms, with hundreds of new graphic medicine titles catalogued and the formation of an international community of graphic medicine enthusiasts.

Citing the unique contribution this genre of comics makes to the understanding of illness and care, Patricia Brennan, the director of the National Library of Medicine (NLM), stated that through graphic medicine, "We now have a different grammar, a new language, to express health." Brennan was speaking at the launch of the NLM collection and exhibit, "Graphic Medicine: Ill-Conceived and Well-Drawn" in March of 2018. The online component of the exhibit includes high school and university level lesson plans.[1]

Why comics?

This relatively quick embrace of comics into the health-care context raises the following questions: Why did comics in health care so quickly find a community around the world? Why was mainstream health care willing to adopt this unusual combination? Why, too, were universities willing to add graphic medicine courses to their graduate and undergraduate curricula?

There are likely many varied answers to these questions. It seems to be the right movement at the right moment; in the twenty-first century we live in visual culture and our digital age is driven by a combination of images and text. More substantially, many of the recent applications of comics in the context of health and illness rely on the medium of comics possessing a unique ability to engage the reader and efficiently convey information.

Comics are particularly adept at conveying information when three factors are present:

1. There is a high density of information to be learned.
2. There is a high level of importance to the information.
3. Learners are in a high-stress situation.

Think of the informational safety cards on planes that tells passengers what to do in the event of an emergency. Those cards are almost universally in comic format. The three factors above are also present in health-care settings, for example, when getting a new diagnosis, as well as the reality of students in demanding educational programs.

Comics can add visual attraction and appeal, making the experience of using them enjoyable, even if the situation they are used in or the content of the comic is not. Brian Fies has said of *Mom's Cancer* that he made the book he wish existed for his family as they were going through a difficult experience. Several graphic medicine creators have similarly echoed this sentiment, reporting that in times of great duress, they were unable to focus on long passages of text, which are common in the informational handouts we so frequently provide our patients and students. Comics offer an alternative yet effective learning modality.

In addition, comics bring a long history beneficial to their use in modern health care. Underground comics have often taken as their subject stigmatized aspects of the human experience. Within health care, this has led to comics that bring light to traditionally stigmatized topics such as living with disability (*The Spiral Cage* by Al Davison), facing dying and death (*Last Things* by Marissa Moss), sexual abuse (*Becoming, Unbecoming* by Una), the lived reality of grieving (*Rosalie Lightning* by Tom Hart), or the struggles of professional and family caregiving (*The Bad Doctor* by Ian Williams, or *Tangles* by Sarah Leavitt).

Comics also have a long history of use in social and political activism. Applied to health care, this has made for insightful comics about racial and gender bias in medicine (as in the work of Whit Taylor and Aubrey Hirsch on *thenib.com*) as well advocacy for health care as a basic human right (as in the collaborative work "Sketches from Outside the Margins: Stories from the Seattle/King County Clinic").

One last "why" for the use of comics in the health humanities is community. Whether bringing together people in real life at academic conferences and comic-cons, or virtual communities online, comics are a medium of social connection. Appreciation for the medium of comics transcends geography, language, social status, and culture. Illness often isolates, and comics by their nature are a potent antidote for both social and physical isolation for creators, readers, scholars, and fans.

Use of comics in the health humanities

As the field expands, graphic medicine is increasingly being used in professional training and in clinical settings. One of the earliest recognitions of the potential for works of graphic medicine was in the training of health professionals. In depicting personal narratives dealing with illness, receiving health care, and death, graphic narratives confront challenging and complex experiences and provide both commentary on and critique of the health-care system. Similar to narrative medicine, the careful reading and discussion of these works has the potential to improve a trainee's understanding of the illness experience, the provider–patient relationship, and ethical and professional dilemmas. Additionally, creating comics as a self-reflective exercise allows trainees to explore their experiences, including professional development and contentious or stigmatizing topics.

Michael Green (2015) has shown that reading and creating comics with medical students can improve important skills such as empathy, communication, clinical reasoning, and attention to non-verbal cues. Additionally, the comics created by students reveal experiences impactful to their professional identity and formation. Joshi et al. (2019) have recently shown that using educational comics with students on a psychiatry clerkship improved their understanding of the material, eased their transition to the clerkship, and found the material more engaging. While the early use of comics in medical education focused on medical students, expanding the use of comics in professional training to other levels of trainees (pre-medical, resident) and to other health professions (such as nursing, social work, and pharmacy) is an exciting new direction for graphic medicine.

Graphic narratives are increasingly being used to engage patients through patient education materials, workshops, and support groups. An analysis (Houts et al., 2006) of the use of pictures in patient education has shown that pictures can improve patient attention, comprehension, recall, and adherence and can be particularly useful for individuals with low literacy skills. Additionally, this analysis indicates that simple drawings, as compared with stick-figures or more realistic images, are more effective at promoting comprehension. Since patients experience their illnesses as a narrative, the combination of simple drawings in a narrative format has the potential to more directly engage patients. Compared with educational materials that are disease-focused, patient education materials that incorporate graphic narrative allow patients to better imagine themselves within an illness narrative, one that can lay out diagnostic and therapeutic considerations as well as simplify complex processes or procedures. The ability to insert oneself into a narrative allows a patient to better contextualize their position within a broader narrative that addresses the challenges of receiving health care. However, challenges to incorporating graphic narrative into patient educational materials include concerns about comics being too juvenile and potentially trivializing a serious matter, that pictures can potentially be too distracting, and in terms of appropriate representation of a diverse patient population.

Similar to the use of reading and creating comics within the health professions, an emerging use of comics within health care is through workshops and activities in which patients use the creation of comics to reflect upon their health and well-being. The embodied process of creating comics allows for deep reflection and neurocognitive processing of living with a condition, receiving health care, and interacting with loved ones and one's community. The medium of comics allows patients to simultaneously express multiple, and sometimes conflicting, feelings and thoughts, providing a rich and complex understanding of their illness experience. The modular nature of comics also allows for patients to build upon their narratives or permit others (e.g., caregivers or providers) to contribute to this narrative. Scholarly approaches to the creation and research of graphic narratives has the potential to better understand the experience of illness and design interventions that better provide for and empower patients. While creating comics about one's own experience enables introspection, reading published graphic narratives by individuals with similar conditions may both broaden an individual's understanding of a condition and create a sense of community. The addition of graphic novels and comics to disease-specific book clubs can engage patients with a medium that is visually appealing and particularly adept at capturing the illness experience and provide the opportunity to discuss concerns, anxieties, and hope with others. However, the benefits of using graphic novels in support groups are unclear and remain an area for future research.

Future of the field

Susan Squier, in announcing the formation of the Graphic Medicine Collective in her 2018 keynote address in White River Junction, Vermont, stated that:

> We choose this name with very deep awareness of its limitations ... We see it as our mission to reframe, expand, and to reclaim both the term graphic and the term medicine to cast the widest net ... Our priorities will expand to facilitate more cross-disciplinary work, mentorship, and research, to focus on patient projects, environmental applications, and social activism. We strive to be intentional about diversity, inclusion, and international outreach, all without losing sight of our core mission which is to work at the intersection of the medium of comics and the discourses of health, illness, caregiving, and disability.
>
> *Comic Nurse, 2018*

In addition to the goals established above, the field of graphic medicine would benefit from developing "best practices" for use within various disciplines. For example, in literature studies we could ask, "What does it mean to closely read a comic about experiences of illness, disability, and/or caregiving?" In bioethics, we ask, "What ethical considerations should guide our use of comics in clinical settings?" In nursing, medicine, and the allied health professions we can explore questions like "When is the best time to give a patient a comic? What comics are best for particular conditions? What are the critical elements of effective educational comics for patients and families?," or even "Which particular comics, though widely considered graphic medicine, might we avoid recommending for use with patients and families?"

For art therapists and cartoonists working with patients and care providers to create graphic narratives about the experience of illness, caregiving, trauma, and disability, we could ask, "What kinds of guidance and support do people need at different stages of the creation of their comics?" For health librarians, "How does one approach development and promotion of a collection of graphic medicine texts?" In health-care–related bench and fieldwork we can ask, "Would our research benefit from sharing our results in comic form? If so, how do we begin to approach this work? How do we partner with a cartoonist who may not have clinical or research experience?" For cartoonists interested in working in this area, questions arise such as, "What logistical and ethical considerations do I need to take into account when making a comic about experiences in health care, both personal stories and those of others?" Answering these questions—and many more—is the future work of the many individuals representing a diversity of disciplines whose work gathers at the intersection of comics and medicine. Doing so will ensure that graphic medicine continues to flourish as an exciting and impactful field within the health humanities.

Note

1 See www.nlm.nih.gov/exhibition/graphicmedicine/index.html

References

Comic Nurse. (2018). "Scaling up Graphic Medicine" – Susan Squier's 2018 Conference Keynote Address. https://www.graphicmedicine.org/scaling-up-graphic-medicine-susan-squiers-2018-confer ence-keynote-address/ (Accessed 8/12/2019).

Czerwiec, M.K., Williams, I., Squier, S.M., Green, M.J., Myers, K.R. and Smith, S.T. (2015). *The Graphic Medicine Manifesto*.University Park, PA: Penn State University Press.

Fies, B. (2006). *Mom's Cancer*. New York: Abrams Image.

Green, M.J. (2015). Comics and Medicine: Peering Into the Process of Professional Identity Formation. *Academic Medicine*, 90(6): 774–779.

Houts, P.S., Doak, C.C., Doak, L.G. and Loscalzo, M.G. (2006). The Role of Pictures in Improving Health Communication: A Review of Research on Attention, Comprehension, Recall, and Adherence. *Patient Education and Counseling*, 61(2): 173–190.

Joshi, A., Hillwig-Garcia, J., Joshi, M., Lehman, E., Khan, A., Llorente, A. and Haidet, P. (2019). Comics as an Educational Tool on a Clinical Clerkship. *Academic Psychiatry*. 43(3): 290–293.

49

HORTICULTURAL ARTS

Jonathan Coope

Introduction

Awareness of the links between gardens and well-being is nothing new: a heavenly garden, intimately associated with the ideal landscape, is found in numerous ancient cultures and religions. With reference to key evidence and theories, this chapter situates the health and well-being benefits of horticultural arts and display within the growing field of social and therapeutic horticulture (STH), and explains how anyone can get started in STH or gardening. You won't even need a garden!

Horticultural display is an important aspect of STH, the commonly used term to describe therapeutic practices that involve working *with* plants or responding *to* plants, gardens, landscapes, and nature. There are two broad approaches to STH: horticulture therapy (HT) and therapeutic horticulture (TH). In HT, a trained therapist uses horticultural activities as part of a therapeutic program with specific clinical outcomes in mind. TH, on the other hand, is geared towards improving well-being more generally, with successful application with a broad range of service users including prison inmates (Baybutt and Chemlal, 2016), people with learning difficulties (Sempik et al., 2014), people with dementia (Hewitt et al., 2013), and people experiencing mental health difficulties (Kamioka et al., 2014).

Awareness of the health and well-being benefits of gardens and landscapes can be been found throughout the historical record. In the twentieth-century post-war era, gardening became a common element in occupational therapy programs and among therapeutic communities. Since the 1980s interest in horticulture's therapeutic aspects has grown considerably. The most prominent STH organization in the United Kingdom is Thrive, whose recent "Garden of Celebration" (designed in conjunction with students and presented at the BBC Gardeners' World Live event in Birmingham, United Kingdom, in June 2018) offers a vivid example of the benefits claimed for horticultural presentation:

> The students have given a huge amount of thought to the use of space, with particular regard to the therapeutic aspects of horticulture, using plants to improve physical and mental health and communication and thinking skills ... The soft stones [and] natural muted colours depict calmness and tranquillity. The path-line softly meanders up through the garden ... allowing the eye to rest before moving back through the garden at a slow rhythm. This circular path offers an easy way to navigate the garden representing how we support our elderly clients, some of whom may be living with dementia. The delicate alpines and succulents represent the diverse range of clients we tailor our care to, all of whom are individuals with

different needs and abilities. Gentle scents are added to the air with herbs and lavender representing our sensory area. (Thrive, 2018)

In terms of access and accessibility, STH can readily take place outdoors or indoors. Planting and potting activities can easily occur on tabletops, inside care homes, with the elderly, and people with dementia or other disabilities.

Overview of evidence

The literature suggests three broad theories for the therapeutic benefits of STH and other "green care" approaches: (1) attention restoration theory; (2) psycho-evolutionary stress reduction theory; and (c) E.O. Wilson's *biophilia* thesis that humans share a natural kinship with the natural world. Each of these three theories focuses on the restorative effects of nature (Clatworthy et al., 2013: 215; Bragg and Atkins, 2016: 85–86). Evidence for health and well-being benefits of gardens and gardening is frequently linked to the broader evidence base regarding health benefits of green spaces, which has reported reductions in health conditions such as cancer and heart disease, as well as greater physical activity, lower obesity rates, and higher self-reported mental health (Buck, 2016).

Evidence for the more specific benefits of gardens and gardening is "diverse and complex" (Buck, 2016: 6). To date, few randomized controlled trials have been conducted (but see Kamioka et al., 2014); however, qualitative and observational studies have reported results consistent with a wide range of mental and physical health benefits (Bragg and Atkins, 2016; Ohly et al., 2016). Well-designed studies indicate gardens in schools can encourage vegetable and fruit consumption, and personal pride and achievement at "growing things"; children with learning or behavioral difficulties are sometimes able to find particular tranquillity within a school's garden (Ohly et al., 2016). Other research has found that allotment gardening improved self-esteem, mood, and cortisol levels compared with matched controls (Berg and Custers, 2011). A range of mental health benefits have been indicated—studies have shown significant reductions in anxiety and depression, together with improved social function (Clatworthy et al., 2013). Nevertheless, there is still a need for better-designed studies to gain a clearer understanding of how gardens and gardening can improve health and well-being (Clatworthy et al., 2013; Pálsdóttir et al., 2018). Less directly, it is evident that gardens can contribute to human health via food production, moderation of pollution and climate, as well as flood reduction.

For many older people, gardens can be important for physical activity, and retaining or developing identity and independence. Some evidence indicates that gardening may help prevent falls in older people by helping them to maintain balance and gait (Buck, 2016). Other studies indicate gardening as beneficial for those with dementia and for dementia prevention (Pálsdóttir et al., 2018). It is also worth noting that recent years have seen a growing use of gardens within the United Kingdom's National Health Service (NHS). One example is Lambeth GP Food Co-op, in which patients with long-term conditions collaborate in growing food that is then sold to King's College Hospital. Gardens are also used to support recovery from illness and research has also pointed to benefits of gardens in care homes and hospices (Buck, 2016).

Significantly, the efficacy and cost-effectiveness of horticulture and green care approaches has attracted growing interest among policy makers. In 2016 the UK government's Natural England commissioned the *Review of Nature-Based Interventions for Mental Healthcare* (Bragg and Atkins, 2016) and the King's Fund's *Gardens and Health: Implications for Policy and Practice* (Buck, 2016).

Case study: "Minding the Garden"

Gary was suffering with obsessive compulsive disorder and anxiety (Vardakoulias, 2013). In his twenties and in receipt of paid benefits, he had been feeling isolated and was struggling to leave his home. With reassurance and support, he attended an informal interview with the "Minding the Garden" project in North Hampshire, set up for people with mental health or learning difficulties.[1]

Gary began as a supported volunteer. As he gained confidence, he soon felt able to travel to the "Minding the Garden" project independently using public transport. His regular attendance and work with the project helped Gary gain the self-assurance to chat and joke with other volunteers and staff. Prior to joining the project, Gary mentioned that he had "felt worthless," but the project had given him a "sense of worth" and also helped with his physical stamina. What Gary most enjoyed about the project, he explained:

> [B]eing active and physical health is very important to me. Seeing the finished garden and the hard work I've put in to transform the garden's appearance and quality is something I enjoy ... you don't have to talk to others if you don't want to ... it's an opportunity to do something worthwhile and valuable and gives you a feel good factor, pride in the work you do and accomplish.

As Gary's confidence grew so too did his skills. With support he began looking for jobs in horticulture, successfully gaining an apprenticeship in horticulture at a local school.

Barriers and opportunities

Safety can always be an issue when gardening, as can back problems, particularly among older clients. Nevertheless, adjustments can be made for those with disabilities. In their survey of STH and other green care approaches, Sempik et al. (2010: 118) found "no reports of adverse reactions or of any negative views."

To promote gardening more widely within the UK health-care system, the 2016 King's Fund report recommends intervening at three levels: strategically, locally, and through implementing and developing the evidence base. At the local level, for example, under-used public sector land could be used for community gardening schemes where appropriate. At the broader policy and strategic level, a joint strategy might be developed among key influencers in health, environment, and horticulture to influence policy and explore the potential of horticulture in supporting key NHS programs such as New Models of Care, Healthy New Towns, and Social Movements for Health.

Getting involved

Those trying gardening for the first time often find it best to begin with modest goals, for example working on tidying one area of an overgrown garden rather than tackling the whole garden. For most of us it is often easier to find the motivation to continue with gardening week after week by arranging to work with others, and on a regular basis.

You don't even need your own garden. Houseplants can be an easy, low-cost way to try out your skills at growing things; there is plenty of information available online about looking after particular plants. Gardening indoors means you get the benefit and delight of nurturing plants, whatever the weather. Furthermore, group horticulture projects can be adapted for people of all abilities, disabilities, and ages. They can be delivered in care homes via table-top sessions as well as gentle outdoor gardening. It is often best to ask for help from a trained STH practitioner at first (e.g., from an organization like Thrive), who can pass on the requisite skills and knowledge to enable and empower you, or other care home staff, to garden with residents and other potential users with confidence.

Resources

- American Horticultural Therapy Association. The US organization for STH; publishes *Journal of Therapeutic Horticulture*. www.ahta.org
- Carry on Gardening. Advice for those with disabilities. www.carryongardening.org.uk
- Enabling Environments Programme. Dementia-friendly design program run by the Association for Dementia Studies at University of Worcester. www.worc.ac.uk/dis cover/ads-enhancing-the-healing-programme.html
- Enhancing the Healing Environment. The King's Fund worked with almost 30 hospitals and 35 hospices to support the design of healing environments and gardens. www.kingsfund.org.uk/projects/enhancing-healing-environment/completed-projects
- Incredible Edible Network. Incredible Edible began with display and growing of fruit, herbs and vegetables around Todmorden in West Yorkshire—providing food to share with anyone who wants to pick it. There are now more than 700 official Incredible Edible groups worldwide. www.incredibleedible.org.uk
- Sensory Trust. Authority on sensory garden design. www.sensorytrust.org.uk
- Social Farms and Gardens. Guidance and advice for community gardens. www.farmgar den.org.uk
- Thrive. The leading UK organization supporting the use of STH. https://thrivelearn. org.uk/portfolio/

Note

1 Gary's case study is explored in Vardakoulias (2013: 19–21).

References

Baybutt, M. and Chemlal, K. (2016). Health-Promoting Prisons: Theory to Practice. *Global Health Promotion*, 23: 66–74.

Berg, A.E. van den, and Custers, M.H.G. (2011). Gardening Promotes Neuroendocrine and Affective Restoration from Stress. *Journal of Health Psychology*, 16(1): 3–11.

Bragg, R. and Atkins, G. (2016). *A Review of Nature-Based Interventions for Mental Healthcare*. Natural England Commissioned Reports, Number 204. London, UK: Natural England.

Buck, D. (2016). *Gardens and Health: Implications for Policy and Practice*. London, UK: King's Fund.

Clatworthy, J., Hinds, J. and Camic, P.M. (2013). Gardening as a Mental Health Intervention: A Review. *Mental Health Review Journal*, 18(4): 214–225.

Hewitt, P., Watts, C., Hussey, J., Power, K. and Williams, T. (2013). Does a Structured Gardening Programme Improve Wellbeing in Young-Onset Dementia? A Preliminary Study. *British Journal of Occupational Therapy*, 76: 355–361.

Kamioka, H., Tsutani, K., Yamada, M., Park, H., Okuizumi, H., Honda, T., Okada, S., Park, S.J., Kitayuguchi, J., Abe, T., Handa, S. and Mutoh, Y. (2014). Effectiveness of Horticultural Therapy: A Systematic Review of Randomized Controlled Trials. *Complementary Therapies in Medicine*, 22: 930–943.

Ohly, H., Gentry, S., Wigglesworth, R., Bethel, A., Lovell, R. and Garside, R. (2016). A Systematic Review of the Health and Wellbeing Impacts of School Gardening: Synthesis of Quantitative and Qualitative Evidence. *BMC Public Health*, 16: 286.

Pálsdóttir, A.M., Sempik, J., Bird, W. and van Den Bosch, M. (2018). Using Nature as a Treatment Option. In M. van Den Bosch and W. Bird, eds, *The Oxford Textbook of Nature and Public Health: The role of nature in improving the health of a population*. Oxford, UK: Oxford University Press: 125–131.

Sempik, J., Hine, R. and Wilcox, D. (2010). *Green Care: A Conceptual Framework. A Report of the Working Group on the Health Benefits of Green Care, COST Action 866, Green Care in Agriculture*. Loughborough, UK: Centre for Child and Family Research, Loughborough University.

Sempik, J., Rickhuss, C. and Beeston, A. (2014). The Effects of Social and Therapeutic Horticulture on Aspects of Social Behaviour. *British Journal of Occupational Therapy*, 77(6): 313–319.

Thrive (2018). *Silver Merit for Thrive celebration garden*. Thrive. www.thrive.org.uk/news/news/news-515. aspx (Accessed 30/8/2018).

Vardakoulias, O. (2013). *The Economic Benefits of Ecominds: a case study approach*. London, UK: NEF Consulting.

50

CHOIRS AND SINGING

Stephen Clift

Introduction

In 1588 the English composer William Byrd gave eight reasons to persuade everyone to sing, believing that singing was beneficial for health. Byrd was remarkably prescient, but it is only four centuries later that his insights have been the subject of scientific enquiry and practical efforts to promote the provision of singing groups to promote health and well-being. The Sidney De Haan Research Centre, Canterbury Christ Church University, United Kingdom, has contributed substantially to these developments. This chapter provides a brief overview of findings from their research program on singing and well-being and the value of singing for people with long-term health conditions.

Prior to 2000 there is virtually no research on singing, well-being, and health, despite the fact that the value of singing for well-being has been well understood for centuries. William Byrd (1588) expressed his insight in the couplet:

Since singing is so good a thing,
I wish all men would learn to sing.

He elaborated this idea with eight reasons including the ideas that singing is good for health, strengthens the muscles of the chest and exercises the lungs, and can help with voice problems including stammering. He was also well aware that if people are to engage positively with singing for such benefits they need the support of a good facilitator and must value the activity.

Even before research can take place on singing and well-being, it is necessary that certain conditions are in place to allow an assessment of the putative benefits. People will engage with singing only if they value the activity, feel it something they are able to do, and have the opportunity to do so. They will continue if the group is convivial and competently facilitated, the material being sung is to their taste, and it involves an appropriate level of challenge giving rise to a sense of achievement.

De Haan Research Centre: singing, well-being, and health

From 2000 onwards there has been a considerable expansion of interest in research on the potential health benefits of singing. The Sidney De Haan Research Centre has played a considerable role in furthering research in this area.

Systematic reviews

Systematic reviewing of available research was a priority from the establishment of the Centre in 2005, and two of the earliest reviews in the field were undertaken in the first few years (Clift et al., 2010). Since then, the Centre has undertaken a comprehensive review of research on singing and older people (Clift et al., 2018), and contributed to a review on singing and chronic obstructive pulmonary disease (COPD) (Lewis et al., 2016), a Cochrane review on the same topic (McNamara et al., 2017), and a review on singing and common mental health conditions (Williams et al., 2017). All of these studies demonstrate that regular group singing can have positive benefits for participants, especially older people with long-term conditions. They also point to some of the limitations of previous research and the need for further larger scale and more robust trials.

Established choirs and choral societies

The Centre has also conducted a major international survey of singers in existing choirs and choral societies in Australia, England, and Germany (Clift et al., 2010), which employed nationally validated forms of the World Health Organization Quality of Life Scale (WHOQoL BREF) to gather comparable data on well-being. Analysis of scores on the psychological well-being scale together with qualitative narratives identified four sub-groups of participants in choirs experiencing challenges to their mental well-being: those with a history or current mental health problems; those coping with partners with mental or physical health problems; participants who were coping with serious physical illness; and those who were recently bereaved. People with lower mental well-being were more likely to express significant appreciation of the value of singing in helping them to cope with life challenges, compared with participants with higher mental well-being scores on the WHO scale (Clift and Hancox, 2010; Livesey et al., 2012). Interestingly, participants varied in their degree of certainty or tentativeness in their views on the physical health benefits of singing, with those people who had experienced problems with their physical health (e.g., respiratory illness) being more confident that singing had helped them (Clift et al., 2009).

A second study involving singers in established choirs surveyed a large network of choirs for women connected with the British Armed Forces, managed by the Military Wives Choirs Foundation (Clift et al., 2016). Participants clearly expressed the value of singing for their mental, social, and physical well-being, especially in the context of the demands placed on wives and partners of men in the military. In addition, however, the study revealed some of the tensions and difficulties that can arise in choirs due to internal politics, personality clashes, and the demands place on members by performance expectations and schedules.

Singing for health groups

Singing and older people living independently

In 2012–2013 the Centre undertook the first pragmatic randomized controlled trial on singing for older people, aged 60 and over, living independently in their community (Coulton et al., 2015; Skingley et al., 2013, 2015). This study demonstrated that three months of weekly singing resulted in measurable improvements in mental well-being and reductions in anxiety and depression, and that the increases in mental health were maintained after a further three months.

Singing and mental health

The Centre has also conducted two studies with participants who have a history of enduring mental health challenges (Clift and Morrison, 2011; Clift et al., 2017). The earlier study conducted in East Kent involved setting up six weekly singing groups and participants were monitored over eight months using the Clinical Outcomes in Routine Evaluation (CORE) questionnaire, widely used in the evaluation of therapeutic interventions in the United Kingdom. Significant reductions occurred in mental distress over this period, and improvements were reflected in narrative accounts gathered from participants. A further replication was untaken in West Kent and Medway, employing both a positive measure of mental well-being (the Warwick Edinburgh Mental Wellbeing Scale) and a short form of the CORE questionnaire (CORE10). In line with the earlier study, significant reductions were found in mental distress, together with significant improvements in mental well-being, abundantly supported by participant testimonies.

Singing and COPD

The Centre has explored the potential value of regular group singing for people affected by the respiratory condition COPD in two feasibility studies. In the first (Morrison et al., 2013; Skingley et al., 2014), six singing groups for people with COPD were established in East Kent and ran for ten months. Assessments of lung function were undertaken at the start and end of the program of singing and participants also completed standardized questionnaires to assess the health-related quality of life. This study revealed significant improvements in self-reported health status and small improvements in lung function. An analysis of written comments from participants revealed clear evidence of the social and personal benefits of group singing for people with COPD.

In a further study in South London (Skingley et al., 2018), four community singing groups for people with COPD and other respiratory challenges were established in Lambeth and Southwark and ran over ten months. This study failed to find the improvements in lung function reported from the earlier project. But qualitative feedback from interviews with participants provided clear evidence again that singing helped people with respiratory illness to manage their condition more effectively and served to improve personal and social well-being.

Conclusion

In line with Byrd's intuitive insights over 400 years ago, research since 2000 has amply confirmed the holistic benefits of singing, especially for older people with long-term conditions. The De Haan Centre has played its part in contributing to the now extensive body of knowledge on singing, health, and well-being. It has also sought to educate and encourage health and social care professionals to see the potential of regular singing as a health-promoting activity that can improve the quality of life and well-being of people affected by long-term conditions and mental health challenges.

But research does not automatically translate into policy and practice, and while "singing for health" groups are widespread now in the United Kingdom, and actively promoted by a number of leading health charities, the opportunities to participate are still very limited and in some areas may be non-existent. Given, for example, that there may be over 3 million people with respiratory illness, including COPD, in the United Kingdom, the challenges of promoting singing for this population and scaling up the provision are abundantly clear. There is still much to do to establish "singing on prescription" as an evidence-based activity to promote health and well-being.

References

Byrd, W. (1588). *Psalms, Sonnets and Song.* Reprint, London: Stainer and Bell, 1965.

Clift, S., Gilbert, R. and Vella-Burrows, T. (2018). Health and Well-Being Benefits of Singing for Older People. In: N. Sutherland, D. Bendrups, N. Leandowski and B. Bartlett, eds, *Music, Health and Well-being: Exploring Music for Health Equity and Social Justice.* London: Palgrave: 97–120.

Clift, S. and Hancox, G. (2010). The Significance of Choral Singing for Sustaining Psychological Well-being: Findings from a Survey of Choristers in England, Australia and Germany. *Music Performance Research,* 3(1): 79–96.

Clift, S., Hancox, G., Morrison, I., Hess, B., Kreutz, G. and Stewart, D. (2009). What Do Singers Say About the Effects of Choral Singing on Physical Health? Findings from a Survey of Choristers in Australia, England and Germany. In: J. Louhivuoiri, T. Eerole, S. Saarikallio, T. Himberg and P-S. Eerola, eds, *Proceedings of the 7th Triennial Conference of European Society for the Cognitive Sciences of Music (ESCOM 2009).* Jyvaskkyla, Finland.

Clift, S., Manship, S. and Stephens, L. (2017). Further Evidence That Singing Fosters Mental Health: Findings from the West Kent and Medway Project. *Mental Health and Social Inclusion,* 21(1): 53–62.

Clift, S. and Morrison, I. (2011). Group Singing Fosters Mental Health and Wellbeing: Findings from the East Kent "Singing for Health" Network Project. *Mental Health and Social Inclusion,* 15(2): 88–97.

Clift, S., Nicols, J., Raisbeck, M., Whitmore, C. and Morrison, I. (2010). Group Singing, Wellbeing and Health: A Systematic Mapping of Evidence. *UNESCO Journal,* 2(1). Available from: www.abp.unim elb.edu.au/unesco/ejournal/.

Clift, S., Page, S., Daykin, N. and Peasgood, E. (2016). The Perceived Effects of Singing on the Wives and Partners of Members of the British Armed Forces. *Public Health,* 138: 93–100.

Coulton, S., Clift, S., Skingley, A. and Rodriguez, J. (2015). Effectiveness and Cost-Effectiveness of Community Singing and Health in the Older Population: A Randomised Controlled Trial. *British Journal of Psychiatry,* 207(3): 250–255.

Lewis, A., Cave, P., Stern, M., Welch, L., Taylor, K., Russell, J., Doyle, A.M., Russell, A.M., McKee, H., Clift, S., Bott, J. and Hopkinson, N.S. (2016). Singing for Lung Health: A Systematic Review of the Literature and Consensus Statement. *Primary Care Respiratory Medicine,* 26. doi: 10.1038/npjpcrm.2016.80. Published online 1 December 2016.

Livesey, L., Morrison, I., Clift, S. and Camic, P. (2012). Benefits of Choral Singing for Social and Mental Wellbeing: Qualitative Findings from a Cross-National Survey of Choir Members. *Journal of Public Mental Health,* 11(1): 10–27.

McNamara, R., Epsley, C., Coren, E. and McKeogh, Z. (2017). *Singing for Adults with Chronic Obstructive Pulmonary Disease (COPD)* (Review). Cochrane Database of Systematic Reviews, 12: CD012296. doi: 10.1002/14651858.CD012296.pub2.

Morrison, I., Clift, S., Page, S., Salisbury, I., Shipton, M., Skingley, A., Burrows, T.V., Coulton., S. and Treadwell, P. (2013). A UK Feasibility Study on the Value of Singing for People with Chronic Obstructive Pulmonary Disease (COPD). *UNESCO Journal,* 3(3). Available from: http://web.educa tion.unimelb.edu.au/UNESCO/pdfs/ejournals/vol3iss3_2013/003_MORRISON_PAPER.pdf (Accessed 19/2/2019).

Skingley, A., Bungay, H., Clift, S. and Warden, J. (2013). Experiences of Being a Control Group: Lessons from a UK-based Randomized Controlled Trial of Group Singing as a Health Promotion Initiative for Older People. *Health Promotion International,* 29(4): 751–758.

Skingley, A., Clift, S., Hurley, S., Price, S. and Stevens, L. (2018). Community Singing Groups for People with Chronic Obstructive Pulmonary Disease: Participant Perspectives. *Perspectives in Public Health,* 1381: 66–75.

Skingley, A., Martin, A. and Clift, S. (2015). The Contribution of Community Singing Groups to the Wellbeing of Older People: Participant Perspectives from the United Kingdom. *Journal of Applied Gerontology,* 35(12): 1302–1324.

Skingley, A., Page, S., Clift, S., Morrison, I., Coulton, S., Treadwell, P., Burrows, T.V., Salisbury, I. and Shipton, M. (2014). 'Singing for Breathing' Groups for People with COPD: Participants' Experiences. *Arts and Health: An International Journal for Research, Policy and Practice*, 6(2): 59–74.

Williams, E., Dingle, G., Clift, S. and Coren, E. (2017). A Systematic Review of Wellbeing Outcomes for Adults with a Mental Health Condition Participating in Group Singing (Protocol). Available from: www.crd.york.ac.uk/PROSPERO/ (Accessed 19/2/2019).

51

ANCIENT TEXTS

Christina Lee

Introduction

The past is a foreign country; they do things differently there.
L. P. Hartley, *The Go-Between* (1953: 5)

In most modern views of the history of medicine pre-Enlightenment era "cures" are regarded as ineffective, if not "backwards." Recent years have witnessed some revaluations of medieval remedies with remarkable results. This chapter explores the potential that such remedies may have for the future of modern pharmacology and medicine. One of the reasons why modern readers often misjudge medieval medicine is because it looks very different from modern healing methods. To understand medieval medicine we also need to understand its culture. Today there is a general expectation that illness is curable or at least may be mitigated through medical intervention. Health in the past may have been defined differently: we find a range of reasons why people get sick. These can range from punishment for sins, to a divine test of faith. In a society that did not define one's worth through participation in work, physical and mental difference may have had less of an impact compared with today.

People in the past had fewer medicines but apparently a wider range of caring options, some that included aspects of narration or the help of chants or "magic." Medieval medicine often works on a more holistic idea of healing in which the patient and healer are part of the healing process, in which prayers or chants accompaning either the application or the preparation of medicine are an integral part of the process. Medieval medicine can be described as being "multimodal," combining remedies with what has been labeled as "charms," including supernatural entities (such as elves and dwarves) but also liturgical elements. Many of these charms, however, are focused on the preparation and administration of remedies and the conceptual understanding of causation and disease (Künzel, 2017; Arthur, 2018). In modern terms: such remedies combine plant biology with etiology, clinical use with patient care. They unite practitioner and patient in rituals of healing. These acts may have a range of purposes: to assure and calm the patient, and give them "something to do" while the doctor is applying the remedy; to teach the application of the remedy and the plants involved; to measure time (in the absence of clocks or watches); or to receive spiritual assistance. In many cases there will have been a combination of factors. The importance of narration and dramatization has been shown in modern research into mental health and well-being (Crawford et al., 2014), but we yet have to examine the importance of narrative in cure in past societies (Lee, 2018).

However, the experience of serious infection is not a new phenomenon. We find a range of different cures in medieval medical manuscripts, which will be the focus of this paper. There is a question whether they had any efficacy, but also whether such texts were used by practitioners. Medieval manuscripts were written on parchments in centers of learning: the sheer effort involved in turning animal hides into writing materials and the fact that not many people had access to such items means that they were always the privilege of an elite. Medical manuscripts were thus either the visible tip of an iceberg of medical knowledge, or a kind of store house for information that was accessible to only a few.

Why research "old" medicines?

The advancement of modern medicine has also made many people forget the problems that bacteria and viruses can bring with them: an over-reliance on medication or worse; forgetting that some conditions that are labeled "childhood diseases" have serious consequences (such as measles, which may lead to severe complications and a weakened immunity for life); and, increasingly, the problem of immunity against important cures, such as antibiotics. The rise of serious complications caused by preventable diseases in the West, largely caused by parents who have chosen to no longer inoculate their children in the erroneous belief that the vaccine is more harmful than the disease, in conjunction with an increase in antibiotic resistance should remind us that conditions that we had been consigned to the history books may easily make a reappearance. Increasing antimicrobial resistance is a serious concern for governments and the World Health Organization; there is now a race to find novel remedies to stem the tide of antimicrobial resistance, but only recently have scholars considered whether ethnopharmacy may also have some potential in the quest to find novel remedies. Scientists have begun to look at indigenous traditions, and one area of focus is the remedies of the past.

Background: medieval medical manuscripts

The earliest Western medical texts come from classical antiquity, and some of this knowledge was incorporated into medieval literature. In England we have medical texts dated as early as Late Anglo-Saxon England (c. 950–1100 CE). While this paper focuses on the early English sources, it should be pointed out that there are medieval medical texts in Latin or vernacular languages from other Europeans areas such as Ireland, Wales, Brittany, and the continent. One of these is the earliest monastic compilation of medical remedies in Northern Europe, the so-called *Lorscher Arzneibuch*, dated to around CE 800, but we can see from its additional entries in Old High German from the ninth and tenth centuries that it was in use for some time. The *Arzneibuch* is remarkable because it begins with a justification for the practice and purpose of medicine before offering a range of remedies. This type of justification suggests that healing through medical intervention was not always the most accepted form of cure.

Much of medieval medicine is based on traditions, either inherited from classical sources or based on "folk" knowledge. In the early medieval period these may be remedies transmitted from classical sources—such as the fourth-century *Pseudo-Apuleius*, a collection of herbal cures, or composite medical texts, such as the so-called *Bald's Leechbook*, which combines native traditions with selected classical sources. (The bulk of the medical texts surviving from Early Medieval England come from a few major compilations: the two "leechbooks," *Lacnunga*, the Old English translation of the *Herbarium and Medicine De Quadrupedibus*). Fragments of medical texts are found in a range of different text types: from the descriptions of a poultice in the *Life of St Cuthbert* (Colgrave, 1940) to various prognostics preserved in the margins of other texts.

Most of these texts were written down in Late Anglo-Saxon England, a period of unprecedented manuscript production. It is unclear just how many medical texts were once in existence—fire and general neglect may have robbed us of a tradition. We also have not much information of who used such texts. Although there are some named physicians, we only have a vague idea of where these individuals practiced their craft. So far we have not found archaeological evidence for surgeries in which these doctors could have practiced, nor places in which remedies could have been made. We do know, however, that monastic institutions had infirmaries and places for the sick, and we can see from the many lay people with visible illnesses buried close to monastic institutions that they will have been visited by people in search of a cure.

Do the drugs work?

For over a century medieval medicine was associated primarily with "superstition" or "placebo" (Cockayne, 1865; Singer, 1917; Grattan and Singer, 1952; Horden, 2000). While Cockayne's translation was an important milestone in making the material available, he also regarded it as not very sophisticated (Van Ardsall, 2002, 2007; see also Meaney, 1992; Pettit, 2001). Most manuscripts were produced in monasteries: these had both the materials and the trained writers who could make such items. We have to assume that, aside from these centers, there may have been other knowledge of healing. The study of the efficacy of medieval medicine is therefore not as straightforward as it may seem. The writers of medieval medical manuscripts may not necessarily have been physicians; instead, these compilers may have been scribes who had little or no medical training. While we can see similarities in some remedies that are copied across texts, the question remains whether scribes understood what they were copying, who asked for these compilations to be made, and to what purpose.

From our surviving texts it is clear that pre-modern medicine at least *tried* to cure a range of conditions—from surgery for the closing of a cleft lip to intestinal diseases, mental illness to toothache—but there is a great abundance of remedies that address infection in wounds. In the past decade there has been a revaluation of traditional medicine, culminating in the award of the 2015 Nobel Prize in Physiology and Medicine to Tu YouYou, who examined traditional Chinese remedies containing artemisinin as effective remedies against malaria. The work of the Quave lab (http://etnobotanica.us/), as well as the work of Freya Harrison and Olivia Cocorran, shows that traditional and historic medical texts can make major contributions to potential drug therapy. This interest has led to the formation of new multidisciplinary teams that require the work of both scientists and specialists who can read and contextualize the languages and text compilations in which remedies are transmitted (Connelly, 2018).

AncientBiotics

In 2013 the multidisciplinary group AncientBiotics formed out of a meeting by colleagues who were interested in whether medieval medicine "works." We did this by looking at a remedy for an "eye-salve" in the so-called *Bald's Leechbook*—a medical text that was copied around the first quarter of the tenth century but is based on an earlier manuscript (Meaney,

1984: 236). The manuscript (BL Royal D12 D xvii) was later bound with other medical texts. *Bald's Leechbook* was possibly written by the same scribe as that of the annular entries of the version of the Anglo-Saxon Chronicle that is known as the "Parker Chronicle" (236). The eye-salve had been identified as "rational medicine" and potentially an effective antimicrobial in Cameron's seminal work on *Anglo-Saxon Medicine* (Cameron, 1991); the remedy had been tested by a US team in 2005 but without result (Brennessel et al., 2005).

A decade later, the AncientBiotics team decided to have a fresh look at this remedy (Harrison et al., 2015). The eye-salve cures what is described as a *wen*: a sty caused by the bacterium *Staphylococcus aureus* that is now increasingly known in its antibiotic-resistant form, MRSA. One of the difficulties of medieval remedies is that they do not mention the quantities of ingredients, and we also had to contend with the fact that one the main ingredients, *cropleac*, has yet to be clearly identified as a plant. The most authoritative translations in the *Dictionary of Old English* (www.doe.utoronto.ca/pages/index.html) and the *Dictionary of Old English Plant Names* (http://oldenglish-plantnames.org/) identify it as an allium species. We therefore decided to produce two batches: one with onion and one with leeks. We found that both combinations did not just kill MRSA *in vitro*, but that they also worked in mouse trials, indicating that the remedy was based on empirical observation. The main ingredients —onion/leek, garlic—have antimicrobial properties, as does the copper vessel in which it should be made or stored. What is significant, however, is that its efficacy is based the combination of ingredients, not the individual components. The knowledge of an ingredient group that "works" makes this remedy less of a chance discovery and more of what we would recognize as a modern drug.

The research of the AncientBiotics team is ongoing.[1] There are a range of remedies with wound-healing potential in medieval manuscripts, but it is important to find a method of finding relevant examples since testing is time-consuming and expensive. To this point, our team is concentrating on certain ingredient combinations and comparing the frequencies with which they appear together. In the future, working with a network analysis derived from a dataset of multiple texts will allow for a more designated approach to exploration. This work, based on knowledge, skills, and methods derived from arts and humanities used in scientific enquiry, is a good example for health humanities. It is important, however, not to reduce this work just to the level of "usefulness" for modern application. While medieval people had apparently effective remedies, they clearly regarded health as much more than the absence of illness.

Medieval remedies are both cultural artefacts and potential allies in the fight against increased antibiotic resistance. These require a new, less colonial view of the medieval past. Our work shows that research into medieval medicine is an important contribution to health humanities: not only does it demonstrate that scientific research can be enhanced by research that at its very foundation requires the knowledge of old languages, literatures, and culture, but also that medieval medicine—with its focus on sound, touch, and interplay between practitioner and patient—may have few more interesting contributions to healing in future. The study of health requires input from science and the humanities to be most effective.

Note

1 A more detailed exploration by the AncientBiotics team has recently been published: F. Harrison and E. Connelly, 'Could Medieval Medicine Help the Fight Against Antimicrobial Resistance?,' in: C. Jones, C. Kostick and K. Oschema, eds, *Making the Medieval Relevant: How Medievalists Are Revolutionising the Present*. Berlin: De Gruyter, 2019: 113–134.

References

Arthur, C. (2018). *Charms, Liturgies and Secret Rites in Early Medieval England*. Woodbridge, Suffolk: Boydell & Brewer.

Brennessel, B., Drout, M. and Gravel, R. (2005). A Reassessment of the Efficacy of Anglo-Saxon Medicine. *Anglo-Saxon England*, 34: 183–195.

Cameron, M. (1991). *Anglo-Saxon Medicine*. Cambridge: Cambridge University Press.

Cockayne, O. ed. (1865). *Leechdoms, Wort Cunning and Starcraft of Early England*. 3 vols. Rolls series 35. London: Longman Green Longman Roberts and Green.

Colgrave, B. ed., and trans. (1940). *Two Lives of St Cuthbert: A Life by an anonymous monk of Lindisfarne and Bede's Prose Life*. Cambridge: Cambridge University Press.

Connelly, E. (2018). A Case Study of *Plantago* in the Treatment of Infected Wounds in the Middle English Translation of Bernhard of Gorden's Lilium Medicinae. In: E. Connelly and S. Künzel, eds, *New Approaches to Disease, Disability and Medicine in Medieval Europe*. Oxford: Archaeopress Archaeology: 126–140.

Crawford, P., Brown B., Baker, C., Tischler, V. and Abrams B. (2014). *Health Humanities*. Houndsmills: Palgrave Macmillan.

Grattan, J. and Singer, C. (1952). *Anglo-Saxon Magic and Medicine Illustrated from the Semipagan Text 'Lacnunga'*. London: Oxford University Press.

Harrison, F., Roberts, A.E.L., Gabrilska, R., Rumbaugh, K., Lee, C. and Diggle, S. (2015). A 1000 Year Old Antimicrobial Remedy with Anti-Staphylococcal Activity. *mBio*, 6(3). http://mbio.asm.org/content/6/4/e01129-15.full.

Horden, P. (2000). What is Wrong with Early Medieval Medicine? *Social History of Medicine*, 24: 2–25.

Künzel, S. (2017). *Concepts of Infectious, Contagious, and Epidemic Disease in Anglo-Saxon England*. PhD, University of Nottingham, 2017.

Lee, C. (2018). Healing Words: St Guthlac and the Trauma of War. In: W. Turner and C. Lee, eds, *Trauma in Medieval Society*. Leiden: Brill: 259–273.

Meaney, A. (1984). Variant Versions of Old English Remedies and the Compilation of Bald's Leechbook. *Anglo-Saxon England*, 13: 235–268.

Meaney, A. (1992). The Anglo-Saxon View of the Causes of Illness. In: S. Campbell, B. Hall and D. Klausner, eds, *Health, Disease and Healing in Medieval Culture*. Basingstoke: Macmillan: 12–33.

Pettit, E. (2001). *Anglo-Saxon Remedies, Charms, and Prayers from British Library Ms Harley 585: The Lacnunga*. 2 vols. Lampeter: Edwin Mellen Press.

Singer, C. (1917). A Review of the Medical Literature of the Dark Ages. *Proceedings of the Royal Society of Medicine*, 10: 107–160.

Van Arsdall, A. (2002). *Medieval Herbal Remedies: The Old English Herbarium and Anglo-Saxon Medicine*. London: Routledge.

Van Arsdall, A. (2007). Challenging the 'Eye of Newt' Image in Medieval Medicine. In: B. Bowers, ed, *The Medieval Hospital and Medical Practice*. Aldershot: Ashgate: 195–205.

52

PHILOSOPHY

Havi Carel

Introduction

Philosophy has been relatively silent on the issue of human health, but has a venerable tradition examining the value of human life. This includes discussions about the good life, well-being, and meaning, and how these can be achieved. When probed, it becomes quickly obvious that human health plays a key role in any attempt to define or evaluate the good life or well-being. Simply declaring that health is the *sine qua non* of the good life is deeply unsatisfactory, given that illness is a part of almost any human life, and flourishing within illness is an increasingly acknowledged possibility and goal in health care.

Some discussion of aging and facing adversity (e.g., in the Stoic tradition, or the Cynic veneration of suffering) is also to be found over the millennia (Seneca, 2004). But a sustained discussion of human health in the context of modern, large-scale medical institutions is a relatively recent phenomenon within philosophy, spanning work from the 1960s onward. Much of the work stems from philosophy of science, where conceptual and definitional questions about health, illness, and disease have garnered attention, as have questions about causation, knowledge, evidence, and the nature of medical entities (medical ontology). A more person- and patient-centered approach has largely been missing from philosophical writing about health and illness until the late 1980s, when S.K. Toombs began using phenomenology to study the experience of illness (Toombs, 1987, 1988).

However, the philosophical study of values has always been key to medical ethics and beyond it to most areas of medicine. In fact, it is difficult to imagine a value-free medical context in which decision making can take place without appeal to any values and hence to a need for their consideration. To emphasize, these are not only ethical values: values can also be existential, aesthetic, and so on. And because the study of values is a foundational philosophical activity, philosophy ought to play a much larger role in health humanities. In other words, it is not possible to practice medicine or health care without some consideration of the following questions (although this is not an exhaustive list):

- How can we evaluate and compare the value of radically different lives?
- What are the conditions for a valuable life and how should we determine these?
- What is human flourishing and how can it be achieved?

- How can we evaluate and compare different stages of life as well as survival and longevity?
- Is it always possible to determine what the best course of action is in medical decision making?
- How do we weigh risk versus benefit of an intervention in a probabilistic framework?

The role of philosophy is to pose and analyze complex questions using the clearest available terms and concepts to do so, or in some cases, developing terms and concepts that are more suitable to the task at hand. Importantly, philosophy does not usually provide a mechanism to resolve practical ethical and other questions, but it does give its practitioner the tools with which to appreciate the complexity of a problem and the concepts required to examine it and propose ways forward. Often in philosophy it is posing the question in sufficient detail and attentiveness to precision, context, and background assumptions that does much of the work. This is not to say that philosophy does not provide answers; it does in some cases. But its main contribution is in providing a robust framework within which a process of inquiry can take place. Philosophical inquiry eschews dogma and authoritarianism, is willing to question all and any presuppositions, and is marked by sincere openness.

In this manner—by providing a framework for questioning and reflection, and adopting a critical stance—philosophy is foundational to any medical ethics or bioethics problem, as well as to many other questions about value, meaning, understanding, interpretation, and articulation of the major issues in reflection about health care and well-being. For example, we can ask: What is important to a patient? How should conflicting values be ranked? What kind of process is illness? And how can we make sense of a life disrupted by illness? These are all key existential questions that are also of crucial importance to the planning and delivery of health care. This is particularly true of chronic illness, which requires significant adaptation to a long period of living with the illness or disability (Carel, 2018).

Some philosophical discussion has been incorporated to some extent into many medical school curricula. But philosophy remains marginal to medical and other health professions' education and training. However, questions of value and meaning will always be core to medical decision making and to our broader societal thinking about health, aging, disability, assisted dying, abortion, quality of life, and many other fundamental areas in health. It is thus important to incorporate an element of philosophical reflection in training and education in order to cultivate reflective practice and an awareness of the inevitability of these issues and the productive role philosophy can play in societal discussions of this kind.

A philosophical toolkit for patients

The example offered here originated from a philosophical toolkit for patients that I developed in 2012 (Carel, 2012). The need for the toolkit arose from observing the medical focus on the dysfunction or disease, to the exclusion of questions about the meaning of illness for the patient. Patients are sometimes offered counseling or psychological treatment to help them cope with being ill, but they are not offered a reflective space in which they can take the time to think about the life events brought about by illness or their responses to these events. Illness causes existential uprooting and demands deep changes to the patient's life, but this "biographical disruption" and abrupt demand to change one's life, routines, habits, and values is not accounted for nor supported by medicine alone. There is a deep and unanswered need for sense making in light of the illness. The toolkit responds to this need.

The toolkit is made up of three steps, designed to provide a space for philosophical reflection on the illness, given the upheaval, suffering, and anxiety it causes. The toolkit stems from an understanding of the importance of philosophical and reflective space for patients, to help them avoid the Scylla of reductive medical jargon and the Charybdis of restrictive social scripts, forcing the ill person into "the sick role," as Talcot Parsons says.

Philosophical patient support does not take an already developed model of illness and present it to patients. Rather, it provides a flexible individual tool that patients can use to develop their own understanding of their illness. Serious illness removes our conventional understandings and expectations of our life, throwing everything into question at once. This is an opportunity to examine and re-evaluate choices, routines, and habits. In illness, such withdrawal becomes possible or is even imposed. This can be an opportunity to philosophically re-examine one's life. The tools of the toolkit are adapted from phenomenology, a philosophical method for studying first-person experience.

The first step is *bracketing* the already given understanding of illness (the experience of being ill) as caused by an underlying physiological process that we call "disease." We usually take the disease entity for granted and posit it as the source of the illness experience. But for the ill person the illness experience comes before the objective disease entity (Toombs, 1987). Once the belief in the objective disease entity is bracketed and we are distanced from our usual way of experiencing, we can begin to explore how illness appears to the ill person, its structure, and its essential features.

The second step in the toolkit is *thematizing* illness. "Thematizing" refers to the act of attending to a phenomenon, which makes aspects of it explicit (Toombs, 1987: 222). A theme for a particular consciousness is that upon which it focuses its attention. But this also takes into account the kind of attentional focus given to an entity. Thematizing may include attending to the cognitive, emotive, moral, or aesthetic aspects of a phenomenon. A patient may thematize her illness as a central feature of her life, attending to her symptoms as pervasive, while the physician may thematize the illness as a "case of cancer," attending to symptoms as diagnostic clues. The understanding that illness is not an objective entity and the exercise of thematizing may help patients because it enables moving away from prescriptive pronouncements toward a descriptive mode.

Thematizing can be used to articulate the multiple perspectives on one's illness that patient, family, health professionals, and others may have, as each will thematize an illness differently. The patient may thematize her illness emotively, while a health professional will tend to thematize it cognitively. A family member may thematize illness as an experience of empathy. Thematizing is useful for uncovering the variety of ways in which illness can appear.

The third step of the toolkit is to take the new understanding of illness and examine how it changes one's *being-in-the-world*. The term "being-in-the-world" is used by Heidegger (1962) to denote the human being in the broadest sense. Being in the world includes the biological entity, the person, and her environment and meaningful connections. The main components of being in the world, for Heidegger, are being-in (inhabiting or dwelling in a place), the world (the meaningful network of entities, practices, and meanings that make up our world), and being, which is the open existence of humans, capable of temporal existence and understanding.

This term provides a rich account of what it means to exist as a human being. The toolkit uses being-in-the-world to capture the pervasive effects that illness may have on one's sense of place, on interactions with the environment and with other people, on meanings and norms, and on the nexus of entities, habits, knowledge, and other people that make up one's world. This term enables us to elaborate on the impact of illness richly and comprehensively. By moving away from a narrow understanding of illness as a biological process, a thick account of illness as a new way of being-in-the-world can be developed by patients.

The toolkit has been used in the United Kingdom and the United States and continues to be developed by practitioners interested in the idea of well-being within illness (see https://narrativedimensions.org/livingwellwithillnessworkshop/). However, the barriers for the toolkit being widely used by patients include: the diverse background of patients, who are not always interested in or open to reflection; the focus on what is seen as the "bread and butter" of health-care provision at the expense of reflective practices; and the emphasis on interventions based on technology and medication, that is, that view illness as an exclusively pathophysiological process.

Public engagement with philosophy

Having presented the barriers, it is also useful to note that philosophy is a cheap and widely available practice that crosses geographical and historical boundaries and requires no specialist training, skills, or abilities. It is a timeless and satisfying form of inquiry that has in recent years been popularized by public philosophers, podcasts, and freely available online material, including philosophy blogs, books, seminars, and course materials. There are also many philosophy lectures that are free and open to the public, given by most academic institutions. It is a powerful practice that can help illuminate concepts, values, ideas, and underlying assumptions we hold as individuals and societally about health.

Resources

- British Philosophical Association: www.bpa.ac.uk
- Philosophy Bites: https://philosophybites.com/
- Talking Philosophy: blog.talkingphilosophy.com
- Microphilosophy: www.microphilosophy.net

References

Carel, H. (2012). Phenomenology as a Resource for Patients. *Journal of Medicine and Philosophy*, 37 (2): 96–113. 10.1093/jmp/jhs008.

Carel, H. (2018). *Illness*. London: Routledge.

Heidegger, M. (1962). [1927] *Being and Time*. Oxford: Basil Blackwell.

Seneca, L.A. (2004). *On the Shortness of Life*. London: Penguin.

Toombs, S.K. (1987). The Meaning of Illness: A Phenomenological Approach to the Patient-Physician Relationship. *Journal of Medicine and Philosophy*, 12: 219–240.

Toombs, S.K. (1988). Illness and the Paradigm of Lived Body. *Theoretical Medicine*, 9: 201–226.

53

CAPOEIRA

Mel Jordan, Edward J. Wright and Aimie Purser

Introduction

Capoeira, defined as a Brazilian martial art and game to be played (Jordan et al., 2018), is now "globalised and taught widely outside Brazil" (de Campos Rosario et al., 2010: 103). What was once a "practice of resistance is now a fashionable activity available worldwide" (Robitaille, 2014: 230); responses to, and experiences of, capoeira play have evolved to embrace "creativity, beauty, and inclusion" (MacLennan, 2011: 158) and the inclusive nature of capoeira is something that is celebrated (Wesolowski, 2007). Indeed, the sense of community evoked by capoeira play is a strong theme in this study. In terms of capoeira classes in the United Kingdom, "men and women train and play together in Britain, where diasporic capoeira is predominantly a non-contact sport" (Delamont and Stephens, 2008: 63). Capoeira play takes place in the *roda*, accompanied by music played on an instrument called the *berimbau*. Briefly, the *roda* constitutes a ring formed of multiple capoeiristas (i.e. players of capoeira), with two capoeiristas playing in the center of this ring; those forming the ring also provide music on the *berimbau*, to which those in the center of the ring play, following its rhythm (Capoeira, 2002). As Downey (2002) states, this music "informs players when to start and stop their matches and how to play, and ties all participants into the ongoing sequence of games" (Downey, 2002: 491).

This research explored how capoeira play might be considered to facilitate connectedness among newly recruited persons, plus any other ramifications of capoeira involvement. A beginners' course of capoeira was provided to participants in an English city in the West Midlands. One-hour capoeira classes ran weekly, free of charge, for participants. Two capoeira leaders ran the classes, and 18 participants joined the study. All those who attended the classes were research participants. The participant group was naturally occurring and self-selecting. Recruitment to this research occurred via traditional methods and social media routes, for example paper flyers and a Facebook page. The study received ethical approval from the School of Sociology and Social Policy at the University of Nottingham. Participant information sheets were provided and consent forms were signed. Thirteen classes were provided. No experience of capoeira was necessary to begin the capoeira classes. Researchers attended classes to collect/construct overt non-participant observation data. In addition, semi-structured interviews were undertaken with the new capoeiristas after the course. The interviews were audio-recorded and then transcribed verbatim by an external transcription company. Pseudonyms are used in publications to ensure participants' confidentiality. The interdisciplinary research team includes expertise in the sociology of sport, social theory, humanities, medical sociology, the mental health-care service user perspective, nursing, and sociology.

As a result of the aforementioned fieldwork and team analysis, capoeira is theorized in a fresh manner that highlights social benefits of capoeira—for example, as an enjoyable and supportive group endeavor that includes elements of social play and community-building—plus benefits for self that can transcend the boundaries of the class (Jordan et al., 2018). Corporeal and discursive boundary empowerment can also be experienced by capoeiristas, fostering positive identity work in the wider world (Jordan et al., 2018). Capoeira can be argued to concurrently acilitate mutuality (e.g., community experience and group work) and egoism (e.g., an individual's identity work) (Jordan et al., 2018). Within this study relevant features of Brazilian life "such as race … samba, and slavery" (Stephens and Delamont, 2006: 323) were introduced to the new capoeiristas by the capoeira course leaders verbally during classes. Further, "the regular switching of practice partners in class" (de Campos Rosario et al., 2010: 111) is an important mechanism for creating social cohesion and appropriate capoeira teaching, and this occurred in this study. Researchers focused on how newcomers to this practice of capoeira negotiated the bodily requirements of capoeira and how this produced not only sweat, but also smiles and laughter, plus elements beyond this bodily-togetherness itself during the class (e.g., narrated health ramifications). It is to these health and welfare elements we now turn.

Capoeira and health

Participants narrated how capoeira has post-class well-being benefits related to health. Delamont (2006: 171) highlights that "capoeira is an energetic physical activity, and everybody sweats." Downey (2002: 490) demonstrates how capoeira is used in diverse contexts including "physical education classes." Fieldwork data from this study also support this claim regarding capoeira as genuine physical exercise:

> The class worked hard on their routines and many seemed out of breath at the end. (Researcher C, Obs. Data)

> The main exercise component of the class lasts approximately 30 minutes from 8pm to 8.30pm and it is clear that the participants are exhausted. (Researcher B, Obs. Data)

> Many of the students are getting too hot and stop to have breaks, go to their bags and drink water. (Researcher C, Obs. Data)

> Towards the end of the class 3 participants looked too tired, breathless. (Researcher F, Obs. Data)

Stephens and Delamont (2006: 319) confirm that "these settings are noisy, full of movement; they are sweaty." Nevertheless, for the participants in this study, health is neither the central purpose of the activity nor merely incidental to capoeira play, but rather a welcome *addition*—their motivation for capoeira practice is not health first and foremost. Further, some of the arguably unhealthy elements occasionally associated with capoeira culture (e.g., tobacco use [Bedendo and Noto, 2015]) are not observed by researchers, or reported by participants, in this study. In the interviews, participants endorse this notion of healthy exercise via the capoeira classes. The perceived physical health benefits of capoeira are important for those who attend this course:

I go as red as a beetroot by the end of it. But in a way that's kind of the point. Because, like I say, I'm trying to lose weight. (Tanya)

I think it's really energetic. (Michelle)

It is as much about looking after my health, because that's become very important to me, I got diagnosed with X [chronic illness]. (Lucy)

It's kind of good to feel like you're getting a workout. (Tanya)

What is novel here, in this study, is that there are *two* forms to this health narrative. Health reasons are, according to interviewees, both reactionary (e.g., weight loss required) and pro-active (e.g., desire for cardiovascular workout). Capoeira is practicing health at two levels: a future-focused level and a contemporary-response level. Health is understood, verbalized, and actioned by capoeiristas at two distinct levels, both of which are perceived by participants as positive for self-welfare.

If we consider the fact that capoeira has already been implemented within school curricula, specifically as physical education (Capoeira, 2002), alongside the atomistic understandings of health above, the work of Wrench (2017) becomes salient. Evidence of such an *individualized* approach to healthy living and health benefit via sport participation does not align well with the work of Wrench (2017) who argues, instead, for the adoption of health and physical education that intentionally and overtly counteracts "hegemonic notions of *individual* responsibility for healthy citizenship" (1). Therefore, the framing of health citizenship along individualistic lines, as participants do so in this study, is not necessarily positive when analyzed at a societal level—arguably because it removes responsibility from the state (and society as a collective) and instead places responsibility upon increasingly unsupported solitary citizens.

Another intriguing element of the data here is that the form of exercise afforded by capoeira is highlighted as positive for health yet somewhat enigmatic. Capoeira play is narrated as enjoyable exercise by the research participants in this study, but also, rather unusually, almost mystical—or at least difficult to explain.

It feels like it's better and more healthier than just running on a treadmill and getting nowhere. (Lindsey)
I think it's magic. (Elliot)

This finding complements, yet develops, some of the extant literature. This can be demonstrated via these two quotes: (1) "Even if [capoeira] novices are fit, capoeira uses different muscles from their normal exercise—in strange ways" (Delamont and Stephens, 2014; 55); and (2) "Learners are attracted by the opportunity to experience something exotic: using their bodies differently" (de Campos Rosario et al., 2010: 116). In this research capoeira is described as definitely different to the more standard, individualistic, gym-based workout, in an awe-inspiring and mysterious sense. Accordingly, many sociological theories of embodiment recognize that actors embody knowledge that cannot be fully articulated; for example, borrowing from Bäckström (2014: 752), it can be said that the body is "un/knowing" and "knowing and not knowing simultaneously." Another way of saying this is that actors become proficient through learning or practice, but are not necessarily able to express fully in words the knowledge predicating action, and the sensational experience of being-in-the-world in this capacity. Therefore, it is perhaps unsurprising that the new capoeiristas experience an element of their mixed martial art involvement, and benefits for self-welfare, that they are unable to easily articulate verbally.

Conclusion

Capoeira's coverage in the mass media is proliferating. Brazilian martial arts (Brazilian jiu-jitsu, capoeira, and to a lesser extent *vale tudo*) are currently popular in and beyond sporting domains, arguably due to the increasing popularity of mixed martial arts in which they are practiced. Capoeira now receives global media coverage. For example, Conor McGregor—a well-known practitioner of mixed martial arts—was interviewed for the popular US-based talk show *Conan*, during which he gave a short capoeira demonstration. This was published on YouTube on the March 3rd, 2016 and has now been viewed over 1.8 million times. A YouTube search for "capoeira" produces 2,180,000 results. The popularity of capoeira at present is noteworthy because it was a factor in recruitment success for this research. Several participants joined the classes because of pre-existing expectations regarding the high level of physical exertion expected from social media representations of capoeira play and/or the heightened general public interest in, and appeal of, martial arts. Therefore, there exists the possibility for capoeira to be enjoyed by an increasing number of people with its potential benefits for self and health.

Acknowledgements

This study was led by Dr Melanie Jordan at the University of Nottingham and was related to an Arts and Humanities Research Council program grant (ref. AH/K003364/1) held by Professor Paul Crawford. The Institute of Mental Health at the University of Nottingham financially supported this research via its Managed Innovation Network scheme. The full research and authorship team from the University of Nottingham included: Andrew Grundy, Emma Joyes, Nicola Wright, Paul Crawford, and Nick Manning.

Resources

- www.cdob.co.uk
- www.capoeiranottingham.co.uk
- https://londonschoolofcapoeira.com/
- https://ich.unesco.org/en/RL/capoeira-circle-00892

Further Reading

Crossley, N. (2006). In the Gym: Motives, Meaning and Moral Careers. *Body and Society*, 12: 25–50.
Delamont, S. and Stephens, N. (2008). Up On The Roof: The Embodied Habitus Of Diasporic Capo-eira. *Cultural Sociology*, 2(1): 57–74.
García, R.C. and Spencer, D.C. (2013). *Fighting Scholars: Habitus and Ethnographies of Martial Arts and Combat Sports*. London: Anthem Press.
Meziani, M. (2018) Social Participation of People with Disabilities in Boxing and Capoeira: A Comparative Ethnographic Multi-Sited Focus. *Sport in Society*, 21(1): 166–178. 10.1080/17430437.2016.1225889.

References

Bäckström, Å. (2014). Knowing and Teaching Kinaesthetic Experience in Skateboarding: An Example of Sensory Emplacement. *Sport, Education and Society*, 19(6): 752–772. 10.1080/13573322.2012.713861.

Bedendo, A. and Noto, A. (2015). Sports Practices Related to Alcohol and Tobacco Use Among High School Students. *Revista Brasileira de Psiquiatria*, 37(2): 99–105.

Capoeira, N. (2002). *Capoeira: Roots of the Dance-Fight-Game*. Berkeley, CA: Blue Snake Books.

de Campos Rosario, C., Stephens, N. and Delamont, S. (2010). I'm Your Teacher, I'm Brazilian! Authenticity and Authority in European Capoeira. *Sport, Education and Society*, 15(1): 103–120.

Delamont, S. (2006). The Smell of Sweat and Rum: Teacher Authority in Capoeira Classes. *Ethnography and Education*, 1(2): 161–175.

Delamont, S. and Stephens, N. (2008). Up On The Roof: The Embodied Habitus Of Diasporic Capoeira. *Cultural Sociology*, 2(1): 57–74.

Delamont, S. and Stephens, N. (2014). Each More Agile than the Other: Mental and Physical Enculturation in *Capoeira Regional*. In:R.S. Garcia and D.C. Spencer, eds, *Fighting Scholars*. London: Anthem: 49–62.

Downey, G. (2002). Listening to Capoeira: Phenomenology, Embodiment, and the Materiality of Music. *Ethnomusicology*, 46(3): 487–509.

Jordan, M., Wright, E.J., Purser, A., Grundy, A., Joyes, E., Wright, N., Crawford, P. and Manning, N. (2018). Capoeira For Beginners: Self-Benefit For, And Community Action By, New Capoeiristas. *Sport, Education and Society*, DOI: 10.1080/13573322.2018.1441145.

MacLennan, J. (2011). "To Build a Beautiful Dialogue": Capoeira as Contradiction. *Journal of International and Intercultural Communication*, 4(2): 146–162.

Robitaille, L. (2014). Promoting Capoeira, Branding Brazil: A Focus on the Semantic Body. *Black Music Research Journal*, 34(2): 229–254.

Stephens, N. and Delamont, S. (2006). Balancing the *Berimbau*: Embodied Ethnographic Understanding. *Qualitative Inquiry*, 12(2): 316–339.

Wesolowski, K. (2007). *Hard Play: Capoeira and the politics of inequality in Rio De Janeiro*, Columbia University: Unpublished Doctoral Thesis.

Wrench, A. (2017). Framing Citizenship: From Assumptions to Possibilities in Health and Physical Education. *Sport, Education and Society*, DOI: 10.1080/13573322.2017.1403314

54

KUNDALINI YOGA

Elvira Perez and Emily Haslam-Jones

Introduction

The Western media image of yoga—its poses and practice more generally—perpetuates the misconception that the goal is to be flexible enough to create specific shapes. In fact, it is the *process* of exploration through movement, in coordination with breath, which harnesses the mind and creates a changed state of being through the yoga practice. The word yoga derives from the Sanskrit *yuj* meaning "to yoke" or "union" (Khalsa, 2012); through the coordinated use of body and breath, the attention of the mind follows, to create a unified or congruent state of breath and movement. Brain imaging studies have shown that yoga and meditation induce changes in areas such as attention, body awareness, higher level cognitive function, and self-perception (Afonso et al., 2017; Gard et al., 2015; Khalsa and Gould, 2012a; Lazar et al., 2005). The somatic connections enabled by yoga practice create new ways into an individual's inner experience, by addressing emotions and cognitions that may previously have seemed inaccessible (Emerson and Hopper, 2011).

Yoga and its therapeutic qualities

Originally conceived of as a preparation for the body for meditation, yoga has become, in modern times, well recognized for its capacity to allieviate stress and improve many mental and physical conditions. Yoga is a non-pharmacological intervention with few, if any, adverse effects (Cramer et al., 2013; Khalsa and Gould, 2012a) and can be practiced both in groups and individually. Yoga is highly versatile and offers a valuable self-help tool that can be adjusted and tailored to individual needs (Vorkapic and Rangé, 2014): from high-energy styles such as Astanga, Vinyasa, and Kundalini, to slow Yin and Restorative and Adaptive yoga. Various styles generally involve very different foci and purposes, from spiritual and religious goals (such as enlightenment and escape from the cycles of incarnation), to a focus on mental health, to enhanced flexibility, cross-training support for a particular sport, or recovery from injury or illness. Within this variability of purpose, it is generally the approach taken that defines the practice as being yoga as opposed to exercise.

The development of an individual's internal and kinesthetic senses is what defines a mastery of yoga. It is that heightened physical and mental awareness that should prevent a practitioner from injury through both self-awareness and trust between teacher and student-practitioner. This awareness can take time to develop, and requires a discerning approach to instruction; alternatively, such internal and kinesthetic senses may come easily if the skills have been developed elsewhere. Not everything that is labeled yoga is always practiced with these self-care and body-preserving principles in mind. Approaching it with a certain mindset causes a striving towards perfect postures just beyond the practitioner's reach, resulting in a feeling of inadequacy rather than self-acceptance.

Growing concerns about mental health especially have resulted in more health-care practitioners attending to these more contemplative "Eastern" practices, including tai chi and meditation. For example, the British National Health Service (NHS) now recommends the practice of mindfulness to treat stress, anxiety, and depression ("Mindfulness," 2018). Cumulative evidence documenting the therapeutic benefits of yoga has grown considerably in the past few years. Not only has the quantity of studies increased, but also the quality of that research has improved to include controlled trials and active control groups (Khalsa, 2004).

The positive health benefits of yoga have been reported in studies tackling depression, sleep disorders, anxiety, and panic disorder (Balasubramaniam et al., 2013; Khalsa, 2013; Varambally and Gangadhar, 2012; Deepak, 2013). The study of yoga as a complementary therapeutic intervention has also been proven successful in the treatment of insomnia (e.g., Larouche et al., 2015) and as a main therapeutic intervention in effectively reducing stress (Esch et al., 2003; Malathi and Damodaran, 1999; Michalsen et al., 2005; Smith et al., 2007), anxiety (Sahasi et al., 1989; Vahia et al., 1973; Sharma et al., 1991; Javnbakht et al., 2009), depression (Michalsen et al., 2005; Oken et al., 2006), and stress-related symptoms such as hypertension and insomnia (Smith et al., 2007). There is also evidence showing additional benefits of yoga among high school students (e.g., improved self-image; Conboy et al., 2013) and adults with post-traumatic stress disorder symptoms (e.g., research on propagation of optimism about life challenges by Clark et al., 2014; Rhodes, 2015).

Kundalini yoga

Kundalini is a dynamic style of yoga with a special focus on breath with movement. The Kundalini style includes some unusual practices such as long arm holds which, according to traditional knowledge claims, assert that these practices have a positive effect on the body's glandular, hormonal, and nervous systems. Yoga Bhajan went to the United States in 1969 claiming that he was now openly sharing a secret lineage of yoga postures; more likely was his introduction of a creative *bricolage* of fast, repetitive physical moves taken from Swami Dhirendra Brahmachari, and the use of sound from Sant Maharaj Virsa Singh (Deslippe, 2012).

Kundalini yoga breaks from the most commonly recognized form of quiet, still postures. Called by Bhajan and followers "the yoga of awareness," Kundalini yoga can include repetitive vocalizations (chanting), breathing exercises (in particular "breath of fire," a powerful belly-pumping breath), dynamic and still yoga postures, and meditations that, in tandem with its energetic movements, aim to actively facilitate a revitalized and relaxed state of mind and body. Kundalini practitioners assert that this approach may be more suitable for those who have high levels of anxiety or trauma: the active movements and breathwork associated with Kundalini yoga provide multiple tasks to focus on, giving "hooks" for the mind to stay present, through the rhythms of the practice. Using embodied sound and movement, as some researchers have concluded, is an effective tool for enhancing connections between the body and the brain, thus facilitating self-regulation (Van der Kolk, 2014). When the nervous system is overstimulated from stress or distress, coming to a quiet, still place can be facilitated by the physical release of combining challenging postures with meditative pauses.

Kundalini yoga, as practiced by the 3HO organization and associated traditions, entails dressing in white, wearing a turban, becoming Sikh, and having a Sikh name. Two of the most prolific scientific researchers on the application and benefits of yoga, David Shannoff-Khalsa and Sar Bir Singh Khalsa, observe these practices. However, adherence of these customs and beliefs is not necessary to gain benefit from the practice—there are an increasing number of practitioners and teachers outside the organization, perhaps the most notable trainer being Gloria Latham in Vancouver, Canada. Kundalini merges traditional mantras with uplifting music, a combination that has been found to improve relationships (e.g., sense of connection to others and self), promote compassionate thinking, and enhance attentional focus. Practiced regularly over an extended period of time, these changes in perception have the potential to affect participants' quality of life in positive and profound ways (de Castro, 2015).

Reaching out: barriers and opportunities

Although yoga practice more broadly has been growing worldwide, with 36.7 million people taking part in the United States alone (*The Guardian*, 2019), it is estimated that only 300,000–460,000 people currently practice yoga on a regular basis in the United Kingdom (Fox, 2019). Barriers, both real and perceived, include time constraints, lifestyle, costs, negative preconceptions (e.g., excessive challenge for people that are not flexible) and negative health effects (e.g., difficulty for people with certain physical conditions) (Atkinson and Permuth-Levine, 2009; Dayandanda et al., 2014; Quilty et al., 2013). Despite the evidence illustrating the physical and mental benefits of yoga practice (Emerson and Hopper, 2011), cost may often be a barrier to the people who would benefit most.

To combat this problem, organizations and charities such as Give Back Yoga Foundation and Yoga Quota are working to make all types of yoga accessible to vulnerable groups. Accessible yoga adapts to the users' needs and can be delivered both chair-based (for participants with mobility difference) and mat-based. Accessible Yoga is a movement dedicated to bringing yoga practice to excluded and underserved communities. The mission of such organizations is to increase awareness of the benefits of yoga and offer information and resources to the general public.

Case study: Kundalini yoga in children's care homes

We, the authors, were involved in an initiative designed to introduce Kundalini yoga in children's care homes (Perez et al., 2016; Vallejos et al., 2016). This research group developed a study to test the feasibility of incorporating a 20-week Kundalini yoga program in a residential setting including children in care (CIC), youth practitioners, and management. This feasibility study was framed under the notion of creative practice as mutual recovery (Crawford et al., 2013), the idea that shared creativity, collective experience, and mutual benefit can promote resilience in mental health and well-being among communities that traditionally have been divided (e.g., children's home staff and CIC). Feasibility was assessed through recruitment and retention rates as well as participants' self-report perceptions on social inclusion, mental health, and well-being, and through semi-structured interview.

This study initially enrolled 100% of CIC (n=9) and 97% (n=29) of eligible staff. Mean age among CIC was 14.78, and among staff 33. Attendance was low with an average rate of four sessions per participant; low attendance was associated with the challenges faced by the children's workforce (e.g., high levels of stress, low status, profile, and pay), as well as insufficient consultation and involvement of stakeholders on the study implementation pro-cess. These results emphasize the need to promote mutual recovery in terms of well-being and mental health in children's homes among CIC as well as staff, and confirms the import-ance of self-care practices, as well as raising the profile, status, and pay of those who work in children's residential care.

Nevertheless, all participants interviewed reported that the study was personally meaning-ful and experienced both individual benefits (e.g., feeling more relaxed) and social benefits (e.g., feeling more open and positive). This study highlighted important implications for policy and practice including the need to engage stakeholders in a co-production process for implementing yoga practice in residential settings to enhance the sense of ownership and engagement.

People in control of their own health

One issue that may be an impediment to a broader uptake of yoga practice is the sense that it is the task of others to look after our own health. However, the principle that people should have a stronger voice in decisions about their health, and that health services should better reflect patient needs and preferences, has been a policy goal of politicians and senior policy makers in health for at least 20 years in the United Kingdom. The evidence shows that when people look after themselves, health decisions are better, health and health out-comes improve, and resources are allocated more efficiently (Foot et al., 2014).

Accordingly, the NHS provides advice, tips and tools to help people make the best choices about their health and well-being through their Live Well online resources. The NHS is now recommending the practice of yoga as a program of exercise to increase physical activity, espe-cially strength, flexibility, and balance, especially for those with high blood pressure, heart dis-ease, aches and pains (including lower back pain), depression, and stress ("A Guide", 2018).

Initiatives are starting to help promote the self-management of health through yoga in the United Kingdom. There are increasing numbers of public, school, and charity-led clas-ses, with the latter focused on working with vulnerable groups. Yoga in the workplace is also starting to gain ground. However, to become integrated into the NHS teachers need more extensive and accredited training to be able to apply this powerful tool in a more complex range of contexts. Yoga is ultimately an experiential practice and it is up to us to engage in the benefits of this powerful practice to understand its potential.

Two exercises

1. *Meditation for when you don't know what to do*
    This is a gentle meditation exercise that can be adapted to do in everyday contexts, such as when you are sitting on a bus—where appropriate, you can focus only on the breathing steps, and save the hand gestures for a more private setting:

    *   Sit comfortably on the floor or in a chair.
    *   Put the palms of your hands open in front of your chest as if you were holding a book. Then put one on top of other (either hand can be on top) and cross the thumbs to make the hands into a slightly more cupped shape.
    *   Focus your gaze on the tip of your nose or, if that is making you dizzy, simply close the eyes.
    *   Make the mouth into an "o" shape.

- Now breathe in through the nose.
- Breath out through the nose.
- Breathe in through the mouth.
- Breathe out through the mouth.
- Keep going.
- Start with a duration of four minutes, and build up to 11 minutes.
- If you get lost, just go back to the first inhale through the nose. The breath will become longer and easier as you go.

2. *The ego eradicator*
   This exercise gives you a taste of where Kundalini yoga works to create an uplifting feeling—one that builds confidence and resilience:

   - Get a timer and set it to three minutes.
   - Sit on the floor or in a chair. If you have your legs crossed (you don't have to, but it helps stability), place one foot in front of the other rather than on top to avoid pins and needles.
   - Start the timer and lift both arms out to the sides but slightly raised up above the shoulder line. To visualize this, your arms will be creating three equal sections of 60° with the floor as your baseline. The thumbs are sticking out, and the fingers are curled in, to rest on the top of the palms.
   - Close your eyes and keep them closed. This increases the effect of the arm lifts (opening your eyes will reduce the sensation you feel at the end).
   - Now breathe through your nose powerfully, rounding out your tummy on the inhalation (think of it as filling the body with air) and then drawing the belly in and a little up on the exhalation (think "air out, belly empty").
   - Relax, particularly the shoulders. The arms remain straight and strong but not tense. Focus on the breath. If your arms drop, try bending slightly forward and then raising them back up instead.
   - When you hear the timer, without opening your eyes, inhale slowly and deeply, exhale and stretch the fingers.
   - Take another deep inhalation, and let it go. Then, with natural breathing and keeping the eyes closed, let the arms slowly circle down until they touch the ground beside you or rest on your lap. Stay with your eyes closed a moment to notice how you feel.

Acknowledgements

Dr. Elvira Perez Vallejos acknowledges the financial support of the NIHR Nottingham Biomedical Research Centre.

Resources

- www.yoganova.co.uk
- www.youtube.com/user/CarolynCowan/videos
- www.nhs.uk/live-well/exercise/guide-to-yoga/
- www.boysofyoga.com
- https://givebackyoga.org/
- https://accessibleyoga.org/
- https://yogaquota.com/charity-partners/

Further reading

Khalsa, S.B.S. and Gould, J. (2012a). *Your Brain on Yoga*. New York: Rosetta Books.
Van der Kolk, B. (2014). *The Body Keeps the Score*. New York: Viking.

References

Afonso, R.F., Balardin, J.B., Lazar, S., Sato, J.R., Igarashi, N., Santaella, D.F., Lacerda, S.S., Amaro E.Jr, and Kozasa, E.H. (2017). Greater Cortical Thickness in Elderly Female Yoga Practitioners—A Cross-Sectional Study. *Frontiers in Aging Neuroscience*, 9(201). DOI: 10.3389/fnagi.2017.00201.

"A Guide to Yoga." National Health Service (UK) (2018). www.nhs.uk/live-well/exercise/guide-to-yoga/. (Accessed 21/1/2019).

Atkinson, N.L. and Permuth-Levine, R. (2009). Benefits, Barriers, and Cues to Action of Yoga Practice: A Focus Group Approach. *American Journal of Health Behavior*, 33(1): 3–14.

Balasubramaniam, M., Telles, S. and Doraiswamy, P. (2013). Yoga on Our Minds: A Systematic Review of Yoga for Neuropsychiatric Disorders. *Frontiers in Psychiatry*, 3. DOI: 10.3389/fpsyt.2012.00117, available at: http://journal.frontiersin.org/article/10.3389/fpsyt.2012.00117/full (Accessed 9/12/2019).

Clark, C.J., Lewis-Dmello, A., Anders, D., Parsons, A., Nguyen-Feng, V., Henn, L. and Emerson, D. (2014). Trauma-Sensitive Yoga as an Adjunct Mental Health Treatment in Group Therapy for Survivors of Domestic Violence: A Feasibility Study. *Complementary Therapies in Clinical Practice*, 20(3): 152–158.

Conboy, L.A., Noggle, J.J., Frey, J.L., Kudesia, R.S. and Khalsa, S.B.S. (2013). Qualitative Evaluation of a High School Yoga Program: Feasibility and Perceived Benefits. *Explore: The Journal of Science and Healing*, 9(3): 171–180.

Cramer, H., Krucoff, C. and Dobos, G. (2013). Adverse Events Associated with Yoga: A Systematic Review of Published Case Reports and Case Series. *PloS One*, 8(10): e75515.

Crawford, P., Lewis, L., Brown, B. and Manning, N. (2013). Creative Practice as Mutual Recovery in Mental Health. *Mental Health Review Journal*, 18(2): 55–64.

Dayananda, H.V., Ilavarasu, J.V., Rajesh, S.K. and Babu, N. (2014). Barriers in the Path of Yoga Practice: An Online Survey. *International Journal of Yoga*, 7(1): 66–71.

de Castro, J.M. (2015). Meditation Has Stronger Relationships with Mindfulness, Kundalini, and Mystical Experiences Than Yoga or Prayer. *Consciousness and Cognition*, 35: 115–127.

Deepak, K.K. (2013). Yogic Intervention for Mental Disorders. *Indian Journal of Psychiatry*, 55(Suppl 3), S340. available at: www.indianjpsychiatry.org/text.asp?2013/55/7/340/116300 (Accessed 9/12/2019).

Deslippe, P. (2012). From Maharaj to Mahan Tantric: The Construction of Yogi Bhajan's Kundalini Yoga. *Sikh Formations*, 8(3): 369–387.

Emerson, D. and Hopper, E. (2011). *Overcoming Trauma Through Yoga: Reclaiming Your Body*. Berkley: North Atlantic Books.

Esch, T., Fricchione, G.L. and Stefano, G.B. (2003). The Therapeutic Use of the Relaxation Response in Stress-Related Diseases. *Medical Science Monitor*, 9(2): RA23–RA34, available at: www.medscimonit.com/download/index/idArt/474 (Accessed 9/12/2019).

Foot C., Gilburt H., Dunn P., Jabbal J., Seale, B., Goodrich, J., Buck, D. and Taylor, J. (2014). *People in Control of their Own Health and Care: The State of Involvement*. London: King's Fund.

Fox, P. (2019). Yoga is Big Business. www.corestrengthyoga.co.uk/PDF%20files/Microsoft%20Word%20-%20Yoga%20is%20big%20business.pdf (Accessed 20/09/19). King's Fund (in association with National Voices).

Gard, T., Taquet, M., Dixit, R., Hölzel, B.K., Dickerson, B.C. and Lazar, S.W. (2015). Greater Widespread Functional Connectivity of the Caudate in Older Adults Who Practice Kripalu Yoga and Vipassana Meditation Than in Controls. *Frontiers in Human Neuroscience*, 16(9): 137.

The Guardian. (2019). The yoga industry is booming – but does it make you a better person? www.theguardian.com/lifeandstyle/2017/sep/17/yoga-better-person-lifestyle-exercise (Accessed 20/09/2019).

Javnbakht, M., Kenari, R.H. and Ghasemi, M. (2009). Effects of Yoga on Depression and Anxiety of Women. *Complementary Therapies in Clinical Practice*, 15(2): 102–104.

Khalsa, S.B. (2004). Yoga as a Therapeutic Intervention: A Bibliometric Analysis of Published Research Studies. *Indian Journal of Physiology and Pharmacology*, 48(3): 269–285.

Khalsa, S.B.S. (2013). Yoga for Psychiatry and Mental Health: An Ancient Practice with Modern Relevance. *Indian Journal of Psychiatry*, 55(Suppl 3), S334. available at: www.indianjpsychiatry.org/text.asp?2013/55/7/334/116298 (Accessed 9/12/2019).

Larouche, E., Hudon, C. and Goulet, S. (2015). Potential Benefits of Mindfulness-Based Interventions in Mild Cognitive Impairment and Alzheimer's Disease: An Interdisciplinary Perspective. *Behavioural Brain Research*, 276: 199–212.

Lazar, S.W., Kerr, C.E., Wasserman, R.H., Gray, J.R., Greve, D.N., Treadway, M.T., McGarvey, M., Quinn, B.T., Dusek, J.A., Benson, H. and Rauch, S.L. (2005). Meditation Experience is Associated with Increased Cortical Thickness. *Neuroreport*, 16(17): 1893–1897.

Malathi, A. and Damodaran, A. (1999). Stress Due to Exams in Medical Students: A Role of Yoga. *Indian Journal of Physiology and Pharmacology*, 43: 218–224.

Michalsen, A., Grossman, P., Acil, A., Langhorst, J., Lüdtke, R., Esch, T., Stefano, G. and Dobos, G. (2005). Rapid Stress Reduction and Anxiolysis Among Distressed Women as a Consequence of a Three-Month Intensive Yoga Program. *Medical Science Monitor*, 11(12): CR555–CR561. available at: www.medscimonit.com/download/index/idArt/438851 (Accessed 9/12/2019).

"Mindfulness." National Health Service (UK). (2018). www.nhs.uk/conditions/stress-anxiety-depression/mindfulness/ (Accessed 21/1/2019).

Oken, B.S., Zajdel, D., Kishiyama, S., Flegal, K., Dehen, C., Haas, M., Kraemer, D.F., Lawrence, J. and Leyva, J. (2006). Randomized, Controlled, Six-Month Trial of Yoga in Healthy Seniors: Effects on Cognition and Quality of Life. *Alternative Therapies in Health and Medicine*, 12(1): 40–47.

Quilty, M.T., Saper, R.B., Goldstein, R. and Khalsa, S.B.S. (2013). Yoga in the Real World: Perceptions, Motivators, Barriers, and Patterns of Use. *Global Advances in Health and Medicine*, 2(1): 44–49.

Rhodes, A.M. (2015). Claiming Peaceful Embodiment Through Yoga in the Aftermath of Trauma. *Complementary Therapies in Clinical Practice*, 21(4): 247–256.

Sahasi, G., Mohan, D. and Kacker, C. (1989). Effectiveness of Yogic Techniques in the Management of Anxiety. *Journal of Personality and Clinical Studies*, 5(1): 51–55.

Sharma, I., Azmi, S.A. and Settiwar, R.M. (1991). Evaluation of the Effect of Pranayama in Anxiety State. *Alternative Medicine*, 3(4): 227–235.

Smith, C., Hancock, H., Blake-Mortimer, J. and Eckert, K. (2007). A Randomised Comparative Trial of Yoga and Relaxation to Reduce Stress and Anxiety. *Complementary Therapies in Medicine*, 15(2): 77–83.

Vahia, N.S., Doongaji, D.R., Jeste, D.V., Kapoor, S.N., Ardhapurkar, I. and Nath, S.R. (1973). Further Experience with the Therapy Based Upon Concepts of Patanjali in the Treatment of Psychiatric Disorders. *Indian Journal of Psychiatry*, 15(1): 32–37.

Vallejos, E.P., Ball, M.J., Brown, P., Crepaz-Keay, D., Haslam-Jones, E. and Crawford, P. (2016). Kundalini Yoga as Mutual Recovery: A Feasibility Study Including Children in Care and Their Carers. *Journal of Children's Services*, 11(4): 261–282.

Varambally, S. and Gangadhar, B.N. (2012). Yoga: A Spiritual Practice with Therapeutic Value in Psychiatry. *Asian Journal of Psychiatry*, 5(2): 186–189.

Vorkapic, C.F. and Rangé, B. (2014). Reducing the Symptomatology of Panic Disorder: The Effects of a Yoga Program Alone and in Combination with Cognitive-Behavioral Therapy. *Frontiers in Psychiatry*, 5: 177.

55

MUSICAL COMPOSITION AND VOCAL EXPRESSION

Brian Abrams

Introduction

Musical composition, musical use of voice, and vocal music expression have long represented aesthetic embodiments of individual and cultural life, within numerous communities and societies. Each are ways in which people have shared artistic constructions of human experience and meaning, across numerous circumstances. Moreover, each has represented ways of promoting health and well-being, both in formal health-care circumstances, as well as in more everyday, community-oriented contexts. This chapter will provide an overview of the literature on the promotion of health and well-being through (1) songwriting and other forms of composition, and (2) use of voice and vocal expression.

Songwriting and composition for promoting health and well-being

Musical composition is the creative act of establishing an enduring, musical model that can be subsequently reproduced, typically represented in the form of visual notation. Composition allows for the construction of aesthetic architecture outside of live, performance time, affording the composer the space for cultivating a musical product that actualizes artistic ideas and aspirations. Compositions are portable and shareable, and can serve as a legacy that transcends the physical and psychological limitations within which the composer may live, as well as the temporal boundaries of the composer's lifespan itself. While there are numerous applications of music composition for promoting health and well-being for persons of all ages (Baker, 2013a), the literature most prominently and pervasively emphasizes the specific endeavor of *songwriting*, typically (but not always) in the context of music therapy, involving one or more trained, qualified professionals playing a role in facilitating the process.

There is an array of musical factors (Baker, 2015), as well as group and sociocultural factors (Baker, 2013b, 2013c), impacting the therapeutic songwriting process. These can be based upon a wide variety of rationales (Schmidt, 1983), clinical goals (Jones, 2006), and practices (Baker and Wigram, 2005; Baker et al., 2008, 2009). Songwriting has been shown to deepen experiences of aesthetic flow and satisfaction, develop sense of self and identity, and facilitate sense of meaningful achievement and ownership of creative products (Baker and MacDonald, 2013, 2014). Musical, professional, and personal learning can also result from collaborative peer songwriting experiences (Baker and Krout, 2012), as can a general sense of meaningfulness (Baker et al., 2018b).

The benefits of songwriting begin early in life. Children engaging in health-focused and therapeutic songwriting in groups may not only experience fun and general enjoyment, but also improvements in personal safety, and other aspects of general well-being (Baker et al., 2018a). More specifically, at-risk youth engaging together in technology-facilitated songwriting (accompanied by experiences of music and video production) can develop a deeper sense of group identity, control of their artistic processes, and safety in channeling creative energy (Smith, 2012). Bereaved children and adolescents who have experienced the loss of significant others can utilize various forms of songwriting to explore and express grief through improvements in the capacity to process the grief (Dalton and Krout, 2005) and by singing their stories (Roberts, 2006). Children with life-threatening conditions can also benefit from songwriting, such as Filipino children with leukemia who experienced alleviation of pain as well as enhanced capacity for coping with the emotional and existential challenges of their illness (Marin, 2014).

Persons who have experienced neurological trauma and who have engaged therapeutic songwriting experiences as part of rehabilitation have shown improvements in functional skills, levels of distress, self-concept, and general sense of well-being (Baker et al., 2017; Roddy et al., 2018b). For people who have had spinal cord injuries (often faced with comorbid depression and suicidality), therapeutic songwriting can promote the rehabilitation and reintegration of identity (Roddy et al., 2018a) across physical, personal, social, relational, and vocational domains of self-concept (Tamplin et al., 2016). These can manifest as various stages of identity development after the accident, such as non-compliance, accepting help, creative engagement, and transfiguration (Viega and Baker, 2017). For persons whose conditions involve cognitive impairments that may limit levels of participation in the creation of songs (or that may limit capacity to articulate feelings related to the creative process), specific, adaptive techniques that engender successful songwriting such as Song Collage can be helpful (Tamplin, 2006).

In psychiatric care and addictions treatment, experiences of aesthetic flow and sense of meaningfulness in songwriting can serve as predictors of therapeutic outcome for adults receiving care (Baker et al., 2016; Silverman et al., 2016). Songwriting can improve the collaborative disposition of persons with schizophrenia (Silverman, 2003), while significantly increasing feelings of acceptance and joy and significantly reducing feelings of guilt, regret, blame, fear, and mistrust for persons with addictions (Jones, 2005).

The benefits of songwriting extend through the latter stages and end of life. For older adults with dementia, co-creative songwriting can motivate participation; enhance confidence to engage with others actively; develop feelings of accomplishment; stimulate engagement in creative, cognitive, language, and learning processes; and enhance feelings of connection, belonging, group cohesion, and self-consciousness (Hong and Choi, 2011; Baker and Stretton-Smith, 2018). At the same time, for caregivers of people living with dementia songwriting can provide enjoyment and distraction from stress, group cohesiveness, therapeutic insight, and deepened aesthetic appreciation (Klein and Silverman, 2012), while engendering empowerment, a community voice, and important insights (Baker and Yeates, 2018). More specifically, caregivers who engage in songwriting can gain opportunities for coping via development of personal identity (Baker, 2017), as well as opportunities for sharing their personal stories with others, resulting in connections with other caregivers, development of group identity, and development of inner strength and personal growth (Baker et al., 2018c). In end-of-life care contexts, songwriting processes shed light on patient experiences of terminal illness, death, and loss (Heath and Lings, 2012).

Voice and vocal expression for promoting health and well-being

Voice and vocal expression in music involve the intimate conveyance of affect and meaning via the unique, profoundly personal instrument that is the human voice. The voice is physically embodied identity (including a unique timbre that helps us recognize one another), and is a symbolic carrier of human will, agency, and power, expressed within a relational context (e.g., "voicing one's perspectives on the matter," "raising our voices, together," etc.). When voice is expressed within the context of aesthetic forms, such as music, it can empower the vocalist by providing a vehicle and container for lived, felt experiences. Singing, specifically together with others, can help provide a sense of mutual support, empathy, and legitimization, while potentially mobilizing shared community resources. Furthermore, singing, and the bridging of singing to other forms of vocal expression (rhythmic chanting, everyday discourse, etc.), has played various roles in the promotion of health and well-being. Again, many of the implementations of singing for health and well-being have been facilitated within the context of clinical music therapy.

There are numerous relationships between vocal expression and well-being, ranging from neurological bases to the ecological benefits of singing in communities (Norton, 2016). Examples of the latter include the choral singers of Beijing's Jingshan Park (Wei, 2013), and the Silver Voices choir (older adults) in Kristiansand, Norway (Balsnes, 2017). Singing together in community contexts can reduce marginalization and promote equality and social justice. One example is an LGBTQI community choir in Wellington, New Zealand, where members establish intergenerational, cross-gender friendships and community; affirm identities in an LGBTQI space; and educate by representing diversity during a period of greater political equity and social assimilation (Bird, 2017). Another example is a choir of homeless men who, through participation in a community choir, experienced positive life transformations and improvements in emotional, social, and mental engagement (Bailey and Davidson, 2003). In psychiatric care, the supportive conditions of group singing have promoted "musical recovery"—a process of regaining healthy relationships with music as part of overall mental health (Bibb et al., 2018). In one particular example, the "Vocal Group," a patient-centered choir, has performed on a regular basis at the hospital where it originated (Merrick and Maguire, 2017).

For persons with neurological conditions, singing may benefit speech rehabilitation (Barnish et al., 2017). For people with Parkinson's disease, or for people who have had a stroke, singing can motivate them to explore self-management options pertaining to the various challenges accompanying their condition, and can lead to improvement in mood, language, respiration, and voice (Fogg-Rogers et al., 2016). Singing as part of speech rehabilitation has also been shown to benefit persons living with conditions such as stuttering and acquired brain lesions, as well as those with speech-based challenges related to the autism spectrum (Wan et al., 2010). Likewise, for people with neurological conditions resulting in aphasia, participation in a choir has been shown to increase confidence, encourage peer support, enhance mood, augment motivation, and improve general communicative capacities (Tamplin et al., 2013). In addition, for persons with neurological conditions, choral singing has proven meaningful on a basic, social level—for example, the positive experiences of community participation in a choir for people with neurological conditions and their significant others, emerging from an initiative of the University of Auckland's Centre for Brain Research (Talmage et al., 2013).

Singing has also provided benefits in pulmonary rehabilitation, for persons with chronic obstructive pulmonary disease (COPD) and other respiratory conditions (Clift et al., 2017;

Goodridge et al., 2013). For example, long-term participation in a community singing group for adults with COPD have resulted in improved exercise capacity and a reduction in anxiety (McNaughton et al., 2017). Singing has also facilitated improvements in breath control, relaxation, motivation to participate in other health-promoting exercises, and general social engagement for persons with respiratory issues (Skingley et al., 2018).

For older adults with dementia, choral singing can serve as an effective music therapy intervention to reduce depressive symptoms (Ahessy, 2015). Specifically, singing in groups for adults with dementia can provide spaces free of judgment and social stigma, simultaneously engendering personal feelings of well-being, enhancing existing relationships, and promoting a sense of mutual understanding and camaraderie with others who share similar life experiences and challenges (Clark et al., 2018). Singing together can hold benefits for older adults on the level of community and culture. For example, community choirs including older adults from diverse ethnic and socioeconomic backgrounds can improve physical, cognitive, and psychosocial well-being (Johnson et al., 2017). In one study, feedback from older adults in community-based singing ensembles in Norway and Japan demonstrated culture-specific developments in self-expression, sense of community, and relationship to music (Kimura and Nishimoto, 2017). Moreover, community-based, intergenerational singing has been shown to cultivate feelings of general well-being, capacity for self-expression, and sense of accomplishment, while developing new relationships and social and community networks (Vaillancourt et al., 2018).

Finally, singing can play a health-promoting role for persons with life-threatening illness and in end-of-life care. Participation in community choirs for persons with cancer—such as through Tenovus Cancer Care's "Sing with Us" choirs in Wales—has led to improved vitality and reduced anxiety, and has developed overall mental health via uplifting musical activity and a supportive community group (Reagon et al., 2017). Singing in community-based choirs at the end of life can establish a non-threatening environment that helps foster self-expression and mutual empathy among participants, while promoting greater awareness of the services provided by the hospice through public performance (Gosine and Travasso, 2018). Furthermore, for bereaved individuals who have lost significant others, participation in group singing can provide a space through which they can process experiences of grief and loss (Young and Pringle, 2018).

Case illustration

As a case illustration that combines both composition and vocal expression in the service of community, Abrams (2015), serving as Director of the Music Therapy Program at the Cancer Center of the University of Pennsylvania, composed an unaccompanied, motet-style choral piece in four parts (S-A-T-B), based upon the poem, *In Time of Daffodils*, by E.E. Cummings, for an annual memorial program to honor the memory of patients of the Cancer Center who had died during the prior year. The poem was chosen based upon consoling images and sentiments that meaningfully reflected certain important aspects of work with patients during the year for various members of the care community—while the unaccompanied choral format would honor both the spirit of the poem while embodying something about the lives of the patients being recognized at the event, on a collective level. The piece was performed at the memorial event by a small ensemble of eight voices (two to a part), consisting of music therapy students from Temple University. Choral singing of the kind described in this case can serve to support and enhance well-being from a *stake-holdership* perspective—that is, a perspective within which an individual's needs exist in the situated context of the mutual interests of a larger community of care, and in which each member's life potentials are better actualized through some form of shared participation in arts-centered experiences. Moreover, members of the community participate together, as both performers and listeners, in the spirit of *participatory community involvement* and *citizen participation*, affording empowerment toward well-being for each stakeholder in attendance, in different ways that humanize the community as a whole. The stakeholder in the performance of an original piece (such as that describe in the case illustration here) can be understood in accordance with certain principles of community music therapy, in ways articulated by those such as Ansdell and Pavlicevic (2004) and Stige (2012).

Conclusion

There are a myriad of approaches to musical composition and vocal expression as part of engendering health and well-being across a wide variety of communities and clinical contexts. A growing body of research and scholarly literature substantiates this developing domain of work, and will almost certainly continue to expand. As it does, it will very likely occupy an increasingly significant space within the larger discourse of the health humanities.

References

Abrams, B. (2015). Time of Daffodils. In: C.A. Lee, A. Berends, and S. Pun, eds, *Composition and Improvisation Resources for Music Therapists*. Dallas, TX: Barcelona: 43–48.

Ahessy, B. (2015). Creating Community Through Song: A Music Therapy Choir for Older Adults. In: S.L. Brookes and C.E. Myers, eds, *The Use of the Creative Therapies in Treating Depression*. Springfield, IL: Charles C. Thomas Publishers: 141–163.

Ansdell, G. and Pavlicevic, M. (2004). *Community Music Therapy*. London: Jessica Kingsley.

Bailey, B.A. and Davidson, J. W. (2003). Amateur Group Singing as a Therapeutic Instrument. *Nordic Journal of Music Therapy*, 12(1): 18–32.

Baker, F. and Krout, R. (2012). Turning Experience into Learning: Educational Contributions of Collaborative Peer Songwriting During Music Therapy Training. *International Journal of Music Education*, 30(2): 133–147.

Baker, F.A. (2013a). Front and Center Stage: Participants Performing Songs Created During Music Therapy. *Arts in Psychotherapy*, 40(1): 20–28.

Baker, F.A. (2013b). Music Therapists' Perceptions of the Impact of Group Factors on the Therapeutic Songwriting Process. *Music Therapy Perspectives*, 31(2): 137–143.

Baker, F.A. (2013c). The Environmental Conditions that Support or Constrain the Therapeutic Songwriting Process. *The Arts in Psychotherapy*, 40(2): 230–238.

Baker, F.A. (2015). What About the Music? Music Therapists' Perspectives on the Role of Music in the Therapeutic Songwriting Process. *Psychology of Music*, 43(1): 122–139.

Baker, F.A. (2017). A Theoretical Framework and Group Therapeutic Songwriting Protocol Designed to Address Burden of Care, Coping, Identity, and Wellbeing in Caregivers of People Living with Dementia. *Australian Journal of Music Therapy*, 28: 16–33.

Baker, F.A., Jeanneret, N., and Clarkson, A. (2018a). Contextual Factors and Wellbeing Outcomes: Ethnographic Analysis of an Artist-Led Group Songwriting Program with Young People. *Psychology of Music*, 46(2): 266–280.

Baker, F.A. and MacDonald, R.A.R. (2013). Flow, Identity, Achievement, Satisfaction and Ownership During Therapeutic Songwriting Experiences with University Students and Retirees. *Musicae Scientiae*, 17(2): 131–146.

Baker, F.A. and MacDonald, R.A.R. (2014). Experiences of Creating Personally Meaningful Songs Within a Therapeutic Context. *Arts and Health: International Journal for Research, Policy and Practice*, 6(2): 143–161.

Baker, F.A., MacDonald, R.A.R. and Pollard, M.C. (2018b). Reliability and Validity of the Meaningfulness of Songwriting Scale with University Students Taking a Popular Songwriting Class. *Arts and Health: International Journal for Research, Policy and Practice*, 10(1): 17–28.

Baker, F.A., Silverman, M.J. and MacDonald, R.A.R. (2016). Reliability and Validity of the Meaningfulness of Songwriting Scale (MSS) with Adults on Acute Psychiatric and Detoxification Units. *Journal of Music Therapy*, 53(1): 55–74.

Baker, F.A., Stretton-Smith, P., Clark, I.N., Tamplin, J. and Lee. Y.C. (2018c). A Group Therapeutic Songwriting Intervention for Family Caregivers of People Living with Dementia: A Feasibility Study with Thematic Analysis. *Frontiers in Medicine*, 5: 151.

Baker, F.A. and Stretton-Smith, P.A. (2018). Group Therapeutic Songwriting and Dementia: Exploring the Perspectives of Participants Through Interpretative Phenomenological Analysis. *Music Therapy Perspectives*, 36(1): 50–66.

Baker, F.A. Tamplin, J., MacDonald, R.A.R., Ponsford, J., Roddy, C., Lee, C. and Rickard, N. (2017). Exploring the Self Through Songwriting: An Analysis of Songs Composed by People with Acquired Neurodisability in an Inpatient Rehabilitation Program. *Journal of Music Therapy*, 54(1): 35–54.

Baker, F.A. and Wigram, T. (2005). *Songwriting: Methods, Techniques and Clinical Applications for Music Therapy Clinicians, Educators and Students*. London: Jessica Kingsley.

Baker, F.A., Wigram, T., Stott, D. and McFerran, K. (2008). Therapeutic Songwriting in Music Therapy, Part I: Who are the Therapists, Who are the Clients, and Why is Songwriting Used? *Nordic Journal of Music Therapy*, 17(2): 105–123.

Baker, F.A., Wigram, T., Stott, D. and McFerran, K. (2009). Therapeutic Songwriting in Music Therapy, Part II: Comparing the Literature with Practice Across Diverse Clinical Populations. *Nordic Journal of Music Therapy*, 18(1): 32–56.

Baker, F.A. and Yeates, S. (2018). Carers' Experiences of Group Therapeutic Songwriting: An Interpretive Phenomenological Analysis. *British Journal of Music Therapy*, 32(1): 8–17.

Balsnes, A.H. (2017). The Silver Voices: A Possible Model for Senior Singing. *International Journal of Community Music*, 10(1): 59–69.

Barnish, M.S., Atkinson, R.A., Barran, S.M. and Barnish, J. (2017). Potential Benefit of Singing for People with Parkinson's Disease: A Systematic Review Updated to 2017. *Journal of Epidemiology and Community Health*, 71(S1): A52–A52.

Bibb, J. and Skewes McFerran, K. (2018). Musical Recovery: The Role of Group Singing in Regaining Healthy Relationships with Music to Promote Mental Health Recovery. *Nordic Journal of Music Therapy*, 27(3): 235–251.

Bird, F. (2017). Singing Out: The Function and Benefits of an LGBTQI Community Choir in New Zealand in the 2010s. *International Journal of Community Music*, 10(2): 193–206.

Clark, I.N., Tamplin, J.D. and Baker, F.A. (2018). Community-Dwelling People Living with Dementia and Their Family Caregivers Experience Enhanced Relationships and Feelings of Wellbeing Following Therapeutic Group Singing: A Qualitative Thematic Analysis. *Frontiers in Psychology*, 9: 1332.

Clift, S., Skingley, A., Page, S., Stephens, L., Hurley, S., Dickinson, J., Meadows, S., Levai, I., Jackson, A., Sullivan, R., Wren, N., McDaid, D., Park, A., Azhar, S., Baxter, N., Rozenthuler, G. and Shah, S. (2017). *Singing for Better Breathing: Findings from the Lambeth and Southwark Singing and COPD project*. Christ Church, New Zealand: Canterbury Christ Church University, Folkestone, Kent: Sidney De Haan Research Centre for Arts and Health.

Dalton, T.A. and Krout, R.E. (2005). Development of the Grief Process Scale Through Music Therapy Songwriting with Bereaved Adolescents. *Arts in Psychotherapy*, 32(2): 131–143.

Fogg-Rogers, L., Buetow, S., Talmage, A., McCann, C. M., Leão S. H., Tippett, L., Leung, J., McPherson, K.M. and Purdy, S.C. (2016). Choral Singing Therapy Following Stroke or Parkinson's Disease: An Exploration of Participants' Experiences. *Disability and Rehabilitation*, 38(10): 952–962.

Goodridge, D., Nicol, J.J., Horvey, K.J. and Butcher, S. (2013). Therapeutic Singing as an Adjunct for Pulmonary Rehabilitation Participants with COPD: Outcomes of a Feasibility Study. *Music and Medicine: An Interdisciplinary Journal*, 5(3): 169–176. 10.1177/1943862113493012.

Gosine, J. and Travasso, R. (2018). Building Community Through Song: The Therapeutic Hospice Choir. *British Journal of Music Therapy*, 32(1): 18–26.

Heath, B. and Lings, J. (2012). Creative Songwriting in Therapy at the End of Life and in Bereavement. *Mortality*, 17(2): 106–118.

Hong, I.S. and Choi M.J. (2011). Songwriting Oriented Activities Improve the Cognitive Functions of the Aged with Dementia. *Arts in Psychotherapy*, 38(4): 221–228.

Johnson, J.K., Gregorich, S.E., Acree, M., Nápoles, A.M., Flatt, J.D., Pounds, D., Pabst, A. and Stewart, A.L. (2017). Recruitment and Baseline Characteristics of the Community of Voices Choir Study to Promote the Health and Wellbeing of Diverse Older Adults. Contemporary Clinical Trials. *Communications*, 8: 106–113.

Jones, J.D. (2005). A Comparison of Songwriting and Lyric Analysis Techniques to Evoke Emotional Change in a Single Session with People Who Are Chemically Dependent. *Journal of Music Therapy*, 42(2): 94–110.

Jones, J.D. (2006). Songs Composed for Use in Music Therapy: A Survey of Original Songwriting Practices of Music Therapists. *Journal of Music Therapy*, 43(2): 94–110.

Kimura, H. and Nishimoto, Y. (2017). Choirs in Two Countries: A Study of Community Music Therapy for the Older Adults in Norway and Japan. *Voices: A World Forum for Music Therapy*, 17(1), https://doi.org/10.15845/voices.v17i1.860.

Klein, C.M. and Silverman, M.J. (2012). With Love From Me to Me: Using Songwriting to Teach Coping Skills to Caregivers of Those with Alzheimer's and Other Dementias. *Journal of Creativity in Mental Health*, 7(2): 153–164.

Marin, M.V. (2014). Exploring Therapeutic Songwriting for Filipino Children with Leukemia. *Music and Medicine*, 6(1): 17–24.

McNaughton, A., Weatherall, M., Williams, M., McNaughton, H., Aldington, S., Williams, G. and Beasley, R. (2017). Sing Your Lungs Out: A Community Singing Group for Chronic Obstructive Pulmonary Disease: A 1-Year Pilot Study. *British Medical Journal*, 7: e014151.

Merrick, I. and Maguire, A. (2017). From Let It Be to It Must Be Love: The Development of a Choir for Patients and Staff at a High Secure Hospital. *Arts and Health: International Journal for Research, Policy and Practice*, 9(1): 73–80.

Norton, K. (2016). *Singing and Wellbeing: Ancient Wisdom, Modern Proof*. New York: Routledge.

Reagon, C., Gale, N., Dow, R., Lewis, I. and Deursen, R. (2017). Choir Singing and Health Status in People Affected by Cancer. *European Journal of Cancer Care*, 26(5): e12568.

Roberts, M. (2006). "I Want to Play and Sing My Story": Home-Based Songwriting for Bereaved Children and Adolescents. *Australian Journal of Music Therapy*, 17: 18–34.

Roddy, C., Rickard, N., Tamplin, J. and Baker, F.A. (2018a). Personal Identity Narratives of Therapeutic Songwriting Participants Following Spinal Cord Injury: A Case Series Analysis. *Journal of Spinal Cord Medicine*, 41(4): 435–443.

Roddy, C., Rickard, N., Tamplin, J., Lee, Y.C. and Baker, F.A. (2018b). Exploring Self-Concept, Wellbeing and Distress in Therapeutic Songwriting Participants Following Acquired Brain Injury: A Case Series Analysis. *Neuropsychological Rehabilitation*, Mar, 21: 1–21. 10.1080/09602011.2018.1448288.

Schmidt, J.A. (1983). Songwriting as a Therapeutic Procedure. *Music Therapy Perspectives*, 1(2): 4–7.

Silverman, M.J. (2003). Contingency Songwriting to Reduce Combativeness and Noncooperation in a Client with Schizophrenia: A Case Study. *Arts in Psychotherapy*, 30(1): 25–33.

Silverman, M.J., Baker, F.A. and MacDonald, R.A.R. (2016). Flow and Meaningfulness as Predictors of Therapeutic Outcome Within Songwriting Interventions. *Psychology of Music*, 44(6): 1331–1345.

Skingley, A., Clift, S., Hurley, S., Price, S. and Stephens, L. (2018). Community Singing Groups for People with Chronic Obstructive Pulmonary Disease: Participant Perspectives. *Perspectives in Public Health*, 138(1): 66–75.

Smith, L. (2012). Sparkling Divas! Therapeutic Music Video Groups with At-Risk Youth. *Music Therapy Perspectives*, 30(1): 17–24.

Stige, B. (2012). *Elaborations Toward a Notion of Community Music Therapy*. New Braunfels, TX: Barcelona Publishers.

Talmage, A., Ludlam, S., Leão, S.H.S., Fogg-Rogers, L. and Purdy, S.C. (2013). Leading The CeleBRation Choir: The Choral Singing Therapy Protocol and the Role of the Music Therapist in a Social Singing Group for Adults with Neurological Conditions. *New Zealand Journal of Music Therapy*, 11: 7–50.

Tamplin, J. (2006). Song Collage Technique: A New Approach to Songwriting. *Nordic Journal of Music Therapy*, 15(2): 177–190.

Tamplin, J., Baker, F.A., Jones, B., Way, A. and Lee, S. (2013). "Stroke a Chord": The Effect of Singing in a Community Choir on Mood and Social Engagement for People Living with Aphasia Following a Stroke. *NeuroRehabilitation*, 32(4): 929–941.

Tamplin, J., Baker, F.A., Macdonald, R.A.R., Roddy, C. and Rickard, N.S. (2016). A Theoretical Framework and Therapeutic Songwriting Protocol to Promote Integration of Self-Concept in People with Acquired Neurological Injuries. *Nordic Journal of Music Therapy*, 25(2): 111–133.

Vaillancourt, G., Da Costa, D., Han, E. and Lipski, G. (2018). An Intergenerational Singing Group: A Community Music Therapy Qualitative Research Project and Graduate Student Mentoring Initiative. *Voices: A World Forum for Music Therapy*, 18(1), 10.15845/voices.v18i1.883.

Viega, M. and Baker, F.A. (2017). Remixing Identity: Creating Meaning from Songs Written by Patients Recovering from a Spinal Cord Injury. *Journal of Applied Arts and Health*, 8(1): 57–73.

Wan, C.Y., Rüber, T., Hohmann, A. and Schlaug, G. (2010). The Therapeutic Effects of Singing in Neurological Disorders. *Music Perception*, 27(4): 287–295.

Wei, S. (2013). A Multitude of People Singing Together. *International Journal of Community Music*, 6(2): 183–188.

Young, L. and Pringle, A. (2018). Lived Experiences of Singing in a Community Hospice Bereavement Support Music Therapy Group. *Bereavement Care*, 37(2): 55–66.

56

STORYTELLING

Alan Bleakley, Mike Wilson and Jon Allard

Introduction: storytelling and its discontents

We tell stories to give meaning to the world, develop mutually supportive social struc-tures, and construct identities. We tell stories of the dead to keep them alive in memory. We are born into "big" stories such as how the world was created: on the one hand, through myth and folklore, and on the other through science. Such big stories carry and express human values and moral dilemmas, forming the basis for a social con-tract, professional conduct, and the law (Bruner, 2003). Within these big, impersonal arcs each person's life course constitutes a local and unique story. Lives are recounted as overarching themes ("I've been a restless soul, and a bad apple"), and particular episodes ("Remember that time when ... ?"), confessed as truth, deliberate invention, or caricature.

But stories are potentially dead game until poached by the storyteller and revived through performance. Then, they have meaning and interest for others; otherwise, for a hungry audience they can be a bland filling, trivial, mere data. Good stories are embodied, or literally have *impact* and are *memorable* even at the level of the jelly of the brain and in the fibres of muscle. For example, reading an impactful novel is accompan-ied by activity in the left temporal cortex of the brain causing neural changes persisting for several days, but also leads to changes in the primary sensory motor region of the brain, leading some authors to speculate that when we read or listen to stories we experience it through a "ghost" muscle rehearsal (Berns et al., 2013). We shadow the action of the gripping drama. Good stories are "sticky" (Zipes, 2006) and then memor-able; or, better, the live teller of the story is the one we remember, where the story is just the vehicle for the performance, turning the spotlight again from the story told to the telling and the teller of the story.

Stories told of illness and heard as catalogues of symptoms

Good stories then twitch the muscles in anticipation and connection with characters and action; they make us laugh, cry, and wrinkle our brows in puzzlement—they are the glue and balm of human contact. But stories too can be sour or acidic, deliberately used to deceive and manipulate, as malignant tales of spite and revenge. Inevitably, stories recount, and reflect upon, sickness and symptom as we try to make sense of ailing bodies and minds in concert with those who treat us or care for us. But our narratives of "illness" may not match their case studies of "disease" (Kleinman, 1989), and this mismatch between *experiences* of illness and *treatment* of disease constitutes a story genre in itself, one of either patients' or health-care professionals' confessions (Bauby, 2006; Kalanithi, 2016).

Aligning the patient's and the clinician's account through dialogue is commonly described as the basis for a humane, "narrative-based" health care. As physician Rita Charon (2011) says: "My job is to pay exquisite attention to stories … to weave multiple, sometimes contradictory narratives [of patient history, symptoms, and diagnostic tests] into a provisional attempt to build something we can act on."

Prior to writing, oral traditions transmitted and re-imagined cultural habits. Storytellers—often shamans and healers—were skilled at memorizing, performing, and re-inventing story according to the audience's response. The ancient Greek epics that shaped a pre-biblical Western consciousness (Homer's *Iliad* and *Odyssey*) have their origins in a highly structured poetry not told, but sung, by experts: *rhapsodes*. The themes of those two stories are, respectively, *kleos* (heroic glory) and *nostos* (familial homecoming). These forms have immediate relevance for modern health care and its tensions and contradictions, where the identities in particular of doctors (especially surgeons) have been shaped by masculine, heroic stories of "cure," those of patients shaped by masculine tales of endurance and triumph over ordeal, while identities in particular of nurses have been shaped by feminine stories of "hospitality" (the same root as "hospital") and "care" (Marshall and Bleakley, 2017). Key martial metaphors, such as "the war on cancer," continue to bolster medicine's heroic image, stigmatize patients, and overshadow "homecoming" and "hospitality" metaphors such as "illness as a journey" (Bleakley, 2017).

Stories can be formulaic, reductive, and rhetorical

No singer of the ancient epics such as the *Iliad* could have remembered or sustained the poem's telling without formulaic structures and short cuts such as repetitive phrases ("the wine dark sea") and recurrent epithets ("cunning" Odysseus). Health care too depends upon reformulating and reducing patients' messy and complex stories to the hardtack of "case notes." Paradoxically, stories may have the biggest impact when they are told informally in "corridor conversations" where dark humour, expletives, and frank honesty give muscle, color, and depth to tales that cannot be told elsewhere as they stretch the bounds of professional and ethical conduct (Piemonte, 2015). In such contexts, and also in research where anonymity is guaranteed, stories can be deliberately rhetorical (Box 56.1).

Box 56.1 **Rhetoric in stories**

In a research project looking at how to improve teamwork in operating theatres, stories were collected from surgical staff (mainly nurses) about "close call" incidents—issues that could have led to an error but were nipped in the bud. Analysis of such stories offers a key way to re-design team practices. Such stories can, however, be deliberately misleading, where rhetoric persuades the reader into a point of view favoring the author. For example, a nurse wrote about a series of incidents during one series of operations in which she cast the surgeon in a poor light, as reactive and antagonistic, but cast herself in a good light, as proactive and agreeable. From further discussions with practitioners this appeared to be a reflection of her own perspective of events, which may have encompassed a construction/telling of the story in a way that allowed her to be perceived in a certain way. Bleakley (2006) describes this as "the

---

rhetorical construction of identity"—specifically, a moral identity ("I am the good person exposing the bad") that may be pious and high-handed. This is consistent with what folklorists call the "looking good principle" in personal storytelling, whereby storytellers cast themselves in a sympathetic light.

From one couch to another

Modern psychological health care begins with Freud's deep interest in storytelling—the client given space and time to allow unconscious material to rise to consciousness—as the catharsis-based "talking cure." Once catharsis clears, insight and interpretation begin. Freud himself was a great storyteller, winning the Goethe Prize for literature. His case studies are beautifully crafted fictions. Psychoanalysis is restricted to private clients paying large fees, but now the public can engage in mass catharsis and subsequent insight through the media of television, for no fee. "Medi-soaps" providing "infotainment" or "edutainment"—such as *ER*, *House MD*, *Casualty*, and *Holby City*—would not grip and entertain if they did not tell compelling stories about the human condition that are also therapeutic by proxy (Box 56.2). Helpline numbers are provided at the end of programs.

Box 56.2 **Confessional, cathartic storytelling is therapeutic**

Research we carried out on how stories might be used collaboratively by doctors, their patients, and patients' carers illustrated the therapeutic value of storytelling. Stories were shared in an online, anonymized forum. Doctors—who are characteristically overworked and stressed, with little in the way of formal opportunity for support or cathartic release—took the opportunity to tell confessional and cathartic stories about their childhoods, siblings, families, and job pressures as if they were on the analyst's couch or playing a role in a TV medi-soap (Allard, Wilson and Bleakley, 2020).

Is there evidence that telling stories has health benefits?

There is not a large body of evidence that can be quoted to defend the claim that stories have healing and restorative value beyond a wealth of anecdote and opinion. Rigorous research in the field is a priority. Two key pieces of evidence for the value of stories are shown below (Box 56.3).

Box 56.3 **Listening to stories has health benefits**

1   Stories can motivate through empathy. Blood tests taken after reading a story about a father and his relationship with a terminally ill son showed increased levels of cortisol (a stress hormone) and oxytocin (a chemical associated with empathy and bonding). When invited to donate to a children's cancer charity,

---

these same study participants with raised cortisol and oxytocin levels were more likely to donate than a control group (Zak, 2013).

2   Storytelling was used to control high blood pressure among a sample of inner city African American individuals, a population vulnerable to hypertension, heart disease, and stroke. In a randomized controlled trial, 230 African Americans with hypertension watched three DVDs of peers telling stories describing how they had learned to interact well with doctors and to develop strategies to increase adherence to prescribed medication. The control group, who had similar baseline blood pressures to the experimental group, watched health-related video topics not related to hypertension. In the words of the researchers: "The storytelling intervention produced substantial and significant improvements in blood pressure for patients with baseline uncontrolled hypertension" (Houston et al., 2011).

When storytelling is pathologized and not sanitized

Let's not be smug about storytelling: it is largely for the able. Dementia, psychosis, aphasia, mutism, autism—all queer the pitch for our sunny account of storytelling's virtues. Also, there are important stains on the well-tempered story: a dislocation of self (e.g., in the narcissistic personality) can lead to the bizarre "flash fiction" illustrated by President Donald Trump's infamous tweet-fests, which, while they may be collectively constructed phenomena, are significant in constructing a political persona.

Enthusiasm for the benefit of stories masks the claim that, for some, "narrativizing" is not a natural way of communicating (Strawson, 2004). In "Against Narrativity," the philosopher Galen Strawson distinguishes between those who prefer the Episodic (having a sense of continuity through time) and those who prefer the Diachronic (not time bound, but more sensitive to space). Strawson's argument is not based on population statistics—he may be talking about a minority of diachronics (including himself), but it is certainly thought-provoking and a reminder that narrativity has, for some, become a faith rather than an exploratory model. Recounting an illness experience for diachronics may not unfold as a story, but as spatial experiences. If you are wedded to temporality, the best way to understand diachronic experience is to read high modern and postmodern literature that refuses conventional plot, such as James Joyce's *Ulysses*, where Dublin's topography plays as important a role as the characters (Seidel, 2014).

More important than whether or not people can be typed as sensitive or insensitive to temporal story is an ethical question of how story is used. Jean-Paul Sartre claims that while narrative life is inevitable, telling stories opens the door to fantasy and distortions of truth. Narrative capacity equates with "bad faith," where stories are used to manage impressions through manipulation or deceit, returning us to the power of rhetoric. A persuasive story involving deception, fabrication, or other ploys allows a nursing, physiotherapy, or medical student to get away with not knowing much on a ward round when quizzed by their seniors.

A highly respected (now retired) surgeon turned storyteller, Henry Marsh (2014), says: "We have a very complicated relationship with patients . . . as soon as we have any interaction with patients, we start lying. We have to. There is nothing more frightening for a patient than an anxious or doubtful doctor." We might, as an antidote to Marsh's cynicism, note the remark of the late celebrated fiction writer Denis Johnson, who says: "It's always been my tendency to lie to doctors, as if good health consisted only of the ability to fool them."

References

Allard, J., Wilson, M. and Bleakley, A. (2020). Digital Storytelling in Mental Health. In A. Bleakley, ed, *Routledge Handbook of Medical Humanities*. London, Routledge, 410–418.

Bauby, J-D. (2006). *The Diving-Bell and the Butterfly*. London: Harper-Collins.

Berns, G. S., Blaine, K., Prietula, M. and Pye, B. E. (2013). Short- and Long-Term Effects of a Novel on Connectivity in the Brain. *Brain Connectivity*, 3: 590–600.

Bleakley, A. (2006). "You Are Who I Say You Are": The Rhetorical Construction of Identity in the Operating Theatre. *Journal of Workplace Learning*, 18: 414–425.

Bleakley, A. (2017). *Thinking with Metaphors in Medicine: The State of the Art*. London: Routledge.

Bruner, J. (2003). *Making Stories: Law, Literature, Life*. Harvard, MA: Harvard University Press.

Charon, R. (2011). TEDx Atlanta: Honoring the Stories of Illness. Online Seminar. Available from www.youtube.com/watch?v=24kHX2HtU3o (Accessed 29/01/2019).

Houston, T.K., Allison J.T., Sussman, M., Horn, W., Holt, C.H., Trobaugh, J., Salas, M., Pisu, M., Cuffee, Y.L., Larkin, D., Person, S. D., Barton, B., Kiefe, C.I. and Hullett, S. (2011). Culturally Appropriate Storytelling to Improve Blood Pressure: A Randomized Trial. *Annals of Internal Medicine*, 154: 77–84.

Kalanithi, P. (2016). *When Breath Becomes Air*. London: Bodley Head.

Kleinman, A. (1989). *The Illness Narratives: Suffering, Healing and the Human Condition*. London: Basic Books.

Marsh, H. (2014). *Do No Harm: Stories of Life, Death, and Brain Surgery*. London: Weidenfield & Nicholson.

Marshall, R. and Bleakley, A. (2017). *Rejuvenating Medical Education: Seeking Help from Homer*. Newcastle: Cambridge Scholars.

Piemonte, N. (2015). Last Laughs: Gallows Humor and Medical Education. *Journal of Medical Humanities*, 36: 375–390.

Seidel, M. A. (2014). *Epic Geography: James Joyce's* Ulysses. Princeton, NJ: Princeton University Press.

Strawson, G. (2004). Against Narrativity. *Ratio*, 17 (4): 428–452.

Zak, P. J. (2013). *The Moral Molecule: The New Science of What Makes us Good or Evil*. London: Corgi.

Zipes, J. (2006). *Why Fairy Tales Stick: The Evolution and Relevance of a Genre*. London: Routledge.

57

APPLIED THEATRE

Gretchen Case and Sydney Cheek-O'Donnell

Introduction

We can apply theater in many different ways in health care. In this chapter, we describe how to use it to improve patient handoffs. Handoffs, or signouts, of patients are necessary at every level of health care, but come with serious risks for error or neglect. The Johns Hopkins University School of Medicine offers a concise definition in its guidelines:

> A handoff is the process of transferring information and authority and responsibility for a patient during transitions of care. Transitions include changes in providers, whether from shift to shift, service to service, or hospital or clinic to home. Transitions also occur when a patient is moved from one location or level of service to another.
>
> *(General Medical Education Committee, 2011: 1)*

The body of research focused on one of the most common handoffs, shift change in an inpatient setting, has shown that it raises the potential for mistakes (Riesenberg, 2012: 4). The move toward procedural checklists in operating rooms responds to the same problem: mistakes made or information lost when a patient arrives for surgery and is transferred from one team to another (Gawande, 2010).

We propose that by building visual and tactile connections with a partner, one can also build empathy for that partner and for others sharing the activity. With shared empathy comes attention and commitment to shared goals. The theater exercises described here are themselves handoffs of leadership and control, and provide a low-stakes environment in which partners must work together to complete the handoff by both giving and receiving in turn.

When we bring an exercise from theater into another discipline, it is vital to remember that the things we take for granted with theater students—interest in the exercise, attention and willingness to participate, trust that no matter how strange the activity there is a point to it—cannot be taken for granted in another setting. Perhaps nowhere is this as true as it is in a room full of students heading toward a career in health care, who have been trained to work in a very different mode in a high-stakes environment.

We find that when working with health-care personnel, it is very helpful to discuss and establish specific learning goals with the group. With health-care learners, goals are most successful when they are explicitly connected to a real-life situation or skill. As you will see in the description below, we have suggested that these exercises connect directly to the perception and expression of empathy, as well as to skills necessary for handoffs. Your group may find additional connections, depending on your individual and shared experiences and the health disciplines for which your learners are preparing.

In addition, because this type of learning activity is sometimes quite foreign to people working in health care, it is important to establish (or reiterate) a set of ground rules or working agreements before beginning. At the very least these agreements should include something along the following lines: (1) everyone will try the exercises; (2) accommodations and adjustments are always possible (give participants a chance to ask for these privately and in advance); and (3) everyone will do their best to make these exercises welcoming and comfortable. This last guideline is important because some participants may feel vulnerable during the exercises. Reassurance that they are in a supportive space can make the difference between a successful and an unsuccessful learning experience.

Exercise 1: mirroring

This fairly simple exercise encourages participants to pay very close attention to and imitate the movements of a partner while holding their gaze. The intimacy and intensity of looking into another person's eyes for an extended period is challenging for many people. However, maintaining appropriate eye contact is cited repeatedly in health communication literature as a fundamental means of conveying empathy (Riess and Kraft-Todd, 2014: 1109–1110).

Interestingly, the secondary task of mirroring the movements of a partner while holding the gaze diffuses some of the tension inherent in unbroken eye contact. In addition to improving direct eye contact, participants learn to use their peripheral vision to keep track of and even anticipate the movements in their partners. While they cannot read each other's minds, the intensive attention partners pay to one another during this exercise leads to the partners moving in sync with one another so fluidly that onlookers cannot tell who is leading and who is following.

We suggest presenting all of the following instructions to participants before beginning the exercise so that they are ready when they hear the call to move to the next part of the activity.

Instructions

- Move into pairs, with learners facing each other, about three feet (one metre) apart. Standing is preferred for range of possible motion, but seated is fine and will not interfere with the goals of the exercise. One learner should volunteer to begin as leader.
- Begin by making eye contact with your partner. Take 60–90 seconds to settle into the discomfort of staring directly into someone else's eyes and get any giggles out of the way. Sustained eye contact is harder than you think. Throughout this entire exercise, you should maintain direct eye contact, no matter what.
- The leader then begins changing their facial expression, slowly enough that the follower can copy that expression, as if a reflection in a mirror. Try for smooth changes between expressions, but still slow enough that the follower can keep up.

- After about two minutes, the instructor should call "switch," and the follower becomes the leader and the exercise continues. Try not to stop for this change in roles, merely let the new leader take over in the middle of whatever expression is being performed at that moment.
- After another two minutes, the instructor calls "same leader, use your body" and the movement can now include more than just facial expressions and extend to all parts of the body. Learners should maintain eye contact at all times.
- After 60–90 seconds, the instructor calls "switch leaders." Again, the switch should be without interruption, and all parts of the body are now in play.
- After 60–90 seconds, the instructor calls "no leader." Without speaking or otherwise signaling, the two learners need to figure out who is leading each gesture or expression. Both should be trying to lead and to follow so that the series of movements is unbroken. This is the hardest part of the activity and also the most significant. This last part of the activity can go on for between two and five minutes, or as long as learners seem fully engaged. If the instructor sees the mirroring begin to falter, they should end the exercise before the connection breaks down.

Once the activity has ended, ask students to discuss it. Some possible questions include:

1. What was the hardest part of this exercise? Why was it hard?
2. When did you feel most uncomfortable? Comfortable?
3. Did you prefer to lead or follow?

Exercise 2: push hands

This exercise comes from a workshop with the British theater group Frantic Assembly. During a workshop with formerly incarcerated adults, one of the authors used this exercise as a means to build trust and teamwork, develop non-verbal communication skills, and improve proprioception.

Instructions

In an open space clear of obstacles, participants should break up into pairs. Pairs should spread themselves out around the room so they have plenty of space to move. Everyone should be standing.

- Have each pair identify one person who will be "A" and one person who will be "1." Have the A's hold out their right hands, palms down. Invite the 1's to place their right hands on top of their partner's right hand. At this point, the 1's should each have their right hand resting, palm down, on top of their partner's right hand, also palm down.
- Now invite the 1's to lead the A's by moving their hand around. The leader is not allowed to hold or grip the follower's hand. Instead, both partners must maintain constant contact by exerting equal and opposite pressure through their hands. This is not a contest of strength, so the pressure should be just what is necessary to maintain contact and direct movement.
- Invite the leaders to explore moving their partners' hands in a variety of directions—up and down, side to side, diagonally, etc.—through different levels—from close to the

floor to as high as the partners can reach. Invite leaders to begin moving so that the followers must change their footing or body position.

- Periodically remind leaders not to grip their partners' hands. It is typical to see a thumb creep down to try to get a grip—they may not even notice they are doing it. This exercise should be conducted with a minimum of talking.
- As the pairs begin to move more fluidly with one another, instruct the leaders to begin moving their partners through the space. It is the leader's responsibility to avoid colliding with other people and objects. But it is also the leader's job to offer some challenge to their follower. You may wish to suggest experimentation with levels, speed, direction, etc.
- Switch leaders and guide participants through this part of the exercise again with the A's leading and the 1's following.
- Once both partners have had the opportunity to lead, take a couple of minutes to discuss the experience with the participants. This does not need to be a long conversation. Just get some basic observations:

    - What was it like to be a leader? A follower?
    - How was it to move around the space?
    - Did you bump into anyone?
    - Any other observations?

Now ask the 1's to lead again, but this time the A's will close their eyes and follow using only the cues they receive through the pressure point on the top of their hands. Remind the leaders that it is their responsibility to keep their partners safe during this exercise—making sure not to run into other people or objects. Have leaders take it slow to begin. Again, remind people not to grip hands—use only gentle opposing pressure to remain in contact.

- When it seems that the pairs are reasonably comfortable, invite leaders to offer a bit more challenge to their partners—perhaps moving a bit more quickly, changing directions, exploring more levels, etc. There may be some laughter and a few nervous comments, but remind participants that this is a silent exercise and that they are communicating with one another only through their sense of touch at this one point of contact.
- Switch leaders again (A's lead, 1's follow with eyes closed) and repeat.
- Once both partners have had the opportunity to lead, have everyone sit in a circle so that you can debrief on the exercise together. The circle is important because it allows everyone to see the person who is speaking, creates a sense of community, and puts everyone in the discussion on equal ground—the facilitator is not the focus. Here are some suggested prompts for discussion:

    - Was it difficult to maintain your point of contact?
    - Were you able to improve the consistency of your contact as you worked? How did that happen?
    - What was it like when you closed your eyes?
    - Was it more or less difficult to follow with eyes closed? Why?
    - How did it feel to lead someone else? Was it different when their eyes were closed?
    - Were you able to keep track of where you were in the room with your eyes closed?

In all theater-based exercises, we find that it is best to "scaffold" activities, by starting with something simple and building up to the more complicated (e.g., do "Push Hands" with eyes open first, then build up to the version with eyes closed). These exercises can and should be adjusted to accommodate a range of abilities and disabilities among participants, including limited mobility. If you have an odd number of participants, a facilitator can partner with a learner.

Facilitating discussion

Following these exercises, we suggest a facilitated discussion to connect participants' experience to the clinical practice of handoffs. Learners who have experienced clinical rotations or other direct patient interaction will be best able to discuss handoffs in detail. Other students will require guidance in understanding what is at stake in a handoff. Thus, the discussion might need to expand to include other team-based aspects of the delivery of health care.

Ask about moments at which leader and follower switched. What mental process did you go through? Was there an emotional or reactive process—that is, did you feel anything about being asked to switch? What did you notice about when it went smoothly? When it did not go smoothly, what did you and your partner do to recover your rhythm? Ask learners to think about non-verbal indicators of handoffs. What would happen if those were named, using words, as a moment of leadership change?

Whether students prefer to lead or follow can be an interesting discussion, and again, answers are unpredictable. Guide this discussion by asking them how their preference in these exercises lines up with their preferences in other team or group situations. Push a bit on people who say they had no preference to try to get them to think about when and why they decide to lead or follow. Talk as neutrally as possible about both terms, so that neither leading nor following is valued more highly. Move into a discussion of how teamwork requires a mix of leading and following by all parties.

One of the ways we connect with other humans is to look at them. Looking into someone's eyes is usually an intimate act, meant to signal a desire for understanding and connection. It may also signal an attempt to get information about someone else (the "windows into the soul" idea). Ask learners to discuss when in their lives they look directly into someone's eyes, and what the barriers to doing so are. Ask them to talk about how they feel about their partner in this exercise after ten minutes or so of staring directly into their eyes. Were they able to see what was going on with the rest of their partner's body, even while maintaining eye contact?

In clinical situations, patients often report wanting direct eye contact, especially during discussions of serious matters. What does direct eye contact do, and why do people want it? How might this differ according to culture of origin? Why might you, as a provider, feel uncomfortable with direct eye contact with a patient or family member? Is it OK to "cheat" and look at their forehead or between the eyes—is there something special about looking directly in the eyes? Learners often report that gender plays a role, although unpredictably so. Perceived hierarchy can also be a factor, especially in a mixed group, and can be a challenge for any learners paired with facilitators. Culture of origin almost certainly affects how comfortable learners are with eye contact; if they do not bring it up, ask them to talk about how they perceive this sort of gaze.

When presented in a supportive atmosphere, learners are willing to discuss the possible applications of this exercise to their clinical experiences, current and future. For example, a group of fourth-year medical students already matched into a variety of residency programs were able to discuss how the quality of eye contact matters between members of a surgical team in an operating room as well as between physician and patient or family member. Because of the practical applications and larger context it can provide, the discussion following may last much longer—and leave greater impact—than the activity itself.

References

Gawande, A. (2010). *The Checklist Manifesto: How to Get Things Right*. New York: Metropolitan Books.

General Medical Education Committee. (2011). *Guidelines for Patient Handoffs Johns Hopkins University School of Medicine Graduate Medical Education Committee*. Baltimore: Johns Hopkins Medicine. www.hopkinsmedicine.org/som/gme/GME_Policies/handoff_%20policy.doc (Accessed 28/9/2018).

Riesenberg, L.A. (2012). Shift-to-Shift Handoff Research: Where Do We Go from Here? *Journal of Graduate Medical Education*, 4: 4–8.

Riess, H. and Kraft-Todd, G. (2014). E.M.P.A.T.H.Y.: A Tool to Enhance Nonverbal Communication Between Clinicians and Their Patients. *Academic Medicine*, 89: 1108–1112.

58

VISUAL ARTS

Victoria Tischler

Introduction

The practice of using visual arts to enhance health-care settings and to benefit patients and residents is not new. Many hospitals have their own art collections, commission creative programs of work, and engage artists-in-residence. Some examples are Chelsea and Westminster Hospital's collection, which includes over 1000 artworks displayed across their clinical sites in London, including Veronese's exceptional painting *The Resurrection* (1850), displayed in the chapel; modern art (e.g., Julian Opie's *Sian Walking* [2010]); and commissioned pieces such as *The Dispensary* (2015), an interactive sculpture by Tabitha Andrews made in collaboration with inpatients living with dementia. The hospital has even developed a self-guided walking tour of its collection, available digitally (CW+, 2018).

The arts and health charity Paintings in Hospitals, established in 1959, holds the United Kingdom's first and only national collection of art that is loaned to clinical and social care settings, aiming to benefit the physical and mental health of patients and staff (Paintings in Hospitals, n.d.). Great Ormond Street Hospital, a specialist children's hospital in London, commissions creative programs through their arts team "GOSH Arts." Projects include Nature Trail, digital interactive wallpaper aiming to calm patients before surgery as they travel to the operating theater (Great Ormond Street Hospital, 2018). The hospice service St. Barnabas, in Sussex, has been running an artist-in-residence program since 2005, offering creative input to encourage self-expression and a sense of purpose for those experiencing life-limiting conditions (Artist in Residence, n.d.).

This chapter outlines a program of work that embeds artists in care home settings. The benefits of visual arts practice for care home residents, as well as for wider health and social care provision are presented, using examples from current practice. Guidance is given about how to establish similar programs, with challenges and barriers to this practice also considered.

What's the evidence?

A growing body of research is emerging in the fields of arts and health, as well as health humanities, that supports the positive impact of visual arts on mental and physical health. A useful overview is contained in *Creative Health* (2017), a wide-ranging analysis of initiatives across art forms, and applications for a diverse range of conditions. Examples from the visual arts include art making and gallery discussion programs for those living with dementia; Arts on Prescription, a general practice referral scheme for patients with a variety of conditions including chronic pain, stroke, and depression, offering creative activities including ceramics, drawing, painting, and mosaics. Given an increase in research evidence, *Creative Health* recommends the expansion of these types of programs for mental and physical health problems. Specific recent findings indicate positive impacts on resilience for people living with dementia in care homes who engage with visual art activities, through enabling creative expression, increased communication, and improved self-esteem (Newman et al., 2018). Additionally, people with dementia who participated in a visual arts program expressed enhanced well-being in domains including interest, attention, pleasure, and self-esteem compared with those undertaking an alternative activity (Windle et al., 2017).

A systematic review found that adults with mental health problems who engaged with visual arts benefited in a variety of ways, including improved self-esteem and self-respect, reduced depression and anxiety, re-engagement with the wider social world, and potential identity re-negotiation via practice-based activities (Tomlinson et al., 2018). The visual arts are beneficial to staff and health-care trainees as well, with exposure reported to increase empathy in medical students (Mangione et al., 2018), while looking at artwork has been noted to enhance nursing and medical students' observational skills (Klugman et al., 2015).

A range of hospital and health-care staff may also benefit from the ways in which art can create a space for reflection and for depicting specific issues such as older age and mental health ("A doctor," 2015). With pressure on health and social care budgets globally, much personal care provided to older people is delivered by health-care assistants. These staff work under challenging conditions and receive minimal remuneration (Bailey et al., 2015; Scales et al., 2017). The rising numbers of older people needing care, combined with structural barriers governing adequate care provision, mean that this staff group are acknowledged to require enhanced training yet are not well supported in practice (Sarre et al., 2018).

Artists in care homes

The value of the visual arts for patients and staff has been demonstrated; however, less work has focused on the potential of creative practitioners to influence the delivery of health and social care. Inspired by the ethos of transdisciplinarity, artist residencies in care homes for people living with dementia aimed to explore the potential of artistic practice, with parity between creative activities and shaping and changing delivery of care.

Transdisciplinarity represents a commitment to working across disciplines, transcending multi- and interdisciplinary approaches by bypassing or abandoning subject boundaries. It is characterized by creative enquiry and intellectual risk-taking (Augsburg, 2014), embracing diversity including socioeconomics, and foregrounds the creation of new knowledge, unconstrained by binary or either/or positions that often constrain disciplinary epistemologies (Bernstein, 2015). The residencies therefore aimed to harness the curiosity, flexibility, and creativity of artists, creating a space for them to respond to, and disrupt, regular provision with a view to changing and enhancing it.

The arts are beginning to be explored as a potential method for training staff and enhancing provision. For example, a play about a dementia ward, *Created Out of Mind*, was found to raise awareness of care needs and to generate practical responses (Schneider, 2017). "Imagination Café" (2018), a touring installation, used artwork created by people with dementia, challenging negative preconceptions about the condition and offering training for artists wishing to work in care settings. Art in Residence (2018), a project involving Ben Uri Arts and Dementia Institute and Nightingale Care Home in South London, represents a long-term collaboration between a cultural institution and a care setting. The project aims to deliver, refine, and compare art discussion and art-making sessions, utilizing high-quality artwork on loan from the gallery partner's (Ben Uri Gallery and Museum) collection. The partnership is sustained through long-term funding, meaning that relationships can be consolidated, nurturing trust and commitment.

One of the most ambitious creative projects to take place in a care setting has been "Moving In," the work of artists Claire Ford and Kate Sweeney who lived in a dementia care home for a month, working and sleeping on the premises (Moving In, 2017). In a film about the project, Ford and Sweeney reflect on the opportunities provided by abandoning their comfort zones and immersing themselves in the care setting. This deepened relationships with staff and residents, and enhanced their creative practice as time constraints were removed. They also witnessed at first hand the commitment of staff and the impact of and creativity in a setting where death and dying is commonplace.

Two artists-in-residence have been placed in dementia care settings—(1) an illustrator in a care home in South West London, and (2) a theater designer in a care home in Surrey—as part of a current program of work focusing on visual arts and dementia care. Both artists have been working in situ for over 12 months, despite the initial brief detailing a three-month residency only. In both cases, the care home managers have committed to exploring the residency as part of routine practice with a particular focus on (1) twice-weekly creative sessions including outings and staff participation, and (2) the design of a 1950s-style tea-room space in a new day center. The artists and the project lead (the author) committed to building and sustaining relationships with the care homes, resulting in the continuation of the project beyond its original scope.

Initial data from (1) indicates that the artist has become embedded in the staff team, her engagement being extended as the residency progressed. In the case of (2), the tea-room, the project was prolonged to include design of space in other areas of the home including a multisensory room containing specially commissioned furniture and tapestries, interactive walls to exhibit photography, and a "street view" garden makeover with a phone box, vintage street signs, and a post box. It is hoped to move this project into other care settings, with the grand ambition being *an artist in every home.*

Advice

For those looking to develop similar programs of work, some key pointers are listed below:

- Build relationships. Take time to get to know partners and collaborators, their priorities, values, and challenges. Make a commitment that has longevity. This includes acknowledging, and working with barriers such as staff resistance, management ambiguity, and power differentials.
- Aim high. You may encounter cultures of mediocrity and health and social care hierarchies that do not value the arts or give them priority. Everyone has the human right to participate in cultural life (UNESCO, 1948). Those with health challenges are part of the global community and deserve the same access to high-quality arts as their fellow citizens.

- Be prepared to change your own views and practice. This is transdisciplinarity in action. The rewards are great: innovation in practice, and personal and professional growth.
- Start small. Focus on developing profound change at a local level before scaling up or outward.
- Secure long-term funding commitment. This enables iterative and reflective practice and sustains collaboration over time.

References

Art in Residence (2018). Ben Uri Gallery's Wellbeing Programme. Retrieved from www.benuri.org.uk/wellbeing-programme/ (Accessed 20/2/2019).

Artist in Residence (n.d.). St Barnabas House. Retrieved from www.stbarnabas-hospice.org.uk/our-care/patients/artist-in-residence/ (Accessed 20/2/2019).

Augsburg, T. (2014). Becoming Transdisciplinary: The Emergence of the Transdisciplinary Individual. *World Futures*, 70(3): 233–247.

Bailey, S., Scales, K., Lloyd, J., Schneider, J. and Jones, R. (2015). The Emotional Labour of Health-Care Assistants in Inpatient Dementia Care. *Ageing and Society*, 35(2): 246–269.

Bernstein, J. H. (2015). Transdisciplinarity: A Review of Its Origins, Development, and Current Issues. *Journal of Research Practice*, 11(1): R1. http://jrp.icaap.org/index.php/jrp/article/view/510/412 (Accessed 20/2/2019).

All-Party Parliamentary Group, Creative Health: The Arts for Health and Wellbeing (2017) *Report of the All-Party Parliamentary Group on Arts, Health and Wellbeing.* Retrieved from www.artshealthandwellbeing.org.uk/appg-inquiry/ (Accessed 30/11/2019).

CW+ Chelsea and Westminster Hospital NHS Foundation Trust Charity (2018). *Art Collection.* Retrieved from www.cwplus.org.uk/our-work/patient-experience/art-collection/

A doctor who is combining art and medicine (2015). Retrieved from www.gponline.com/gp-life-doctor-combining-art-medicine/article/1367362 (Accesssed 20/2/2019).

Great Ormond Street Hospital for Children (2018) Art Collection. Retrieved from www.gosh.nhs.uk/parents-and-visitors/gosh-arts/art-collection

Imagination Café (2018). *The Imagination Café.* Retrieved from www.cultureand.org/projects/the-imagination-cafe/ (Accessed 20/2/2019).

Klugman, C.M. and Beckmann-Mendez, D.B. (2015). One Thousand Words: Evaluating an Interdisciplinary Art Education Program. *Journal of Nursing Education*, 54(4): 220–223.

Mangione, S., Chakraborti, C., Staltari, G., Harrison, R., Tunkel, A.R., Liou, K.T., Cerceo, E., Voeller, M., Bedwell, W.L., Fletcher, K. and Kahn, M.J. (2018). Medical Students' Exposure to the Humanities Correlates with Positive Personal Qualities and Reduced Burnout: A Multi-Institutional US Survey. *Journal of General Internal Medicine*, 33(5): 628–634.

Moving In (2017). Claire Ford and Kate Sweeney's artist residency at Northbourne Care Home. Retrieved from https://movingintocare.blogspot.com/p/film.html (Accessed 20/2/2019).

Newman, A., Goulding, A., Davenport, B. and Windle, G. (2018). The Role of the Visual Arts in the Resilience of People Living with Dementia in Care Homes. *Ageing and Society*, 39 (11): 2465–2482. https://doi.org/10.1017/S0144686X18000594

Paintings in Hospitals (n.d.). Retrieved from www.paintingsinhospitals.org.uk (Accessed 20/2/2019).

Sarre, S., Maben, J., Aldus, C, Schneider, J., Wharrad, H., Nicholson, C. and Arthur, A. (2018). The Challenges of Training, Support and Assessment of Healthcare Support Workers: A Qualitative Study of Experiences in Three English Acute Hospitals. *International Journal of Nursing Studies*, 79: 145–153.

Scales, K., Bailey, S., Middleton, J. and Schneider, J. (2017). Power, Empowerment, and Person-Centred Care: Using Ethnography to Examine the Everyday Practice of Unregistered Dementia Care Staff. *Sociology of Health and Illness*, 39(2): 227–243.

Schneider, J. (2017). Evaluation of the Impact on Audiences of *Inside Out of Mind*, Research-Based Theatre for Dementia Carers. *Arts and Health*, 9(3): 238–250.

Tomlinson, A., Lane, J., Julier, G., Duffy, L. B., Payne, A., Mansfield, L., Kay, T., John, A., Meads, C., Daykin, N., Ball, K. Tapson, C., Dolan, P., Testonis, S. and Victor, C. (2018). *A Systematic Review of the Subjective Wellbeing Outcomes of Engaging with Visual Arts for Adults ("Working-Age", 15–64 years) with Diagnosed Mental Health Conditions.* What Works Wellbeing. Retrieved from https://whatworkswell being.org/blog/visual-arts-mental-health-and-wellbeing-evidence-review/ (Accessed 24/2/2018).

Universal Declaration of Human Rights (1948). Article 27. Retrieved from www.un.org/en/universal-declaration-human-rights/ (Accessed 24/2/2019).

Windle, G., Joling, K. J., Howson-Griffiths, T., Woods, B., Hedd Jones, C., van de Ven, P. M., Newman, A. and Parkinson, C. (2017). The Impact of a Visual Arts Program on Quality of Life, Communication, and Wellbeing of People Living with Dementia: A Mixed-Methods Longitudinal Investigation. *International Psychogeriatics*, 30(3): 409–423.

59

KNITTING

Betsan Corkhill

Introduction

The activity of knitting has been around for centuries, although there is no consensus on when knitting, as we know it today, was first performed. The first garments were likely to have been caps or stockings created purely for practical benefit by men and women. Knitting as a therapeutic tool is alluded to in Tolstoy's *War and Peace* (1869) as the countess Natasha Rostova knitted stockings beside the deathbed of Prince Andrei: "There was something soothing about knitting." There are also sketchy reports of knitting being used to calm hysteria in Victorian women.

Knitting took off during World War I. Women reported that while being useful for the war effort it also calmed their nerves and made them feel better to know that their hand-knitted items would be comforting to soldiers and loved ones. There is pictorial evidence of soldiers suffering from shell shock being treated with knitting at the Walter Reed Memorial Hospital in Washington (1918) following World War I (Time Life Pictures, 1918). Many soldiers knitted to cope with the trauma of war and long periods of bed rest. At this time, boys were taught to knit in school. It was often used to keep boys who might nowadays be called hyperactive calm. There are reports that Charles Montague Fletcher (1911–1996), the epidemiologist behind the Royal College of Physicians' report on the hazards of smoking (1962), used knitting to stop smoking.

As health care became more scientific, knitting as a tool in clinical settings was discarded. The idea was rekindled in 2005 when I stumbled across a large number of stories about its benefits from people of different backgrounds and cultures. These were profound tales of life-changing experiences, so I set about exploring the possible science behind their claims.

The first major barrier was to get clinicians and academics to see beyond the word "knitting." Resistance was so strong at first that I was forced to call knitting a "Bilateral Rhythmic Psychosocial Intervention." This opened the door and enabled me to prime the conversations before introducing the "K" word. Knitting is perceived as a "soft" or "woolly," simple activity performed by older women. As such, stories that emerge from its practice can be regarded as the antithesis of hard scientific facts required for evidence-based practice.

When we look behind the word we find a number of benefits that are closely entwined and are best summarized in the Knitting Equation (Figure 59.1).

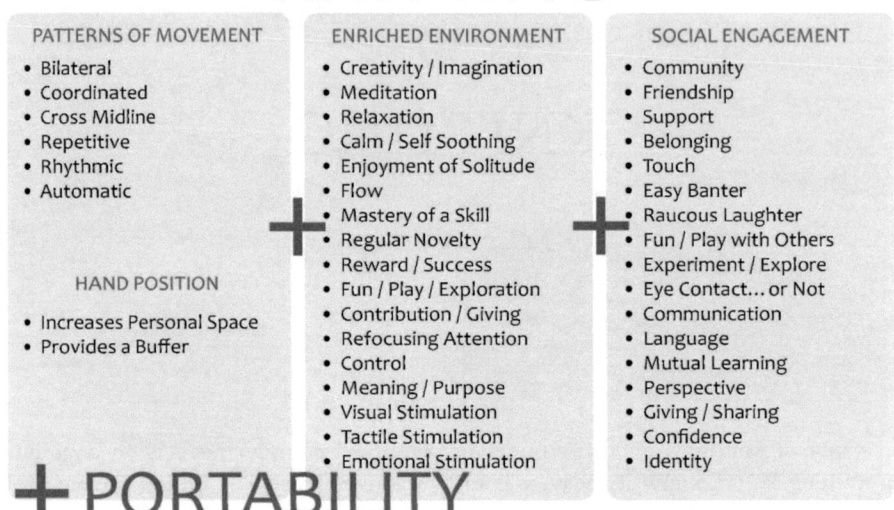

KNITTING =

PATTERNS OF MOVEMENT	ENRICHED ENVIRONMENT	SOCIAL ENGAGEMENT
• Bilateral	• Creativity / Imagination	• Community
• Coordinated	• Meditation	• Friendship
• Cross Midline	• Relaxation	• Support
• Repetitive	• Calm / Self Soothing	• Belonging
• Rhythmic	• Enjoyment of Solitude	• Touch
• Automatic	• Flow	• Easy Banter
	• Mastery of a Skill	• Raucous Laughter
	• Regular Novelty	• Fun / Play with Others
HAND POSITION	• Reward / Success	• Experiment / Explore
	• Fun / Play / Exploration	• Eye Contact... or Not
• Increases Personal Space	• Contribution / Giving	• Communication
• Provides a Buffer	• Refocusing Attention	• Language
	• Control	• Mutual Learning
	• Meaning / Purpose	• Perspective
	• Visual Stimulation	• Giving / Sharing
	• Tactile Stimulation	• Confidence
	• Emotional Stimulation	• Identity

+ PORTABILITY

Figure 59.1 Knitting equation

I soon realized that knitters could learn to enhance these benefits to deliberately improve well-being, so I began to develop the idea of therapeutic knitting. Therapeutic knitting is the combination of knitting and knowledge: knowledge about how to enhance the benefits to manage day-to-day stresses and life's challenges, plus knowledge about any medical condition and how to use knitting to manage symptoms to complement and enhance treatment.

All the issues listed in the Knitting Equation are beneficial for well-being. The benefits of knitting alone are different from those of knitting in a group. You will find those issues outlined in columns two and three in other creative activities. However, the nature of the movements (column one) and its portability set knitting apart from other activities.

When both hands are involved in a complex pattern of precise movement that crosses the midline of the body, it takes up a lot of brain capacity in the moment, leaving little room to focus on anything else. Most stories tell of rhythmic movements enabling a meditative-like state, a sense of deep calm.

The nature of meditative state can change according to the project knitted. A complex stitch combination facilitates a state of focused attention to distract the knitter and break into negative thought cycles. An easy project encourages a state of effortless presence or daydreaming. All of these give the mind a break and are beneficial for well-being in many ways. You can also choose to knit mindfully. Knitting is a great way of enabling a meditative state and learning what this feels like without needing to understand or undertake the prolonged practice of achieving this mind state.

Combine this instantaneous calm with portability and you have an effective tool you can access any time, anywhere, in the middle of the night, on your commute to work, or even on your lunch break.

The most significant finding from a study I was involved in of over 3500 knitters from 31 countries was that the more frequently people knit (more than three times a week), the happier and calmer they reported feeling. A total of 81% felt happier, while 54% felt happy or very happy during and after knitting. This translated across to respondents with clinical depression, with fewer than 1% remaining sad (Riley et al., 2013).

The automatic nature of the movement appears to be important too. I have observed that when the brain is given a background automatic task, it somehow frees up thoughts, breaks into rumination, and enables people to speak more freely and deeply. In addition, the hand position protects personal space. This gives a sense of security and can be used to help those who find public transport, social contact, or attending a group stressful.

There is an increasing realization that well-being and health need to be addressed from a whole-person perspective. It is not enough to treat symptoms alone for longer term success.

Therapeutic knitting gives us an effective, accessible, portable tool with which we can encourage and grow creative ability, curiosity, and sense of exploration. Knitters learn that mistakes are not catastrophic, everyone makes them, and it's the best way of learning. Confidence and self-esteem rise as knitters build a positive sense of self and identity. Other life skills are learned alongside. These include patience, perseverance, planning, computer skills, and social skills.

A knitting group provides a rich source of social contact with people from a range of backgrounds, education, ages, and cultures. This rich social context expands the experience base, and exposes the knitter to a wide range of knowledge, opinions, and conversations, the diversity of which is difficult to access in modern-day life. Most of us tend to socialize with those of similar interests. It provides a level playing field where those less advantaged can shine regardless of circumstance. Knitters report feeling more confident and socially aware, and it can be used to deliberately nurture these qualities. Importantly, the group provides a safe space for people to laugh, play with creativity, have fun, and make friends.

The field of therapeutic knitting is still in its infancy. It can be used to manage stress and life's inevitable challenges, or be taken a step further to manage a range of medical issues. It enables the knitter to switch off, which is increasingly important for good mental health in our 24/7 society. It allows space to stop, heal, and recover from the pressures of life.

Specific issues can be addressed too. Knitting for 20 minutes or so before sleep can stop whirring thoughts and prepare the mind for sleep. A simple project can be kept by the bed if waking in the early hours is a problem.

Knitting can be used to deliberately raise mood. This can be enhanced by an informed choice of color and texture. Our study found that texture was twice as effective as color for affecting mood (Riley et al., 2013). Touching something good makes you feel good.

We can explain therapeutic knitting from the biological perspective of pain. The rhythmic, calming nature and benefits listed in the Knitting Equation all contribute towards biasing the complex conversation that can result in pain, toward not making pain.

We are coming full circle. We heard earlier that Charles Montague Fletcher used knitting to stop smoking. "Knit to Quit" groups exist specifically for this purpose. Knitters report conquering other addictions including alcohol, binge eating, even hard drug addiction. Knitting keeps the hands and mind occupied in a unifying, calming way.

Stories from knitters tell of symptoms of post-traumatic stress disorder (PTSD) significantly improving a long time after the event. They speak of being able to think through dark or traumatic thoughts while knitting, not becoming stressed by them. They talk of this as somehow enabling safe "filing" of these memories and reducing flashbacks as a result.

Other peer-reviewed studies to date include a pilot conducted in an inpatient eating disorder unit (Clave-Brule et al., 2009). The authors concluded that engaging in knitting can alter routines seen in eating disorder patients, helping to decrease their focus on anxious, preoccupying thoughts.

As part of a 12-month therapy program, a knitting group in a drug and alcohol rehabilitation center used knitting as a self-soothing and affect management tool (Duffy, 2007). Participants reported knitting as calming, helping with concentration, instilling a sense of safety and hope that things could change, and increased self-esteem.

A study of knitting in homeless teen mothers had similar findings in terms of personal well-being (Rebmann, 2006). Other motivators to knit were creativity, being productive, a sense of pride, and the benefits of social support and friendship. Therapeutic knitting also benefits clinicians. A knitting education program on burnout among oncology nurses reported that they found the rhythm of knitting soothing and bonded over the activity (Anderson et al., 2016).

One of my most memorable cases is a lady who suffered physical abuse throughout life. Her anxiety and fear were so overwhelming she was unable to be around people. She carried the history of trauma around like a weight and inevitably suffered from pain, anxiety, panic disorder, and intense loneliness. We knitted side by side, once a week for a year, before she felt able to attend a group. One of the benefits of knitting is that it is perfectly acceptable to sit and knit quietly if you wish so at first she did just that, listening to the banter around her.

Ten years on, with the help of a supportive new partner, she is unrecognizable. She is comfortable in a range of different environments, teaches knitting within the group, and is a published designer. She describes herself as happy and recovered from long-term pain. She just has the normal aches and pains we all experience from time to time. Her anxiety and panic responded well to therapeutic knitting. She carried a small project around with her, so when she felt anxiety rising she would sit and knit quietly to tap into the instantaneous sense of calm.

Knitting's accessibility is key in its development as a health-care tool. It is not messy and can be done from an armchair or bed. There remains a reluctance and some resistance to look beyond the "K" word, particularly in men, but we are seeing a gradual change, with more men becoming involved and speaking out.

Projects need to be chosen with care to match and gently push skill levels to avoid frustration. The focus should be on enjoyment of process with no deadline as knitting to tight deadlines negates the benefits.

Getting involved in knitting and knitting groups is easy for most. Most towns have more than one group. Universities often have social knitting groups and an increasing number have groups linked to student well-being services. Online groups are popular too. The online platform Ravelry (www.ravelry.com) has millions of members and is growing. It provides a directory of patterns, yarn, and forums through which knitters around the world can connect online.

- Stitchlinks (www.stitchlinks.com) started by myself in 2005 has pioneered the idea of therapeutic knitting and provides information for those wanting to learn more as well as guidance on how to set up therapeutic knitting groups.
- UK Hand Knitting (www.ukhandknitting.com) is a source of valuable information including knitting lessons and a list of United Kingdom-based groups. The Craft Yarn Council (www.craftyarncouncil.com) in the United States has similar information.

For those wanting to learn how to knit there are numerous books, such as *The Knitting Bible* by Clare Crompton (2004), and YouTube videos. Real-time videos on YouTube can be particularly helpful when learning or encountering new techniques.

- *The Mindfulness of Knitting: Meditations on Craft and Calm* by Rachael Matthews (2016) is a beautiful little book that does what it says on the tin.
- *Knit for Health and Wellness: How to Knit a Flexible Mind and More* by Betsan Corkhil (2014) pulls together my work on therapeutic knitting and will enable you to get started on knitting to improve your well-being.

References

Anderson, L. W., Gustavson, C. U. and Pehlivanova, M. (2016). Combatting Compassion Fatigue Among Oncology Nurses: An Exploration of the Impact of a Knitting Intervention. *Clinical Journal of Oncology Nursing*, 20(1): 102–104.

Clave-Brule, M., Mazloum, A., Park, R. J., Harbottle, E. J. and Birmingham, C. L. (2009). Managing Anxiety in Eating Disorders with Knitting. *Eating and Weight Disorders*, 14: e1–e5.

Corkhill, B. (2014). *Knit for Health and Wellness. How to Knit a Flexible Mind and More*. Bath, UK: FlatBear Publishing.

Crompton, C. (2004). *The Knitter's Bible*. Exeter, UK: David & Charles.

Duffy, K. (2007). Knitting Through Recovery One Stitch at a Time: Knitting as an Experiential Teaching Method for Affect Management in Group Therapy. *Journal of Groups in Addiction and Recovery*, 2: 67–83.

Matthews, R. (2016). *The Mindfulness in Knitting*. Brighton, UK: Leaping Hare Press.

Rebmann, H. (2006). Warning – There's a Lot of Yelling in Knitting: The Impact of Parallel Process on Empowerment in a Group Setting. *Social Work with Groups: A Journal of Community and Clinical Practice*, 29: 5–24.

Riley, J., Corkhill, B. and Morris, C. (2013). The Benefits of Knitting for Personal and Social Wellbeing in Adulthood: Findings from an International Survey. *British Journal of Occupational Therapy*, 76: 50–57.

Time Life Pictures. (1918). *Bedridden Wounded Soldiers Lying in Beds*. The LIFE Picture Collection, Getty Images. www.gettyimages.co.uk/license/50596909 (Accessed 24/2/2019).

Tolstoy, L. (1869). *War and Peace, Book Four*. Moscow: The Russian Messenger.

60

THERAPEUTIC FILMMAKING

J. Lauren Johnson

Introduction: the history of film and video in health and culture

Film and video have played an important role in technological cultures since their early days. Some of the earliest uses of motion pictures were to answer questions (i.e., when a racehorse breeder financed a photographic experiment by Eadweard Muybridge to determine whether horses lift all four hooves off the ground when galloping), to entertain (i.e., Thomas Edison's early "peephole machines" that played vaudeville acts on short loops for paying customers), and to document (i.e., the Lumiere brothers' early newsreel footage documenting both ordinary and extraordinary aspects of human life) (Sklar and Cook, 2018). Over time, film and video became important mass media that were used to spread information and ideas through cinema and television, providing media through which culture-defining stories could be spread far and wide. Film and video have been implicated in significant cultural phenomena, including the global dominance of the English language and the spread of American culture through the worldwide popularity of Hollywood cinema (Movies and Culture, 2016).

It is apparent that film and video are influential media on a worldwide scale, but it is worthwhile to recognize how influential they can be on an individual person's thoughts and behaviors as well. Popular films have the capacity to change the way people think about and act upon issues of social importance and personal health. For example, studies have demonstrated at least temporary behavior changes reported by audience members following screenings of films such as the climate change documentary *An Inconvenient Truth* (Cook, 2016) and the food industry documentary *Food, Inc.* (Blakley et al., 2016). Furthermore, change can occur not just through watching films, but also creating them, with art therapists and psychologists using film and video as expressive arts media for therapeutic purposes for decades (e.g., Arnott and Gushin, 1976). Given all this, it is clear that film and video have the potential to inform and engage people in a variety of ways, and that this potential can be used therapeutically in the fields of health and medicine.

In this chapter I intend to provide some information about how I have used the powerful media of film and video to elicit therapeutic change in my work as a psychologist. In particular I will discuss the use of filmmaking as a therapeutic tool in the context of working in psycho-oncology (i.e., my psychological practice with cancer patients and their families). Before I discuss how I have used filmmaking as a therapeutic tool with cancer patients, I will first briefly provide some information about what therapeutic filmmaking is and what it involves.

The history of therapeutic filmmaking

I currently work as a psychologist in a large northwestern Canadian city, although I began my education with a Bachelor of Fine Arts degree in Film and Video Production. As I transitioned into the field of psychology, I reflected on the therapeutic role my own personal filmmaking played in my psychological development, and following this I combined my interests in film/video and psychology to complete a pilot study on the use of therapeutic filmmaking as a treatment modality for my Master's thesis (Johnson and Alderson, 2008). However, I was certainly not the first person to use film- or video-making as a therapeutic tool, as it has been used by various others in the fields of psychology, counselling, and art therapy for decades. Nevertheless, there appeared to be a dearth of published research on the mechanisms and efficacy of this modality at the time, and since then there has been ever-growing evidence to indicate that therapeutic filmmaking is indeed a valuable psychological tool. For example, the handbook *Video and Filmmaking as Psychotherapy: Research and Practice* (Cohen et al., 2015) highlights research on how film- and video-making have been used to reduce symptoms of post-traumatic stress disorder (PTSD) in combat veterans, reduce symptoms of distress in grieving children following a loss, and improve connection and promote social wellness for the family member of someone suffering from schizophrenia.

In the present chapter, I intend to highlight the use of therapeutic filmmaking with a cancer patient. I will provide a brief overview of the client case, and then provide some methods of how we engaged in therapeutic filmmaking in our work together. This chapter will end with a discussion of other ways therapeutic filmmaking can be used, along with some ideas for further exploration and reading.

The case: an unexpected cancer diagnosis

People often think and speak in stories, and the stories that we develop about ourselves and the world around us can help us make sense of our pasts, guide how we live our current lives, and shape the futures we choose to live into (Habermas and Bluck, 2000; McAdams, 2008). Jessica (pseudonym) had a particular story about herself: she was a Canadian farm girl who grew up to get an education, move to the city, and marry a handsome young man who was the love of her life. She became a mother in her early twenties, fulfilling a lifelong dream of hers to have children of her own, and began settling peacefully into the life she had built for herself as a wife and young mother.

Before her baby was born, she began noticing changes in her breasts that did not feel like a normal part of her pregnancy. She followed up about these with her doctor, who reassured her that changes in women's breasts are quite common during pregnancy, and she had nothing to worry about. Her pregnancy progressed without complication and she gave birth to a beautiful baby girl. As she adjusted to life with a new baby, she noticed her body changing in both expected and unexpected ways, and her attention once again returned to the changes in her breast that had persisted throughout her pregnancy and transition into breastfeeding. She once again followed up on her concerns with her doctor, and to ease her mind he suggested she complete some basic breast screening procedures.

Jessica was in the living room playing with her baby on a play mat on the floor when she got the call. It was the doctor; the screening tests had come back positive. She had cancer. While Jessica tried to comprehend this information, her mind went blank as the doctor kept talking, and information about next steps to stage and treat the cancer and setting up numerous appointments with all kinds of different specialists seemed to pour out of the phone and pool onto the floor below. Nothing stuck with her. She was frozen.

Luckily, Jessica had a very strong support system, and her family swooped in to help her get through this shock. They were able to follow up with the doctor and get the information Jessica had missed, and with a speed that surprised her she was able to get her cancer staged, meet with an oncologist to develop a treatment plan, and begin treatment. Being connected with the cancer hospital for her medical treatment, Jessica learned that she could reach out to the psychology department for psychological support as well, and shortly after she began her first round of chemotherapy she was connected with me.

Jessica informed me that she was struggling to make sense of her cancer. She did not have any of the risk factors: no family history, no lifestyle risk factors, she ate well and exercised, and didn't smoke or drink. She was a young mother from the farm, after all, raised on fresh food and clean air. "What did I do wrong?," she wondered; "How am I going to get through this?" I assessed her psychological functioning and needs and determined that she was doing quite well under the circumstances, but she was experiencing a bit of traumatic distress associated with the shock of her diagnosis and the terror of having a serious illness. Although her prognosis was good and she had a very good chance of survival, she was still facing the prospect of going through many months of medical (chemotherapy), surgical, and radiation therapy, which represented a significant existential threat to her. In discussing the kind of work we could do together, one option we discussed was engaging in therapeutic filmmaking, which piqued her interest. As such, we decided to proceed with this approach in our work together.

What we did: the methods of therapeutic filmmaking

Over the course of the next several months, I led Jessica through the process of therapeutic filmmaking that I follow with most clients, which roughly corresponds to the five stages of commercial filmmaking: development, pre-production, production, post-production, and distribution/exhibition. Beginning with development, Jessica and I discussed the story she wanted to tell about herself, her life as a whole, and how cancer fitted into that story. This part of the process took the longest, as it often does. During this stage, we engaged in creative prompting, brainstorming, developing and adjusting stories about her life, and contemplating what she hoped her future would look like. As we engaged in these activities over the course of multiple sessions, Jessica began developing a greater sense of hope for her future, and she was able to use this hope for a healthy future to help her bear the difficulties she faced going through her treatments.

In pre-production, we engaged in the process of preparing to shoot the footage she would need for her video. As such, we discussed what visual elements she wanted to populate her story with, which involved her going through existing materials such as photographs and videos, and coming up with new visual ideas such as scenes she would like to shoot and visual metaphors she would like to include in her video. For example, Jessica identified her early life growing up on the farm as a source of great comfort and strength for her, and so visual elements representing the farm held special meaning for her. For example, she chose to represent her new understanding of her own resilience with the visual metaphor of shafts of golden wheat bending in the wind and then returning to their full height, indicating their flexibility and capacity to withstand storms. We also identified some audio elements she wanted to include, as well, such as particularly meaningful music and the sounds of her infant daughter cooing in her arms.

Once this was completed, we moved on to production, or the image-creation stage, wherein we used a small digital video camera to capture new images, gathered existing materials, and used online image searches to download other visual and audio media that she wanted to include. As often happens with therapeutic filmmaking, this stage took the least amount of time to complete. We then moved on to post-production, which involved editing together all the various media elements we had gathered into one cohesive whole. As such, using the structure of the story we created during development, I guided Jessica through the process of using a non-linear video-editing system to stitch together the audio and visual media we had shot, downloaded, or obtained from other sources. In this process, we continually checked the emerging story against the original plan and against how she felt now, and we adjusted the project whenever a new insight or development arose. In doing so, Jessica was continually assessing her experience of going through cancer treatment and finding new ways to think about it, feel about it, and integrate it into her life, while never losing sight of the vision for her future, which involved surviving to see her daughter grow up.

Finally, once the video was completed, Jessica and I discussed what she wanted to do with it: who she would want to share it with, who she would like to keep it private from, and how she might want to share it with selected others. This marked our entry into the final stage, distribution/exhibition, during which the client/filmmaker determines how to share their video (i.e., screening party at home versus posting it on Facebook, etc.), and with whom (i.e., selected friends and family, large groups, support communities like a breast cancer advocacy group, etc.). This stage of therapeutic filmmaking often involves conversations about the need for privacy and confidentiality, and how important it is for a given client to be able to maintain control over the finished product (i.e., it may be possible for a stranger to obtain the video, download it, and share it elsewhere if it is posted online). In the end, Jessica chose to keep her video fairly private, so she chose to burn it to a DVD and host an intimate screening at her home with her close family and friends. After this we were able to meet again and debrief this experience together, and shortly thereafter we were able to conclude our therapeutic work together.

Therapeutic filmmaking elsewhere

Although I am a psychologist who works directly with individuals seeking psychological support, individuals may be able to appreciate the therapeutic benefit of filmmaking without the support of a psychologist. Indeed, there are a number of ways that people can engage in filmmaking for the purposes of self-expression and self-discovery by making themselves or their concerns the subjects of their own films. Further, people can use the influential mass media power of film and video to engage in education and/or advocacy around a particular topic. As technology has advanced, film and video cameras have become more user friendly and affordable, and non-linear editing software is more accessible than ever, with some of these, such as Apple's iMovie software, even included as standard applications in some new computers. With the advent of video-sharing platforms, such as Vimeo, YouTube, Vine, and others, there are many opportunities to watch, create, and share film and video projects for personal and social benefits.

Resources

For further information about using film and video for mental health and wellness, I encourage anyone who is interested in this topic to explore some of the following websites and books:

- *www.cinematherapy.com* provides a great deal of information about watching widely available films for therapeutic effect.
- *www.pattonveteransproject.org* is a website with a great deal of information on the use of therapeutic filmmaking with veterans and includes sample films and information on upcoming workshops (primarily in the United States).
- *https://workmanarts.com* is the website for a collaborative arts and mental health organization that showcases artistic collaborations and artworks, and also hosts the annual Rendezvous With Madness film festival in Toronto, Ontario (Canada).
- *Video and Filmmaking as Psychotherapy: Research and Practice* (2015) is an edited foundational book on film- and video-based therapies with a variety of chapters on a wide range of topics written by authors from across the world that provides a good overview of how film and video is being used in mental health today.
- *The Handbook of Art Therapy and Digital Technology* (2018) is a more recent book that provides an excellent overview of various ways that digital technologies are being used in mental health treatment and promotion, including the use of video, digital storytelling, animation, and virtual reality.

References

Arnott, B. and Gushin, J. (1976). Filmmaking as a Therapeutic Tool. *American Journal of Art Therapy*, 16(1): 29–33.

Blakley, J., Huang, G., Nahm, S. and Shin, H. (2016). *Changing Appetites and Changing Minds: Measuring the Impact of Food, Inc.* Los Angeles, CA: USC Annenberg Norman Lear Center.

Cohen, J., Johnson, J.L. and Orr, P. (2015). Introduction. In J. Cohen and J.L. Johnson eds, *Video and Filmmaking as Psychotherapy: Research and Practice*. New York: Routledge: 3–12.

Cook, J. (2016). Ten Years On: How Al Gore's An Inconvenient Truth Made Its Mark. *The Conversation*. Retrieved from: http://theconversation.com/ten-years-on-how-al-gores-an-inconvenient-truth-made-its-mark-59387 (Accessed 24/2/2019).

Habermas, T. and Bluck, S. (2000). Getting a Life: The Development of the Life Story in Adolescence. *Psychological Bulletin*, 126: 748–769.

Johnson, J.L. and Alderson, K.G. (2008). Therapeutic Filmmaking: An Exploratory Pilot Study. *Arts in Psychotherapy*, 35(1): 11–19.

McAdams, D. P. (2008). Personal Narratives and the Life Story. In O. John, R. Robins and L. Pervin eds, *Handbook of Personality: Theory and Research* (3rd ed.). New York: Guilford Press: 242–264.

Movies and Culture. (2016). *Understanding Media and Culture: An Introduction to Mass Communication*. University of Minnesota Libraries Publishing. Retrieved from: https://doi.org/10.24926/8668.2601 (Accessed 24/2/2019).

Sklar, R. and Cook, D.A. (2018). History of the Motion Picture. Encyclopaedia Britannica. Retrieved from: www.britannica.com/art/history-of-the-motion-picture (Accessed 24/2/2019).

61

COOKING

Danny George and Tomi D. Dreibelbis

Introduction

Recent decades have witnessed a global rise in non-communicative chronic diseases that are directly linked to lifespan nutritional habits (World Health Organization, 2003). As health-care systems across the world grapple with how to train health professionals capable of educating patients about nutrition in a competent and culturally sensitive manner, there would seem to be a natural role for the health humanities in building curricular experiences that assist in educating a skilled workforce. Not only can a health humanities lens provide an important critique of the social, political, and economic forces that have shaped food environments and eating behaviors over time and across cultures, it can also deepen appreciation for the rich aesthetics of the culinary arts.

Applied activities like food cultivation, food preparation, and the creation of community partnerships and local infrastructure that address socioeconomic aspects of unhealthy eating and chronic disease (e.g., food insecurity and food deserts) can further build teamwork, skills in project management, passion for community organizing, and an intimate understanding of social justice issues enmeshed with food. In undertaking such inquiry, there would seem to be a particularly "fruitful" role for humanities-based modalities such as literature, philosophy, creative and reflective writing, comics, visual arts, film, theater, narrative, and other expressive art forms that yield insight into the complex human relationships with food.

Such interdisciplinarity has already been embraced by food studies, a young and emerging field that critically examines food from the perspective of biology, art, history, society, and ethics (Weissman et al., 2012). Presently more of an "academic movement" than an established discipline (Nestle and McIntosh, 2010), the raison d'etre of food studies is to go beyond the mere consumption and production of food, examining such subjects as the ecological dimensions of food, systems of oppression, and food and identity. In this sense, perspectives from the health humanities can be viewed as highly complementary. Scholars who bring creative methods to bear in facilitating deep learning experiences centered around nutrition that integrate the humanities and arts can, in turn, foster fundamental lessons in professionalism, ethical discernment, communication with patients, community organizing, and creative problem solving in the context of improving population health. In this chapter, we will articulate an applied role for the health humanities in the education of future health professionals, sharing specific "culinary medicine" and "food as medicine" strategies we have used with students at Penn State College of Medicine (PSCOM).

Overview of evidence

In the twenty-first century, chronic diseases have become the leading causes of death and disability worldwide. The four most prominent non-communicable diseases—cardiovascular diseases, cancer, chronic obstructive pulmonary disease, and type 2 diabetes—are accelerating across every region and pervading all socioeconomic classes (World Health Organization, 2002). As Western health-care systems have endeavored to reduce rates of these illnesses and lower costs, medical schools in North America and beyond have adapted their curricula accordingly to prepare physicians to more effectively guide patients towards healthier eating habits. Whereas medical education curricula have traditionally neglected nutrition, with an average of only 14.3 hours committed to nutritional content (Adams et al., 2015), a new field called "culinary medicine" (CM) has emerged in the last decade to address this shortfall. By blending culinary arts and social science with biomedical nutrition science, CM is aimed at training students to help coach at-risk patients in consistently accessing and eating high-quality meals that prevent and treat chronic disease and restore well-being (La Puma, 2016).

Within this movement, the Goldring Center for Culinary Medicine at Tulane University has been a leading force, having launched in 2014 the first dedicated teaching kitchen within a medical school to address lack of nutrition education. In recent years, Tulane has expanded to involve the local community, creating opportunities for students to teach low-income, food-insecure patients how to improve their diets and cooking skills and thereby their health (Goldring Center, 2019). The model has been replicated at nearly 50 medical schools, including at PSCOM, where we started a fourth-year CM elective in 2016. Research across these institutions suggests that student participation in CM courses can significantly increase their readiness to improve patients' health outcomes particularly for cardiovascular disease (Monlezun et al., 2018).

Along with the adoption of CM programs as a model for building student aptitude in addressing chronic disease burden, teaching hospitals have also found value in strategic partnerships with local agriculture and food production initiatives. For instance, research has shown a growing number of farmers' markets (n=92) (George et al., 2011) and community gardens (n=110) (George et al., 2015) located on hospital campuses in the United States. Such spaces not only provide greater access to healthy foods for patients, but also serve as a staging area for medical, nursing, physician assistant, dietetic, nutrition, public health, and other health trainee students to interface with the community, apply nutrition education principles, and make other conceptual and aesthetic contributions centered around food issues (George et al., 2017).

At PSCOM, students in a "Food as Medicine" advocacy group have worked with humanities faculty to establish a farmers' market and community garden on our hospital campus, and have also implemented "prescription produce" programs that allow clinicians within the health system to socially "prescribe" fruits and vegetables from the market and garden to at-risk, low-income patients. Students have developed other community partnerships enabling distribution of produce from the market and community garden to consistently reach food insecure populations. For instance, students have partnered with the hospital's driving instructor to deliver weekly harvest from the garden to clients at local food pantries and to migrant workers in local horse stables who live in food deserts within the hospital's service area. These student-led, humanities-informed models aimed at culturally sensitive engagement with patients and populations affected by chronic disease via addressing food insecurity have proven feasible (George et al., 2016b), have demonstrated preliminary efficacy in improving patient outcomes (Trinkkeller et al., 2019), and have given students opportunities for professional development and improved patient- and self-care (George et al., 2016b, 2016c). We describe both our CM and "Food as Medicine" programs below in greater detail.

Case presentation

Culinary medicine

Given that we lack teaching kitchen facilities at PSCOM, our CM course was established in partnership with a center for older adults near the medical school, which offered its kitchen facilities as a venue for the class. Consequently, medical students have been able to teach and learn among area elders who participate in the course, adding a dynamic intergenerational component to the traditional curriculum (Dreibelbis and George, 2017a; 2017b). More recently, the course formed a second partnership with the teaching kitchen of a local food bank and expanded to include community members from a drug and alcohol rehabilitation center and a domestic abuse shelter.

The course is taught using an interdisciplinary pedagogical method by an executive chef from the hospital system, a nutritionist/health education specialist, a nutritional biochemist, and a humanities faculty member over an intensive month with eight three-hour sessions. In the first hour, students learn the advanced nutritional science behind disease states through case-based discussions geared towards chronic illness. In the second hour, students are joined by community members and work collaboratively in the kitchen to prepare recipes pertaining to the day's lesson (e.g., discussing the advantages of adhering to a Mediterranean diet and then cooking whole-wheat spaghetti with vegetables and lentil sauce). This involves students and community members practicing basic cooking skills and discussing the interpersonal and socioeconomic aspects of meal planning, shopping, and eating on a budget. In the third hour, students and their partners taste-test their recipes, share sensorial impressions of prepared foods, and revisit nutritional concepts from the first hour.

Advancing beyond the teaching of traditional biomedical nutrition science and integrating humanities-oriented content into the sessions (e.g., intergenerational narrative exchange, culinary aesthetics, discussion of social determinants of health, etc.) has enabled richer and deeper learning opportunities. For instance, community partners frequently share favored food preparation techniques with students, but also offer poignant personal stories (e.g., being affected by eating disorders, not being able to afford produce, etc.) and exhortations (e.g., to be more aware of nutritional limitations faced by low-income individuals) that help put the curriculum's nutritional science in a distinctly human context. In particular, collaborating around the aesthetics of food during the third hour has consistently allowed relationships to grow as more sensorial exchange (i.e., tasting, smelling, and visually reacting to prepared foods) enables new ways for people to communicate and connect. Because we initially observed such rich exchange happening during the third hour, we quickly adapted the course to allow students and community members to bring in recipes of personal, familial, or cultural importance and take turns teaching the group on preparation. Generally speaking, this modification reflects the larger opportunities for the health humanities to integrate its methods with conventional food sciences curricula to more deeply explore and contextualize the rich human-oriented dimensions of food. In our experience, allowing students to explore issues of identity, ethnicity, and cultural specificity in the context of nutritional science has dramatically enriched their personal investment in the course.

Indeed, students consistently identify the experiential, community-based aspect of the course as important to their professional identity formation. As one student wrote: "It's my favorite part of the course. For us to interact with different community members and get a better sense for how future patients may approach cooking and enact the recommendations they are given in clinic—it's invaluable." This formative experience has appeared to carry over from the course into other aspects of students' training. One student expressed that she has "already started to apply what I have learned in the CM elective to patient care through speaking with some patients on my next rotation about making healthier choices and what substitutions can be made as part of their diets—just as we discussed in class."

Food as medicine

The aforementioned "Food as Medicine" group of medical students has played a role in the CM course, contributing produce grown in their hospital's community garden plot for teaching kitchen recipes, and hosting fourth-year students and elders for on-site visits to learn about food production and the history of medicinal plants. Under the supervision of a faculty member in the PSCOM Humanities Department, "Food as Medicine" students work outside the formal curriculum to collectively manage this 400-square-foot plot during the growing season, weeding, watering, and harvesting produce that, as alluded to above, is donated to food-insecure populations in rural and urban underserved areas. Students also help tend a medicinal plant plot that cultivates over 40 species of herbal and folk medicines, and collaborate in running plots used in patient care with cancer survivors and teenagers affected by eating disorders. This work in a community garden has not only generated rich, hands-on service learning for students vis-à-vis patients and with vulnerable populations, but has also yielded publications, including essays about culinary and horticultural arts in the "Art of Medicine" section in *The Lancet* (George et al., 2016a).

Students also partner with the hospital's farmers market and multiple other markets in the area as collaborators in the aforementioned "prescription produce" program. Building on the traditional "prescription produce" model (Wholesome Wave, 2017), students have developed a variation on the program they call "Prevention Produce" whereby at-risk patients are "prescribed" vouchers for fruits and vegetables that can be redeemed at farmers' markets and additionally receive month-long, one-on-one weekly mentorship by medical students at the market (George et al., 2016b). Through this relationship, students gain a deep understanding of their patients' lives, learn to appreciate the complex personal, familial, and socioeconomic barriers to healthy eating and the social determinants of health that affect food-insecure patients, and sharpen their preventive health-coaching skills.

This clinical program has recently expanded into the community to include other at-risk populations in Prevention Produce (George et al., 2016c). For the last several years, the group has arranged weekly meetings at a farmers' market in inner-city Harrisburg with women living in transitional housing and over a dozen recently resettled refugee families from Syria. Students have used these food-based relationships as a means of coaching at-risk populations to improve nutritional habits and have also found that the rich cultural exchange in a community (non-clinical) setting helps ground a sense of professional identity. As one student wrote, "In the beginning of med school, and as part of our oath, we made a pledge to be the voice for the vulnerable and those without voice. So by working with Syrian families to address food insecurity I am not doing anything that I shouldn't be doing as a med student." Students have recently undertaken qualitative research to examine the challenges of refugees transitioning to new food environments, have begun learning Arabic, and have organized fundraising dinners where Syrian families have prepared authentic cuisine for hospital employees. Such cross-cultural experiences confer humility, increase knowledge, empathy, and curiosity, and powerfully inform students' sense of professional identity and responsibility (Bouhmam et al., 2017).

Engaging the public

In our work, we have found that food can be a starting point for a deeper commitment to one another. In other words, because food is at the intersection of so many cultural forces it is a universal starting point that can facilitate relationships, insights, and ideas that build naturally from medicine/academia into the community and empower student learning and action. The organizations that we have brought together in our efforts—medical schools, centers for older adults, chefs, farmers' markets, community gardens—are present in many communities across the country, and stakeholders all share a common interest in attaining better health through better diets. Such approaches evoke the ancient wisdom that access to nutritious foods is foundational to individual and community health (e.g., Hippocrates' instruction to "Let thy food be thy medicine").

In general, attempts to align modern health-care systems with local agriculture present fruitful opportunities, creating demand for local producers while ensuring that food-insecure populations have access to healthy foods. Indeed, in the United States, where the Affordable Care Act has incentivized hospitals contributing to population health via compulsory "community health needs assessments" submitted annually, many institutions are increasingly observing high-yield outcomes through nutrition-oriented partnerships (George et al., 2017). There is also an emerging trend towards health systems developing the infrastructure to provide daily medically tailored meals to chronically ill, low-income patients as a means of reducing costs and improving outcomes (Brown, 2018; Gurvey et al., 2013). Such large-scale trends point to major opportunities for the health humanities to play a role in preparing students as thought leaders within these movements.

As we reflect on our applied efforts thus far, we see greater opportunities for dissemination of humanities-informed works in CM and Food as Medicine programming—for instance using social media, writing op-eds in local newspapers, or creating public or digital installations that further empower students and participants to give voice to their experiences via artistic expression that is shared with the broader community. There is also, in our experience, a clear benefit to students with respect to greater self-care habits (e.g., healthier eating, exercising, etc.) that emerges through participation in our CM and food-as-medicine programming, and this dynamic deserves further attention and inquiry. We also see great potential in having students actively train community members to lead CM courses and programs such as "Prevention Produce," thereby creating greater reach of health humanities programming into local communities and empowering community members as peer educators. Moreover, community sites like farmers' markets and gardens can serve as venues for public engagement around humanities, for instance book clubs, film screenings, roundtables, or speaker series that engage in a cross-disciplinary way around timely food issues. Lastly, there would seem to be potential opportunities to extend the CM experience to undergraduate students in pre-med studies.

Ultimately, while relatively little work has been done within the health humanities involving food, it is an area that leads quite naturally to scholarly inquiry and community-level action in the service of building critically important skill sets in students in the health professions. Learning experiences that integrate humanities and arts in the area of food/cookery may provide subtle but formative lessons for students in professionalism, ethical discernment, awareness of social determinants of health, and communication with patients in their care, which ultimately may lead to greater joy in one's practice and the delivery of more empathic and effective care.

Resources

- Tulane's Culinary Medicine website: https://culinarymedicine.org/
- Wholesome Wave: www.wholesomewave.org
- YouTube video of the Culinary Medicine course: www.Youtube.Com/Watch? V=Zkrw2hdsj5s
- Rodale Institute: https://rodaleinstitute.org

Further reading

La Puma, J. (2016). What Is Culinary Medicine and What Does It Do? *Population Health Management*, 19(1): 1–3.

Miller D. (2013). *Farmacology*. New York: William Morrow.

Pollan, M. (2009). *In Defense of Food*. New York: Large Print Press.

References

Adams, K.M., Butsch, W.S. and Kohlmeier, M. (2015). The state of nutrition education at US medical schools. *Journal of Biomedical Education*, 2015: 1–7.

Bouhmam, H., Boothe, D. and George D.R. (2017). Hosting Syrian Refugees: Resources Exist in Our Communities. *American Journal of Public Health*, 107(7): 1013.

Brown, P.L. (2018). Cod and 'Immune Broth': California Tests Food as Medicine. *New York Times*, May 11, 2018. Available at: www.nytimes.com/2018/05/11/health/food-as-medicine-california.html?rref=collection%2Fsectioncollection%2Fhealthandaction=clickandcontentCollection=healthandregion=rankandmodule=packageandversion=highlightsandcontentPlacement=5andpgtype=sectionfront (Accessed 7/1/2019).

Dreibelbis, T.D. and George, D.R. (2017a). An Intergenerational Teaching Kitchen: Reimagining a Senior Center as a Shared Site for Medical Students and Elders Enrolled in a Culinary Medicine Course. *Journal of Intergenerational Relationships*, 15(2): 174–180.

Dreibelbis, T.D. and George, D.R. (2017b). Integrating Intergenerational Mentoring into a Culinary Medicine Curriculum. *Medical Science Educator*, 27(4): 575–576.

George, D.R., Beachy, W., Chan, J., Forbes, C., Trinkkeller, J. and Gonzalo, J. (2016c). Teaching Population Health: Using the Classroom as a Bridge to the Community. *Medical Teacher*, 38(11): 1182–1183.

George, D.R., Hanson, R., Gilman, F. and Edris, W. (2016a). Medicinal Plants: The Next Generation. *Lancet*, 387: 220–221.

George, D.R., Kraschnewski, J., Rovniak, L., Hanson, R. and Sciamanna, C. (2015). A Growing Opportunity: Community Gardens Associated with US Hospitals and Academic Health Centers. *Preventive Medicine Reports*, 2: 35–39.

George, D.R., Kraschnewski, J.L. and Rovniak, L.S. (2011). Public Health Potential of Farmers' Markets on Medical Center Campuses: A Case Study from Penn State Hershey Medical Center. *American Journal of Public Health*, 101(12): 2226–2236.

George, D.R., Manglani, M., Minnehan, K., Chacon, A., Gunderson, A., Dellasega, C. and Kraschnewski, J. (2016b). Examining Feasibility of Mentoring Families at a Farmers' Market and Community Garden. *American Journal of Health Education*, 47(2): 94–98.

George, D.R., Rovniak, L. and Snyder, G. (2017). The Role of Nutrition-Related Initiatives in Addressing Community Health Needs Assessments. *American Journal of Health Education*, 48(1): 58–63.

Goldring Center for Culinary Medicine at Tulane University. Available at https://culinarymedicine.org/ (Accessed 7/1/2019).

Gurvey, J., Rand, K., Daugherty, S., Dinger, C., Schmeling, J. and Laverty, N. (2013). Examining Healthcare Costs Among MANNA Clients and a Comparison Group. *Journal of Primary Care and Community Health*, 4(4): 311–317.

La Puma, J. (2016). What Is Culinary Medicine and What Does It Do? *Population Health Management*, 19(1): 1–3.

Monlezun, D.J., Dart, L., Vanbeber, A., Smith-Barbaro, P., Costilla, V., Samuel, C., Terregino, C.A., Abali, E.E., Dollinger, B., Baumgartner, N. and Kramer, N. (2018) Machine learning-augmented propensity score-adjusted multilevel mixed effects panel analysis of hands-on cooking and nutrition education versus traditional curriculum for medical students as preventive cardiology: multisite cohort study of 3,248 trainees over 5 years. *BioMed Research International*, 2018: 5051289. doi:10.1155/2018/5051289.

Nestle, M. and McIntosh, W.A. (2010). Writing the Food Studies Movement. *Food, Culture and Society*, 13(2): 159–179.

Trinkkeller, J., Forbes, C., Lehman, E. and George, D.R. (2019). Prevention produce: Integrating medical student mentorship into a fruit and vegetable prescription program for an at-risk patient population. *Permanente Journal*, 23: 64–69.

Weissman, E., Gantner, L. and Narine, L. (2012). Building a Food Studies Program: On-the-Ground Reflections from Syracuse University. *Journal of Agriculture, Food Systems, and Community Development*, 2(3): 79–89.

Wholesomewave.org [Internet]. Wholesome Wave: Fruit and Vegetable Prescription Program Fact Sheet; c2010-2017. [cited 2017 Aug 4]. Available from: www.wholesomewave.org/sites/default/files/network/resources/files/FVRx%20Factsheet_Updated_5_18_17.pdf

World Health Organization. (2002). *The World Health Report 2002: Reducing Risks, Promoting Healthy Life*. Available at: www.who.int/whr/2002/en/(Accessed 24/2/2019).

World Health Organization. (2003). *Diet, Nutrition and the Prevention of Chronic Diseases. Report of the Joint WHO/FAO Expert Consultation*. WHO Technical Report Series, No. 916 (TRS 916). Available at: www.who.int/nutrition/publications/obesity/WHO_TRS_916/en/ (Accessed 24/2/2019).

62

AESTHETICS OF SPACE

Hilary Moss

Introduction

As the new director of a national arts and health center, situated within a large university teaching hospital, I faced the task of transforming an aesthetically deprived environment. There were long, white, empty corridors without a single artwork; absolutely no music could be heard (only radio and TV channels in the background of many areas); and waiting and treatment rooms were devoid of color, photographs, or plants. Everything about the environment was professional, clean, and functional, but the effect was a sterile, clinical environment lacking warmth and humanity. The research and practice that grew out of the work of the center highlighted how the arts can enrich hospital spaces, but also provided evidence on how the arts are a neglected resource.

The Arts Council of Ireland list of art forms include music, dance, visual art, sculpture, film, literature, theater, circus, street theater, and many more. Our hospital arts program embraced all art forms depending on suitability and appropriateness for the people served from cradle to grave by a diverse clinical workforce. In advancing the arts in the hospital I worked in, it was clear from the start that I needed to work with the creative skills and resources of the whole community: patients, family members, and clinicians. I found that within the walls of the hospital, there were hundreds of artists and creators, people who played musical instruments, attended art classes, sang in choirs, or were active members of book or film clubs. I began to see that the community had the resources to reverse the aesthetic deprivation in the hospital. I just needed to tap into their creative lives.

So began a journey of research and practice to improve the aesthetic space of the hospital and telling a story of how simple changes to hospital spaces can make a huge difference to the impression, welcome, efficiency, and quality of care in hospital.

Setting the scene: the aesthetics of hospital space

The relationship between aesthetics, well-being, and heath is emerging as an important area of study (Cold, 2001; Cuypers et al., 2011). It is unfortunate that planners, politicians, architects, and builders regularly neglect the aesthetic, especially in public buildings and health-care settings, where the predominant concerns are health and safety concerns and efficiency. The result can be ugly, hostile, unpleasant, and unhealthy environments:

It would appear as if we are more focused on diseases than sick people's recovery, more on productivity than the well-being of employees, more on cars, comfort and speed than aesthetically pleasant places, more on quantity than quality, more on rational and intellectual matters than sensuous and emotional ones (Cold, 2001: 3).

The hospital space is often a space of anxiety. In attending hospitals, patients and their families often enter a strange, unknown, clinical space. The arts can welcome and support anxious people attending hospital; they can also support staff to do their job efficiently, reduce stress and tension in the environment, and contribute to improving quality of care. However, a study of 86 hospitals in Norway indicated that very few concrete guidelines or directions for the aesthetic dimension of the hospital are included in written documents. Caspari et al. provide robust evidence that hospitals give little attention to aesthetics and patients are often dissatisfied with their choices in this regard (Caspari et al., 2006, 2007). The role of aesthetics in health-care facilities appears to be a neglected or undervalued field. It is possible that our current health system, with its emphasis on efficiency and measurement, has difficulty in quantifying aesthetic values. Moreover, there is limited current evidence to support its use in health care settings. Those planning health care tend to neglect the idea of beauty:

> Are the arts ... merely window dressing or institutional vanity distracting us from the real concerns of service users? Do they take money and resources away from more deserving areas? Do the arts make a difference? Do they merely pander to the preferences of a select and intellectual elite? (Gallagher, 2007: 424)

The elite perception of the arts in contemporary society adds further to the neglect of the aesthetic in hospitals. Many hospital staff lack confidence in owning the arts in hospital, preferring to lean into the "expertise" of the artist or arts manager in the building. The professional hierarchies that are firmly entrenched in health-care settings play out in the choice of art on the walls, for example, where arts managers, senior clinicians, and managers may be the only staff willing to decide which art to display. While the live classical music program in our hospital atrium is a popular feature of the arts performance program, the most successful event by far is a 1970s cover band, which draws hundreds of staff and patients to the atrium, creating a motivating, uplifting atmosphere. One of the most important features of the hospital arts program is engaging staff at all levels of the organization in decision making and selection of the arts, to ensure that any notions of "proper" or "appropriate" art are mediated by the stakeholders who engage with them.

Case examples

Create-While-You-Wait

This initiative was a visual art project created to support children as they enter the waiting areas of the hospital on their way to the outpatient clinic, emergency care, or day procedure. Some children must attend a series of clinicians (e.g., the nurse, doctor, speech therapist, phlebotomist, and psychologist) so the day can be long and stressful. In collaboration with nurse managers, a team of professional artists set to work on enhancing this waiting area. They stocked an art trolley with artistic materials and resources, converting a section of the waiting area into a creative zone. Activities included puppet making, mask making, playing, and painting. Sometimes a music therapist joined the children and sang songs with the puppets. Children could gather at the table to participate, or just watch, as they wished. Parents and siblings could also participate. Many children returned to the table after attending their appointment to finish creative work that they had started. Others took their artwork with them to their appointment. In evaluating the project, nurse managers reported that the creative intervention resulted in much lower stress and tension in the waiting room, and fewer complaints from parents in periods of art activity. Also, clinicians reported on how the artwork or puppets that the children take with them into various consultation rooms provide a bridge between child and clinician, presenting a talking point and ice-breaker. Importantly, parents remarked on how the activity made the visit more positive for their children, reducing their fears and tears. Indeed, some struggled to bring their children home as the children wanted to continue making art!:

> My son enjoyed it very much. It made him very happy and occupied. It makes the idea of coming to the hospital easier as he wants to come back to finish his work. He says himself that it makes him less nervous about seeing the doctor. (Parent feedback 1)

> It helped my daughter to share and pass time without any tantrums … she had a chance to express her creativity instead of having to sit still and wait for her turn. (Parent feedback 2)
>   Ava arrived at the Emergency Department sleepy and poorly but when the session started she got involved and seemed to become more alert. It was also fantastic to distract her sister from the unexpected trauma she had witnessed; and to give her something to do while waiting for her sister to have treatment. (Parent feedback 3)

> We have found that once the children are distracted and happy then the parents are contented also regardless of the waiting time. This then spreads throughout the department, an atmosphere that was once tense disappears as the children interact with your [arts] team. (Clinical Nurse Manager)

In this space, the arts act as diversion—they welcome children and create positive, hopeful associations with coming to hospital. The space is unthreatening and somewhere children can play and express themselves. This simple adjustment can have a huge impact on compliance with treatment, engagement with clinicians, and the quality of relationships key to developing positive health outcomes.

The Bathroom Project

This project developed arts engagement further, transforming a space simply and cheaply using artistic expertise, but also providing specialized therapeutic support to distressed young people.

The teenagers on a children's unit were not receiving appropriate recreational, social, or psychological support while in hospital, and these needs warranted attention. Activities on offer in the playroom were too "young" for them, and yet they needed to engage, be stimulated, and have space to express worries and fears. Some teenagers were seriously disturbed following self-harm. At times, staff struggled to engage with the teenage population and it was clear that there were few opportunities for the young people to express their feelings in a safe way. An opportunity to improve the emotional quality of the environment came about with a decision to upgrade the bathroom on the unit and the appointment of an art therapist to find the best solution. Working with nursing staff and play specialists, the art therapist decided to initiate a collaborative mural project to meet the needs of young people aged 12–17 who were inpatients in the hospital.

A designer drew the murals for the bathroom and the art therapist then took over, using her artistic skills to transfer this design onto its walls. Each week she invited two or three teenage patients to join in with painting the bathroom. She set up a music system, so they could listen to their favorite sounds and together, gradually, they transformed the space (Figure 62.1). Sessions were informal and teenagers could come and go, having as much engagement as they wanted. Meeting the teenagers in an informal space and engaging in a non-verbal creative activity enabled them to talk as much or as little as they wanted, bonding over safe topics such as what music they liked and how to paint the bathroom, while developing a therapeutic relationship of trust. This enabled the young people to talk, share concerns, and experience a sense of achievement while in hospital. In all, the creative venture led to three clear wins: (1) upgraded facilities; (2) creative, social, and emotional engagement for the teenagers; and (3) resources to distract and comfort very young children during wound cleaning.

> The art therapy service brings a lot of laughter, togetherness and joy to all in the hospital. I am constantly asked if the Art Therapist is available to do art with the children. I could say so much more about the importance of art therapy for children in hospital and the value of it. (Play Specialist)

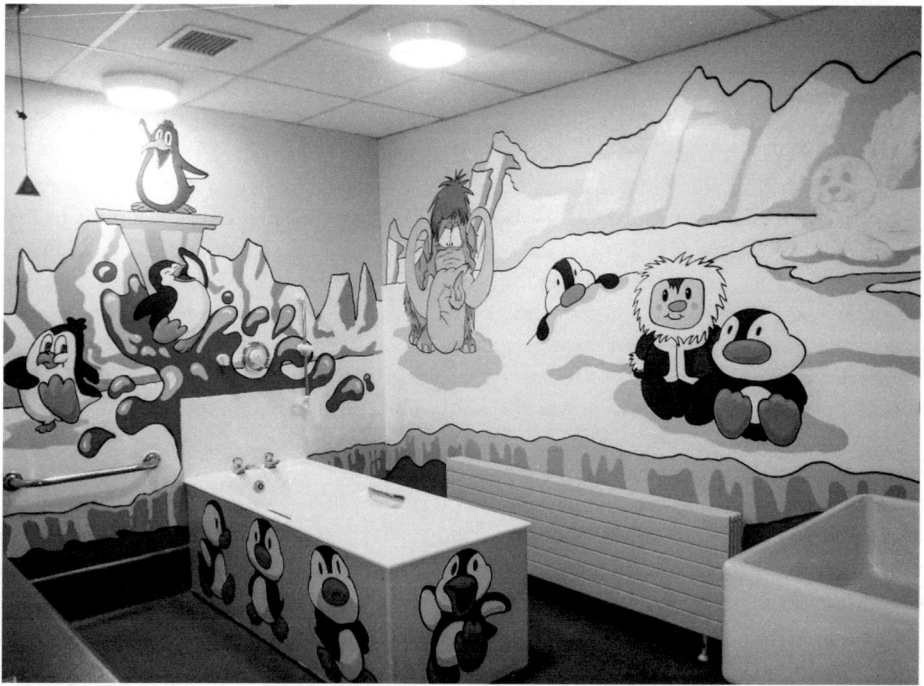

Figure 62.1 The Bathroom Project

I loved getting out of my room and having something to do while I was staying in hospital. Painting the mural and listening to music with other patients was fun and way better than just staying in your room all the time. (Young adult inpatient, paediatric ward)

It's such a wonderful initiative to have the patients involved in a project like this and something they can be really proud of. [My daughter] really enjoyed herself, and the bathroom is now cheerful and fun for future patients to enjoy. (Parent of young adult, inpatient paediatric ward)

Issues and barriers to artistic activity in hospital

The two projects described above were simple, low-cost initiatives that transformed hospital spaces. They brought the arts to service users in an accessible, appropriate way, and provided a solution to real problems experienced by clinicians and managers. However, the artistic quality of these interventions would have been lost had the team involved not argued for professional resources. At one point, management wanted to staff the service with volunteers and provided little space for storage of materials. Project delivery had a number of hurdles in this risk-averse medical context, not least in requiring the artists involved to be trained in health and safety, infection control, and confidentiality issues. In the Bathroom Project, the art therapist had to make the case for the additional time spent completing the upgrade while engaging with young people in the process. Overall, the main barrier to artistic solutions in the hospital was the value managers and clinicians gave to perceived risks. At times, this led to excessive concern around health and safety for young people, such as raised concerns about involvement of a child with difficulty in standing taking part in the mural painting.

Final thoughts

Personalized, individualized, high-quality arts interventions add much to the hospital space. Trained professionals are important, whether arts therapists or experienced arts practitioners, and aims for any work or intervention must be clearly articulated and meet the needs of patients. Co-creation of artistic interventions is the best way to ensure tailoring of the resources to recipient populations. To date, few theorists have addressed the importance of everyday aesthetics and the neglect of the aesthetic in hospital settings. Saito (2007) observes that the aesthetic quality of the bedlinen and crockery in hospital might be a more important aesthetic experience for patients than access to "high" art such as classical music or visual art. Theorists also argue that the aesthetic impression of a hospital can give a sense of health and moral attitude. In a way, aesthetic appeal acts as an advertisement of quality. For example, the design of a nursing home, from gardens to curtains and décor, give a clue as to whether it meets the well-being of residents. A clinic that has been designed in haste and carelessly (e.g., an untidy area, lacking in color or attention to detail) can give an impression of insensitivity or indifference to the patients attending a clinic. There is a body of research about "sick" buildings, which have poor ventilation, lighting, and air quality and which can increase staff absenteeism and poorer recovery rates (Lawson and Phiri, 2003; Ulrich, 1984, 1992; Ulrich et al., 2010, 2008).

As researchers, it is important that we move away from trying to "prove the benefit" of the arts—an uphill task of combining scientific rigor and the subjective realm of artistic participation—and instead focus our work on showing evidence that the *absence* of the arts in our normal environment can and does impact negatively on our health and well-being. "It is tempting to drop the talk about beauty altogether and steer the discussion toward more quantifiable matters: cost, sustainability, economic benefits, and so forth" (Parsons, 2010: 19–20). The most important aspects of curating hospital spaces are to offer service users control and choice over their space wherever possible, to collaborate and consult all stakeholders throughout the process of integrating arts into the hospital space, and to be open to both the benefits and disbenefits of the creativity of art.

Resources

- National Alliance for Arts, Health and Wellbeing, United Kingdom www.artshealthand wellbeing.org.uk
- Arts and Health Forum, Republic of Ireland www.artsandhealth.ie
- National Center for Creative Ageing, United States https://creativeaging.org/

Acknowledgements

The author would like to thank all the artists, staff, management, and service users at Tallaght University Hospital, Dublin, who contributed to these projects. In particular Aimee O'Neill, an art therapist, who created the case examples described above. Funding comes from many sources, but in particular thanks to the National Children's Hospital Foundation and The Meath Foundation for support of the projects described.

References

Caspari, S., Eriksson, K. and Naden, D. (2006). The Aesthetic Dimension in Hospital: An Investigation into Strategic Plans. *International Journal of Nursing Studies*, 43: 851–859.

Caspari, S., Eriksson, K. and Naden, D. (2007). Why Not Ask the Patient? An Evaluation of the Aesthetic Surroudings in Hospitals by Patients. *Quality Management in Healthcare*, 16: 280–292.

Cold, B. ed. (2001). *Aesthetics, Wellbeing and Health. Essays Within Architecture and Environmental Aesthetics.* Aldershot, UK: Ashgate Publishing.

Cuypers, K., Krokstad, S., Holmen, T. L., Knudtsen, M., Bygren, L. O. and Holmen, J. (2011). Patterns of Receptive and Creative Cultural Activities and Their Association with Perceived Health, Anxiety, Depression and Satisfaction with Life Among Adults: The Huntstudy, Norway. *Journal of Epidemiology and Community Health Online*, 10.1136/jech.2010.113571.

Gallagher, A. (2007). Review of 'The Role of the Arts in Mental Health Nursing: Emperor's New Suit or Magic Pill'? *Journal of Psychiatric and Mental Health Nursing*, 14: 424–429.

Lawson, B. and Phiri, M. (2003) *The Architectural Healthcare Environment and Its Effect on Patient Outcomes.* London: Stationery Office.

Parsons, G. (2010). Beauty and Public Policy. *People and Places*. London: Commission for Architecture and the Built Environment.

Saito, Y. (2007) *Everyday Aesthetics*. Oxford: Oxford University Press.

Ulrich, R. (1984). View Through a Window May Influence Recovery from Surgery. *Science*, 224: 420–421.

Ulrich, R. (1992). How Design Impacts Wellness. *Healthcare Forum Journal*, 35: 20–25.

Ulrich, R.S., Berry, L.L., Quan, X. and Parish, J.T. (2010). A Conceptual Framework for the Domain of Evidence-Based Design. *Health Environments Research and Design*, 4: 95–114.

Ulrich, R. S., Zimring, C., Barch, X. Z., Dubose, J., Seo, H. B., Choi, Y. S., Quan, X. and Joseph, A. (2008). A Review of the Research Literature on Evidence-Based Healthcare Design. *Health Environments Research and Design*, 1: 61–125.

63

LAW

Lydia Bracken

Introduction

Law comprises rules that regulate all aspects of our lives. These rules reflect a consensus within society about how we should behave and create structures to ensure that standards of behavior are maintained. Criminal law, for example, prohibits citizens from taking certain actions and imposes punishments where crimes are committed. Constitutional law establishes the functions and responsibilities of State bodies and (usually) protects against any abuse of power by the State. Contract law establishes the rules that govern written and oral agreements between individuals. Many more divisions in the law exist. Common across all legal subjects is the creation and enforcement of normative rules and standards to control and regulate the conduct of society. The broad area of health is no different.

Health law covers all areas in which law and health intersect. In doing so, it engages many otherwise distinct areas of law such as constitutional law, criminal law, human rights, children's rights, family law, property law, and many more (Herring, 2016). Law has a vital role in regulating health and health care. Laws are required: to establish the entitlements of patients; to regulate the role of the health-care professional; to control the use of medicines; and to recognize the roles of formal and informal carers. Importantly, the law must also place obligations on the State. Although individuals have primary responsibility for protecting their own health and the health of their family, the State must ensure that appropriate laws are in place to regulate the provision of health care. A good standard of health is only achievable where the law supports the provision of appropriate care.

This chapter discusses the role of law in human health and society, with an emphasis on the application of human rights law as an advocacy tool in the health-care sphere. Human rights have their origins in documents such as the Magna Carta, which was drafted in 1215, but the widespread recognition of human rights began in earnest after World War II when a number of international organizations, such as the United Nations and the Council of Europe, were established. The aim of these organizations was to promote international co-operation and to prevent the human rights atrocities of the war from re-occurring. Member States of the organizations were required to sign international conventions that establish universal rights and freedoms for citizens. Thus, human rights transcend national boundaries and are applicable to all human beings in all aspects of life, including health care.

The vital role of law in health care

The legal regulation of health care protects the interests of all stakeholders. Laws define the relationship between the patient and the healthcare professional and, in doing so, protect both. The emergence of human rights law has also had a significant impact on human health (Lombard, 2018). International human rights norms establish that patients have rights relevant to all health-care contexts such as: the right to bodily integrity; freedom from torture and inhuman or degrading treatment; the right to non-discrimination; access to information; freedom of expression; and many more. Recognition of these rights has an important effect on the provision of health care by imposing obligations (positive rights) or by preventing any restriction of the right (negative rights).

Human rights law also has a vital role in establishing the right *to* health. The right to health is recognized in numerous international conventions including the Universal Declaration of Human Rights (Article 25), the International Covenant on Economic, Social and Cultural Rights (Article 12.1), and the United Nations Convention on the Rights of the Child (Article 24).[1] Acknowledgement of the right to health recognizes that health is an essential prerequisite for the exercise of all other rights; that it is crucial to the human experience. Thus, the value of law in health cannot be understated. Laws serve to protect all stakeholders and, when appropriately applied,[2] can ensure that the health-care system functions in a way that maximizes the quality of our existence. Human rights operate to humanize the legal regulation of health care.

Human rights do not, however, provide the "answer" to every health-care dilemma. Often a balancing of rights is necessary and there might not always be a clear solution. This explains why many health-care decisions come before the courts for judges to determine and balance the legal arguments on both sides. It must also be acknowledged that the extent to which human rights are protected and understood differs from country to country according to the constitutional, political, and social context. Human rights are universal, but their legal application and interpretation is not always consistent (Zanichelli, 2014). These issues are apparent in many areas where law interacts with health and well-being, including the regulation of assisted reproduction, as discussed in the case study example below.

Case study: assisted human reproduction

Assisted human reproduction (AHR) refers to the process whereby medical treatment is used to achieve a pregnancy. It includes techniques such as donor insemination (where donor sperm is used to achieve the pregnancy) and *in vitro* fertilization or IVF (where eggs are fertilized outside the womb and later transferred back to the woman's uterus).

AHR disrupts normative conceptions of "the family" as a number of adults will be involved in the child's conception and the intended parents, who initiate the process and intend to subsequently raise the child, might not have any genetic connection to the child. As a result, there is no consensus between countries on how or if AHR processes should be legally regulated. Lawmakers must grapple with difficult moral and ethical questions, such as: deciding who should be recognized as a legal parent where a child is conceived using donated gametes (sperm and/or egg); whether the parents should be required to tell the child that he or she is donor-conceived; and whether the gamete donors should be allowed to remain anonymous if they so wish. There are no easy answers to these questions. In addressing them, lawmakers must consider the rights of all stakeholders as well as general public policy considerations concerning the nature of the legal family and intimate relationships.

The stakeholders in AHR include the intended parents, the donor(s) of genetic material, the child, and health-care professionals. Balancing the rights of these individuals is not always a straightforward exercise. Take, for example, the question of whether the donors of genetic material should be allowed to donate anonymously. On the one hand, the donor has a right to reproductive autonomy to make his or her own reproductive choices. The donor also has a right to privacy. Hence, if the donor's free and informed decision is that they wish to assist another person in their desire to have a child and to remain anonymous in doing so, should we not respect those views? This argument might be strengthened when we consider the rights of the intended parents in circumstances where they agree that the donor should remain anonymous. The intended parents may fear that the security of their family unit would be jeopardized if the child was to learn that one intended parent is not a genetic parent. Hence, the intended parents' rights to privacy and reproductive autonomy might also demand that the desire for anonymity should be respected.

However, the child also has rights that must be considered (Bracken, 2016). The child has the right to identity, the right to information, the right to health, and the right to have his or her best interests considered in the development of health-care policy, among others. Information about the donor may be required for medical purposes or to discover if the child is susceptible to an inheritable disease. Information about the donor may also be required to foster the child's sense of personal identity and psychological development. Research suggests that the earlier donor-conceived children learn about the nature of their conception, the better their outcomes are in terms of identity formation and development of family relationships. Secrecy as to the child's genetic background is generally associated with negative outcomes for the child (Blyth et al., 2017). Thus, the detriment to the child of allowing anonymous donations appears to be much greater than the detriment to the donor and intended parents of prohibiting anonymity. As a result, many legal systems around the world prohibit anonymous gamete donation in order to secure the rights and interests of children. For example, anonymous donations are legally prohibited in the United Kingdom, Ireland, Sweden, Switzerland, the Netherlands, Norway, and New Zealand among others. That said, the question of whether anonymous donations should be permitted or prohibited will be for each individual country to determine after its lawmakers have considered and balanced the rights of all stakeholders within their specific domestic context. As such, not every country prohibits anonymous donations.[3]

Examples of public engagement

Public engagement has a positive, transformative effect on legal policy. Law reform bodies frequently invite members of the public to engage in consultations on certain matters. For example, the Law Commission of England and Wales is currently undertaking a review of surrogacy laws following public consultation on the matter.[4] The consultation process gives citizens an opportunity to have a say in shaping law reform proposals and ensures that any recommendations made by that body reflect the will of the people. The government may also consult with members of the public in developing laws and legal policy. The participation of members of the public in these consultations is designed to give them a voice in the development of laws in order to strengthen the democratic legitimacy of law making. However, a drawback of the consultation processes is that the citizen must usually wait for the consultation to be initiated and advertised before they can engage.

The public engagement activities of third-level institutions offer another way for members of the public to engage with the law. University law schools frequently run public lectures, seminars, and workshops on various legal topics, often free of charge. These events are attended by academics, students, practitioners, non-governmental organizations (NGOs), and others and are designed to facilitate knowledge exchange between the expert speaker and the audience on topical legal issues. Some university law schools also run community law initiatives that are specifically designed to engage members of the public in legal scholarship.[5]

There is also scope for members of the public to become involved in campaigns run by NGOs that seek to effect legal change in a particular area. NGOs work to defend or promote a particular cause. Many are involved in advocacy and human rights work. Public engagement in an NGO campaign might involve the person signing a petition, sending an email to a politician on a particular issue, participating in a survey, or volunteering to assist the NGO in another way. This type of engagement facilitates the advocacy role of the NGO.

Social media also allows for public engagement in various aspects of the law and provides an accessible way of learning about the latest research undertaken by legal academics, the work of NGOs, legal information campaigns, and information on upcoming lectures and workshops.

Conclusion

This chapter has outlined the important role of human rights law in health care. Although law is created and regulated by State institutions, individual citizens have a role in shaping the law through litigation, lobbying for legal reform, engagement with law reform bodies, and other types of activism. It is therefore important that we are all aware of how the law operates and interacts with health care and what our legal entitlements are within that sphere.

Resources

- Amnesty International: www.amnesty.org/en/get-involved/take-action/
- Equality and Human Rights Commission: www.equalityhumanrights.com/en
- Law Commission: www.lawcom.gov.uk
- Law Reform Commission (Ireland): www.lawreform.ie
- United Nations Human Rights Office of the High Commissioner, Stand Up 4 Human Rights: www.standup4humanrights.org/en/take-action.html
- UNICEF: www.unicef.ie/get-involved/youth-engagement/advocacy/

Notes

1 See also the International Convention on the Elimination of All Forms of Racial Discrimination of 1965, Article 5 (e) (iv) and the Convention on the Elimination of All Forms of Discrimination against Women of 1979, Articles 11.1 (f) and 12.
2 The World Health Organization notes that "law is not always an unmitigated social good, but can actually stand in the way of progress in health and human rights." See World Health Organization (2017: xvi).
3 For example, in many parts of the United States, anonymous donations are legally permitted.
4 See Law Commission, "Surrogacy," www.lawcom.gov.uk/project/surrogacy/ (accessed 2/2/19).
5 For example, the School of Law at the University of Limerick engages with the community through various initiatives such as Advanced Lawyering Projects, UL Engage practicums and community law lectures. See, for example, https://ulsites.ul.ie/law/node/18261 (accessed 2/2/19).

References

Blyth, E., Crawshaw, M., Rodino, I. and Thorn, P. (2017) Donor-Conceived People Do Benefit from Being Told About Their Conception. *Bionews*, 30 May 2017. www.bionews.org.uk/page_845387. asp.

Bracken, L. (2016). In the Best Interests of the Child? The Regulation of DAHR in Ireland. *European Journal of Health Law*, 23(4): 391–408.

Herring, J. (2016). *Medical Law and Ethics*. 6th edition. Oxford: Oxford University Press.

Lombard, J. (2018). *Law, Palliative Care and Dying: Legal and Ethical Challenges*. London: Routledge.

World Health Organization. (2017). *Advancing the Right to Health: The Vital Role of Law*. Geneva: World Health Organization.

Zanichelli, M. (2014). Humanity Beyond Rights: Proximity as a Normative Principle. *Law and Humanities*, 8(2): 290–303.

64

QUILTING

Jacqueline M. Atkinson

Introduction

Quilting has a long history and, together with other textile crafts, has been predominantly associated with women. Although quilting has a specific meaning (the process of sewing through three layers—the top, batting, and backing), it is also used to encompass patchwork (both piecing and appliqué) and will be used in this generic sense here. It is frequently seen as a "thrift" craft and associated with poorer communities, whether this is the pioneer women moving westward across America piecing fabric scraps into quilts, or Japanese peasants patching old clothes and bedding in the traditional boro technique. The functionality of such quilting was of economic importance for the families where women's contribution was largely within the home.

Where thrift was not an issue, more decorative forms of quilting developed, such as the highly embellished patchwork of the Victorian era. In many instances the main "purpose" of the item was to demonstrate that women had sufficient leisure time and skill to make the item and could afford the materials used. The Industrial Revolution saw a decline in the economic importance of sewing skills, which became mainly confined to the home. The introduction of the domestic sewing machine freed up much of women's functional sewing time within the family.

There was a decline in interest in quilting at the start of the twentieth century but the Rural Industries Bureau promoted interest in the 1920s and a general revival in crafts in the late 1960s and 1970s included quilting. Although many people quilt as a solitary occupation, traditionally it has been associated with sociability and women's groups. The quilting bee has been depicted in many popular American films and novels. As well as an important meeting place for women who might otherwise be fairly isolated, quilting gave women an outlet for their creative sensibilities and a way of expressing individuality. Thus, almost inadvertently, quilting was contributing to both the family's as well as the woman's well-being.

Quilting in relation to well-being, health, and health care

The research evidence looking at the impact of quilting on health and well-being is variable but nonetheless supports its positive impact. Much of the research is qualitative, such as interviews with quilters who report its positive effects (e.g., Burt and Atkinson, 2012).

Supplemented by the stories of individuals and groups in books, magazines, and internet blogs, where the weight of anecdote must be seen as evidence, the support becomes strong (MacDowell et al., 2017). Three groups of variables need to be taken into account when considering the research: the nature or process of quilting itself, the characteristics of the quilters, and the outcomes measured. This can be problematic as it creates very specific conditions and may not be amenable to manipulation in research.

The process

One important factor may be whether the quilting is done by hand or machine. Other variables mentioned in interviews include the use of color, pattern, and texture, and the design process. Many quilters mention focus or "flow" as an important part of the process. The time commitment also seems to have importance. Another aspect is whether the quilting is a solitary occupation, carried out in a group, or both. The product of the quilting may also have relevance: whether the item is for the person themselves, a gift for others (e.g., to mark a life transition or as thanks) or a charity, for use by individuals, to fundraise, or part of a public educational project.

The quilter

The main difference between quilters is likely to be whether they are experienced or a novice quilter. A sub-division of experienced quilters would be professional and hobbyist. The motivation for quilting might be important. Although the research suggests that many quilters have found a positive impact on their well-being, some people take up quilting in response to trauma or difficult personal circumstances. This might be as part of a rehabilitative process provided by health-care services or a personal decision. The objective measurement of these is, however, often missing.

Outcomes

What, and how, to measure the impact of quilting is not straightforward. Qualitative research makes it clear that quilters believe it contributes to the maintenance of general well-being and mental health. It also reportedly contributes to: reducing and managing stress and anxiety; helping work through personal and family problems, including health issues; loss, whether through bereavement or divorce; a sense of achievement or altruism through making quilts for others; establishing connections with others in similar circumstances; and public education and advocacy (MacDowell et al., 2017).

The impact of quilting

Bringing these variables together is a complex task. Some things stand out, however, through either the weight of qualitative evidence or the few quantitative studies and is comprehensively reviewed by MacDowell et al. (2017). In describing the calming or restorative effects of quilting, in physical conditions such as cancer, multiple sclerosis, migraines, and arthritis, as well as mental health and well-being, people refer to distraction, repetition, focus, flow and, latterly, mindfulness. The Slow Stitching Movement highlights these beneficial aspects.

Not to be underestimated is the potential time-consuming nature of quilting. This can help provide structure and productively fill days that might otherwise be empty, with the added benefit of a sense of achievement and pride in completing a goal. Where hopelessness is a concern the time involved can contribute to thinking positively about the future, whether this is working through an issue or living long enough to complete the quilt (Reynolds, 2008).

Commemorative and memorial quilts can be made in relation to coping with or overcoming illness or loss. These can include fabric and embellishments from the clothing or household items of the deceased person, or materials used in treatment and therapy. The American quilter Ricky Tims commemorated his triple bypass surgery with the quilt "The Beat Goes On."

One experimental study considered the role of learning quilting compared with digital photography or both (Park et al., 2014). Participants were given five hours' formal instruction and engaged in the activity for nearly 17 hours a week for three months. In the quilt group this meant learning to design a quilt and sew it using a computerized sewing machine and learning the software. The main outcome measures were on memory. Episodic memory was improved in all groups, but not significantly in the quilting-only group. What appeared to be important was that the participants were learning something new, particularly the computing aspects, which were even more prominent in the photography group. Thus, although this study is important for having objective outcomes, it is for a very specific group of participants and learning conditions. How much can be extrapolated to other quilters and conditions is unknown.

The social aspects of quilting in groups is important not just for those who might otherwise be isolated, but also because it can bring together people in similar circumstances, whether through formal rehabilitation groups, in community groups arising to deal with a disaster or other event, or to make quilts to support a cause or charity.

Case presentation

Linus quilts are well known to most people who quilt. The now international project started in the United States in 1995, in response to a newspaper article on how much comfort a quilt had brought to a child with cancer. Originally made for children and adolescents with terminal or life-long conditions they are now made for any child "in need of a hug," including refugee children, those taken into care, and children involved in disasters. Although individuals make them, many are made as part of a group activity. The charity began in the United Kingdom in 2000 and approximately 3,500 quilts are delivered each month. The website gives details of what is required and local co-ordinators.

Facilitators and barriers to quilting

Quilting is both highly accessible and diverse and some form can be found to suit most potential quilters, whether in a domestic or health-care environment. Only basic sewing skills and equipment are needed to start. Internet tutorials give an introduction and quilt teachers can be found in many areas along with quilt groups. Quilting has the advantage of being easily carried out in the home as the need for specialist equipment is limited, certainly for the beginner. Machine quilting is very popular and sewing machines are available across a wide price range. These machines can be useful for people with limited hand dexterity. Hand sewing has the advantage of being portable, easy to work on in short periods of time, and able to be carried out while still being with the family.

Although associated with thrift, the cost of quilting can be as little or as much as suits the individual pocket. Recycled fabric may be good to learn on but if a lot of time is spent on making a functional quilt that will get repeated washing (e.g., a cot quilt), new, good quality fabric might be preferable. There are few barriers to quilting, although some people find the idea of the time commitment off-putting.

Public and community quilting

Much public and community quilting will be for others or charity, whether local or global. Groups can arise spontaneously in response to a crisis or established groups might respond to the same, or to a perceived ongoing need, such as Linus quilts, or "fidget quilts" made for people living with Alzheimer's disease or other forms of dementia. These lap quilts have many textures and embellishments for sensory and tactile stimulation that can be fingered by the recipient and seem to help calm someone who is agitated. Women's charities are popular too, and heart-shaped quilted pillows are helpful to support the arm after mastectomy and during treatments.

Groups may come together to make a quilt to both educate and commemorate. One example is the AIDS memorial quilt, made in a number of countries, to commemorate those lost in the early days of the AIDS epidemic. The NAMES Project AIDS Memorial Quilt in Washington DC provides a well-known example of quilting as a memorial (in this case, to celebrate the lives of people who have died of AIDS-related causes). As well as helping those involved in managing grief and depression, such quilts have provided an effective means of public health education. Students who visited the exhibitions changed their perceptions about people with AIDS and through associated discussions may have reduced risky behavior (Krause and Austin, 1999).

Resources

- Quilters' Guild of the British Isles: www.quiltersguild.org.uk
- Linus Quilts: projectlinus.org.uk
- Slow Stitching Movement: www.slowstitiching.com

References

Burt, E.L. and Atkinson, J.M. (2012). The Relationship Between Quilting and Wellbeing. *Journal of Public Health*, 34(1): 54–59.

Knaus, C.S. and Austin, G.W. (1999). The AIDS Memorial Quilt as Preventative Education. *AIDS Education and Prevention*, 11(6): 525–540.

MacDowell, M., Luz, C. and Donaldson, B. (2017). *Quilts and Health*. Indiana: Indiana University Press.

Park, D.C., Lodi-Smith, J., Drew, L., Haber, S., Hebrank, A., Bischof, G.N. and Aamodt, W. (2014). The Impact of Sustained Engagement on Cognitive Function in Older Adults. *Psychological Science*, 25 (1): 103–112.

Reynolds, F. (2008). Textile Art Promoting Wellbeing in Long-Term Illness. *Journal of Occupational Science*, 11(2): 58–67.

65

SENSORY DESIGN AND SMART TEXTILES

Jenny Tillotson

Introduction

This chapter examines wearable technology concepts that amplify the human senses with digital fragrances to improve self-care, mood, well-being, and sleep hygiene, and to prevent chronic mental ill-health from escalating. "Sensory design" is a growing discipline that seeks to understand the interfaces between human senses, design, architecture, haptic environments, "futurescapes," and immersive technologies. It is matched by society's growing desire for "multisensory" experiences in both the commercial and public spheres. The term also extends to "intelligently aware" jewelry, clothing, and textiles that register and adapt to the emotions and needs of the inhabitants through artificial intelligence, machine learning, and deep learning.

Sensory design considers sensations beyond the traditional five senses such as pressure, vibration, and temperature, with a view to impacting human health and influencing lifestyle. Here, wearable, connected devices and sensor-induced fragrance released in response to shifts in mood and behavior can work to improve both individual and social well-being. Through an appealing intervention for personalized management of mental health care, research presents the convergence of the digital health care and scent revolutions with novel, wearable devices that leverage disparate biological data sources to discover more accurate health-related correlations linked to the olfactory sense.

Everything in nature has a circadian rhythm dictated by day and night, but these patterns are often affected by signals in the environment. The sense of smell is an important means of communication and one of the last scientific frontiers to be explored in the modern world. As humans in modern society, we have grown to underuse our senses, including our sense of smell: our most evocative and direct sense. We may not be fully aware of using our sensitive olfactory system as it has been replaced by the more dominant audio and visual senses. The people of pre-historic time relied greatly on what we underuse: cognition and imperceptible changes in light, smell, color, touch, and sound kept them alive. Their sensory appreciation taught them where there was danger, which diseases they had, what foods to avoid, when females were ovulating, and when it was time to sow and reap. Animals still rely on personally discriminating those precise changes. We humans have not lost those faculties but have grown to rely on data presented in other ways. By learning from our ancestors, it is possible to "re-invent" our sensory faculties by amplifying our sense of smell through advances in sensory design, deep learning, wearable technology, and the power of fragrance ingredients on the limbic system in the human brain.

Through earlier Arts and Humanities Research Council–funded research on "Smart Second Skin" and "eScent," a multisensorial approach to both fashion and biomedical designs has emerged, resulting in a practical ongoing project to miniaturize wearable fragrance delivery systems for health and well-being. "Smart Second Skin" was a conceptual garment that illustrated a "smart" sensory fabric interacting with human emotions, whereby the aroma dimension is an integral part of the user's sensory experience (Figure 65.1). This award-winning project was installed at the Victoria and Albert Museum as part of the "Touch Me" exhibition in 2006 and demonstrated how a future AI-powered sensory garment could interact with the wearer's changing moods by releasing the appropriate aroma in response to different human emotional triggers (Tillotson, 2009).

This led to an Innovation Award on eScent inspired by the defence mechanism in animals and insects, and resulted in jewelry that emitted picoliter droplets of fragrance in response to a

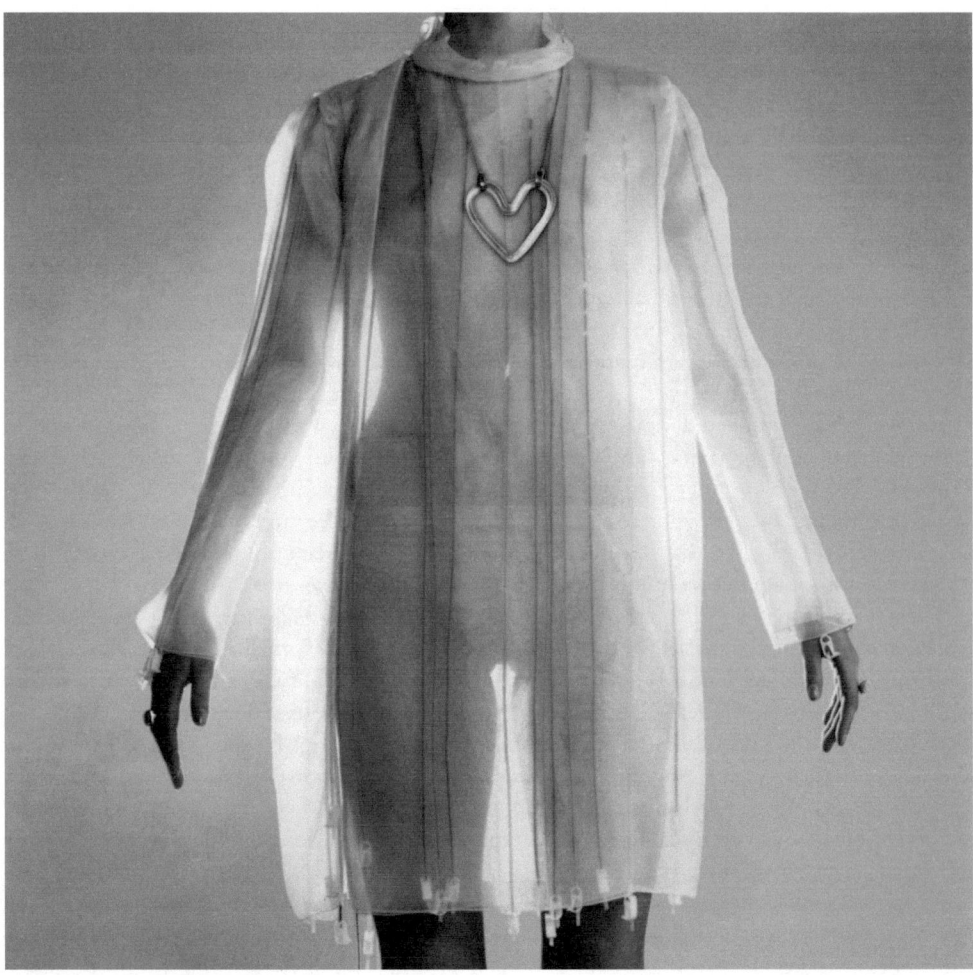

Figure 65.1 "Smart Second Skin" dress (funded by Arts and Humanities Research Council)

biometric or environmental stimulus (Jenkins et al., 2006). Subsequent patents were filed and awarded on wearable liquid-delivery and sensor systems for digitally managed, scent-based treatments that detect and act upon context and mental health status (Jenkins and Tillotson, 2006, 2007, 2010, 2018). The arts and humanities projects proved that it was possible to create "emotionally responsive" garments and jewelry that harnessed the power of the senses and heightened design's impact to respond to biosignals, blood pressure, pulse, sound, light, temperature, humidity, skin, conductance, sweat, and even the buzzing sound of biting insects. The two projects made way for a new approach to a data-driven scent intervention and next-generation sensor system that triggers the release of counteractive well-being scents to combat stress. The patents paved the way for a platform technology that combines sensing and dispensing any "liquid" for multiple health-care and experiential applications, beyond essential oils and perfumes, including insect repellent, food/flavor-replicating liquids, deodorant, hydrating mist, anti-UV/pollution mist, and other liquids including hormones, pheromones, pharmaceutical, cannabinoids (e.g., CBD), nootropics, cognitive-enhancing drugs, and microdosing psychedelic medicine (e.g., psilocybin) for therapeutic applications.

Much background work has been completed on the eScent dispenser so that sensory detectors and fragrance emitters will eventually be miniaturized and invisibly integrated into "smart" embroidery pieces, jewelry, garments, and textiles to highlight the importance of smell as an untapped opportunity for emotional self-regulation, self-awareness, circadian rhythms, and the sleep/wake cycle. This has led to development work by Sensory Design and Technology (the entity commercializing the eScent patents) to establish and maintain a localized "sphere" of detectible levels of scent dependent upon user context and environment, and a patent employing machine learning techniques and voice-assistive wearable scent-delivery systems (Tillotson and Temple, 2019).

Overview of evidence

Recent scientific research shows that our sense of smell is much more important than we realize in our emotional lives, with evidence suggesting that fragrance can help with sleep and mood regulation. Odors drive our emotions, cause social bonding, change physiology, improve cognitive performance, influence body chemistry, and drive behavior on an instinctive and subconscious level. Using reasonably good methods to test the impact of aroma on mood, a study on both men and women undergoing a stressful procedure showed a decreased state of anxiety and a more positive mood when exposed to orange oil (Lehrner et al., 2005). Further studies have shown lavender to include sedative properties with the potential to reduce stress, improve a sense of well-being in everyday living, and help in relaxation (Fismer and Pilkington, 2012). Other studies have found lavender beneficial in fighting insomnia (Hwang. and Shin, 2015), while also providing stress-alleviating and sleep-enhancing scents to improve sleep quality (Sarris and Byrne, 2011). Certain aromas have also been used to reduce behavioral and psychological symptoms of dementia in the elderly population (Fung et al., 2012).

In recent years there has been a move towards scent-infused products for the home that appeal to consumer needs by engaging with the senses, and improve their standard of living (Krishna, 2012). This growing trend in scented air care products opens new horizons for sensor-induced aroma treatments worn on the body. Essentials oils used for clinical aromatherapy applications, coupled with connected sensors and artificial intelligence, have the potential to create biofeedback scent solutions for preventative health care, informed by psychology and neurology studies that show the benefits of aromas and the influence of certain fragrances on affective, as well as cognitive, states in humans.

eScent: a case study of wearable scent dispenser for enhanced health and well-being

Despite the complexity of miniaturizing liquid-delivery systems, the controlled release of fragrances offers a substantial technological breakthrough for the next generation of wearable technology, and one which could bring with it considerable opportunities for health care. eScent is at the cutting edge of sensory, aroma, and medical work, and the basis for a new behavior change platform technology. It is a context-responsive wearable device that detects emotions and sends a personalizable "scent bubble" to the user's nose, underpinned by sophisticated mathematics (Tillotson and Temple, 2019). It combines sensing and dispensing aromatics for immersive experiences and multiple health benefits, including enhancing human cognition and reducing anxiety, and presents an empowering, sensory intervention and resilience builder that emits mood-enhancing aromas in a controllable way, depending on biofeedback.

The advantage of essential oils merged with AI and connected sensors (e.g., intelligent tracking and smart home devices) could lead to a new palette of mood-enhancing and sleep-inducing aromas, triggered by biometric and/or environmental stimuli (i.e., localized noise, blue light, and social media pollution from smartphones and iPads). In response to real-time dynamic changes in vital signs, voice characteristics, body odor signature, behavior, lifestyle, sleep, and social media patterns, wearable items worn near the nose dispense fragrances that are relevant to the health situation, context, or location of the user, augmenting how we as humans interact with the digital and physical world around us. Fragrances are therefore bio-synchronized to an individual's emotional, mental, and physical state, and algorithmically filtered in real time to mitigate and relieve high levels of stress, anxiety, or circadian dysfunction, as depicted in the AI process diagram (Figure 65.2). The user's mood is therefore lifted, and the body's internal clock is realigned, thus promoting quality sleep and self-care, and preventing the risk of a serious mental ill-health relapse (such as clinical depression or elevated or low mood for bipolar disorder).

Closure of the loop of wearable scent-delivery systems requires an innovative, creative, and collaborative approach, crossing many disciplines in psychology-related sciences, biotechnology, industrial design, liquid engineering, and design. Testing such hypotheses in translational human studies is a matter of future research and clinical trials that could lead to valuable interventions for psychiatric disorders, neurodegenerative disorders, and pain relief for cancer care. Given the increasing numbers of people affected by poor mental health and the reported lack of willingness to seek support, the research on eScent could lead to valuable strategies for enhancing well-being and assisting with the day-to-day management of affective disorders and other mental health conditions. With the exploration of multiple health-care and well-being applications in eScent's product pipeline, the delivery of fragrance under software control can be used to calm children with autism spectrum disorder or recall autobiographical memories and encourage appetite in individuals with early-stage dementia. Alternatively, if pulsed intermittently, it can be used to test our smelling capabilities and potentially help diagnose the early stages of Huntington's or Alzheimer's disease since olfactory dysfunction is an early preclinical feature to predict the onset of such neurodegenerative diseases (Hawkes and Doty, 2009).

eScent could also potentially change human behavior, especially for individuals who are anxious about speaking in public. It could lead to new immersive scent applications and

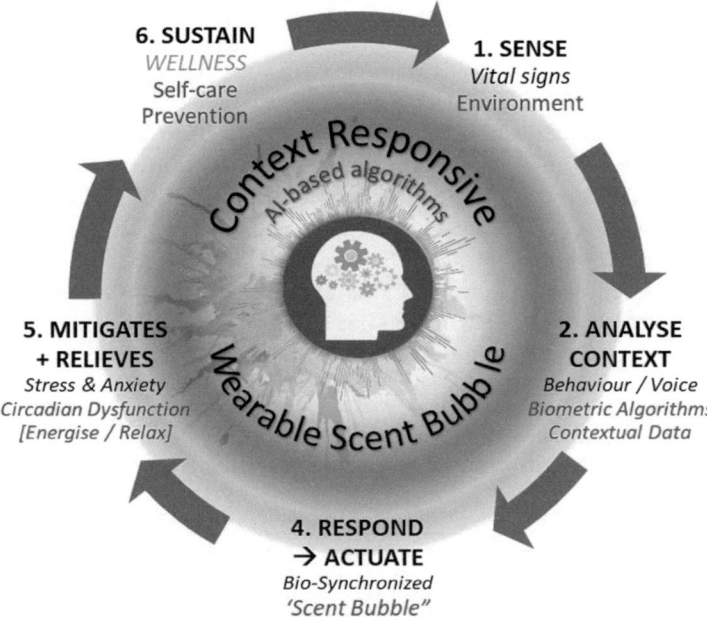

Figure 65.2 AI process behind the eScent Biofeedback Intervention Dispenser

sensory exercises to enhance current research on virtual reality for cognitive behavioral therapy treatments or complement therapeutic sound therapy techniques using voice and rhythmic instruments (Figure 65.3). As a mindfulness meditation tool, it can be used to create a deeper, richer experience to bring more awareness to live in the moment, while also invigorating, refueling, and empowering the user, or acting as a tool to retain memory.

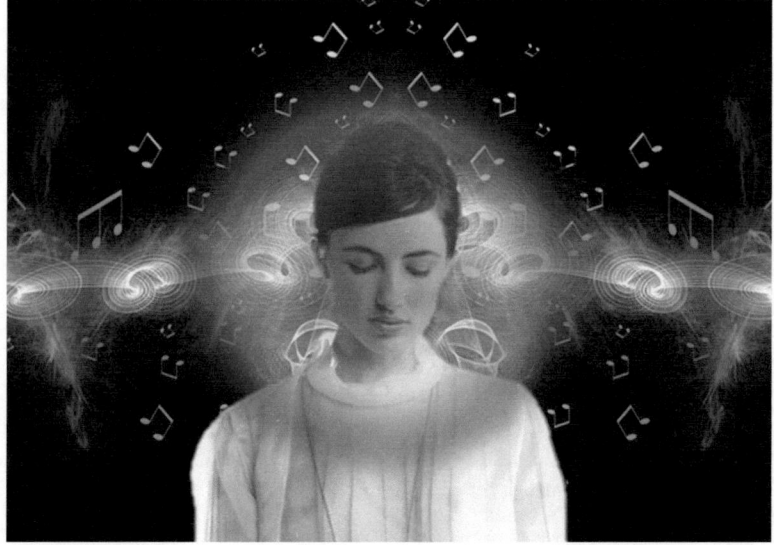

Figure 65.3 Scent release for therapeutic immersive experiences and sound therapy

Examples and methods for engagement in this wearable scent dispenser

Effective engagement methods for this research have included focus groups, film launches, surveys, advisory group meetings, market intelligence studies, fellowships, and numerous presentations at national/international conferences and seminars (for example, the Centre for Fashion Enterprise, Cambridge Neuroscience, Research Institute for Fragrance Materials, London Science Museum, Tate Modern, STEM, RCUK, TEDx, Pitch@Palace, Mental Health Foundation, Winston Churchill Memorial Trust, In-Part University Platform, University of Cambridge, Anxiety Festival, SIGGRAPH, Cambridge Science Festival, Royal Society of Medicine, and Cambridge International Conference on Mental Health). The results have provided insights into the ongoing development of eScent and digital aroma-based technologies by introducing new sensory solutions to prevent the escalation of chronic mental ill-health.

London Fusion user experience study

A market intelligence scent diffusion study, undertaken in collaboration with Goldsmiths College, University of London, and funded by an ERDF "London Fusion" award, has helped design key elements of the eScent device. Ten participants using evidenced-based aromatherapy oils diffused from a device attached to a mobile phone handset showed that "resilience" was the prevalent emotion related to controlled scent release, divided into three different emotions: happiness, energy, and calm. The three emotions indicated where the delivery of scent "on demand" allowed the user to change their behavior or feeling or sense of self. The results found that dispensing lavender as a personalized and localized "scent bubble," as and when required, subtly changed the mood of the user from anxious anticipation to a sense of calm. Participants also expressed positive benefits for using scent in public spaces in terms of individual well-being, its impact on other people, and wanting more self-regulation capabilities over what scent they used and when it was applied (Barth and Brauer, 2014).

Churchill Fellowship

The results of a Churchill Fellowship awarded in 2013, and based on "lived experiences" (20 years living with a bipolar disorder diagnosis), found that using aroma-based stress management strategies as an intermittent "scent bubble" could reduce anxiety and stress levels through the controlled-release of fragrances for people suffering with affective disorders. Interviews conducted with psychiatrists and psychologists at US medical institutes (UCSF, UCSD, and John Hopkins University) expressed positive feedback on the concept, indicating that eScent could be used as a valuable "prodromal scent intervention" to help individuals manage triggers by recognizing, learning, avoiding, and therefore preventing the risk of an acute bipolar disorder episode from escalating. It was noted that eScent would potentially interest the pharmaceutical industry and could be beneficial as an enhancement for practicing mindfulness meditation techniques. It was also considered a favorable tool to reduce stigma; just as the pink ribbon has de-stigmatized breast cancer, eScent can be a de-stigmatizing fashion item that could benefit all mental health conditions and is easy to integrate into everyday items.

Resources

- eScent website: www.escent.ai
- Exploring mental health and wellbeing report, AHRC (2017): https://ahrc.ukri.org/documents/project-reports-and-reviews/mental-health-and-wellbeing/
- Supporting Good Mental Health in the Workplace, Mental Health Foundation, Winston Churchill Memorial Trust (2017): www.wcmt.org.uk/sites/default/files/reports/WCMT%20Supporting%20mental%20health%20in%20the%20workplace%20booklet.pdf
- "The Scent of Things To Come," case study, AHRC 10th Anniversary Brochure and article: https://ahrc.ukri.org/documents/publications/10th-anniversary-brochure/ and https://ahrc.ukri.org/research/readwatchlisten/features/the-scent-of-things-to-come/
- Perfumery and Flavorist: The Juice (2016): http://perfumerflavorist.texterity.com/perfumerflavorist/august_2016?folio=8andpg=10#pg10
- Science Fiction: Scented Healthcare Reality, Pitch@Palace (2016): http://pitchatpalace.com/science-fiction-scented-healthcare-reality/
- In Part (Technology Insights): Beating the Zika buzz with wearable technology (2016): https://in-part.com/blog/beating-the-zika-buzz-with-wearable-technology/
- CEB (University of Cambridge) Focus 17 (2016): www.ceb.cam.ac.uk/news/ceb-focus/ceb-focus-17-january-2016
- eScent—A New Dimension (2015): www.escent.ai/escent-new-dimension-2015
- Sensory Fashion (2014): www.escent.ai/sensory-fashion-2014
- TED x Granta: Women Shaping the Future, (2010) www.youtube.com/watch?v=OEQiuWrCRss
- Scentsory Design (2005): www.escent.ai/scentsory-design-2005
- Cambridge Neuroscience (Jenny Tillotson, Visiting Scholar, University of Cambridge): www.neuroscience.cam.ac.uk/directory/profile.php?scentsory
- Research Institute for Fragrance Materials (2014): www.rifm.org/events-detail.php?id=151#.WHOx2_mLTIU
- Creativeworks London, case study London Fusion Collaborative Award (ERDF and AHRC funded) on the collaboration with Goldsmiths College, University of London (2014): www.creativeworkslondon.org.uk/wp-content/uploads/2015/01/Sensory-Design-Technology.pdf
- Future Morph, Interactive Fragrance Technology: www.futuremorph.org/my-future-finder/fashion-textiles/interactive-fragrance-technology/
- Patent Published Feb 2019: https://patentscope.wipo.int/search/en/detail.jsf?docId=WO2019025763&redirectedID=true
- Churchill Fellowship Report (PDF): www.wcmt.org.uk/sites/default/files/report-documents/Tillotson%20J%20Report%202013%20Final.pdf

References

Barth, J. and Brauer, C. (2014). *Making Scents of Wearable Technology and Social Wellbeing, User Experience Case Study*. [online]. www.escent.ai/london-fusion (Accessed 12/1/2019).

Fismer, K.L. and Pilkington, K. (2012). Lavender and Sleep: A Systematic Review of the Evidence. *European Journal of Integrative Medicine*, 4(4): 436–447.

Fung, J., Tsang, H. and Chung, R. (2012). A Systematic Review of the Use of Aromatherapy in Treatment of Behavioral Problems in Sementia. *Geriatrics Gerontology International*, 12(3): 372–382.

Hawkes, C.H. and Doty, R.L. (2009). *The Neurology of Olfaction.* Cambridge: Cambridge University Press.

Hwang. E. and Shin, S. (2015). The Effects of Aromatherapy on Sleep Improvement: A Systematic Literature Review and Meta-Analysis. *Journal of Alternative and Complementary Medicine,* 21(2): 61–68.

Jenkins, G., Manz, A. and Tillotson, J. (2006). Scent Whisper. *IET Seminar MEMS Sensors and Actuators*: 97–104, 10.1049/ic:20060451.

Jenkins, G. and Tillotson, J. (2006). *A System and Method For Dispensing Fluid In Response To A Sensed Property,* GB2423075B, 16th August 2006 GB2423075B.

Jenkins, G. and Tillotson, J. (2007). *A System and Method For Dispensing Fluid In Response To A Sensed Property,* CN101155510B, 23rd July 2007.

Jenkins, G. and Tillotson, J. (2011). *A System and Method For Dispensing Fluid In Response To A Sensed Property,* US9675987B2, 8th February 2010.

Jenkins, G., Tillotson, J. (2018) *A System And Method For Dispensing Fluid In Response To A Sensed Property,* US 2018/0093288 A1, 8th April 2018.

Krishna, A. (2012). An Integrative Review of Sensory Marketing: Engaging the Senses to Affect Perception, Judgment and Behavior. *Journal of Consumer Psychology,* 22(3): 332–351.

Lehrner, J., Marwinski, G., Lehr, S., Johren, P. and Deecke, L. (2005). Ambient Odors of Orange and Lavender Reduce Anxiety and Improve Mood in a Dental Office. *Journal of Physiology and Behaviour,* 86(1–2): 92–95.

Sarris, J. and Byrne, G.J. (2011). A Systematic Review of Insomnia and Complementary Medicine. *Sleep Medicine Reviews,* 15(2): 99–106.

Tillotson, J. (2009). Scentsory Design, 2009, A "Holistic" Approach to Fashion as a Vehicle to Deliver Emotional Wellbeing. *Fashion Practice: The Journal of Design, Creative Process and the Fashion Industry,* 1(1): 33–61.

Tillotson, J. and Temple, S. (2019) *Liquid dispensing system creating and maintaining a personalised bubble with a defined radius and concentration,* PCT/GB2018/052097, 7th February 2019.

INDEX

Page numbers: Figures are given in *italics* and tables in **bold**.